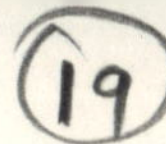

AF553274

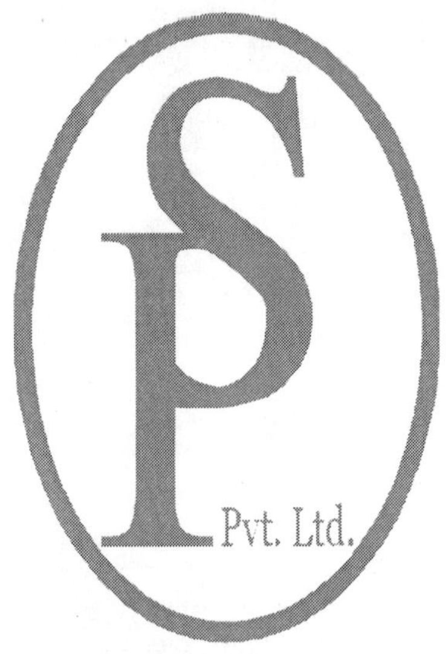
SP
Pvt. Ltd.

Recent Advances in the Molecular Mechanism of Flavonoids

K. Pandima Devi
Department of Biotechnology
Alagappa University, Karaikudi
Tamil Nadu – 630 004

2018

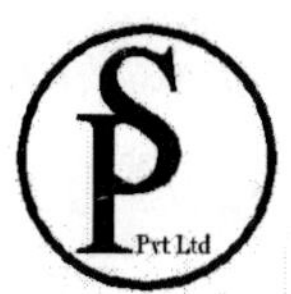

Studium Press (India) Pvt. Ltd.

Recent Advances in the
Molecular Mechanism of Flavonoids

© 2018

This book contains information obtained from authentic and highly regarded sources. Reprinted material is quoted with permission, and sources are indicated. A wide variety of references are listed. Reasonable efforts have been made to publish reliable data and information, but the editor and the publisher cannot assume responsibility for the validity of all materials or for the consequences of their use.

All rights are reserved under International and Pan-American Copyright Conventions. Apart from any fair dealing for the purpose of private study, research, criticism or review, as permitted under the Copyright Act, 1956, no part of this publication may be reproduced, stored in a retrieval system or transmitted, in any form or by any means–electronic, electrical, chemical, mechanical, optical, photocopying, recording or otherwise–without the prior permission of the copyright owner.

ISBN: 978-93-85046-21-6

Published by:

Studium Press (India) Pvt. Ltd.
4735/22, 2nd Floor, Prakash Deep Building
(Near Delhi Medical Association),
Ansari Road, Darya Ganj, New Delhi-110 002
Tel.: + 91-11-43240200-15 (15 lines); Fax: 91-11-43240215
E-mail: studiumpress@gmail.com

Printed at India

About the Editor

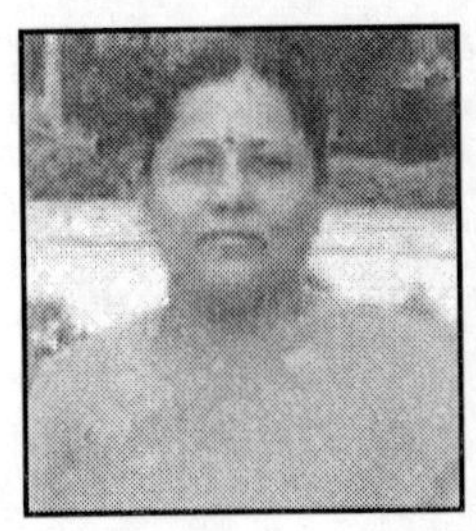

The Editor **Dr. K. Pandima Devi** is currently working as Associate Professor at Department of Biotechnology, Alagappa University, Karaikudi, Tamil Nadu. After obtaining her PhD in Biochemistry from University of Madras in the year 2001, she did her Post Doctoral Research at National Institute of Immunology, New Delhi on expression of human sperm specific proteins and then in CSIC-CID, Spanish National Research Council, Barcelona, Spain on synthesis and applications of peptides for diagnosis of Rheumatoid arthritis. After joining as Faculty in Alagappa University, Karaikudi in 2003, she is mainly focusing on isolation of bioactive compounds from marine plants like seaweeds and mangroves to be used as promising drugs for combating Alzheimer's disease and lung cancer. She is also concentrating on nanotechnology based delivery systems of the bioactive compounds, which will provide a novel medical strategy to combat these diseases. She has published over 75 scientific papers and review articles and nearly 12 chapters in books. She is a life member of BRSI, SBC, ISCA and Proteomics Society, India. She was conferred with the "Tamil Nadu Young Women Scientist Award" for the year 2010 by the Department of Higher Education, Government of Tamil Nadu, and Women Scientist Award for the year 2014 by Biotech Research Society of India (BRSI), for her significant contributions in the field of Natural Product Pharmacology.

Acknowledgements

I am grateful to all the authors of this book for contributing appropriate chapters for this book, which contains up to date scientific data on the relevant topics. I am indebted to all my research scholars who gave me suggestions for designing the book. Above all, I owe my special thanks to Studium Press for accepting our proposal and for providing technical assistance in compiling the book.

Preface

This book has been written to give a detailed insight on the molecular mechanisms of flavonoids identified for the treatment of various diseases of human being. The primary audiences for this book are researchers doing advance research in delineating the pharmacological applications of flavonoids and also the postgraduate students who can use it for reference purpose. As a researcher working on many natural compounds for the past 20 years, I realized that books explaining the molecular mechanisms of natural compounds like flavonoids with appropriate illustrations are very less, which prompted me to edit this book. There are many books available in the market which superficially reviews the pharmacological properties of flavonoids. But this book is distinct since it is framed to centre around the detailed molecular mechanisms of flavonoids, focusing on almost all the major diseases of human like cancer, neurodegenerative disorders, diabetes, infectious diseases and so on. The content and structure of all the chapters have been framed to contain details regarding the effectiveness of flavonoids in interfering with the signaling pathways which are observed to be defective in different diseases. I want to emphasize that appropriate illustrations are included in all the chapters to enable the readers to understand the concepts easily. I hope that the book will be worth reading for scientists interested in understanding the pharmacological mechanisms of flavonoids and to do research in this aspect.

K. Pandima Devi

Table of Contents

1

Flavonoids and Their Anti-Cancer Effect Targeting the Major Signaling Pathways Involved

K. PANDIMA DEVI[1*] AND D. JAYA BALAN[1]

ABSTRACT

Cancer which is a class of diseases that occurs due to uncontrolled growth of cells, is caused by various factors ranging from genetic mutations to different lifestyle factors like exposure to chemicals, radiations, tobacco usage, lack of physical exercise and so on. According to the GLOBOCON worldwide cancer report, more than 100 types of cancers have been identified so far, the most common cause of cancer death being lung, liver and stomach cancers. Though several treatment options are available for cancer like surgery and therapies using radiation, chemical drugs, stem cells and so on, these treatment options can only reduce the symptoms of the disease, and complete cure cannot be expected. Mostly the cancer cells which remain / survive after the treatment options like surgery and radiation are killed by using chemotherapeutic drugs. While these chemical drugs are powerful in killing the cancer cells, they cause many undesirable side effects ranging from nausea and vomiting to causing damage to the vital organs of the system like kidney, heart and lung. Hence, one of the promising treatment options for reducing the side effects and to increase the effectiveness of the chemotherapeutic drugs is to use natural products, which have been used historically for the treatment of various types of cancers. Flavonoids which are a class of phytochemicals, interferes with the expression of many proteins in the cell and influences the various molecular mechanisms of the cell. The current review focuses on the molecular mechanism of the flavonoids in the treatment of different types of cancer.

[1] Department of Biotechnology, Alagappa University, Karaikudi – 630 004, Tamil Nadu, India

**Corresponding author*: E-mail: devikasi@yahoo.com

Key words: Cancer, Flavonoids, Signaling mechanism, Molecular effect.

1. INTRODUCTION

Cancer which is a group of diseases begins in the cells and leads to uncontrolled growth of cells. The incidence of cancer is increasing at a faster rate, that the global cancer burden is predicted to rise to more than 15 million by the year 2020, with deaths predicted to increase to nearly 12 million (Kanavos, 2006). It is very alarming to note that, nearly 60% of the cancer cases are expected to be from developing countries along with lesser survival rates (López-Gómez *et al.,* 2013). Though more than 100 types of cancers have been identified so far, according to the International Agency for Research on Cancer which published the GLOBOCAN report, the most common type of cancer, which caused more number of mortality are lung, stomach and liver cancers (Ferlay *et al.,* 2010). Since cancer is also a disease of aging, and as the aging population is increasing, not only the incidence of cancer, the expected cost for cancer care is also predicted to increase overmore than 20% by the year 2020 (Mariotto *et al.,* 2011). Not only aging, the other major risk factors for cancer includes genetic factors, overweight, lack of physical activity, smoking and the changes associated with the urbanization (Torre *et al.,* 2015). Obesity which is associated with increased adiposity contributes to more than 3% of the cancers worldwide (Byers and Sedjo, 2015).

There are many treatment options available for cancer including surgery, hormonal therapy, radiation therapy, chemotherapy and so on. Of these different types, chemotherapy is a type of cancer treatment where anti-cancer drugs are used for inducing cytotoxic effect to the cancer cells. These cytotoxic drugs kills the cancer cells through different mechanism like interference with cell cycle or induction of apoptosis by either interfering with DNA or changing the expression pattern of the proteins involved in cell division (Fernando and Jones, 2015). In the search for cytotoxic agents, natural products have continued to serve as a source of new anti-cancer agents over the past 30 years. Analysis of the chemical nature of many of the clinically approved anti-cancer drugs reveal that more than 60% of the drugs have originated from nature *i.e.,* they are either natural products or a derivative of the natural compound (Demain and Vaishnav, 2011). Examples of natural compounds which were introduced before 1997 as anti-cancer drugs and still in current use includes actinomycin, vinca alkaloids, campotothecin, taxoids, anthracyclines and so on. From 1997 till 2007, natural products were not considered for anti-cancer drug research and more focus was given only for targeted therapy. However, after realizing the importance of natural products, there was a re-emergence of natural products in anti-cancer drug discovery, and after 2007 many natural drugs including rapamycin were approved for cancer treatment (Basmadjian *et al.,* 2014).

Over the past few decades, plants have continued to serve as an important source of compounds for drug development. Many chemical compounds termed as secondary metabolites are naturally present in plants like flavonoids, alkaloids, terpenes and so on. Though these secondary metabolites do not support the growth and development of the plants, they do help the plants to survive in the changing environment. However human beings have exploited these secondary metabolites as flavouring agent or more importantly as drugs. Of these secondary metabolites, flavonoids are important polyphenolic compounds produced by plants which exhibit various pharmacological actions due to their antioxidant property. Flavonoids comprise of a collection of pigments which includes anthocyanidines, anthocyanides, flavonoles, iso-flavonoles, flavones, iso-flavones, flavanols, iso-flavanols, flavanes, iso-flavanes, aurones, benzo-furones and coumarins. Though it is difficult to exactly calculate the daily dietary intake of flavonoids, since these compounds are ubiquitously present in many plants, it has been estimated by nutritionist that on a normal diet, humans consume nearly 1-2 g of flavonoids per day (Havsteen, 2002). Due to the antioxidant property of the flavonoids, they have been observed to exhibit many pharmacological properties like anti-microbial, anti-inflammatory, anti-diabetic, anti-mutagenic, anti-cancer and so on. With reference to its anti-cancer effect, flavonoids interfere with many process like blocking cell cycle, inhibiting angiogenesis process and inducing apoptosis, so that the cancer cells are stopped further from propagating (Ravishankar *et al.*, 2013). The current review focuses on the molecular mechanisms exhibited by flavonoids in mediating their anti-cancer activity, with special reference to the signaling pathways involved in cancer.

2. MAJOR SIGNALING PATHWAYS OF CANCER

Cancer cells are characterized by a variety of signaling pathways, the network of which is believed to regulate the homeostatic pathways of cancer cells and play a major role in the development of cancer (Yap *et al.*, 2013). Since tumour cells depend on these various signaling pathways for controlling their growth and differentiation, the currently developed anti-cancer drugs are mainly targeted at the signaling molecules involved in these pathways. Designing of molecular targeted therapy is possible by using either single or a combination of drugs which targets these different signaling pathways in the tumour cell (Sebolt-Leopold and English, 2006).

2.1. Apoptosis Signaling in Cancer

Apoptosis is the critical processes that carry out programmed cell death and it is important for the development of an organism and maintaining the homeostatic condition in tissues. Deficiency in apoptosis leads to cancer or autoimmunity (Plati *et al.*, 2011). Apoptotic signaling consists of death receptor mediated extrinsic pathway or mitochondria mediated intrinsic pathway. Extrinsic pathway consists of cell surface death receptors which are TNF family of proteins and include TNF-receptor 1 (TNF-R1, p55, CD120a), Fas (CD95, APO-1) and TNF-related apoptosis-inducing ligand receptors (TRAIL-R1, DR4; TRAIL-R2, DR5, APO-2). The death receptor get activated by TNF-α, Fas ligand (CD95/APO1) or TRAIL and lead to the formation of death-inducing signaling complex (DISC) which contains a death receptor, the adapter protein FADD, caspase 8 and 10, which subsequently activate the downstream caspases leading to apoptosis (Bortner *et al.*, 2014; Hassan *et al.*, 2014). The activation of intrinsic pathway is usually achieved by anticancer drugs, toxins, growth factor deprivation, oxidants, Ca^{2+} overload, oncogene activation, DNA-damaging agents, microtubule targeting drugs and radiation, which alter the mitochondrial membrane property leading to the release of cytochrome c and second mitochondria-derived activator of caspase. The released cytochrome c combines with procaspase- 9, the adapter protein Apaf-1to form apoptosome. The formation of apoptosome subsequently activates downstream caspases which leads to cell death (Hassan *et al.*, 2014, Huang *et al.*, 2015) (Fig. 1). Evading apoptosis is one of the hall mark of cancer cell which is achieved by increasing the expression of anti-apoptotic genes or decreasing the expression of pro-apoptotic genes. Cancer cell can also modify the anti-apoptotic or pro-apoptotic proteins post translationally such as phosphorylation to avoid cell death. There are multiple mechanisms that

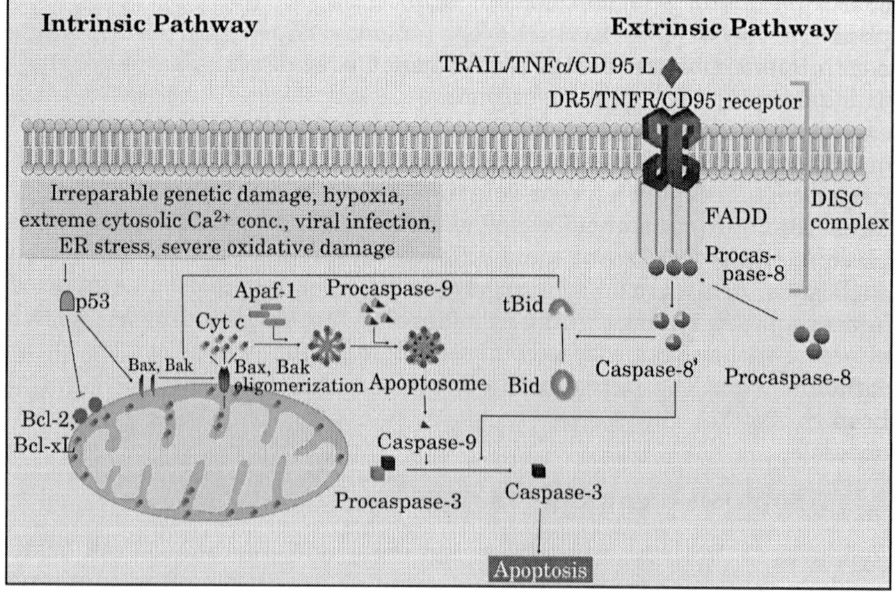

Fig. 1: Schematic diagram of apoptosis signaling pathway.

could be followed by cancer cells to evade apoptosis (Hassan *et al.,* 2014). Taken together, targeting of apoptotic pathway is the most important therapeutic strategy in cancer research.

2.2. Nf-κB Signaling and Cancer

NF-κB(nuclear factor-κB) is the important transcription factor that regulates the gene expression for immune and inflammatory responses, besides the genes determining developmental processes, cell growth and apoptosis (Hoesel *et al.,* 2013). There are five related proteins present in NF-κB family such as p50 (NF-κB1) and p52 (NF-κB2), p65 (RelA), RelB and c-Rel (Rel). Normally these proteins occur as dimers, either homo or heterodimers and through the 300 amino acid long N-terminal Rel homology domain (RHD) it makes direct contact with DNA to regulate gene transcription by the recruitment of co-activators and co-repressors, respectively (Tieri *et al.,* 2012). Certain inhibitors of κB proteins also are found that includes IκBα, IκBβ, IκBε, IκBζ, BCL-3, IκBns and two precursor proteins p100 (NF- κB2) and p105 (NF-κB1). These two precursor proteins contain multiple ankyrin repeat domain to bind with NF-κB dimmers. IκB proteins can inhibit and augment transcriptional responses through binding with NF-κB dimers in the cytoplasm and nucleus (Hayden *et al.,* 2014). The activation of NF-κB involves proteasomal degradation of IκB molecules or by cleavage of inhibitory ankyrin repeat domains of p100 and p105. In general, there are two types of NF-κB pathways, the canonical and non-canonical pathway. The canonical pathway accounts for the inflammatory cues which recruits NEMO-IKK2 (NEMO-IKKβ) kinase complex for the phosphorylation of inhibitory IκB proteins. This leads to the proteasomal degradation of IκBs and release of NF-κB protein dimers like RelA: p50. The released protein dimers enter into the nucleus for activating the expression of pro-inflammatory chemokine and cytokine genes and also its own inhibitor IκBα, for the proper attenuation of the inflammatory responses. Whereas the non-canonical pathway involves cell-differentiating cues that recruit NIK and IKK1 (NIK-IKKα) for the inhibitor phosphorylation and subsequent proteasomal degradation to generate RelB:p52 NF-κB dimer from RelB:p100 complex for the expressions of organogenic chemokine genes in the nucleus (Banoth *et al.,* 2015) (Fig. 2). NF-kB signaling is the major signaling pathway responsible for the inflammatory cancers including Hepatocellular carcinoma (HCC). It has been well documented that the upregulation of NF-kB signaling occur in chronic liver diseases and hepatocarcinogenesis (Marquardt *et al.,* 2015). Further, in most cancer cases the activation of NF-κB promotes anti-apoptosis signaling pathways which allow the proliferation, invasion and metastasis of cancer cells (Tong *et al.,* 2015). Hence the suppression of NF-κB signaling pathway will be a most potent therapeutic target for the treatment of cancer.

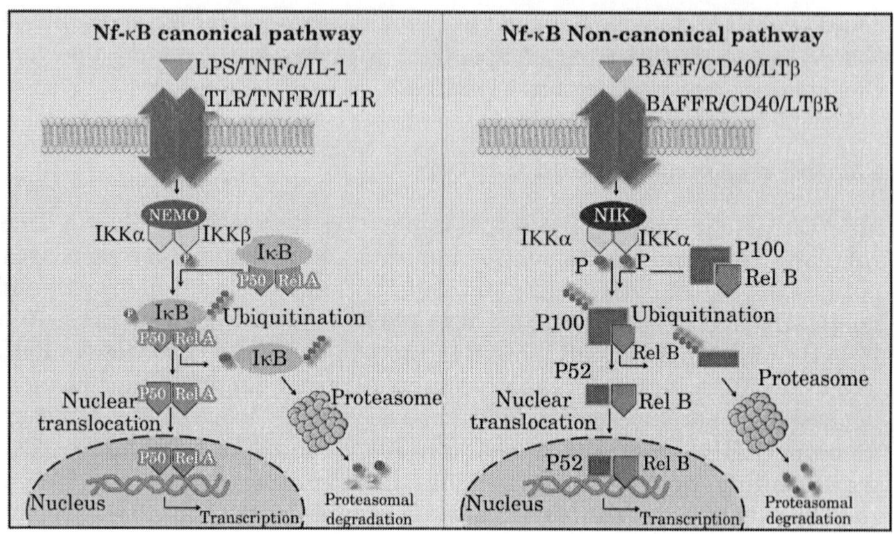

Fig. 2: Schematic diagram of *Nf-kB* signaling pathway.

2.3. Nrf 2 Signaling and Cancer

The Nuclear factor erythroid 2-related factor 2 (Nrf2) is a conserved basic leucine zipper containing transcription factor (Jaramillo *et al.,* 2013). Initiation of Nrf2 pathway in response to oxidative and xenobiotic stress plays an important role in protecting the DNA from damage (Geismann *et al.,* 2014). Oxidative stress and other toxic substances are sensed by Kelch-like ECH-associated protein 1 (KEAP1) which is a cytosolic protein containing large number of cysteine residues (Kim *et al.,* 2016). When the cells make contact with substances that induce oxidative damage and other toxic effects, it leads to the modification of cysteine residues in Kaep1 cytosolic protein. Subsequently Keap1 releases Nrf2 which enter into the nucleus and heterodimerize with Maf proteins. The complex recognizes the Antioxidant Response Elements (AREs), which is located in regulatory regions of genes for cellular defence enzymes and induce their expression (Sparaneo *et al.,* 2016) (Fig. 3a).The environmental stress conditions and metabolic dysfunction cause excess release of reactive oxygen species (ROS). These proactive ROS molecules induce cellular senescence, carcinogenesis and cell death. Various scientific reports implies that the level of ROS increases in cancer when compared to normal cells. Since NrF2 pathway reduces the cancer favoring environment and prevent the tumorogenesis process (Ryoo *et al.,* 2016), activation of Nrf2 might be a promising strategy to block carcinogenesis.

2.4. EGFR Signaling and Cancer

EGFR (epithelial growth factor receptor) is one among the four members of the HER family of receptor tyrosine kinases which includes EGFR, HER2,

HER3, and HER4 (Tetsu *et al.,* 2016). It regulates the growth and maintenance of epithelial tissues and the cancer cells which have been frequently found with EGFR dysregulation or hyper activation (Han *et al.,* 2015). Scientific reports evidenced that the angiogenesis, epithelial–mesenchymal transition, cellular proliferation are influenced by the *EGFR* signaling pathways (Fang *et al.,* 2014). EGFR binding ligands are EGF, transforming growth factor-α, and heparin binding EGF-like growth factor. Binding of any of these ligands with EGFR will initiate the EGFR signaling. Many pathways like PLC-γ–PKC, Ras-Raf-MEK, PI-3K-Akt-mTOR and JAK2-STAT3 are activated upon the stimulation of EGFR. Numerous signaling molecules such as PLC-γ, Ras, PI-3K and JAK2 are recruited, phosphorylated and get activated upon the activation of EGFR followed by the dimerization of STAT3 (signal transducer and activator of transcription-3 is activated by EGFR through phosphorylation). STAT3 dimer further enter into the nucleus for gene regulation (Fig. 3b). EGFR can also be activated independent of kinase, where it gets activated by interacting with proteins physically (Han *et al.,* 2012; Normanno *et al.,* 2006). Overexpression of EGFR is associated with the transformation of solid tumors for metastasis (Chong *et al.,* 2013). Therefore, the suppression of EGFR signaling promotes good results in cancer treatment.

2.5. RAF-ERK Signaling in Cancer

Raf-ERK is the intracellular signaling pathway which includes extracellular signal-regulated protein kinase 1 and 2 (ERK1/2), c-Jun N-terminal kinase (JNK) and p38 pathways. Initiation of this pathway occurs by the protein known as Raf-1 which subsequently phosphorylates MAP kinase/ extracellular signal-regulated kinase kinase 1 and 2 (MEK1/2) (Cao *et al.,* 2011). The extracellular signal-regulated kinase (ERK) is one of the subfamily members of MAPK. This MAPK is activated by MAPKKK (Raf)/ ERK kinase (MEK) in response to growth stimuli. Activation of MAPKKK (Raf) is by dismissing its auto inhibition that is achieved through phosphorylation by Src kinase (Tian *et al.,* 2009).The complex is activated when Raf kinases bind to activated Ras which is present in the plasma membrane. The activated Raf complex phosphorylates and activates MEK 1/2 (Mitogen activated Protein Kinase-/Extracellular Signal Regulated Kinase-Kinase). And these subsequently phosphorylate and activate ERK1/ 2 followed by the transport of activated ERKs into nucleus for transcription factor modification which can influence gene expression (Martin *et al.,* 2010) (Fig. 3c). Since ERK pathway play a role in the alteration of nuclear transcription factors there by regulating cell proliferation or differentiation, impairment in the regulation of Raf/ERK pathway leads to development of cancerous condition. Moreover Raf/ERK pathway is considered as one of the oncogenic pathways (Du *et al.,* 2015). Hence targeting the Raf/ERK pathway for inhibition is the promising strategy for cancer therapeutics.

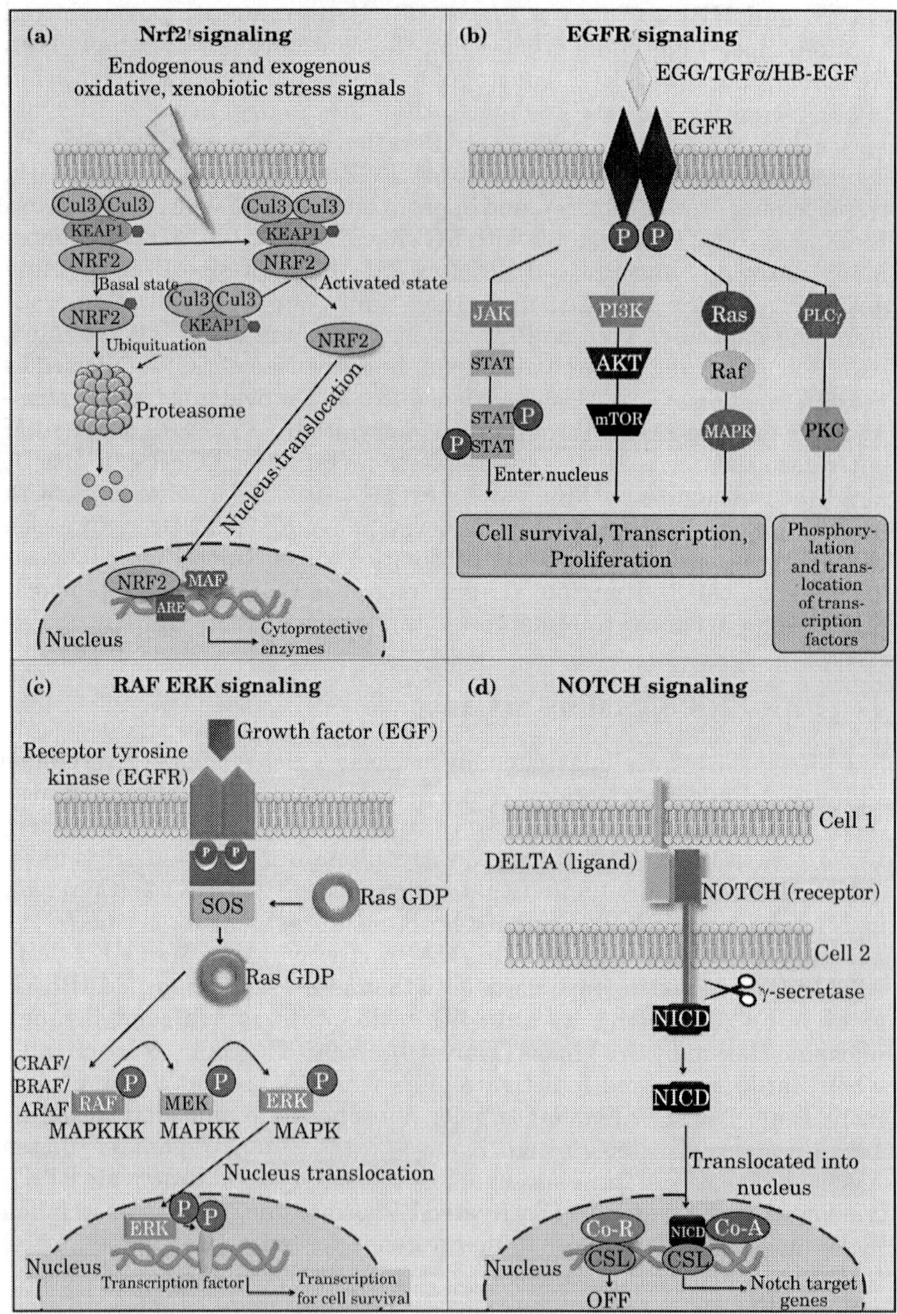

Fig. 3: Schematic diagram of *Nrf2* signaling pathway (a), EGFR signaling pathway (b), RAF- ERK signaling pathway (c), Notch signaling pathway (d).

2.6. Notch Signaling in Cancer

Notch signaling pathway is highly conserved evolutionarily, which plays an important role in a variety of cellular processes like proliferation, differentiation, and apoptosis. In human, four Notch receptors are found such as Notch 1, 2, 3, and 4 and their ligands are Delta-Like 1, 3, and 4 and Jagged 1 and 2 (Brzozowa-Zasada *et al.,* 2016). The interaction between receptor and ligand of two neighbouring cells will initiate the Notch signaling pathway. On binding with the ligand, Notch receptors are subjected to proteolytic cleavage which is catalyzed by γ-secretase. The cleaved Notch intracellular domain is subsequently translocated into nucleus and heterodimerizes with the DNA-binding protein CSL (CBF1, Suppressor of Hairless, Lag-1) in order to activate the transcription of genes containing CSL binding sites. This CSL inhibits Notch-targeting genes in the absence of Notch intracellular domain (Huang *et al.,* 2016) (Fig. 3d). One of the commonly activated signaling pathways in cancer is notch signaling pathway and abnormal activation plays a significant role in cancer. The function of Notch pathway in tumor development is highly variable. Depending on the cellular context, it can act as tumor suppressive or pro-oncogenic (Capaccione *et al.,* 2013). Recently, it has been reported that the notch signaling plays dual role in cancer development either as a tumor suppressor or tumor promoter in human prostate cancer (Lefort *et al.,* 2016). One of the cancer therapeutic strategies is blocking the cleavage of Notch at the cell membrane which is achieved by inhibiting the γ-secretase using γ-secretase inhibitors (Brzozowa-Zasada *et al.,* 2016). But depending on the cell types, Notch cascade activation exerts oncogenic or tumor suppressive function in various type of cancers. Hence, targeting the Notch signaling varies according to the cancer types

2.7. Wnt/β-Catenin Signaling and Cancer

Wnt signaling plays a vital role in the regulation of various processes including cell proliferation, survival, migration and polarization, embryonic development, specification of cell fate and stem cell self-renewal (Liu *et al.,* 2016). The two pathways involved in Wnt signaling are catenin dependent canonical pathway and catenin independent non-canonical pathway (Sherwood and Victoria, 2015). These pathways begin with the binding of Wnt ligands (glycoproteins) to the multiple transmembrane receptors such as 10 members of the frizzled (FZD) family of G-protein-coupled receptors. In canonical pathway, the absence of Wnt stimulation leads to the degradation of β-catenin employed by the destruction complex containing adenomatous polyposis coli (APC), glycogen synthase kinase 3b (GSK3b), and Axin. This degradation of β-catenin further induces the expression of β-catenin-repressed target genes c-Myc, cyclin D1. However in the presence of Wnt signal, it binds to its own receptors that prevent the destruction of β-catenin by activating the dishevelled protein. This result in the accumulation of β-catenin in cytoplasmic regions and it enter into nucleus where it act as a coactivator of T cell transcription factor (TCF) and lymphoid enhancer factor for the transcription of genes which promotes the change in cell proliferation, survival, and differentiation (Tai *et al.,* 2015) (Fig. 4). The abnormal activation of Wnt signaling may lead to various malignancy conditions. The role of Wnt signaling in intestinal stem cell maintenance is very crucial. The suppression of negative regulators like adenomatous polyposis coli (APC) in Wnt signaling leads to the development of colon cancer (Novellasdemunt *et al.,* 2015). Notably, the tumorigenicity of cancer stem cells (CSCs) is contributed by the constant activation of Wnt signaling without any negative regulation (Le *et al.,* 2015). It has been reported that the helicobacter infection and inactivation of Wnt inhibitors mainly causes gastric cancer (Chiurillo *et al.,* 2015). In this case, the development of antagonist to control the constitutive expression of Wnt signaling will be the best therapeutic strategy for the cancer treatment.

2.8. P13/Akt/mTOR Pathway

The PI3K/Akt/mTOR (Mammalian target of rapamycin) pathway is an important cellular pathway which regulates cell growth, proliferation, and survival (Murugan *et al.,* 2013). The mTOR signaling begins in response to

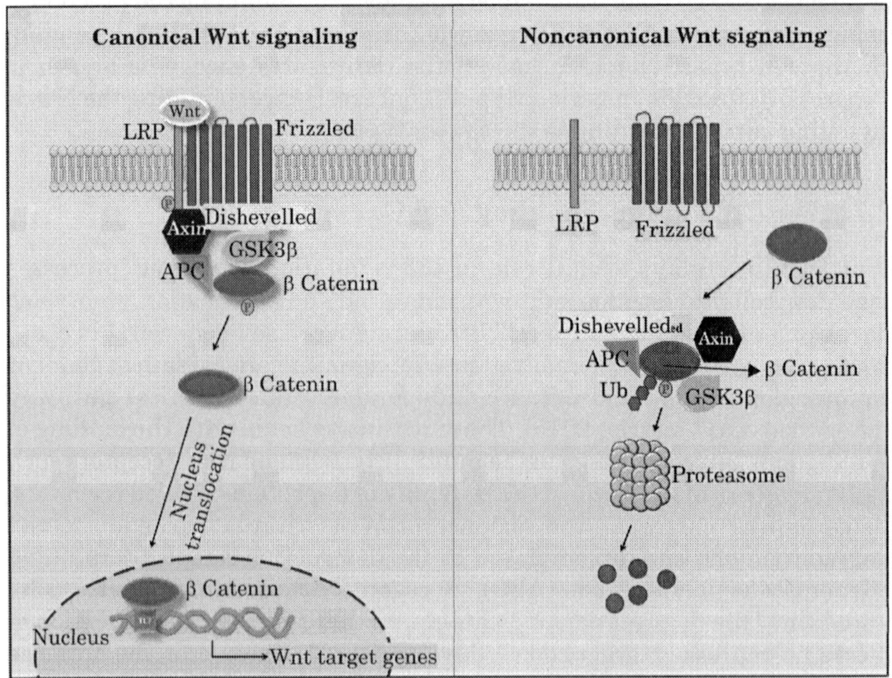

Fig. 4: Schematic diagram of *Wnt/β-catenin* signaling pathway.

extracellular stimuli, including insulin, insulin-like growth factor-1 (IGF-1), epidermal growth factor (EGF) and fibroblast growth factor (FGF). Upon binding of the stimulating factor like insulin, it leads to the phosphorylation of insulin receptor substrate 1 (IRS1) at tyrosine sites. This further activates phosphatidylinositol-3 kinase (PI3K) that converts phosphatidylinositol-4,5-bisphosphate (PIP2) into phosphatidylinositol-3,4,5-trisphosphate (PIP3). Then Akt is recruited to the membrane by PIP3, where Akt is phosphorylated by the enzyme PDK1 at Thr308 and by rictor-bound mTOR complex 2 at Ser473 for complete activation. Finally the Akt activates raptor-bound mTOR complex 1 that mediates phosphorylation of 4E-BP1 and p70S6K (S6K) (Li *et al.,* 2014). mTOR is a serine-threonine kinase that contains two different signaling complexes, mTORC1 and mTORC2. These complexes are composed of some common subunits like mTOR, mLST8, DEPTOR and unique subunits such as PRAS40 and regulatory associated protein of mTOR (RAPTOR) which are specific to mTORC1. The mTORC2 contains RICTOR, mSIN1, and PROTOR1/2. The mTORC1 regulates anabolic metabolism and inhibit catabolic pathways, however mTORC2 regulates actin cytoskeleton, cell-cycle progression, and cellular survival (Xu *et al.,* 2016) (Fig. 5a). The aberrant activation of mTOR-signaling pathway favours tumor development. PI3K/Akt and mTOR signaling are interconnected because mutations in the PI3K/Akt pathway lead to the activation of mTORC2. Also, it controls the activation of mTORC1 through TSC1/TSC2 inhibition which is depending on Akt. PI3K amplification/mutation, PTEN loss of function, overexpression of Akt, and overexpression of S6K1, 4EBP1 and eIF4E are common in cancer (Moschetta *et al.,* 2014). Hence the therapeutic drugs which promotes the regulation of PI3K/Akt is necessary to control the mTOR-signaling pathway.

2.9. MAPK Signaling in Cancer

Mitogen-activated protein kinase (MAPK) or extracellular signal–regulated kinase (ERK) pathway is the evolutionarily conserved pathway that controls cell growth, differentiation, embryogenesis and death (Chakraborty *et al.,* 2016). MAPK signaling is the signaling by sequential phosphorylation. MAPK pathway begins when epidermal growth factor and bind to its receptor followed by the formation of a complex containing Shc/Grb2/SOS. A small GTP binding protein called Ras interact with SOS there by it attain its active conformation by exchanging its GDP for GTP and recruiting Raf to the cell membrane and thus leading to the sequential phosphorylation of the Raf/MEK/ERK signaling cascade by serine/threonine protein kinases which are highly conserved evolutionarily (ArkunandYaman, 2016). The extracellular stimuli for the activation of MAPK are environmental stress, growth factors and cytokines. The sequential phosphorylation involves activation of MAPKK kinases (MAP3K) which phosphorylate MAPK kinases (MAP2K), which in turn phosphorylate MAPKs and this continues until the final substrate/target

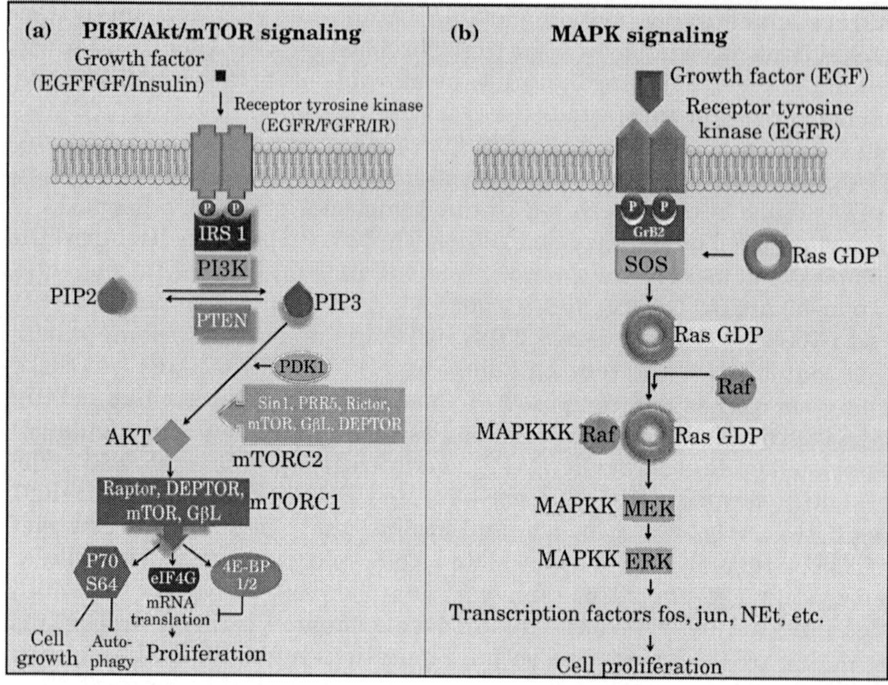

Fig. 5: Schematic diagram of *P13/Akt/mTOR* pathway(a) and *MAPK* signaling pathway(b).

is activated (Fig. 5b). The conventional MAPK member includes extracellular signal-regulated kinases1/2 (ERK1/2) and ERK5, c-Jun amino (N)-terminal kinases1/2/3 (JNK1/2/3), and the p38 isoforms (p38a, p38b, p38g, and p38d) (Rodríguez-Carballo *et al.,* 2016). It has been reported that the p38 MAPKs activation can give epithelial-mesenchymal transition property that helps for the migration of tumor cells. The inhibition of p38 MAPKs make tumor cells to resist anoikis which allow the cancer cell to survive without any contact with another cell and extra cellular matrix (Koul *et al.,* 2013). Hence the proper regulation of MAPKs pathway will indisputably be helpful for the cancer treatment.

3. TARGETING OF THE MAJOR SIGNALING PATHWAYS OF CANCER BY FLAVONOIDS

Many research reports have shown that flavonoids modulate many of the tumour related signaling pathways, which will be discussed in this review.

3.1. Targeting Apoptosis Signaling by Flavonoids

Apoptosis is the programmed cell death which is characterised by various phenotypic conditions like necrosis, membrane blebbing, cell shrinkage, nuclear fragmentation, chromatin condensation and apoptotic body formation. This apoptotic process occurs through both caspase dependent or independent manner. The flavonoid scutellarin present in the medicinal plant *Scutellaria barbata* induced pro-apoptotic effect in the human colon cancer cells HCT-116 which was revealed by the TUNEL staining, reduction in the expression level of Bcl-2 (B cell lymphoma 2, the anti-apoptotic protein) and increase in the expression of the Bax (Bcl 2 associated X apoptosis regulator) and caspase-3 proteins. The flavonoid also enhanced the phosphorylation of p53 protein and induced apoptosis in the cells (Yang *et al.,* 2017). The flavonoid astragalin which is a 3-o-glucoside of kaempferol induced apoptosis in Non-small cell lung carcinoma cells (when treated at 20 mg/ml) through activation of the caspase enzymes 9 and 3 to nearly 4.6 and 5.8 fold respectively. The flavonoid induces apoptosis through caspase-dependent mitochondrial pathway since the ratio of Bax: Bcl-2 was also increased. Astragalin inhibited the activation of PI3K/Akt signaling (which inhibits apoptosis), decreased p38 and ERK phosphorylation and inhibited the cell survival inducing NF-κB signaling in the cancer cell lines (Chen *et al.,* 2017). Since development of multitargeted approach is considered as an alternative strategy to increase the efficacy of anti-cancer drugs, flavonoids like taxifolin was tested for its anti-cancer efficacy in HeLa cells in combination with the diterpenoid andrographolide. The cells which were treated with both andrographolide and taxifolin (at 50 μM and 100 μM respectively) increased the cleaved PARP (poly (ADP-ribose) polymerase) and caspase 7 (which cleaves PARP). The formation of these products is considered as a hallmark of apoptosis process (Alzaharna *et al.,* 2017). Fisetin, a flavonol (at a concentration of 50 mM) induced apoptosis in the human oral cancer cells SSC-4 by increasing the activities of caspase 3,8 and 9 and the expression of the apoptosis associated proteins like calpain 1 and 2, Bax, AIF (Apoptosis inducing factor) and cytochrome c. Since fisetin induced a loss of mitochondrial membrane potential, it is suggested that the flavonoid could induce apoptosis in the cells through intrinsic/mitochondrial signaling pathway (Su *et al.,* 2017).

3.2. Targeting EGFR Signaling by Flavonoids

The epidermal growth factor receptor (EGFR) which is a transmembrane protein is a family of RTK (receptor tyrosine kinase) which gets activated upon binding by the peptide growth factors. Upon stimulation in a cancer cell, the EGFR sends a growth stimulating signal to the cells and promotes tumor growth, invasion, and metastasis. Hence drugs which target EGFR is considered as an alternate therapeutic approach for cancer (Sasaki *et al.,* 2013). Naringin, a flavonoid present in citrus fruits reduced the phosphorylation of EGFR by nearly 50% in the HeLa and A549 cancer cells, when treated at a concentration of 400 mM. The flavonoid also decreased the phosphorylation of ERK (Extracellular signal-regulated kinases), which is one of the down-stream signaling molecule in the EGFR pathway. Since ERK is a key molecule involved in promoting cell growth and survival, inhibition of the EGFR/ERK pathway could be the mechanism for cell growth inhibition by naringin (Yoshinaga *et al.,* 2016). Treatment of the squamous cell carcinoma (KYSE150 and Eca109 cells) with the bioflavonoid kaempferol reduced the expression of EGFR and also caused an inhibition in the phosphorylation of the down-stream proteins ERK1/2 and Akt. Histopathological analysis also revealed the reduced expression of EGFR in the tumour tissues. The results show that high dietary intake of kaempferol could be used for the treatment of esophagus carcinoma patients since overexpression of EGFR has been observed in nearly 62.8% of the carcinoma patients (Yao *et al.,* 2016). Quercetin was able to reduce both EGFR and p-EGFR protein expression levels in the prostrate cancer induced rats. It was also able to regulate the 2 signaling pathways of EGRF namely PI3K/Akt and MAPK/ERK. Quercetin acted as a potential inhibitor of P13 andp-ERK1/2 and down regulated the levels of p-Akt in the prostate cancer animals. The inhibition of Akt phosphorylation is associated with the inhibition of cell cycle progression, since the proteins controls the inhibition of cyclin D1 protein expression (Firdous *et al.,* 2014).

3.3. Targeting RAS/RAF/MEK/ERK Signaling by Flavonoids

Ras is a small GTP binding protein and the Ras gene (originally discovered in Rat sarcoma) has been commonly mutated to nearly 33% in different types of human cancers. Upon activation, it activates the downstream Raf/ MEK/ERK cascade and mediates the oncogenesis process. Hence the Ras/ Raf/MEK/ERK signaling pathway is considered as a better target for treatment of cancer with Ras mutations (Roberts and Der, 2007). This signaling mechanism may be modulated by drugs that upregulate the RKIP (Raf kinase inhibitor protein) which interacts with both Raf-1 and MEK and disrupts the Raf/MEK/ERK cascade. The flavonoid didymin isolated from *Origanum vulgare* protected against liver cell carcinoma by increasing the expression of RKIP and inhibiting the phosphorylation of MEK and ERK (Extracellular Regulated Kinase). Apart from its effect on RKIP, the flavonoid also inhibited the P13K/Akt pathway and induced apoptosis (Wei *et al.,* 2017). The main active compound of the traditional Chinese medicinal plant *Carthamus tinctorius* L is the flavonoid hydroxysafflor yellow A, which also protected the hepatocellular carcinoma cells by decreasing the expression of p-c-raf and p-ERK (phosphorylated forms) and further reducing the levels of angiogenic factors (Yang *et al.,* 2015).

3.4. Targeting Notch Signaling by Flavonoids

Notch is a transmembrane receptor, which gets cleaved upon binding with its ligand. On activation, it releases the NICD (Notch intracellular domain) protein which translocates to the nucleus and helps in the transcription of proteins required for cell proliferation, inhibition of apoptosis and metastasis (like cIAPs-cellular inhibitor of apoptosis, survivin, Bcl-2, cyclin D1). Since Notch signaling promotes malignant phenotype in many types of cancers, it is considered as a good target for drug development. In the gastric cancer cells (Hs-746T and MKN28), the flavonoid luteolin blocked the Notch signaling and exhibited anti-cancer effect mainly by increasing apoptosis of the cancer cells and inhibiting proliferation and migration of the cells (Zang *et al.,* 2017). The mRNA of the Notch receptor is blocked by the micro RNA miR34a, which reduces the Notch protein expression, downregulates the Notch signaling and thus acts as a tumour suppressor. Rhamnetin, which is an O-methylated flavonol reduced the expression of Notch 1 mRNA in the liver cancer cell line HepG2, by increasing the level of miR34a. Apoptosis was further promoted by rhamnetin by reducing the expression of its down-stram targets cIAP and surviving (Jia *et al.,* 2016).

3.5. Targeting Wnt/β-Catenin Signaling by Flavonoids

The canonical Wnt pathway which involves the β-catenin protein plays an important role in the initiation and progression of different types of cancers. Hence inhibition of the Wnt/β-catenin signaling is considered as a better therapeutic intervention for cancer treatment. The breast cancer MDA-MB-231 cells treated upto 40 μmol/L concentration of baicalein isolated from *Scutellaria* species suppressed the expression of the ligand Wnt1 which activates the Wnt/β-catenin signaling. It also caused inhibition of β-catenin transcription and its downstream targets Cyclin D1 and Axin2, which shows that the flavonoid protects against breast cancer by interfering with the Wnt/β-catenin pathway (Ma *et al.,* 2016). The flavonoid wogonin isolated from the same genus protected the MCF-7 breast cancer cells by interfering with the Wnt/β-catenin pathway. Similar to baicalein, this flavonoid also decreased the levels of the ligand Wnt3a and reduced the levels of β-catenin by promoting its phosphorylation, so that it can undergo degradation by the proteasomes (Huang *et al.,* 2016). Isoquercetin which is a derivative of quercetin inhibited the Wnt/ β-catenin signaling in Xenopus embryo and also in the colon cancer cells DLD, SW480, and HCT116 by affecting the phosphorylation of β-catenin (Amado *et al.,* 2014).

3.6. Targeting STAT3 by Flavonoids

The transcription factor STAT3 (Signal transducer and activator of transcription 3), gets phosphorylated by the JAK tyrosine kinase at tyr 705 in response to the external stimuli, and mediates the transcription of proteins involved in cell survival. Hence inhibition of STAT3 is linked with a protective mechanism in cancer cells, since it is oncogenic and gets constitutively activated in the tumour cells. The flavonoid luteolin present in pepper, celery and lemon, downregulated the expression of STAT3 and also its pro-survival proteins survivin, Bcl-xl (B-cell lymphoma-extra large) and Mcl-1 (myeloid cell leukemia 1) in the gastric cancer cells. It was observed that treatment of luteolin caused dephosphorylation of STAT3 by preventing the binding of SHP-1 (Src homology region 2 domain-containing phosphatase-1; a tyrosine-specific protein phosphatase) to STAT3 (Song *et al.,* 2017). The breast cancer cell lines MDA-MB435 express STAT3 constitutively and contribute for resistance to chemotherapeutic drugs. The flavonoid silibinin isolated from milk thistle, caused a suppression in the level of pSTAT3 (phosphorylated) in MDA-MB435 cells and promoted apoptosis by activating the ERK and AKT signaling pathways and also by increasing the levels of caspase 3. The ERK and AKT pathways are involved in promoting cell proliferation and are constitutively expressed in many types of cancers. Hence the inhibition of these pathways by silibinin makes it a better alternative for treating drug resistance in breast cancer (Molavi *et al.,* 2017).

3.7. Targeting Nf-κB and Nrf2 Signaling by Flavonoids

Activation of both Nrf2 and Nf-κB protect the cancer cells from the anti cancer drugs by activating the cancer cell survival pathways. Nf-κB is the major contributor for the development of multi drug resistance since they enhance the expression of the anti-apoptotic proteins and causes the secretion of pro-inflammatory cytokines. Since Nrf2 also promotes chemoresistance, anti-cancer drugs which are Nf-κB and Nrf2 inhibitors will have more efficiency in eliminating cancer cells. Treatment of the CMl cells (Chronic myelogenous (or myeloid or myelocytic) leukemia cells) with the flavonoid wogonin isolated from the roots of the medicinal plant *Scutellaria baicalensis* inhibited both Nrf2 and STAT3 (by preventing the tyr 705 phosphorylation) signaling mainly mediated through the inhibition of NF-κB signaling (Xu *et al.,* 2017). The flavonoid baicalein (at 40 μM) isolated from the roots of *Scutellaria baicalensis* and *Scutellaria lateriflora* stabilises the Nrf2 in the colon cancer HCT 116 cells and translocates it into the nucleus. The release of Nrf2 into the nucleus favours the expression of the antioxidant enzymes in the cells (Havermann *et al.,* 2016). Citrus fruits contain the flavonoid diosmetin which inhibited NF-κB in HepG2 cells by inactivating the IKKα and IKKβ and downregulating the Notch3 and cleaved Notch3 levels. The inhibition of Nf-κB pathway by diosmetin resulted in activation of apoptosis pathway through upregulation of the apoptotic proteins Bax and PARP (poly (ADP-ribose) polymerase) and downregulation of the anti-apoptotic protein Bcl-2 (Qiao *et al.,* 2016).

3.8. Targeting P13/Akt/mTOR and MAPK Signaling by Flavonoids

Since this signaling pathway mediates cell proliferation, many small molecules are developed which can act as inhibitors of the P13/Akt/mTOR signaling mechanism. Naringenin which is a phytoestrogen present in orange and grapes downregulated the P13/Akt signaling in the PC3 prostate cancer cells. Apart from inhibiting the P13/Akt signaling, naringenin also caused an inhibition of the ERK1/2, JNK-1 and P38 MAPK signaling mechanism, which is also involved in inducing cell proliferation. Blocking of JNK-1 by naringenin might probably induce apoptosis in the prostate cancer cell by increasing the cleavage of the procaspase 3 and 8. Since naringenin has a regulatory action on both PI3K/AKT and MAPKs pathways, it may be considered as a therapeutic agent for the treatment of prostrate cancer (Lim *et al.,* 2016). The flavonoid fisetin present in grapes, onion and cucumber prevented digestive cancer, as observed by its effect to activate the caspase cascade (caspase 3/7) in HepG-2, Caco-2 and Suit-2 cell lines. Identification of molecular targets through microarray and western blot revealed that fisetin could be used either alone or in combination to treat tumour since it has an effect on multiple signaling pathways in the cancer cells like Nrf2 (nuclear factor erythroid 2), ERK/ MAPK, CDK5 (cyclin-dependent-like kinase 5), GADD45A and B (Growth arrest and DNA damage inducible Alpha and Beta), TOP2a (DNA Topoisomerase Type IIα), CCNB2 (Cyclin B2) and so on (Youns and Abdel Halim Hegazy, 2017).

A small population of the cancer stems that is responsible for tumour relapse are the cancer stem cells (CSC). Since these cells cause the recurrence of cancer, drugs are specifically designed to eliminate these CSCs. Apigenin most commonly present in celery and chamomile tea significantly enhanced the anti-cancer activity of cisplatin in the PCa prostate cancer cells by causing a downregulation of survivin, sharpin, Bcl-2 and NF-κB, an upregulation in expression of Apaf 1, p53 and caspase 8 and reducing the phosphorylation of p-PI3K and p-Akt. The flavonoid mainly targeted the CSC in the prostate cancer cells and mediated its therapeutic effect (Dragu *et al.,* 2015). In the lung cancer cell line A549 also, apigenin modulated the PI3K/Akt signaling pathway and exhibited chemopreventive effect by decreasing the expression and activation of Akt and inhibiting the expression of its downstream targets matrix metalloproteinases-9, glycogen synthase kinase-3β, and HEF1 (Human Enhancer of Filamentation 1) (Zhou *et al.,* 2017) .

4. CONCLUSIONS AND FUTURE PERSPECTIVES

Plants contain different types of flavonoids which possess strong antioxidant properties. Hence dietary intake of flavonoids has been associated with the prevention of various types of oxidative stress disorders like cancer. Since a complex signaling network operates in the cancer cells, molecular targeted therapeutics are very much needed for the effective treatment of cancer. The flavonoids which are ubiquitously present in plants interferes with many tumour related signaling pathways like NF-κB, Nrf2, EGFR,

RAF-ERK, Notch, Wnt/β-catenin, P13/Akt/mTOR, MAPK, apoptosis signaling and so on. Some of the flavonoids like quercetin targets multiple signaling pathways and blocks the growth of cancer cells. Since flavonoids exhibit promising effect towards cancer treatment, the future perspective on flavonoid research should focus on evaluation of anti-cancer efficacy of combination of more than one flavonoid and also combining flavonoids with the standard drugs.

5. ACKNOWLEDGEMENT

The authors gratefully acknowledge the Bioinformatics Infrastructure Facility provided by the Alagappa University (funded by Department of Biotechnology, Government of India; Grant No. BT/BI/25/015/2012)

REFERENCES

Alzaharna, M., Alqouqa, I. and Cheung, H.Y. (2017). Taxifolin synergizes andrographolide-induced cell death by attenuation of autophagy and augmentation of caspase dependent and independent cell death in HeLa cells. *PloS ONE,* 12(2): e0171325.

Amado, N.G., Predes, D., Fonseca, B.F., Cerqueira, D.M., Reis, A.H., Dudenhoeffer, A.C., Borges, H.L., Mendes, F.A. and Abreu, J.G. (2014). Isoquercitrin suppresses colon cancer cell growth *in vitro* by targeting the Wnt/β-catenin signaling pathway. *Journal of Biological Chemistry*, 289(51): 35456–67.

Arkun, Y. (2016). Dynamic modeling and analysis of the cross-talk between insulin/ AKT and MAPK/ERK signaling pathways. *PloS ONE*, 11(3): e0149684.

Banoth, B., Chatterjee, B., Vijayaragavan, B., Prasad, M.V., Roy, P. and Basak, S. (2015). Stimulus-selective crosstalk *via* the NF-κB signaling system reinforces innate immune response to alleviate gut infection. *Elife*, 4: e05648.

Basmadjian, C., Zhao, Q., Bentouhami, E., Djehal, A., Nebigil, C.G., Johnson, R.A., Serova, M., De Gramont, A., Faivre, S., Raymond, E. and Désaubry, L.G. (2014). Cancer wars: Natural products strike back. *Frontiers in Chemistry,* 2: 20.

Bortner, C.D. and Cidlowski, J.A. (2014). Ion channels and apoptosis in cancer. *Phil. Trans. R. Soc. B.*, 369(1638): 20130104.

Brzozowa-Zasada, M., Piecuch, A., Dittfeld, A., MielaD czyk, A ., Michalski, M., Wyrobiec, G., Harabin-SB owiD ska, M., Kurek, J. and Wojnicz, R. (2016). Notch signaling pathway as an oncogenic factor involved in cancer development. *Contemp. Oncol.* (Pozn), 20(4): 267–72.

Byers, T. and Sedjo, R.L. (2015). Body fatness as a cause of cancer: Epidemiologic clues to biologic mechanisms. *Endocrine-Related Cancer*, 22(3): R125–34.

Cao, L., Xu, C.B., Zhang, Y., Cao, Y.X. and Edvinsson, L. (2011). Secondhand smoke exposure induces Raf/ERK/MAPK-mediated upregulation of cerebrovascular endothelin ET A receptors. *BMC Neuroscience*, 12(1): 109.

Capaccione, K.M. and Pine, S.R. (2013). The Notch signaling pathway as a mediator of tumor survival. *Carcinogenesis,* p. 127.

Chakraborty, C., Sharma, A.R., Patra, B.C., Bhattacharya, M., Sharma, G. and Lee, S.S. (2016). MicroRNAs mediated regulation of MAPK signaling pathways in chronic myeloid leukemia. *Oncotarget.*, 7(27): 42683–97.

Chen, M., Cai, F., Zha, D., Wang, X., Zhang, W., He, Y., Huang, Q., Zhuang, H. and Hua, Z.C. (2017). Astragalin-induced cell death is caspase-dependent and enhances the susceptibility of lung cancer cells to tumor necrosis factor by inhibiting the NF-:κB pathway. *Oncotarget*.

Chiurillo, M.A. (2015). Role of the Wnt/β-catenin pathway in gastric cancer: An in-depth literature review. *World Journal of Experimental Medicine*, 5(2): 84.

Chong, C.R. and Jänne, P.A. (2013). The quest to overcome resistance to EGFR-targeted therapies in cancer. *Nature Medicine,* 19(11): 1389–400.

Demain, A.L. and Vaishnav, P. (2011). Natural products for cancer chemotherapy. *Microbial Biotechnology*, 4(6): 687–99.

Dragu, D.L., Necula, L.G., Bleotu, C., Diaconu, C.C. and Chivu-Economescu, M. (2015). Therapies targeting cancer stem cells: Current trends and future challenges. *World Journal of Stem Cells*, 7(9): 1185.

Du, W., Pang, C., Xue, Y., Zhang, Q. and Wei, X. (2015). Dihydroartemisinin inhibits the Raf/ERK/MEK and PI3K/AKT pathways in glioma cells. *Oncology Letters*, 10(5): 3266–70.

Fang, S. and Wang, Z. (2014). EGFR mutations as a prognostic and predictive marker in non-small-cell lung cancer. *Drug Des. Devel Ther.*, 8: 1595–611.

Ferlay, J., Shin, H.R., Bray, F., Forman, D., Mathers, C. and Parkin, D.M. (2010). Estimates of worldwide burden of cancer in 2008: GLOBOCAN 2008. *International Journal of Cancer,* 127(12): 2893–917.

Fernald, K. and Kurokawa, M. (2013). Evading apoptosis in cancer. *Trends in Cell Biology,* 23(12): 620–33.

Fernando, J. and Jones, R. (2015). The principles of cancer treatment by chemotherapy. *Surgery* (Oxford), 33(3): 131–5.

Firdous, A.B., Sharmila, G., Balakrishnan, S., RajaSingh, P., Suganya, S., Srinivasan, N. and Arunakaran, J. (2014). Quercetin, a natural dietary flavonoid, acts as a chemopreventive agent against prostate cancer in an *in vivo* model by inhibiting the EGFR signaling pathway. *Food & Function,* 5(10): 2632–45.

Geismann, C., Arlt, A., Sebens, S. and Schäfer, H. (2014). Cytoprotection "gone astray": Nrf2 and its role in cancer. *Onco. Targets Ther.*, 7: 1497–518.

Han, F., He, J., Li, F., Yang, J., Wei, J., Cho, W.C. and Liu, X. (2015). Emerging roles of microRNAs in EGFR-targeted therapies for lung cancer. *BioMed Research International,* 2015.

Han, W. and Lo, H.W. (2012). Landscape of EGFR signaling network in human cancers: Biology and therapeutic response in relation to receptor subcellular locations. *Cancer letters,* 318(2): 124–34.

Hassan, M., Watari, H., AbuAlmaaty, A., Ohba, Y. and Sakuragi, N. (2014). Apoptosis and molecular targeting therapy in cancer. *BioMed Research International,* 2014.

Havermann, S., Chovolou, Y., Humpf, H.U. and Wätjen, W. (2016). Modulation of the Nrf2 signaling pathway in Hct116 colon carcinoma cells by baicalein and its methylated derivative negletein. *Pharmaceutical Biology*, 54(9): 1491–502.

Havsteen, B.H. (2002). The biochemistry and medical significance of the flavonoids. *Pharmacology & Therapeutics,* 96(2): 67–202.

Hayden, M.S. and Ghosh, S. (2014). Regulation of NF-κB by TNF family cytokines. In Seminars in immunology. Academic Press. 26(3): 253–266.

Hoesel, B. and Schmid, J.A. (2013). The complexity of NF-κB signaling in inflammation and cancer. *Molecular Cancer,* 12(1): 86.

Huang, C. and Freter, C. (2015). Lipid metabolism, apoptosis and cancer therapy. *International Journal of Molecular Sciences*, 16(1): 924–49.

Huang, T., Zhou, Y., Cheng, A.S., Yu, J., To, K.F. and Kang, W. (2016). Notch receptors in gastric and other gastrointestinal cancers: Oncogenes or tumor suppressors? *Molecular Cancer*, 15(1): 80.

Huang, Y., Zhao, K., Hu, Y., Zhou, Y., Luo, X., Li, X., Wei, L., Li, Z., You, Q., Guo, Q. and Lu, N. (2015). Wogonoside inhibits angiogenesis in breast cancer *via* suppressing Wnt/β-catenin pathway. *Molecular Carcinogenesis*.

Jaramillo, M.C. and Zhang, D.D. (2013). The emerging role of the Nrf2–Keap1 signaling pathway in cancer. *Genes & Development,* 27(20): 2179–91.

Jia, H., Yang, Q., Wang, T., Cao, Y., Jiang, Q.Y., Sun, H.W., Hou, M.X., Yang, Y.P. and Feng, F. (2016). Rhamnetin induces sensitization of hepatocellular carcinoma cells to a small molecular kinase inhibitor or chemotherapeutic agents. *Biochimicaet Biophysica Acta (BBA)-General Subjects,* 1860(7): 1417–30.

Kanavos, P. (2006). The rising burden of cancer in the developing world. *Annals of Oncology,* 17(suppl 8): viii15–23.

Kim, J. and Keum, Y.S. (2016). NRF2, a key regulator of antioxidants with two faces towards cancer. *Oxidative Medicine and Cellular Longevity*, 2016.

Kondratskyi, A., Kondratska, K., Skryma, R. and Prevarskaya, N. (2015). Ion channels in the regulation of apoptosis. *Biochimicaet Biophysica Acta (BBA)-Biomembranes*, 1848(10): 2532–46.

Koul, H.K., Pal, M. and Koul, S. (2013). Role of p38 MAP kinase signal transduction in solid tumors. *Genes & Cancer,* 4(9–10): 342–59.

Le, P.N., McDermott, J.D. and Jimeno, A. (2015). Targeting the Wnt pathway in human cancers: Therapeutic targeting with a focus on OMP-54F28. *Pharmacology & Therapeutics,* 146: 1–1.

Lefort, K., Ostano, P., Mello-Grand, M., Calpini, V., Scatolini, M., Farsetti, A., Dotto, G.P. and Chiorino, G. (2016). Dual tumor suppressing and promoting function of Notch1 signaling in human prostate cancer. *Oncotarget*, 7(30): 48011.

Li, T. and Wang, G. (2014). Computer-aided targeting of the PI3K/Akt/mTOR pathway: Toxicity reduction and therapeutic opportunities. *International Journal of Molecular Sciences*, 15(10): 18856–91.

Lim, W., Park, S., Bazer, F.W. and Song, G. (2017). Naringenin-induced apoptotic cell death in prostate cancer cells is mediated *via* the PI3K/AKT and MAPK signaling pathways. *Journal of Cellular Biochemistry.*

Liu, L.J., Xie, S.X., Chen, Y.T., Xue, J.L., Zhang, C.J. and Zhu, F. (2016). Aberrant regulation of Wnt signaling in hepatocellular carcinoma. *World Journal of Gastroenterology*, 22(33): 7486.

López-Gómez, M., Malmierca, E., de Górgolas, M. and Casado, E. (2013). Cancer in developing countries: The next most preventable pandemic. The global problem of cancer. *Critical Reviews in Oncology/Hematology,* 88(1): 117–22.

Ma, X., Yan, W., Dai, Z., Gao, X., Ma, Y., Xu, Q., Jiang, J. and Zhang, S. (2016). Baicalein suppresses metastasis of breast cancer cells by inhibiting EMT *via* downregulation of SATB1 and Wnt/β-catenin pathway. *Drug Design, Development and Therapy*, 10: 1419.

Mariotto, A.B., Yabroff, K.R., Shao, Y., Feuer, E.J. and Brown, M.L. (2011). Projections of the cost of cancer care in the United States: 2010–2020. *Journal of the National Cancer Institute.*

Marquardt, J.U., Gomez-Quiroz, L., Camacho, L.O., Pinna, F., Lee, Y.H., Kitade, M., Domínguez, M.P., Castven, D., Breuhahn, K., Conner, E.A. and Galle, P.R. (2015). Curcumin effectively inhibits oncogenic NF-κB signaling and restrains stemness features in liver cancer. *Journal of Hepatology*, 63(3): 661–9.

Martin, C., Chen, S., Heilos, D., Sauer, G., Hunt, J., Shaw, A.G., Sims, P.F., Jackson, D.A. and Lovri , J. (2010). Changed genome heterochromatinization upon prolonged activation of the Raf/ERK signaling pathway. *PloS ONE*, 5(10): e13322.

Molavi, O., Narimani, F., Asiaee, F., Sharifi, S., Tarhriz, V., Shayanfar, A., Hejazi, M. and Lai, R. (2017). Silibinin sensitizes chemo-resistant breast cancer cells to chemotherapy. *Pharmaceutical Biology*, 55(1): 729–39.

Moschetta, M., Reale, A., Marasco, C., Vacca, A. and Carratù, M.R. (2014). Therapeutic targeting of the mTOR-signaling pathway in cancer: Benefits and limitations. *British Journal of Pharmacology*, 171(16): 3801–13.

Murugan, A.K., Alzahrani, A. and Xing, M. (2013). Mutations in critical domains confer the human mTOR gene strong tumorigenicity. *Journal of Biological Chemistry,* 288(9): 6511–21.

Normanno, N., De Luca, A., Bianco, C., Strizzi, L., Mancino, M., Maiello, M.R., Carotenuto, A., De Feo, G., Caponigro, F. and Salomon, D.S. (2006). Epidermal growth factor receptor (EGFR) signaling in cancer. *Gene*, 366(1): 2–16.

Novellasdemunt, L., Antas, P. and Li, V.S. (2015). Targeting Wnt signaling in colorectal cancer. A review in the theme: Cell signaling: Proteins, pathways and mechanisms. *American Journal of Physiology-Cell Physiology,* 309(8): C511–21.

Plati, J., Bucur, O. and Khosravi-Far, R. (2011). Apoptotic cell signaling in cancer progression and therapy. *Integrative Biology,* 3(4): 279–96.

Qiao, J., Liu, J., Jia, K., Li, N., Liu, B., Zhang, Q., Zhu, R. (2016). Diosmetin triggers cell apoptosis by activation of the p53/Bcl-2 pathway and inactivation of the Notch3/ NF-κB pathway in HepG2 cells. *Oncology Letters,* 12(6): 5122–8.

Ravishankar, D., Rajora, A.K., Greco, F. and Osborn, H.M. (2013). Flavonoids as prospective compounds for anti-cancer therapy. *The International Journal of Biochemistry & Cell Biology,* 45(12): 2821–31.

Roberts, P.J. and Der, C.J. (2007). Targeting the Raf-MEK-ERK mitogen-activated protein kinase cascade for the treatment of cancer. *Oncogene*, 26(22): 3291–310.

Rodríguez-Carballo, E., Gámez, B. and Ventura, F. (2016). p38 MAPK signaling in osteoblast differentiation. *Frontiers in Cell and Developmental Biology*, 4.

Ryoo, I.G., Lee, S.H. and Kwak, M.K. (2015). Redox modulating NRF2: A potential mediator of cancer stem cell resistance. *Oxidative Medicine and Cellular Longevity*, 2016.

Sasaki, T., Hiroki, K. and Yamashita, Y. (2013). The role of epidermal growth factor receptor in cancer metastasis and micro-environment. *BioMed Research International*, 2013.

Sebolt-Leopold, J.S. and English, J.M. (2006). Mechanisms of drug inhibition of signaling molecules. *Nature,* 441(7092): 457–62.

Sherwood, V. (2015). WNT signaling: An emerging mediator of cancer cell metabolism? *Molecular and cellular biology*. 35(1): 2–10.

Song, S., Su, Z., Xu, H., Niu, M., Chen, X., Min, H., Zhang, B., Sun, G., Xie, S., Wang, H. and Gao, Q. (2017). Luteolin selectively kills STAT3 highly activated gastric cancer cells through enhancing the binding of STAT3 to SHP-1. *Cell Death & Disease,* 8(2): e2612.

Sparaneo, A., Fabrizio, F.P. and Muscarella, L.A. (2016). Nrf2 and Notch signaling in lung cancer: Near the crossroad. *Oxidative Medicine and Cellular Longevity,* 2016.

Su, C.H., Kuo, C.L., Lu, K.W., Yu, F.S., Ma, Y.S., Yang, J.L., Chu, Y.L., Chueh, F.S., Liu, K.C. and Chung, J.G. (2017). Fisetin-induced apoptosis of human oral cancer SCC-4 cells through reactive oxygen species production, endoplasmic reticulum stress, caspase-, and mitochondria-dependent signaling pathways. *Environmental Toxicology*.

Tai, D., Wells, K., Arcaroli, J., Vanderbilt, C., Aisner, D.L., Messersmith, W.A. and Lieu, C.H. (2015). Targeting the WNT signaling pathway in cancer therapeutics. *The Oncologist,* 20(10): 1189–98.

Tetsu, O., Hangauer, M.J., Phuchareon, J., Eisele, D.W., McCormick, F. (2016). Drug resistance to EGFR inhibitors in lung cancer. *Chemotherapy*, 61(5): 223–35.

Tian, H.P., Huang, B.S., Zhao, J., Hu, X.H., Guo, J. and Li, L.X. (2009). Non-receptor tyrosine kinase Src is required for ischemia-stimulated neuronal cell proliferation *via* Raf/ERK/CREB activation in the dentate gyrus. *BMC Neuroscience*, 10(1): 139.

Tieri, P., Termanini, A., Bellavista, E., Salvioli, S., Capri, M. and Franceschi, C. (2012). Charting the NF-κB pathway interactomemap. *PloS ONE*, 7(3): e32678.

Tong, L., Yuan, Y. and Wu, S. (2015). Therapeutic microRNAs targeting the NF-kappa B signaling circuits of cancers. *Advanced Drug Delivery Reviews*, 81: 1–5.

Torre, L.A., Bray, F., Siegel, R.L., Ferlay, J., Lortet-Tieulent, J. and Jemal, A. (2015). Global cancer statistics, 2012. CA: A cancer. *Journal for Clinicians,* 65(2): 87–108.

Wei, J., Huang, Q., Bai, F., Lin, J., Nie, J., Lu, S., Lu, C., Huang, R., Lu, Z. and Lin, X. (2017). Didymin induces apoptosis through mitochondrial dysfunction and up-regulation of RKIP in human hepatoma cells. *Chemico-Biological Interactions*, 261: 118–26.

Xu, J., Pham, C.G., Albanese, S.K., Dong, Y., Oyama, T., Lee, C.H., Rodrik-Outmezguine, V., Yao, Z., Han, S., Chen, D. and Parton, D.L. (2016). Mechanistically distinct cancer-associated mTOR activation clusters predict sensitivity to rapamycin. *The Journal of Clinical Investigation,* 126(9): 3526–40.

Xu, X., Zhang, X., Zhang, Y., Yang, L., Liu, Y., Huang, S., Lu, L., Kong, L., Li, Z., Guo, Q. and Zhao, L. (2017). Wogonin reversed resistant human myelogenous leukemia cells *via* inhibiting Nrf2 signaling by Stat3/NF-κB inactivation. *Scientific Reports,* 7.

Yang, F., Li, J., Zhu, J., Wang, D., Chen, S. and Bai, X. (2015). Hydroxy safflor yellow A inhibits angiogenesis of hepatocellular carcinoma *via* blocking ERK/MAPK and NF-κB signaling pathway in H22 tumor-bearing mice. *European Journal of Pharmacology*, 754: 105–14.

Yang, N., Zhao, Y., Wang, Z., Liu, Y. and Zhang, Y. (2017). Scutellarin suppresses growth and causes apoptosis of human colorectal cancer cells by regulating the p53 pathway. *Molecular Medicine Reports,* 15(2): 929–35.

Yao, S., Wang, X., Li, C., Zhao, T., Jin, H. and Fang, W. (2016). Kaempferol inhibits cell proliferation and glycolysis in esophagus squamous cell carcinoma *via* targeting EGFR signaling pathway. *Tumor Biology*, 37(8): 10247–56.

Yap, T.A., Omlin, A. and de Bono, J.S. (2013). Development of therapeutic combinations targeting major cancer signaling pathways. *Journal of Clinical Oncology,* 31(12): 1592–605.

Yoshinaga, A., Kajiya, N., Oishi, K., Kamada, Y., Ikeda, A., Chigwechokha, P.K., Kibe, T., Kishida, M., Kishida, S., Komatsu, M. and Shiozaki, K. (). Neu3 inhibitory effect of naringin suppresses cancer cell growth by attenuation of EGFR signaling through GM3 ganglioside accumulation. *European Journal of Pharmacology*, 782: 21–9.

Youns, M. and Hegazy, W.A. (2017). The natural flavonoid fisetin inhibits cellular proliferation of hepatic, colorectal, and pancreatic cancer cells through modulation of multiple signaling pathways. *PLoS ONE,* 12(1): e0169335.

Zang, M.D., Hu, L., Fan, Z.Y., Wang, H.X., Zhu, Z.L., Cao, S., Wu, X.Y., Li, J.F., Su, L.P., Li, C., Zhu, Z.G., Yan, M. and Liu, B.Y. (2017). Luteolin suppresses gastric cancer progression by reversing epithelial-mesenchymal transition via suppression of the Notch signaling pathway. *Journal of Translational Medicine,* 15(1): 52.

Zhou, Z., Tang, M., Liu, Y., Zhang, Z., Lu, R. and Lu, J. (2017). Apigenin inhibits cell proliferation, migration, and invasion by targeting Akt in the A549 human lung cancer cell line. *Anti-Cancer Drugs,* 28(4): 446–56.

2

Molecular Mechanisms of the Antimicrobial Effect of Natural Flavonoids Against Human Pathogens

Ali Esmail Al-snafi[1]*

ABSTRACT

Flavonoids generally possess a broad spectrum of anti microbial activity such as antiviral antibacterial and antifungal activity. Regarding the antibacterial effects, flavonoids have the killing ability against both Gram positive and Gram negative bacteria. Furthermore, synergy between naturally occurring flavonoids and antibacterial agents against resistant strains was also recorded. The antibacterial mechanisms of action of various flavonoids included inhibition of nucleic acid synthesis (especially DNA-gyrase), inhibition of cytoplasmic membrane function, inhibition of energy metabolism and many other anti virulence mechanisms. Regarding the anti-fungal activity of flavonoids, they covalently bind to the catalytic site of fatty acid synthase and disrupt the condensation reaction of acetyl-COA and malonyl-COA, thus inhibiting the biosynthesis of fatty acids and sterols in fungi. In addition, flavonoids also affect the fungal DNA and cell cycle, and many virulent factors. The mechanisms of antiviral activity of flavonoids included antiinfective, antireplicative, inhibitory activity of reverse transcriptase, or RNA-directed DNA polymerase, antiintegrase and antiprotease and many other molecular activities. This article will highlight the antiviral, antibacterial and antifungal effects of various flavonoids and the mechanism of action of flavonoids against different pathogens.

***Key words*:** Flavonoids, Antibacterial, Antiviral, Antifungal, Mechanism.

[1] Department of Pharmacology, College of Medicine - Thi Qar University, Iraq
**Corresponding author*: E-mail: aboahmad61@yahoo.com

1. INTRODUCTION

Flavonoids are polyphenolic compounds isolated from different parts of the plants. The basic structural unit of flavonoid compounds consist of 2-phenyl-benzo α-pyrane or flavane nucleus, which is further composed of two benzene rings (A and B) that are linked by a heterocyclic pyrane ring (C). Flavonoids possess a wide range of pharmacological effects including anticancer, antioxidant, antidiabetic, immunological, antiinflammatory, antipyretic, antibacterial, antifungal, antiviral, antiulcer, antiosteoporotic, endocrine, hepatoprotective, vasorelaxant, antiatherosclerotic, antithrombogenic, cardioprotective, anxiolytic and many other effects (Kumar and Pandey, 2013, Lopez-Lazaro, 2009). This article highlights the molecular mechanism of antibacterial, antifungal and antiviral effects of flavonoids.

2. FLAVONOIDS WITH ANTIBACTERIAL EFFECTS

Preliminary studies showed that natural flavonoids, flavones, flavonol glycosides, isoflavones, flavanones, and chalcones showed potent antibacterial activity (Table 1).

2.1. Synergy of Flavonoids with Each Other and with Antibacterial Drugs

Recently, it appeared that when flavonoids were applied in combinations with other flavonoids or antibiotics, they produced synergistic effects. Bovine isolated methicillin-resistant *S. aureus* (MRSA) showed susceptibility to a combination of quercetin and naringenin (Lee *et al.*, 2013). Flavonoid derivatives such as quercetin-5'- sulfonic acid and the sodium salt of Morin-5'-sulfonic acid showed antimicrobial effect against extended-spectrum beta-lactamase producing (ESBL) *E. coli* strains (Woz nicka *et al.*, 2013; Amin *et al.*, 2015). A combination of flavonoids with a wide variety of antibiotics, to which bacteria were gaining resistance, decrease the MIC of flavonoids and antibiotics (Amin *et al.*, 2015; Alvarez *et al.*, 2006). Synergism was observed between baicalein and penicillins against penicillinase-producing *Staphylococcus aureus* (Qian *et al.*, 2015). Morin with β-lactam antibiotics (Mun *et al.*, 2015), luteolin, quercetin, scutellarin and apigenin (Su *et al.*, 2014), genistein and diosmetin in combination with norfloxacin (Wang *et al.*, 2014), diosmetin with erythromycin (Chan *et al.*, 2013), epigallocatechin gallate and oxytetracycline (Novy *et al.*, 2013), baicalin with oxytetracycline and tetracycline (Novy *et al.*, 2011), rhamnoside with ampicillin, levofloxacin, ceftazidime and azithromycin (An *et al.*, 2011) were effective against methicillin-resistant *Staphylococcus aureus*. Baicalein with ciprofloxacin were effective against NorA over-expressed methicillin-resistant *Staphylococcus aureus* (Chan *et al.*, 2011). Apigenin and ceftazidime had anti microbial activity against ceftazidime-

Table 1: Flavonoids Possessing Antibacterial Activity

Source	*Flavonoids*	*Bacteria*	*Activity*	*Ref*
Artocarpus anisophyllus and *Artocarpus lowii*	2',4'-Dihydroxy-4-methoxy-3'-prenyldihydrochalcone; 4-Hydroxyonchocarpin; Isobavachalcone; 2',4'-dihydroxy-3,4(2",2"-dimethyl chromeno)-3'-prenyldihydro chalcone; 5,7-dihydroxy-4'-methoxy-6-prenylflavanone; 5-hydroxy-6,7-(2, 2-dimethyl chromano)-4'-methoxy flavanone; 4',5-dihydroxy-6,7-(2, 2-dimethylchromeno)-2'-methoxy-8-γ, γ-dimethylallyl flavone; artocarpin; yranocycloartobiloxanthone A and cycloheterophyllin	*Staphylococcus aureus, Bacillus cereus, Escherichia coli* and *Pseudomonas putida*	All flavonoids showed inhibitory activity towards selected bacteria. Artocarpin showed strong antimicrobial activity towards all bacteria with inhibition zone diameter more than 11 mm and minimum microbicidal concentration value of 0.45 mg/mL. Isobavachalcone exhibited strong antibacterial activity towards Gram positive bacteria with minimum microbicidal concentration value of 0.45 mg/mL	Jamil *et al.*, 2014
Bartramia pomiformis, D. scoparium, P. affine, P. cuspidatum, Hedwigia ciliata	Bartramiaflavone (*Bartramia pomiformis*); apigenin-7 -O-triglycoside and luteolin-7-O-neohesperidoside (*D. scoparium*) ; apigenin and vitexin (*P. affine*) saponarine (*P. cuspidatum)*	*Enterobacter cloaceae, E. aerogenes* and *Pseudomonas aeruginosa*	Enterobacteriaceae showed the greatest sensitivity to the flavonoids. Neither *Staphylococcus aureus* nor *Proteus vulgaris* showed any sensitivity to the substances tested	Basile *et al.*, 1999
Cassia sophera	5,7,3',4'-Tetrahydroxy-3-methoxyflavone-5-O- -L-rhamnopyranosyl-7-O- -D-glucopyranosyl (1 3)-O- -D-xylopyranoside	*Bacillus coagulas, Staphylococcus aureus, Escherichia coli.* and *Pseudomonas aerugenosa*	Its diameter of inhibition at a concentration of 100% ranged between 9.8mm against *Pseudomonas aerugenosa* and 18.3 mm against *Staphylococcus aureus*	Nema *et al.*, 2012
Citrus bergamia	Neohesperidin, hesperetin, neoeriocitrin, eriodictyol, naringin and naringenin	*Escherichia coli, Pseudomonas putida, Salmonella enteric, Listeria innocua,*	The minimum inhibitory concentrations of the neohesperidin, hesperetin, neoeriocitrin, eriodictyol, naringin and naringenin were found	Mandalari *et al.*, 2007

Table 1: *(Contd...)*

Table 1: *(Contd...)*

Source	*Flavonoids*	*Bacteria*	*Activity*	*Ref*
		Bacillus subtilis, Staphylococcus aureus and *Lactococcus lactis*	to be in the range 200 to 800 μg/mL	
Cnidium monnieri	Rutin, naringin and baicalin	*Staphylococcus aureus, Shigella flexneri, Salmonella typhi, Escherichia coli* and *Pseudomonas aeruginosa*	At the dose of 128 mg/l, the flavonoids (rutin, naringin and baicalin) inhibited 25% or less of *P. aeruginosa* and only baicalin was active against *S. aureus.*	Ng *et al.*, 1996
Combretum erythrophyllum	Apigenin; genkwanin; 5-hydroxy-7, 4′-dimethoxy flavone, rhamnocitrin; kaempferol; quercetin-5, 3′-dimethylether; rhamnazin	*Vibrio cholera, Enterococcus faecali* and *Micrococcus luteus*	All compounds had good activity against *Vibrio cholerae* and *Enterococcus faecalis*, with MIC values in the range of 25–50 μg/mL. Rhamnocitrin and quercetin-5, 3′-dimethylether also inhibited *Micrococcus luteus* and *Shigella sonei* at 25 μg/mL	Maritini *et al.*, 2004
Dalbergia melanoxylon	3-Hydroxyiso flavanones	*M. tuberculosis* H37Rv strains	Inhibited the growth of *M. tuberculosis* H37Rv strains	Mutai *et al.*, 2013
Dodonaea viscose	3, 5, 7-Trihydroxy-4'-methoxyflavone; 5, 7, 4'-trihydroxy-3, 6-dimethoxy flavone; 5, 7-dihydroxy-3, 6, 4'-trimethoxy flavone (santin); and 5-hydroxy -3, 7, 4'-trimethoxyflavone	*Staphylococcus aureus, Enterococcus faecalis, Escherichia coli* and *Pseudomonas aeruginosa*	The minimum inhibitory concentration varied from 16 μg/mL to more than 250 μg/mL. 3,4',5,7-tetrahydroxy flavone (kaempferol) was the most active against all the test organisms with MIC values between 16 and 63 μg/mL. 5, 7, 4'-trihydroxy-3, 6-dimethoxyflavone was the second most active and was the only isolated compound with reasonable activity	Teffo *et al.*, 2010

Table 1: *(Contd...)*

Table 1: *(Contd...)*

Source	***Flavonoids***	***Bacteria***	***Activity***	***Ref***
			against *P. aeruginosa*. 3, 5, 7-trihydroxy -4'-methoxyflavone had the best activity (23 µg/mL) against *E. faecalis*, but had very low activity against the other organisms. 5, 7-dihydroxy-3, 6, 4'-trimethoxyflavone (santin) had poor activity against all the test organisms (MIC between 63 and 125 µg/mL) and 5-hydroxy -3, 7, 4'-trimethoxyflavone had no activity at the highest concentration tested (250 µg/mL).	
Dorstenia barteri	Isobachalcone, kanzanol C, 4-hydroxylonchocarpin, stipulin and amentoflavone	*M. tuberculosis* H37Rv and *M. smegmatis*	They showed antimycobacterial activity against *M. tuberculosis* H37Rv and *M. smegmatis* with the MIC values were the range of 2.44-30 µg/m	Kuete *et al.*, 2010
Dorstenia barteri and *D. dinklagei.*	6,8-Diprenyleriodictyol; isobavachalcone; 6-prenylapigenin and 4-hydroxylonchocarpin	*Staphylococcus aureus* including methicillin resistant *S. aureus* (MRSA) strains	6,8-diprenyleriodictyol; isobava-chalcone and 6-prenylapigenin showed signifiant antibacterial activity against *S. aureus* including MRSA strains, with MICs values ranged between 0.5-16 µg/mL.	Sichel *et al.*, 1991
Eucalyptus maculate	2,6-Dihydroxy-3-methyl-4-methoxy-dihydrochalcone; eucalyptin and 8-desmethyl-eucalyptin	*Staphylococcus aureus, Bacillus cereus, Enterococcus faecalis, Propionibacterium acnes* and *Escherichia coli*	All compounds possessed inhibitory activities against the tested bacteria with MIC ranging from 1.0 to 31 mg. 2, 6-dihydroxy-3-methyl-4-methoxy-dihydrochalcone less active antibacterial than eucalyptin and 8-desmethyl-eucalyptin.	Takahashi *et al.*, 2004
Euphorbia hirta	(-)-Epicatechin 3-gallate	*Pseudomonas aeruginosa*	It demonstrated significant minimum inhibitory concentration of	Perumal *et al.*, 2015

Table 1: *(Contd...)*

Table 1: *(Contd...)*

Source	*Flavonoids*	*Bacteria*	*Activity*	*Ref*
			31.3 µg/mLl	
Galium fissurense, Viscum album ssp. album and *Cirsium hypoleucum*	5,7-Dimethoxyflavanone-4'-O-β-D-glucopyranoside, 5,7-dimethoxy-flavanone-4'-O-[2''-O-(5'''-O-trans-cinnamoyl)-β-D-apiofuranosyl]-β-D-glucopyranoside, naringenin-7-O-β-D-glucopyranoside, 5,7,3'-trihydroxy-flavanone-4'-O-β-D-glucopyranoside, rutin, and nicotiflorin	extended-spectrum β-lactamase producing multidrug-resistant *Klebsiella pneumoniae*	All the flavonoids showed *in vitro* antimicrobial activity against all the isolated strains of *K. pneumoniae* similar to the control antibacterial (ofloxacin) at the concentrations of 32-64 µg/ mL	Özçelik *et al.*, 2008
Glycyrrhiza inflata	Licochalcones A and C	*Staphylococcus aureus* and *Micrococcus luteus*	licochalcone A inhibited incorporation of radioactive precursors into macro-molecules (DNA, RNA, and protein)	Haraguchi *et al.*, 1998
Heritiera littoralis	Cinnamolyglico flavonoids 3-cinnamoyltribuloside, afzein and stilbin	*Mycobacterium species, M. madagascarience* and *M. indicus pranii*	The MIC values were the range of 1.6-0.8 mg/mL	Christopher *et al.*, 2014
Indigofera secundiflora	Quercetin; quercetin 3-O-methylether and quercetin 3,31,41-trimethylether	*Staphylococcus aureus, Bacillus subtilis, Escherichia coli* and *Pseudomonas aeruginosa*	Quercetin showed the least activity, quercetin-3-O-methylether possessed significant activity against *Staphylococcus aureus*, while quercetin 3,3′,4′-trimethylethe showed activity against all the tested pathogens	Ahmadu *et al.*, 2011
Leucaeana leucocephala	Quercetin - 3-O-(2''-trans-*p*-coumaryl)-α-rhamnopyranosyl-(1'''→6'')-β-glucopyranoside; quercetin-3-O-α-rhamnopyranosyl-(1'''→2'')-β–glucopyranoside; quercetin-7-O-α–rhamnopyranosyl-(1'''→2'')-β-glucopyrano side and quercetin-3-O-	*Bacillus cereus, Staphylococcus aureus, Escherichia coli, Pseudomonas aeruginosa* and *Salmonella typhimurium*	All tested flavonoids exhibited significant inhibition against *Salmonella typhimurium* and *E coli* (97.74, 95.49, 81.85, 84.10 %) and (88.34, 83.74, 69.78, 86.04 %) respectively. Only(quercetin-3-O-(2''-trans-*p*- coumaryl)-α-	Mohammed *et al.*, 2015

Table 1: *(Contd...)*

Table 1: *(Contd...)*

Source	*Flavonoids*	*Bacteria*	*Activity*	*Ref*
	β–glucopyranoside		rhamnopyranosyl-(1'''→6'')-β-glucopyranoside) was effective compound against *Pseudomonas*	
Mangifera indica	(–)-Epicatechin-3-O-β-glucopyranoside; 5-hydroxy-3-(4-hydroxylphenyl) pyrano [3,2-g]chromene-4(8H)-one; 6-(p-hydroxy benzyl) taxifolin-7-O-β-D-glucoside (tricuspid); quercetin-3-O-α-gluco pyranosyl-(1→2)-β-glucopyranoside; and (–)-epicatechin (2-(3,4-dihydroxy phenyl)-3,4-dihydro-2H-chromene-3,5,7-triol)	*Lactobacillus sp., Escherichia coli, Azospirillium lipoferum* and *Bacillus sp.*	Different concentrations of these compounds decreased bacterial growth by 52–96 %. (–)-epicatechin-3-O-β-glucopyranoside exhibited the lowest antibacterial activity, resulting in a 7–75 % reduction in the growth of the different bacterial species. (–)-epicatechin(2-(3,4-dihydroxy phenyl)-3,4-dihydro-2H-chromene-3,5,7-triol) showed the greatest antibacterial activity and the different concentrations reduced the bacterial growth by 45–99.9 %.	Kanwal *et al.*, 2009
Mangifera indica	Cyanidin-3- glycosides and quercetin-3-rutinoside (rutin)	*Pseudomonas* and *Staphlococcus*	Rutin and cyanidin-3- glycosides showed antibacterial activity against *Pseudomonas* and *Staphlococcus.*	Sami and Shakoori, 2011
Mentha longifolia	Quercetin3-O-glycoside, apigenin, luteolin-7-O-glucoside, luteolin-7,3'-O-diglucoside and kaempfero-3-O-glucoside	*E. coli, S. aureus, B. cereus, P. aeruginosa* and *B. subtilis*	Flavonoids identified gave an inhibition of all the species with MICs varying between 0.095 mg/mL and 0.025 mg/mL. Only the luteolin-7-O-glucoside and the luteolin-7,3'-O-diglucoside did not have an action on the growth of *E. coli* and *P. aeruginosa,*. The synergism between the three most active identified flavonoids gave a best antimicrobial activity with 0.050 mg/mL for *E. coli*, 0.070 for *S. aureus*,	Akroum *et al.*, 2009

Table 1: *(Contd...)*

Table 1: *(Contd...)*

Source	*Flavonoids*	*Bacteria*	*Activity*	*Ref*
			0.045 mg/mL for *B. cereus*, 0.040 mg/mL for *P. aeruginosa* and 0.010 mg/mL for *B. subtilis.*	
Mimusops elengi	2,3-Dihyro-3,3'4'5,7-pentahydroxyflavone and 3,3',4',5,7-pentahydroxyflavone	*Escherichia coli* ATCC 25922, *Bacillus subtilis* ATCC 6633 and *Salmonella typhi* ATCC 6539	The compounds showed strong inhibitory activity against Gram positive and Gram negative bacteria	Hazra *et al.*, 2007
Morus alba, Morus mongolica, Broussnetia papyrifera, Sophora flavescens and *Echinosophora koreensis*	Papyriflavonol A, kuraridin, sophora-flavanone D, sophoraisoflavanone A, Kuwanon C, mulberrofuran G, albanol B, kenusanone A, sophoraflavanone G, Morusin, sanggenon B, kazinol B, kurarinone, kenusanone C, broussochalcone A and isosophoranone	*Escherichia coli, Salmonella typhimurium, Staphylococcus epidermis* and *S. aureus*	Papyriflavonol A, kuraridin, sophoraflavanone D and sophoraiso-flavanone A exhibited strong antibacterial activity. Kuwanon C, mulberrofuran G, albanol B, kenusanone A and sophoraflavanone G showed strong antibacterial activity with 5-30 microg/mL of MICs. Morusin, sanggenon B and D, kazinol B, kurarinone, kenusanone C and isosophoranone were effective to only gram positive bacteria	Sohn *et al.*, 2004
Murraya paniculata	3',4',5',7-Tetramethoxyflavone	*Porphyromonas-gingivalis* (ATCC33277)	Diameter of zone of inhibition was 13 against *Porphyromonas gingivalis*	Rodanant *et al.*, 2015
Oncoba spinosa	Kaempferol, quercetin, apigenin-7-O-β-D-glucuronopyranoside, quercetin 3-O-β-D-galactopyranoside and quercetin 3-O-α-L-rhamnopyranosyl (1→6) β-D-glucopyranoside	*Enterobacter aerogenes, Escherichia coli, Klebsiella pneumonia* and *Staphylococcus*	Quercetin 3-O-α-L-rhamnopyranosyl (1→6) β-D-glucopyranoside and quercetin were the most active compounds against bacteria (MIC= 8–64 µg/mL) and fungi (MIC=64 – 128 µg/mL) respectively	Djouossi *et al.*, 2015

Table 1: *(Contd...)*

Table 1: *(Contd...)*

Source	*Flavonoids*	*Bacteria*	*Activity*	*Ref*
		aureus		
Polyalthia longifolia	Rutin and chrysin	*Escherichia coli, Klebsiella aerogenes, Proteus vulgaris, Pseudomonas aeruginosa, Serratia marcescenes, Salmonella typhi, Shigella flexneri, Bacillus subtillis, Streptococcus pyogenes* and *Staphylococcus aureus*	All tested bacteria were sensitive with diameter of inhibition of 11-21mm for rutin	Sampath and Vasanthi, 2013
Polygonum equisetiforme	Quercetin	*Enterobacter aerogenes* and *Escherichia coli*	It had a narrow antibacterial spectrum of activity	Ghazal *et al.*, 1992
Portulaca oleracea	Apigenin	*Pseudomonas aeruginosa, Salmonella typhimurium, Proteus mirabilis, Klebsiella pneumoniae* and *Enterobacter aerogenes*	Among all the bacterial strains, *Salmonella typhimurium* 17.36±0.18 and *Proteus mirabilis* 19.12 ±0.01 have shown maximum diameter of inhibition zone	Nayaka *et al.*, 2014
Praxelis clematides	5.7.4'-trimethoxyflavone	*Staphylococcus aureus* - ATCC 13150, *Staphylococcus aureus* - ATCC 25923, *Staphylococcu-sepidermidis* 12228, *Bacillus subtilis*	5.7.4'-trimethoxyflavone showed a significant inhibitory effect against *Staphylococcus aureus, Pseudomonas aeruginosa* and *Escherichia coli,* with MIC value equal to 128 µg/mL for both (Gram + and Gram - bacteria). However, the flavonoid has no effect on the	Filho *et al.*, 2013

Table 1: *(Contd...)*

Table 1: *(Contd...)*

Source	*Flavonoids*	*Bacteria*	*Activity*	*Ref*
		ATCC 6633, *Pseudomonas aeruginosa*-P03, *Pseudomonas aeruginosa*-ATCC 25853, *Escherichia coli* –ATCC 25922, *Escherichia coli* – 5, *Salmonella enterica* ATCC 6017, *Salmonella enterica* LM08 and *Shigella sonnei*	species *Staphylococcus epidermidis*, *Bacillus subtilis*, *Salmonella enteric* and *Shigella sonnei.*	
Psidium guajava	Morin-3-*O*-lyxoside, morin-3-*O*-arabinoside, quercetin, and quercetin-3-*O*arabinoside	*Bacillus stearothermophilus*, *Brochothrix thermosphacta*, *Escherichia coli* O157:H7, *Listeria monocytogenes*, *Pseudomonas fluorescens*, *Salmonella enterica*, *Staphylococcus aureus* and *Vibrio cholera*	Studies on inhibitory effects of the flavonoids on spoilage and foodborne pathogenicbacteria revealed that they had bacteriostatic mode of action against all tested spoilage and foodborne pathogenic bacteria	Rattana-chaikunsopon and Phumkhachorn, 2010
Retama raetam	Licoflavone C and derrone	*Escherichia coli* ATCC 25922, *Pseudomonas aeruginosa* ATCC 27950, *Enterococcus faecalis*	Both compounds showed antibacterial activity against *S. aureus*, *P. aeruginosa* and *E. faecalis*. Licoflavone C manifested the best antibacterial activity against *Escherichia coli* with an inhibition zone	Edziri *et al.*, 2012

Table 1: *(Contd...)*

Table 1: *(Contd...)*

Source	*Flavonoids*	*Bacteria*	*Activity*	*Ref*
		ATCC 29212 and *Streptococcus aureus* ATCC 25923	of 22 mm. It inhibits the growth of *E. faecalis* and *P. aeruginosa* with an inhibition zone of 20 mm.	
Spondias mombin	Mombinrin, mombincone, mombinoate, and mombinol	*M. tuberculosis*	Exhibited anti-tubercular inhibition against *M. tuberculosis* strain a lower dose of 40 M/mL concentrations	Olugbuyiro and Moody *et al.*, 2013
Tagetes erecta	Patulitrin	*Alcaligens faecalis, Bacillus cereus, Campylobacter coli, Escherchia coli, Klebsiella pneumoniae, Pseudomonas aeruginosa, Proteus vulgaris, Streptococcus mutans* and *Streptococcus pyogenes*	possesses antibacterial activity against all the tested strains with a zone of inhibition ranged from 21mm against *Pseudomonas aeruginosa* to 29.50 mm against *Kiebsiella pneumoniae*.	Rhama *et al.*, 2011
Viscum album ssp. *Album*	5,7-Dimethoxyflavanone-4′-*O*-β-D-glucopyranoside and 5, 7-dimethoxyflavanone-4′-*O*-[2″-*O*-(54-*O*-*trans*-cinnamoyl)-β-D-apiofuranosyl]-β-D-glucopyranoside	*Escherichia coli, Pseudomonas aeruginosa, Proteus mirabilis, Klebsiella pneumoniae, Acinetobacter baumannii, Staphylococcus aureus, Enterococcus faecalis and Bacillus subtilis*	All tested compounds (32–128 μg/mL) showed strong antimicrobial activities	Orhan *et al.*, 2010
Withania somnifera	7, 3', 4'-Trihydroxy flavone-3-O-rhmnosyl, Quercetin -3-O-galactosyl and 5, 7, 4'-	*Bacillus subtilis, Escherichia coli,*	7, 3', 4'-trihydroxy flavone-3-O-rhmnosyl exhibited a moderately	Bashir *et al.*, 2013

Table 1: *(Contd...)*

Table 1: *(Contd...)*

Source	*Flavonoids*	*Bacteria*	*Activity*	*Ref*
	triahydroxy-methyl-3-O-galactosyl flavonol	*Neisseria gonorrhoeae*, *Pseudomonas aeruginosa* and *Staphylococcus aureus*.	inhibition against all five organisms but less than their crude extract of the plant. Quercetin -3-O-galactosyl showed weak inhibition against all organisms. 5, 7, 4'- triahydroxy-methyl -3-O-galactosyl flavonol exhibited high inhibition against all organisms accept *Pseudomonas aeruginosa*.	
Zea mays	2″-O-α-L-rhamnosyl-6-C-(6-deoxyxylo-hexos-4-ulosyl)-luteolin(maysin) and 2″-O-α-L-rhamnosyl-6-C-(6-deoxy-xylo-hexos-4-ulosyl)-luteolin-3′-methyl ether (maysin-3′-methyl ether)	*Bacillus cereus*, *Bacillus subtilis*, *Staphylococcus aureus*, *Pseudomonas aeruginosa*, *Enterobacter aerogenes*, *Salmonella typhi*, *Salmonella paratyphi*, *Escherichia coli*, *Shigella sonnei*, *Shigella flexneri*, *Proteus vulgaris* and *Proteus mirabilis*	Flavonoid glycosides showed wider range of activity towards gram-positive and gram-negative bacteria. Comparatively, maysin exerted highest antibacterial activity towards gram positive bacteria than maysin-3′-methyl ether	Nessa *et al.*, 2012
Zingiber spectabile	Spectaflavoside A: Kaempferol -3-O-(3",4"-di-O-acetyl)-a-L-rhamnopyranoside: Kaempferol-3-O-(2",3"-di-O-acetyl)-a-L-rhamnopyranoside; Kaempferol-3-O-(2",4"-di-O-acetyl)-a-L-rhamnopyranoside; Kaempferol-3-O-(4"-Oacetyl)-a-L-rhamnopyranoside; Kaempferol.	*B. cereus* (ATCC 10876), *B. licheniformis* (ATCC 12759), *S. aureus* (ATCC 12600), *E. coli* (ATCC 25922), *P. vulgaris* and *V. parahaemolyticus* (ATCC 17802)	The y showed mild antibacterial effects especially against Gram negative bacteria	Sivasothy *et al.*, 2013

resistant *Enterobacter cloacae* (Eumkeb and Chukrathok, 2013). The other effective combinations were luteolin and amoxicillin (against amoxicillin-resistant *Escherichia coli)* (Eumkeb *et al.*, 2012), galangin, kaempferide and kaempferide-3-O-β-d-glucoside with amoxicillin combinations (against amoxicillin-resistant *Escherichia coli)* (Eumkeb *et al.*, 2012), epigallocatechin gallate with imipenem (against imipenem-resistant *Klebsiella pneumonia)* (Cho *et al.*, 2011), baicalein and gentamicin (against vancomycin-resistant Enterococcus) (Chang *et al.*, 2007) and kaempferol with erythromycin or clindamycin (against *Propionibacterium acnes)*[(64)].

2.2. Structure Activity Relationships and Anti-bacterial Activity of Flavonoids

Thirty eight flavonoids (flavones, flavonols, and flavanones) were tested for activity against strains of methicillin resistant *S. aureus* (MRSA). The growth of MRSA was inhibited by only the aglycones of the flavonols and flavones. The presence of at least one hydroxyl group in rings A or B at C-3, 5, 7 was important for activity. Compounds without hydroxyl groups in ring B (pinocembrin, chrysin, galangin) or compounds in which the hydroxyl was replaced with a methoxy group (kaempferide, tamarixetin) turned out to be inactive. Substitution of aglycones with glycones, (myricetin glucoside, quercetin glucoside) resulted in a loss of activity against the strains of the tested bacteria (Xu *et al.*, 2001).

The flavonoids which possessed antibacterial activity against extended-spectrum β-lactamase producing multidrug-resistant *Klebsiella pneumonia* contained an obligatory C–4 keto group and hydroxyl group substitutions at C–5 and have at least one hydroxyl group on ring B. The compounds having methoxyl group substitutions at C-5 and C-7 were also effective antibacterial flavonoids (Özçelik *et al.*, 2008). The sites and number of hydroxyl groups on the phenol group were thought to be related to the relative toxicity of flavonoids to microorganisms, with evidence that increased hydroxylation results in increased toxicity. The mechanisms responsible for toxicity to microorganisms include enzyme inhibition by the oxidized compounds, in which the hydroxyl groups determine the affinity to bind with the enzyme active sites, possibly through reaction with sulfhydryl groups or through more nonspecific interactions with the proteins (Shehadi *et al.*, 2014). 5-hydroxyflavanones and 5- hydroxyisoflavanones with one, two, or three additional hydroxyl groups at the 7, 2 and 4 positions possessed strong inhibitory effects on the growth of *S. mutans* and *Streptococcus sobrinus* (Osawa *et al.*, 1998).

Kaempferol and quercetin showed the highest antibacterial ability, and quercetin exhibited stronger inhibitory activity than luteolin, with the only structural difference between these 2 compounds being that quercetin has a hydroxyl group at position 3 in the C ring, while luteolin has none. This indicated that hydroxyl group at position 3 in the C ring was important to the antibacterial activity of flavonoids (Wu *et al.*, 2013; Sichel *et al.*, 1991). The 5,7-dihydroxylation of the A ring and 2,4-or 2,6-dihydroxylation of the B ring in the flavanone structure was important for anti-MRSA activity (Haraguchi *et al.*, 1998). A hydroxyl group at position 5 in flavanones and flavones was important for flavonoid activity against MRSA. Substitution with C8 and C10 chains may also enhance the antistaphylococcal activity of flavonoids belonging to the flavan-3-ol class (Alcaraz *et al.*, 2000). However, the methoxyl group at C-8 in the A ring appears to increase antibacterial activity. Tangeritin showed higher activity than 5,6,7,42-tetramethoxyflavone, both having a similar structure except for the methoxyl group at C-8 in the A ring (Wu *et al.*, 2013).

The antimicrobial activity of flavonoids could be linked to varying degrees of methylation of the -OH groups of these compounds. A hydroxyl was required at C-7 for antibacterial activity and a hydroxyl group was required at C-4 for activity against *P. aeruginosa* but this was apparently not the case with *S. aureus*. It did not seem that substitution at C-6 plays an important role (Teffo *et al.*, 2010). The C atom at position 3 in the C ring has a major role in hydrophobicity which represented the ability of drugs to interact with biological membranes, the factor which play an essential role in antibacterial activity of flavonoids (Wu *et al.*, 2013).

2.3. Molecular Mechanism of Antibacterial Effects of Flavonoids

Flavonoids can exert antibacterial activities through multiple mechanisms, such as disruption of cytoplasmic membrane, inhibition of nucleic acid synthesis, inhibition of energy metabolism, inhibition of folic acid synthesis, inhibition of cell membrane synthesis and function, and anti-virulence mechanisms (Fig. 1).

2.3.1. *Effect on cellular membrane structure and functions*

The membrane interactivity of flavonoids was evaluated by fluorescent probe 1,6-diphenyl- 1,3,5-hexatriene (DPH) polarization and compared with the controls. An increase in fluorescence polarization values (FP) indicated a decrease of membrane fluidity. Flavonoids rigidified the model membrane, in the order: kaempferol < chrysin < quercetin< baicalein < luteolin. The membrane interaction effects of flavonoids were influenced by the number and the position of hydroxyl groups. The hydroxyl group at C-3 in the C ring was important for decreasing membrane fluidity. There was a significant positive correlation between antibacterial capacity and membrane rigidification effect of the flavonoids ($r = 0.921$), indicating that flavonoids exert part of their antibacterial action by reducing membrane fluidity. Kaempferol, located deeply in the hydrophobic core of the lipid

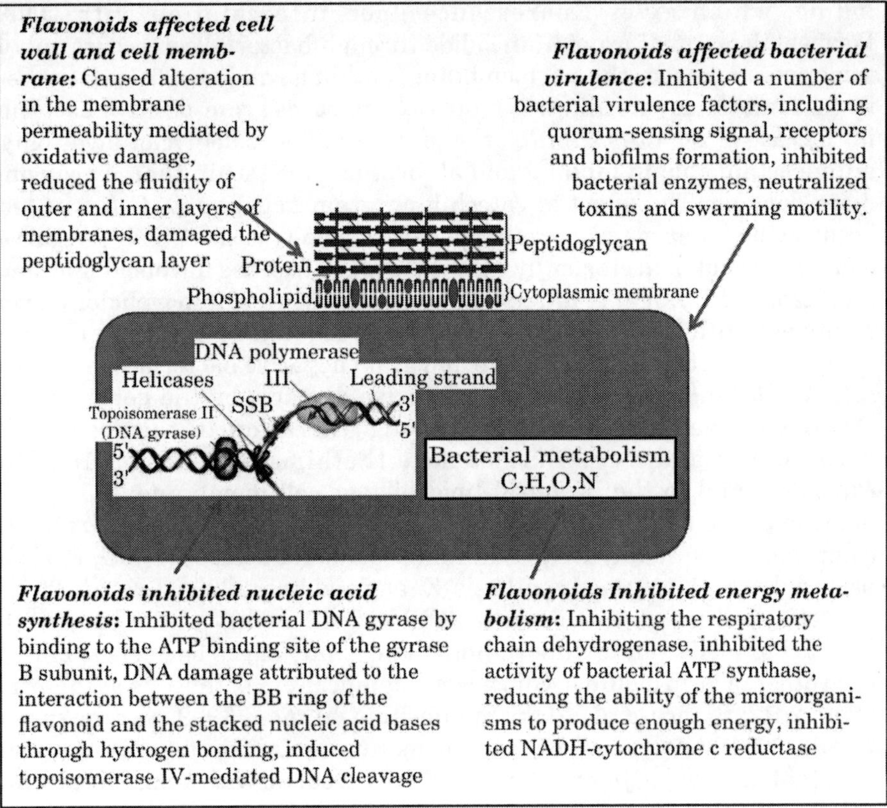

Fig. 1: Mechanisms of Antibacterial Effects of Favonoids

bilayer, decreased the membrane fluidity and exhibiting the highest antibacterial capacity. Functions of membrane enzymes and receptors, as well as the reaction efficacy of membrane components were modulated by fluidity changes, leading to disturbances in multiple membrane functions (Wu *et al.*, 2013).

The sensitive cyanine dye DiS-C3-(5) (3,3'-dipropylthiadicarbocyanine iodide) was used to study the effects of flavonoids (6,8-diprenyleriodictyol; isobavachalcone; 6-prenylapigenin and 4-hydroxylonchocarpin) isolated from *Dorstenia barteri* and *Dorstenia dinklagei* on membrane potential of *Staphylococcus aureus*. Depolarization of membrane was observed in *Staphylococcus aureus* when treated with these flavonoids. At 5-fold minimum inhibitory concentration, compounds caused lysis of *Staphylococcus aureus* (Sichel *et al.*, 1991). Assessment of toxicity of catechin against *Bacillus subtilis* and *Escherichia colii* as model organisms showed that the inhibitory mechanism of catechin was mediated by oxidative damage through membrane permeabilization. The cell membrane integrity and permeabilization were studied using the fluorescent dye propidium iodide, which gives fluorescence upon intercalation with DNA. Permeabilization of propidium iodide through bacterial cell occurs only if some agent damages the cell membrane (Fathima and Rao, 2016). However, it was found that catechin was more toxic towards gram-positive bacteria, in the case of *Bacillus subtilis*, the presence of peptidoglycan layer plays an important role in binding and absorption of catechin thereby causing more damage. The effect of catechin on gram negative *E. Coli* was less because the outer membrane (lipopolysaccharide) with repulsive negative charge does not bind efficiently with the OH group of the flavonoid (Fathima and Rao, 2016; Ikigai *et al.*, 1993). The changes in cell morphology upon treatment with catechin were further documented by scanning electron microscopy. In both gram positive and gram negative bacteria, the mode of action of killing was found to be oxidative damage, by the generation of reactive oxygen species (ROS) causing alteration in the membrane permeability and membrane damage (Fathima and Rao, 2016). Tea catechins bind to the bacterial lipid bilayer cell membrane and causes damage to the membrane (Sirk *et al.*, 2008; Sirk *et al.*, 2009). Green tea components (especially EGCG) inhibit specific reductases (FabG, FabI) in bacterial type II fatty acid synthesis (Zhang and Rock, 2004; Li *et al.*, 2006). Bacterial cell membrane damage inhibited the ability of the bacteria to bind to host cells and further inhibited the ability of the bacteria to bind to each other to form biofilms, which were significant in pathogenesis (Sharma *et al.*, 2012; Blanco *et al.*, 2005; Sugita-Konishi *et al.*, 1999; Sakanaka and Okada, 2004). Analysis of the outer membrane protein profiles of imipenem-resistant *Klebsiella pneumoniae* cultures treated with epigallocatechin gallate revealed unique changes in outer membrane proteins. In addition, scanning electron microscopic analysis showed that bacteria appeared with wrinkled surfaces containing perforations and irregular rod-shaped forms (Cho *et al.*, 2011).

The effect of sophoraflavanone G on membrane fluidity was studied using liposomal model membranes and compared with naringenin. Sophoraflavanone G increased the fluorescence polarisation of the liposomes significantly which indicated that sophoraflavanone G reduced the fluidity of outer and inner layers of membranes. Naringenin also exhibited the same effect but at higher concentrations. The correlation between antibacterial activity and membrane effect sconfirmed that flavonoids possessed their antibacterial activity by reducing membrane fluidity of bacterial cells (Tsuchiya and Iinuma, 2000). Galangin flavonoids also caused marked morphological damage to amoxicillin-resistant *Escherichia coli*, which included loosening or detachment of the OM, possibly resulting from damage to the internal peptidoglycan layer. Some of the bacteria exhibited electron transparent areas devoid of ribosomes in the cytoplasm. Most of the treated bacteria also appeared considerably larger than the control bacteria (Eumkeb *et al.*, 2012). Methicillin resistant *Staphylococcus aureus* clinical isolate treated with (“)-epicatechin gallate and 3-*O*-octanoyl-(+)-catechin, exhibited highly increased levels of labelling with the selectively permeable fluorescent stain propidium iodide (Stapleton *et al.*, 2004).

2.3.2. *Inhibition of nucleic acids synthesis*

DNA gyrase was a type II topoisomerase that can introduce negative supercoils into DNA at the expense of ATP hydrolysis. It was essential in all bacteria but absent from higher eukaryotes, making it an attractive target for antibacterials. DNA topoisomerases are divided into two types, I and II, depending on whether they catalyse reactions involving the transient breakage of one (type I) or both (type II) strands of DNA (Collin *et al.*, 2011).

In general, previous studies showed that quercetin and genistein inhibited topoisomerase type II. Myricetin, quercetin, fisetin, and morin inhibited both topoisomerase I and II, while kaempferol inhibited opoisomerase II only (Constantinou *et al.*, 1995; Talalay *et al.*, 1995; Moskaug *et al.*, 2004). Quercetin inhibited supercoiling activity of bacterial gyrase and induced DNA cleavage. Quercetin jointed to the 24 kDa fragment of gyrase B of *Escherichia coli* with a K (D) value of 15 microM and inhibited ATPase activity of gyrase B. Its binding site overlaps with ATP binding pocket. Quercetin inhibited gyrases through two different mechanisms based either on interaction with DNA or with ATP binding site of gyrase (Plaper *et al.*, 2003). Quercetin also effectively docked with subunit B of DNA gyrase in *M. tuberculosis* and *M. smegmatis* and effectively inhibited the bacilli growth *in vitro* (Suriyanarayanan *et al.*, 2013).

DNA damage caused by catechin to the bacteria can be attributed to the interaction which takes place between the BB ring of the flavonoid and the stacked nucleic acid bases through hydrogen bonding. The presence of open circular form of DNA in the catechin-treated *B. subtilis* clearly reveals the role of catechin as restriction enzymes, which is not seen in the case of catechin-treated *E. coli* DNA (Fathima and Rao, 2016). Catechins inhibited bacterial DNA gyrase by binding to the ATP binding site of the gyrase B subunit. Specific binding to the N-terminal 24 kDa fragment of gyrase B was determined by fluorescence spectroscopy and confirmed using heteronuclear two-dimensional NMR spectroscopy of the EGCG"15N-labeled gyrase B fragment complex. Protein residues affected by binding to EGCG were identified through chemical shift perturbation. Molecular docking calculations suggest that the benzopyran ring of EGCG penetrated deeply into the active site while the galloyl moiety anchored it to the cleft through interactions with its hydroxyl groups, which explained the higher activity of EGCG and ECG (Gradisar *et al.*, 2007).

3,7-diacylquercetin; quercetin 6"-acylgalactoside; and quercetin 2",6"-diacylgalactoside analogues inhibited *Escherichia coli* DNA gyrase and

Staphylococcus aureus topoIV. Most of the investigated compounds exhibited pronounced inhibition with MIC values ranging from 0.13 to 128 μg/mL toward the growth of multidrug-resistant Gram-positive methicillin-resistant *S. aureus*, methicillin sensitive *S. aureus*, vancomycin-resistant enterococci (VRE), vancomycin intermediate *S. aureus*, and *Streptococcus pneumoniae* bacterial strains (Hossion *et al.*, 2011). Radiolabeled thymidine, uridine, and methionine were used to evaluate the effect of flavonoids (6,8-diprenyleriodictyol; isobavachalcone; 6-prenylapigenin and 4-hydroxylonchocarpin) isolated from *Dorstenia barteri* and *Dorstenia dinklagei* on the biosynthesis of DNA, RNA, and proteins. Inhibition of DNA, RNA, and proteins synthesis were observed in *S. aureus* when treated with these flavonoids. At 5-fold minimum inhibitory concentration, the compounds reduced rapidly the bacterial cell density (Sichel *et al.*, 1991). However, it was found that *E. coli* DNA gyrase was inhibited to different extents by seven flavonoids including quercetin, apigenin and 3,6,7,3,4-pentahydroxyflavone (Ohemeng *et al.*, 1993; Wu *et al.*, 2013).

DNA synthesis was predominantly inhibited by the flavonoids in *Proteus vulgaris*, whereas RNA synthesis was inhibited in *Staphylococcus aureus*. DNA synthesis was also inhibited with fragmentation when *E. coli, Staphylococcus aureus* and *Klebsiella pneumonia* were exposed to flavonoids (Mori *et al.*, 1987; Anandhi *et al.*, 2014). On the other hand, with using the enzyme (SOS chromotest), it appeared that rutin selectively promoted *E. coli* topoisomerase IV-dependent DNA cleavage, inhibited topoisomerase IV-dependent decatenation activity and induced the SOS response of the *E. coli* strain. Topoisomerase IV was essential for cell survival, rutin-induced topoisomerase IV-mediated DNA cleavage and caused growth inhibition of *E. coli* cells (Bernard *et al.*, 1997). Green tea flavonoids also inhibited the dihydrofolate reductase in bacteria and effectively blocked the ability of the microorganisms to synthesize folate (Navarro-Martinez *et al.*, 2005; Navarro-Martinez *et al.*, 2006).

2.3.3. *Inhibition of energy metabolism*

Flavonoids also inhibited the respiration of *E. coli, Staphylococcus aureus* and *Klebsiella pneumonia* by inhibiting the respiratory chain dehydrogenase (Anandhi *et al.*, 2014). Bioflavonoids inhibited the activity of bacterial ATP synthase, reducing the ability of the microorganisms to produce enough energy (Chinnam *et al.*, 2010). Licochalcone A and C from the roots of *Glycyrrhiza inflate* showed inhibitory activity against *S. aureus* and *Micrococcus luteus*, by interfering with energy metabolism which is required for uptake of various metabolites and for biosynthesis of macromolecules. Licochalcones inhibited oxygen consumption in *M. luteus* and *S. aureus* but not in *E. coli*, which correlated well with its spectrum of antibacterial activity. Licochalcones A and C effectively inhibited NADH-cytochrome c reductase, but not cytochrome c oxidase or NADH-CoQ reductase. The authors suggested that the inhibition site of these flavonoids was between CoQ and cytochrome c in the bacterial respiratory electron transport chain (Haraguchi *et al.*, 1998). Licochalcone A also produced the same effects in methicillin-resistant *Staphylococcus aureus* and vancomycin-resistant *Enterococcus faecium*. As a result of interference with energy metabolism, it subsequently inhibited RNA, DNA, cell wall and protein synthesis (Salvatore *et al.*, 1998).

2.3.4. *Anti-virulence mechanisms*

In addition to direct antibacterial activities, flavonoids inhibited a number of bacterial virulence factors, including quorum-sensing signal receptors, enzymes and toxins. Evidence of these molecular effects at the cellular level include *in vitro* inhibition of biofilm formation, inhibition of bacterial attachment to host ligands, and neutralisation of toxicity towards cultured human cells (Cushnie and Lamb, 2011). Flavonoids formed complex with proteins through nonspecific forces such as hydrogen bonding and hydrophobic effects, as well as by covalent bond formation. Thus, their mode of antimicrobial action may influence their ability to inactivate microbial adhesins, enzymes, cell envelope transport proteins, and so forth (Kumar and Pandey, 2013). Quercetin inhibited the induced bioluminescence in *V. harveyi* and biofilm formation in *E. coli, V. harveyi,* MRSA and MSSA, and reduced the expression of genes involved in quorum-sensing and virulence of *S. aureus* (Vikram *et al.*, 2010; Lee *et al.*, 2013).

(–)-catechin inhibited violacein production in *C. violaceum*, pyocyanin, and elastase production by *P. aeruginosa*, it also reduced biofilm formation and downregulated quorum-sensing genes expression in *P. aeruginosa* (Vandeputte *et al.*, 2010). (–)-epicatechin increased AHL production and decreased biofilm formation in *E. coli*, enhanced biofilm formation and inhibited elastase activity in *Pseudomonas aeruginosa* and inhibited violacein production in *C. violaceum* (Vandeputte *et al.*, 2010; Plyuta *et al.*, 2013; Borges *et al.*, 2014). (-)-epigallocatechin gallate inhibited quorum-sensing in *E. coli* and *P. putida*, reduced biofilm formation and swarming motility of *B. cepacia* and inhibited biofilm formation in *Eikenella Corrodens* (Matsunaga *et al.*, 2010; Huber *et al.*, 2003). (–)-gallocatechin, (–)-epigallocatechin, (–)-catechin gallate, (–)-epicatechin gallate, (–)-gallocatechin gallate, (-)-epigallocatechin gallate inhibited biofilm formation in *Eikenella Corrodens* bacterium (Matsunaga *et al.*, 2010).

Flavonoids that consist of a 2-phenyl-1,4-benzopyrone (flavone) backbone represented natural products as anti-virulence agents in a *S. aureus* infection. However, isorhamnetin, chrysin and puerarin decreased RNAIII expression and subsequently hla expression which successfully protected the host from pneumonia caused by both MRSA and MSSA. The Agr quorum-sensing system is the regulator of virulence determinant production in *S. aureus*. The production of vital *S. aureus* toxins such as α-, β- and γ-hemolysins, toxic-shock syndrome toxin-1 (TSST-1), enterotoxin B, D, and C, exfoliatin A and B and PVL were positively regulated by the Agr system. In addition to toxins, the secretion of various *S. aureus* enzymes such as serine protease, V8 protease, staphylokinase, glycerol ester hydrolase, nuclease, lipase, PI-phospholipase C and fibrinolysin were also shown to require a functional Agr system for maximal expression. A significant reduction in agr A and hla transcript levels was detected in post-exponential *S. aureus* culture upon treatment with sub-inhibitory concentrations of flavonoids. In addition, naringenin also reduced the production of α-hemolysin and protected mice from *S. aureus*-provoked pneumonia (Jiang *et al.*, 2016; Wang *et al.*, 2011; Tang *et al.*, 2014; Zhang *et al.*, 2013).

Tea catechins neutralized cholera enterotoxin and protected against experimental infection by *V. cholera* (Toda *et al.*, 1991a; Toda *et al.*, 1991b). Catechin polymers and epicatechin neutralize endotoxin of *Vibrio vulnificus*, genistein possessed a protecting effect against *Vibrio vulnificus* toxins in CD-1 mice. (Lopez-Lazaro, 2009). Incubating LPS with the flavonoids resulted in decrease in the amount of lipopolysaccharides (LPS) attached to beads that was coated with binding agent (Vlietinck *et al.*, 1998). Flavonoids also blocked the interaction between LPS (lipopolysaccharides) and its receptors TLR4/MD2 (Lopez-Lazaro, 2009). Anthrax lethal factor (LF) produced by *B. anthracis* was strongly inhibited by ECGC (epigallocatechin-3-gallate) (Dell'Aica *et al.*, 2004). Neurotoxin of botulinum was blocked by the arubigin fraction of black tea. The arubigin also protected mouse from paralysis with *Clostridium tetani* neurotoxin (tetanospasmin) (Satoh *et al.*, 2002a; Satoh *et al.*, 2002b). *Helicobacter pylori* produced vacuolating cytotoxin VacA results in gastritis and ulceration. VacA induced gastritis in rats was effectively inhibited by high molecular weight polyphenols that are extracted from hop bracts (Yahiro *et al.*, 2005).

3. FLAVONOIDS WITH ANTIFUNGAL EFFECTS

Superficial fungal infections are among the most common diseases seen in daily practice. These infections affect the outer layers of the skin, the nails and hair. The main groups of fungi causing superficial fungal infections are dermatophytes, yeasts and moulds. The dermatophytes that usually cause only superficial infections of the skin are grouped into three genera: Microsporum, Trichophyton, and Epidermophyton. Dermatophytes grow on keratin and therefore cause diseases in body sites wherein keratin is present, the skin surface, hair and nail (HO and Cheng, 2010). Candida species are the major human fungal pathogens that cause both mucosal and deep tissue infections. Candida species belong to the normal microbiota of an individual's mucosal oral cavity, gastrointestinal tract and vagina, and are responsible for various clinical manifestations from mucocutaneous overgrowth to bloodstream infections. These yeasts are commensal in healthy humans and may cause systemic infection in immunocompromised situations due to their great adaptability to different host niches (Shao *et al.*, 2007; Eggimann *et al.*, 2003).

The incidence of fungal infections is increasing at an alarming rate, presenting an enormous pressure and challenge to healthcare professionals for their diagnosis and treatment. Emerging fungal infections is also the cause of significant morbidity and mortality. This emergence is directly related to the growing population of immune-compromised individuals. Patients with conditions such as granulocytopenia, advanced HIV infection, bone marrow and solid organ transplantation, cancer, diabetes mellitus, severe burn and trauma and severe malnutrition are among many others predisposing factor for low immunity (Kaur *et al.*, 2015).

Several recent studies have shown that flavonoides possessed antifungal activity against dermatophytes and yeasts as a single treatment or combined with other antifungal agents (Table 2) and can be applied as an alternative antifungal agent for fungal species resistant to traditional drugs.

Table 2: Flavonoids Possessing Antifungal Activity

Source	*Flavonoids*	*Fungi*	*Ref.,*
Aster yomena	Isoquercitrin	*C. albicans, C. parapsilosis, M. furfur, T. rubrum* and *T. beigelii*	Yun *et al.*, 2015
Adina cordifolia	3,4',5,7-Tetraacetyl quercetin	*A. fumigatus* and *Cryptococcus neoformans*	Rao *et al.*, 2002
Alpinia officinarum	Flavons	*C. albicans, Aspergillus niger, Trichophyton rubrum, Trichophyton mentagrophytes,* and *Epidermophyton floccosum*	Dixit *et al.*, 2012; Ray *et al.*, 1976; Ray *et al.*, 1975
Anemopaegma arvense	Quercetin 3-*O*-α-L-rhamnopyranosyl-(1→6)-β-Dglucopyranoside and quercetin 3-*O*-α-L-rhamnopyranosyl-(1→6)-β-D-galactopyranoside	*Trichophyton rubrum*	Costanzo *et al.*, 2013
Aquilegia vulgaris	4-Methoxy-5, 7-dihydroxyflavone 6-Cglucoside (isocytisoside)	*A. niger*	Bylka *et al.*, 2004
Artemisia giraldi	6,7,4Ttrihydroxy-3, 5-dimethoxy flavones; 5,5- dihydroxy-8,2,4-trimethoxyflavone and 5,7,4- trihydroxy-3,5-dimethoxyflavone	*Aspergillus flavus*	Zheng *et al.*, 1996

Table 2: (*Contd...*)

Table 2: *(Contd...)*

Source	*Flavonoids*	*Fungi*	*Ref.,*
Artocarpus anisophyllus and *Artocarpus lowii*	2',4'-Dihydroxy-4-methoxy-3'-prenyldihydrochalcone; 4-Hydroxyonchocarpin; Isobavachalcone;2',4'-dihydroxy-3, 4(2",2"-dimethylchromeno)-3'-prenyldihydrochalcone; 5,7-dihydroxy-4'-methoxy-6-prenylflavanone; 5-hydroxy-6,7-(2,2-dimethylchromano)-4'-methoxyflavanone; 4',5-dihydroxy-6,7-(2,2-dimethylchromeno)-2' -methoxy-8-γ, γ-dimethylallylflavone; artocarpin; yranocycloartobiloxanthone A and cycloheterophyllin	*Candida albicans* and *Candida glabrata*	Jamil *et al.*, 2014
Artocarpus nobilis	2',4',4-Trihydroxy-3'-geranylchalcone; 2',4',4-trihydroxy-3'-[6-hydroxy-3,7-dimethyl-2 (E), 7-octadienyl]chalcone; 2',4',4-trihydroxy-3'-[2-hydroxy-7-methyl-3-methylene -6-octaenyl] chalcone; 2',3,4,4'-tetrahydroxy-3'-geranylchalcone and 2',3,4,4'-tetrahydroxy -3'-[6-hydroxy-3, 7-dimethyl-2 (E), 7-octadienyl]chalcone	*Cladosporium cladosporioides*	Jayasinghe *et al.*, 2004
Ballota inaequidens	5-Hydroxy-3,7,4'-trimethoxyflavone; retusin; pachypodol and 5-hydroxy-7,3', 4'-trimethoxyflavone	*Candida albicans,* and *Candida crusei*	Citoglu *et al.*, 2005
Blumea balsamifera	Luteolin	*T. mentagrophytes, A. niger* and *C. albicans*	Ragasa *et al.*, 2005
Camptotheca acuminate	Trifolin and hyperoside	*Alternaria alternata, Epicoccum nigrum, Pestalotia guepinii, Drechslera spp.* and *Fusarium avenaceum*	Li *et al.*, 2005
Cassia alata	2,5,7,4′- Tetrahydroxyisoflavone and 3,5,7,4′- tetrahydroxy flavones	*Trichophyton schoenleinii, Trichophyton longifurus, Pseudallescheria boydii, Candida albicans, Aspergillus niger, Microsporum canis* and *Trichophyton mentagrophytes*	Rahman *et al.*, 2008

Table 2: *(Contd...)*

Table 2: *(Contd...)*

Source	*Flavonoids*	*Fungi*	*Ref.,*
Castanea sativa, Filipendula ulmaria, Rosa micrantha, Cytisus multiflorus, and *Cistus ladanifer*	Catechin, luteolin, quercetin	*Candida tropicalis, Candida parapsilosis, Candida glabrata* and *Candida albicans*	Alves *et al.*, 2014
Citrus species	Naringin, hesperidin and neohesperidin	*Aspergillus parasiticus* and *Aspergillus flavus,*	Salas *et al.*, 2011
Combretum zeyheri	5-hydroxy-7, 4'-Dimethoxy-flavone	*Candida albicans*	Mangoyi *et al.*, 2015
Dorstenia barteri	6,8-Diprenyleriodictyol; isobavachalcone and 4-hydroxylonchocarpin	*C. neoformans*	Dzoyem *et al.*, 2013
Erythrina latissima	7,3-Dihydroxy-4-methoxy-5-(Y,Y-dimethylallyl) isoflavone (erylatissin A); 7,3-dihydroxy -6, 6-dimethyl-4, 5-dehydro-pyrano [2,3: 4,5] isoflavone (erylatissin B); (")-7, 3-dihy-droxy-4-methoxy -5-(Y,Y-dimethylallyl) flavanone (erylatissin C)	*Candida mycoderma*	Chacha *et al.*, 2005
Eucalyptus maculata	2,6-Dihydroxy-3-methyl-4-methoxy-dihydrochalcone; eucalyptin and 8-desmethyl-eucalyptin	*Trichophyton mentagrophytes*	Takahashi *et al.*, 2004
Eysenhardtia texana	5,7,4-Trihydroxy-8-methyl-6-(3-methyl-[2-butenyl])-(2*S*)-flavanone	*Candida albicans*	Wachter *et al.*, 1999
Galium fissurense, Viscum album and *Cirsium hypoleucum*	5,7-Dime-thoxyflavanone-40-O-b-D-glucopyranoside; 5, 7-di-methoxy-flavanone-40-O-[2-O-(5-O-trans-cinnamoyl) -b-D-apiofuranosyl]-b-D-glucopyranoside; 5,7,30-trihydroxyflavanone-4-O-β-D-glucopyranoside; naringenin -7-O-β-D-glucopyranoside; rutin; and nicotiflorin	*Candida albicans*	Özçelik *et al.*, 2008
Kaempferia parviflora	3,5,7,4'-Tetramethoxyflavone and 5,7,4'-trimethoxyflavone	*Candida albicans*	Yenjai *et al.*, 2004
Leucaena leucocephala	Quercetin - 3-O-(2"-trans-*p*-coumaryl)-α-rhamnopyranosyl-(1'"→6")-β-glucopyranoside; quercetin-3-O-α-rhamno-pyranosyl-(1'"→2")-β–gluco-pyranoside; quercetin-7-O-α–	*Candida albicans* and *Asperagillus niger*	Mohammed *et al.*, 2015

Table 2: *(Contd...)*

Table 2: *(Contd...)*

Source	***Flavonoids***	***Fungi***	***Ref.,***
	rhamnopyranosyl-(1'''→2'')- β-glucopyrano side and quercetin-3-O-β–glucopyrano-side		
Mangifera indica	(-)-Epicatechin-3-O-β-glucopyranoside; 5-hydroxy-3-(4-hydroxylphenyl) pyrano [3,2-g]chromene-4(8H)-one; 6-(p-hydroxybenzyl) taxifolin-7-O-β-D-glucoside (tricuspid; quercetin-3-O-α-glucopyranosyl-(1 → 2)-β-D-glucopyranoside; and (-)-epicatechin (2-(3,4-dihydroxyphenyl)-3, 4-dihydro-2H-chromene-3,5, 7-triol	*Aspergillus fumigatus, Aspergillus niger*	Kanwal *et al.*, 2010
Miliusa sinensis	Pashanone and 5-hydroxy-6, 7-dimethoxyflavanone	*C. neoformans*	Lee *et al.*, 2016
Monanthotaxis littoralis	3, 5 Dihydroxy-7-methoxy anthocynidines and 3,7,5 trihydroxy anthocynidines	*A. niger, A. ochraceus, A. fumigatus, A. flavipes, A. flavus*	Clara *et al.*, 2014
Morus alba, Morus mongolica, Broussnetia papyrifera, Sophora flavescens and *Echinosophora koreensis*	Papyriflavonol A, kuraridin, sophora-flavanone D, sophoraisoflavanone A, broussochalcone A	*Candida albicans*	Sohn *et al.*, 2004
Oncoba spinosa	Kaempferol, quercetin, apigenin-7-O-β-D-glucuronopyranoside, quercetin 3-O-β-D-galactopyranoside and quercetin 3-O-α-L-rhamnopyranosyl (1→6) β-D-glucopyranoside	*Candida albicans, Candida parapsilosis* and *Cryptococcus neoformans*	Djouossi *et al., 2015*
Petalostemum purpureum	Pelalostemumol	*Trichophyton mentagrophytes*	Hufford *et al.*, 1993
Praxelis clematidea	5,7,4´Trimethoxflavone	*Candida albicans*	Filho *et al.*, 2016
Retama raetam	Licoflavone C and derrone	*Candida glabrata, Candida albicans, Candida parapsilosis* and *Candida kreusei*	Edziri *et al.*, 2012
Scutellaria baicalensis	Baicalein	*Candida albicans, Candida tropicalis* and *Candida parapsilosis*	Serpa *et al.*, 2012
Selaginella tamariscina	Isocryptomerin and 7-Hydroxy-3, 4-(methylene dioxy)	*Candida albicans*	Lee *et al.*, 2009;

Table 2: *(Contd...)*

Table 2: *(Contd...)*

Source	*Flavonoids*	*Fungi*	*Ref.,*
	flavan 5,4'-dihydroxy-3, 7-dimethoxyflavone (kumatakenin)		Hwang *et al.*, 2012
Terminalia bellerica	5,7-Dimethoxyflavanone-4'-*O*-β-D-glucopyranoside;	*Candida albicans*	Valsaraj *et al.*, 1997
Varthemia iphionoides	5,7-dimethoxyflavanone-4'-*O*-[2''-*O*-(5'''-*O*-*trans*-cinnamoyl)-β-D-apiofuranosyl]-β-D-glucopyranosid;	*Candida tropicalis*	Afifi *et al.*, 1991
Viscum album ssp. *Album*	5,7,3'-trihydroxy-flavanone-4'-*O*-β-D-glucopyranoside; Naringenin-7-*O*-β-D-glucopyranoside; Rutin and Nicotiflorin	*Candida albicans*	Orhan *et al.*, 2010
Vitex negundo	flavone glycoside	*Trichophyton mentagrophytes* and *Cryptococcus neoformans*	Sathiamoorthy *et al.*, 2007
Waltheria americana	5,2',5'-trihydroxy-3,7, 4'-trimethoxyfllavone	*C. albicans, A. niger* and *T. mentagrophytes*	Ragasa *et al.*, 1997

3.1. Molecular Mechanism of Antifungal Effects of Flavonoids

The antifungal effects of flavonoids were mediated by many mechanisms which are explained below:

3.1.1. *Effect on membrane*

Flavonoids were generally known to cause membrane disturbance resulting in the loss of membrane integrity (Wink, 2013). It appeared that the C atom at position 3 in the C ring has a major role in hydrophobicity which represented the ability of drugs to interact with biological membranes. Tennatural phenolic compounds inhibited the growth of *Fusarium verticillioides*, the results revealed that the antifungal activity increased with hydrophobicity (Wu *et al.*, 2013). The membrane damage was analyzed by monitoring the influx of propidium iodide. Propidium iodide, a DNA-staining fluorescent probe, was impermeable to the cell membrane and only penetrates the cell if there were severe lesions on the membrane, which resulted in an increase in fluorescence intensity (Pina-Vaz *et al.*, 2004; Pinto *et al.*, 2006). The percentage of propidium iodide influx following exposure to isoquercitrin was 54.5% and that of the control was 18.1%. Isoquercitrin induced membrane lesions, decreasing membrane integrity and increasing membrane permeability. Furthermore, the flavanoid increased the membrane permeabilization as estimated by potassium ion release assay. After treatment with the flavonoid, the potassium ion concentration outside the cell was increased. Fungal cells treated with isoquercitrin for 20 min showed a 37.0% release of potassium ions, as compared to untreated cells 10.0% (Yun *et al.*, 2015).

Potassium ion is generally essential for the maintenance of the membrane potential. Potassium ions gets released from the cell when the membrane is disturbed, and contributes to the change in membrane potential and subsequent deterioration of membrane functions leading to the death of cell (Bolintineanu *et al.*, 2010). The disruption of membrane induced by catechin *Candida albicans* and *Trichophyton mentagrophytes* was studied *via* electron microscopy. The results indicated that catechin may act by lysing the cell membrane (Hirasawa and Takada, 2004; Toyoshima *et al.*, 1994). The exposure of fluconazole-resistant strains to fluconazole did not cause a reduction in the number of viable cells compared to that for the control. However, in fluconazole-resistant *C. tropicalis* strains, changes in cell size/ granularity were observed after 24 h of exposure to fluconazole (16 μg/mL) in combination with flavonoids. Yeast cells treated with fluconazole in combination with the flavonoids for 24 h showed a significant increase ($p < 0.05$) in the population with membrane damage (39.43% ± 2.41% for catechin hydrate, 19.52% ± 1.27% for quercetin hydrate, and 13.61% ± 1.45% for epigallocatechin gallate) compared to the population with membrane damage in the control group (1.7% ± 0.58%) (da Silva *et al.*, 2014).

On the other hand, the antifungal activity of amphotericin B against *Cryptococcus neoformans* was enhanced if it is combined with quercetin or rutin. The antifungal effect of flavonoids on *Cryptococcus neoformans* were also related to damaging of membrane structures of these fungi (Faria *et al.*, 2011). Furthermore flavonoids also inhibited the synthesis or assembly of the fungal cell wall polymers. Sorbitol is an osmotic protector used to stabilize fungi protoplasts. Fungal cells protected with sorbitol can grow in the presence of fungal cell wall inhibitors, whereas growth would be inhibited in the absence of sorbitol, this effect was documented by increases in the MIC value of antifungals as observed in medium with sorbitol as compared to the MIC value in medium without sorbitol. The MIC values of flavonoids against *Trichophyton rubrum* when sorbitol was added to the medium, were increased, which indicated that the antifungal effects of flavonoids were mediated by inhibiting fungal cell wall synthesis (Frost *et al.*, 1995; Svetaz *et al.*, 2007; Bitencourt *et al.*, 2013).

Flavonoids were tested to investigate its ability to form complexes with ergosterol, the principal sterol present in yeasts and filamentous fungi, which are necessary for the growth and normal function of the fungal cell membrane and contribute to the proper functioning of enzymes bound to the membrane. MIC of flavonoids was increased in the presence of exogenous ergosterol in relation to the control assay, which indicated that the mechanism of action of flavonoids involved complexation with ergosterol (Bitencourt *et al.*, 2013; Alves *et al.*, 2013).

A reduction in ergosterol content of 33.54% (wild type) and 56.15% (mutant) was observed for two *Trichophyton rubrum* strains cultured in the presence of the MIC of quercetin when compared to untreated cells. This result was comparable to the reduction caused by MICs of fluconazole and cerulenin, which ranged from 40 to 61.5% (Bitencourt *et al.*, 2013). The effect of flavonoid compounds on ergosterol biosynthesis in *Candida albicans* was investigated by quantifying the amount of ergosterol produced by *Candida albicans*in the presence and absence of the test flavonoid compound at time intervals *in vitro*. 5-Hydroxy-7, 4'-dimethoxy flavones caused time dependent decrease in ergosterol synthesis [91. 6 and 63 % at 16 and 24 hrs respectively, at the tested concentration (50% of MIC)] (Mangoyi *et al.*, 2015).

3.1.2. *Effects on DNA and cells cycle*

To investigate how flavonoids ' inhibited the progressive change of fungal cells within a physiological state, cell cycle analysis was performed based on DNA content. The results revealed a reduction in the cell populations by about 10% (from 26.69 to 13.50%) compared with the non-treated cells in the G2/M phase of the cell division cycle. On the other hand, the S phase population significantly increased from 12.37 to 36.47% of the total cell population which reflected that flavonoids induced cell cycle arrest within the S-phase in yeast cells by their biological effects on the intracellular condition (Jung *et al.*, 2007).

The analysis of single cells regarding the distribution of grades of DNA damage, of fluconazole plus (-)-catechin hydrate, quercetin hydrate, or (-)-epigallocatechin gallate on strains of *C. tropicalis* resistant to fluconazole showed that *C. tropicalis* coexposure to fluconazole and the flavonoids for 24 h resulted in a significant increase ($p< 0.05$) in DNA strand break levels. Cells treated with fluconazole in combination with the flavonoid (-)-catechin hydrate, quercetin hydrate, or (-)-epigallocatechin gallate for 24 h exhibited damage index values (arbitrary units) of 64.38 ±2.15, 74.62 ± 3.15, and 61.48 ± 2.56, respectively, and damage frequencies of 36.95% ± 3.17%, 31.83% ± 0.21%, and 29.42% ± 0.10%, respectively (da Silva *et al.*, 2014). Green tea flavonoids also inhibited the dihydrofolate reductase in yeast and effectively blocked the ability of the microorganisms to synthesize folate (Navarro-Martinez *et al.*, 2005, Navarro-Martinez *et al.*, 2006).

3.1.3. *Effects on fungal antioxidant enzymes*

Candida albicans has evolved enzymatic antioxidant (SOD, CAT, GST, GPx, GR and G6PD) defense mechanisms in order to minimise the damaging effects of ROS produced by phagocytes during an infection. Antioxidant enzymes have a role in the protection of *C. albicans* against oxidative stress, thus, inhibition of these enzymes by 5-hydroxy-7, 4'-dimethoxyflavone represented a new target for antifungal flavonoids. The results showed that flavonoids caused complete inhibition of the activity for all the tested enzymes except for catalase (Mangoyi *et al.*, 2015). The combination of flavonoids with fluconazole promoted exposure of the phosphatidylserine in the plasma membrane, changes in cell size/granularity, mitochondrial membrane depolarization, intracellular ROS accumulation, and DNA fragmentation in fluconazole-resistant strains of *C. tropicalis*. The combination of flavonoids with fluconazole induced apoptotic cell death in *C. tropicalis*, in which the generation and intracellular accumulation of reactive oxygen species seem to act as stimulators of early apoptosis signaling, in addition to directly damaging the mitochondria and the nuclear DNA (da Silva *et al.*, 2014; Lee*et al.*, 2011).

3.1.4. *Inhibition of fungal biofilm*

The adherence of *Candida albicans* to each other and to various host and biomaterial surfaces is an important prerequisite for the colonization and pathogenesis of these organisms. Cells in established biofilms exhibited different phenotypic traits and were inordinately resistant to antimicrobial agents. Many flavonoids extracted from the medicinal plants such as *Moringa oleifera*, *Dalea elegans*, green and black tea and Citrus flavonoids induced candida biofilm inhibition (Onsare and Arora 2015; Kobric *et al.*, 2012; Peralta *et al.*, 2015; Evensen and Braun 2009). Black and green tea flavonoids possessed candida biofilm inhibitory effect. Cultures treated with 1.0 μM – (–) epigallocatechin-3-gallate (EGCG), the most abundant polyphenol, displayed a 75% reduction of viable cells during biofilm formation. Established biofilms treated with EGCG were also reduced, by 35 80%, as determined through XTT colorimetric assays. Epigallocatechin (EGC) and epicatechin-3-gallate (ECG) demonstrated similar biofilm inhibition (Peralta *et al.*, 2015; Braun *et al.*, 2009).

4. ANTIVIRAL EFFECT OF FLAVONOIDS ON HUMAN VIRUSES

Human viral infections are significant health problem worldwide. Although much effort has been made, the effective and safe antiviral drugs are relatively rare. Moreover, it is becoming more and more difficult to treat viral infections due to the emergence of drug-resistant strains and the chronic infections. The approved antiviral drugs are mostly for HIV therapy and fewer is available against the other viral infections (Antonelli and Turriziani 2010). Natural compounds are an important source for the discovery and the development of novel antiviral drugs because of their availability and expected low side effects. Naturally occurring flavonoids showed antiviral activity against wide range of viruse (Table 3).

Table 3: Flavonoids Possessing Antiviral Activity

Source	*Flavonoids*	*Viruses*	*Ref.,*
Bauhinia longifolia	Quercetin and quercetin 3-O-glycosides	Mayaro virus (Togaviridae, Alphavirus)	dos Santos *et al.*, 2014
Camellia sinensis	(-)-Epigallocatechin-3-gallate	Hepatitis B virus	Huang *et al.*, 2014
Camellia sinensis	(-)-Epigallocatechin-3-gallate (EGCG)	HIV	Fassina *et al.*, 2002
Camellia sinensis	Epicatechin (-)-gallate and (-)-epigallocatechin gallate	HIV	Nakane and Ono 1990
Camellia sinensis	Epigallocatechin gallate	HCV	Fukazawa *et al.*, 2012
Carica papaya	Quercetin	Dengue virus 2	Senthilvel *et al.*, 2013
Carpolepis laurifolia	Quercetin; 6-methylapigenin-7-methylether; avicularin; quercitrin and hyperoside	Dengue virus	Coulerie *et al.*, 2014
Chrysanthemum morifolium	Apigenin 7-O-beta-D-(4'-caffeoyl) glucuronide	HIV-1	Lee *et al.*, 2003
Chrysanthemum morifolium	Acacetin-7-O-beta-D-galactopyranoside	HIV-1	Wang *et al.*, 1998
Citrus paradise	Naringenin	HCV	Jonathan 2010
Citrus reticulata	Tangeretin and nobiletin	Respiratory syncytial virus (RSV)	Xu *et al.*, 2014
Cleome droserifolia	Isorhamnetin-3-0-B glucopyranosyl-7-0-L-rhamnopyranoside and quercetin -3-0-B – glucopyranosly-7-0-L rhamnopyranoside	Influenza virus	El-kosy *et al.*, 2005
Cynodon dactylon	Luteolin and apigenin rich fraction from the ethanolic extract	Chikungunya virus	Murali *et al.*, 2015
Deschampsia caespitosa and Calamagrostis epogeios	7, 3'-Dimetoxyquercetin and 5,7,3',4'- Tetramethoxyqeercetin	Influenza 1 and herpetic virus	Palchykovska *et al.*, 2013
Embelia ribes	Quercetin	Hepatitis C virus	Bachmetov *et al.*, 2012
Eucalyptus citriodora	Quercetin-3-*O*-α-l-rhamnoside	Respiratory syncytial virus	Zhou *et al.*, 2014
Euphorbia grantii	3-Methylquercetin	polio-, coxsackie- and rhinoviruses	Van Hoof *et al.*, 1984
Ficus benjamina	Quercetin 3-O-rutinoside; kaempferol 3-O-rutinoside and kaempferol 3-O-robinobioside	HSV-1 and HSV-2	Yarmolinsky *et al.*, 2012

Table 3: *(Contd...)*

Table 3: *(Contd...)*

Source	***Flavonoids***	***Viruses***	***Ref.,***
Galium fissurense, Viscum album and *Cirsium hypoleucum*	Rutin, 5,7-dimethoxy flavanone-4′-*O*-β-d-glucopyranoside and 5,7, 3′-trihydroxy-flavanone-4′-*O*-β-d-glucopyranoside	Parainfluenza -3	Orhan *et al.*, 2010
Galium fissurense, Viscum album and *Cirsium hypoleucum*	5,7-Dimethoxy-flavanone -4′-*O*-[2″-*O*-(5‴-*O*-*trans*-cinnamoyl)-β-d-apiofuranosyl]-β-d-glucopyranoside	Herpes simplex virus Type-1 (HSV-1)	Orhan *et al.*, 2010
Hovenia acerba	Kaemperol; quecetin; myricitin; laricetin; (2*R*, 3*R*)-dihydrokaemperol; (2*R*,3*R*)-3,5,7,3′, 5′-pentahydro flavanone; (2*R*,3*R*)-dihydro myricitin; hovenitin; (+) -eriodictyol; (-)-gallocatechin; spinosin; 6‴-acetyl-spinosin; 6‴-*p*-hydroxy-cinnamoylspinosin; 6‴-feruloylspinosin; and 6‴-sinapoylspinosin.	Respiratory syncytial virus	Song *et al.*, 2016
Juglans mandshurica	Taxifolin (dihydroquercetin)	HIV	Min *et al.*, 2002
Kalanchoe daigremontiana	Kaempferol-3-O-β-D-xylopyranosyl (1→2) α-L-rhamnopyranoside; quercetin-3-O-β-D-xylopyranosyl (1→2) α-L-rhamnopyranoside	HSV-1 and HSV-2	Ürményi *et al.*, 2016
Kummerowia striata	Chrysin and apigenin-7-O-beta-D-glucopyranoside	HIV	Wang *et al.*, 1988
Lagerstroemia speciosa	Quercetin-7-glucoside	Human rhinovirus 2	Song *et al.*, 2013
Laggera pterodonta	Chrysosplenetin and pendulentin	Enterovirus 71	Zhu *et al.*, 2011
Larix sibirica	Dihydroquercetin	Coxsackievirus B4	Galochkina *et al.*, 2016
Marrubium peregrinum	Ladanein	HCV	Haid *et al.*, . 2012
Morus alba	Moralbanone, Eudraflavone B hydroperoxide and leachianone G	Herpes simplex type 1	Ahmad *et al*, 2015; Du *et al.*, 2003
Mosla scabra	5-Hydroxy-7, 8-Dimethoxy-flavone, apigenin and acacetin	Influenza virus	Wu *et al.*, 2010; Kirchmair *et al.*, 2012
Mosla scabra	apigenin A	HCV	Ashfaq and Idrees, 2014

Table 3: *(Contd...)*

Table 3: *(Contd...)*

Source	***Flavonoids***	***Viruses***	***Ref.,***
Ocotea notate	Isoquercitrin, reynoutrin, miquelianin, quercitrin, afzelin, catechin, epicatechin, quercetin and kaempferol	Herpes simplex virus type 1 (HSV-1) and type 2 (HSV-2)	Garrett *et al.*, 2012
Paulownia tomentosa	Apigenin	Enterovirus 71	Ji *et al.*, 2015
Pistacia chinensis	Diosmetin and Apigenin	HCV	Rashed *et al.*, 2014
Pithecellobium clypearia	7-O-galloyltri-cetifavan and 7, 4'-di-O-galloyl-tricetifavan	Respiratory syncytial virus (RSV)	Li *et al.*, 2006
Polygonum perfoliatum	Quercetin-3-O-β-D-glucu-ronide	Influenza A virus	Fan *et al.*, 2011
Polygonum perfoliatum	Crude flavonoid extract	Herpes simplex virus 1	Zhang *et al.*, 2014
Psiadia dentate	3-Methylkaempferol	Poliovirus	Robin *et al.*, 2001
Rhododendron ungernii	Quercetin, isoquercitrin, quercitrin, (+)-catechin, (-)-epicatechin	HSV-1	Kemertelidze *et al.*, 2007
Rhus succedanea and *Garcinia multiflora*	Robustaflavone; hinoki-flavone; amentoflavone; agathisflavone; morello-flavone; GB-1a; GB-2a and morelloflavone	HIV	Lin *et al.*, 1997; Tripathi and Rastogi 1981
Rumex acetosa	Epicatechin-3-O-gallate-(4β→8)-epicatechin-3'-O-gallate	Influenza A virus	Derksen *et al.*, 2014
Scutellaria baicalensis	Tetrahydroxyflavone	Influenza virus	Nagari *et al.*, 1992
Scutellaria baicalensis	5,7,4'-Trihydroxy-8-methoxyflavone	Influenza virus	Nagai *et al.* 1990; Nagai *et al.*, 1995a; Nagai *et al.*, 1995b
Scutellaria baicalensis	Baicalin	HIV	Kitamura *et al.*, 1998; Li *et al.*, 2000
Scutellaria baicalensis	7-D-Glucuronic acid-5, 6-dihydroxy-flavone (Baicalin)	HIV-1	Li *et al.*, 1993
Scutellaria baicalensis	Baicalin	Enterovirus 71	Li *et al.*, 2015
Trollius chinensis	Orientin and Vitexin	Para influenza type 3 virus	Pang *et al.*, 2013; Ahmad *et al.*, 2015
Wikstroemia indica	4'-Methoxyda-phnodorin E	Respiratory syncytial virus (RSV)	Huang *et al.*, 2012

4.1. Structure Activity Relationships and Anti-viral Activity of Flavonoids

It was evident that a structure-activity relationship existed between various flavonoids and their antiviral activity. Quercetin, morin, rutin, dihydroquercetin (taxifolin), apigenin, catechin, and hesperidine have been reported to possess antiviral activity against 11 types of viruses. The antiviral activity appears to be associated with the nonglycosidic compounds, and hydroxylation at the 3-position is apparently a prerequisite for antiviral activity (Selway, 1986). Out of twenty eight flavonoids tested, the flavans were generally more effective than flavones and flavonones in the selective inhibition of HIV-1 and HIV-2 or similar immunodeficiency virus infections (Gerdin and Srensso, 1983). Flavonoids in their glycon form were more inhibitory to rota virus infectivity than were flavonoids in their aglycon form (Bae *et al.*, 2000).

Flavonoids with free hydroxyl groups at C-5, C-7, C-3', C-4' and additionally at C-3 showed the highest anti-herpes simplex virus (HSV-1) activity (Wleklik *et al.*, 1988).

Comparative studies with flavonoids, revealed that the presence of both the unsaturated double bond between positions 2 and 3 of the flavonoid pyrone ring, and the three hydroxyl groups introduced on positions 5, 6 and 7, (*i.e.* baicalein) were required for the inhibition of reverse transcriptase activity. Removal of the 6-hydroxyl group of baicalein required the introduction of three additional hydroxyl groups at positions 3, 3' and 4' (quercetin), to afford a compound still capable of inhibiting the reverse transcriptase activity. Quercetagetin which contained the structures of both baicalein and quercetin, and myricetin which has the structure of quercetin with an additional hydroxyl group on the 5' position also proved strong inhibitors of reverse transcriptase activity (Ono *et al.*, 1990). Catechin group (EGCG, ECG, EGC, EC) were characterized in part, by the flavan-3-ol backbone skeleton. Importantly, these molecules became structurally discrete by location and differences in substituent side groups on the rings designated B and C. Specifically, the galloyl moiety bound to the EGCG and ECG at the benzopyrene-2 position (position C3 of the benzopyrene molecular component), appeared to be associated with the increased anti-RTV activity (Lipson, 2013). Structure–activity relationship studies with 4-hydroxy-3-methoxy flavones revealed that the 3-methoxyl and 4-hydroxyl groups of the flavone skeleton, in addition to a substitution at the 5-position and a polysubstituted A ring, were necessary for strong antiviral activity (De *et al.*, 1991).

4.2. Mechanism of Antiviral Action of Flavonoids

Flavonoids possessed complementary and overlapping antiviral mechanisms of action (Fig. 2), including inhibition of the formation of viral DNA or RNA and inhibition of the viral infectivity.

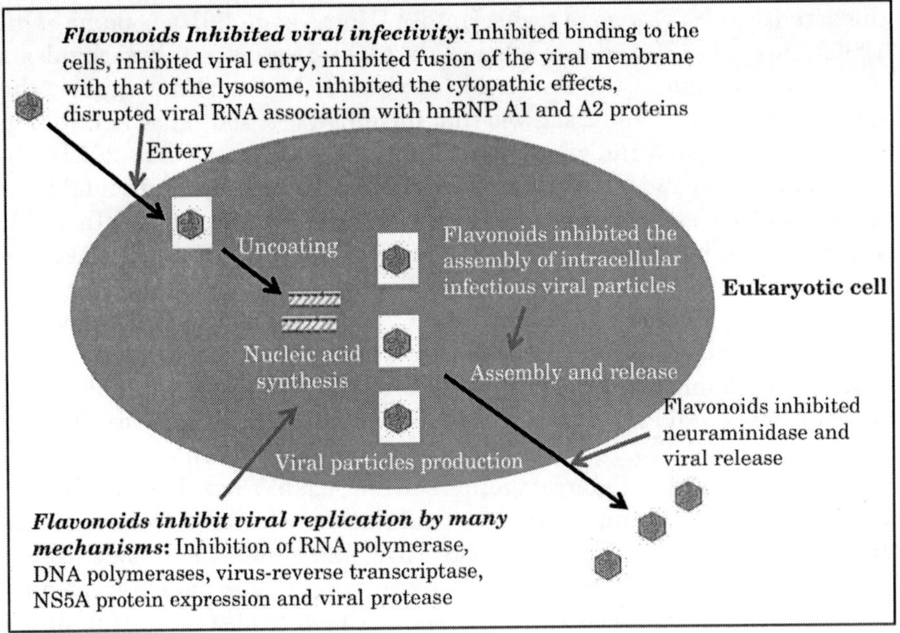

Fig. 2: Mechanisms of Antiviral Effects of Flavonoids

4.3. Inhibition of Viral Replication

Several naturally occurring dietary flavonoids including quercetin, hesperetin, and catechin were previously studied *in vitro* in cell culture monolayers using viral plaque reduction technique and proved to be effective on the infectivity and replication of HSV-1, poliovirus type 1, parainfluenza virus type 3 (Pf-3), and respiratory syncytial virus (RSV). Quercetin caused a concentration-dependent reduction in the infectivity of each virus. Hesperetin had no effect on infectivity but it reduced intracellular replication of each of the viruses. Catechin inhibited the infectivity but not the replication of RSV and HSV-1 and had negligible effects on the other viruses (Kaul *et al.*, 1985). 3-methylkaempferol isolated from *Psiadia dentata* inhibited the genomic RNA synthesis of poliovirus (Robin *et al.*, 2001). Quercetin 3-(63 -(E)-p-coumaroylsophoroside)-7-rhamnoside inhibited replication of dengue virus *via* RNA-dependent DNA polymerase inhibition (Anusuya *et al.*, 2016). Quercetin and luteolin inhibited HCV replication *via* the same mechanism (Luo *et al.*, 2000; Gonzalez *et al.*, 2009). The three-dimensional quantitative structure–activity relationship (3D-QSAR), comparative molecular field analysis (CoMFA), and comparative molecular similarity indices analysis (CoMSIA) were conducted on a series of 44 flavonoid compounds which exhibited *in vitro* avian myeloblastosis virus-reverse transcriptase (AMV-RT) inhibitory activity. The flavonoids with good AMV-RT inhibitory activity showed good binding energies with HIV 1-RT (Phosrithong *et al.*, 2012). However, many flavonoids inhibited the activity of HIV reverse transcriptase (Kuete *et al*, 2010; Nakane *et al*, 1990; Ono *et al*., 1990; Phosrithong *et al*., 2012). Studies on the mechanisms of antiviral action of the flavonoid fraction of *Ocotea notate* against the herpesvirus types 1 and 2 showed that flavonoid fraction caused inhibition of different steps of the virus replication cycle (Garrett *et al*., 2012). (")-epigallocatechin and quercetin exerted their antiviral effects *via* inhibition of cellular RNA polymerases and formation of the complex with RNA. Sylimarin inhibited hepatitis C virus replication by inhibiting the activity of viral RNA polymerase. Quercetin also inhibited dengue virus type-2 (DENV-2) replication and the significant reduction in the DENV specific RNA indicated that quercetin may also target the virus replication machinery *via* inhibiting the RNA polymerase (Shinozuka *et al*., 1988; Nafisi *et al*., 2009; zandi *et al*., 2011). Four flavonoids, 5,6,7-trihydroxyflavone (baicalein), 3,3',4',5,7-pentahydroxyflavone (quercetin), 3,3',4',5,6,7-hexahydroxyflavones (quercetagetin) and 3,3',4',5,5',7-hexahydroxyflavone (myricetin), were found to be potent inhibitors of reverse transcriptases from Rauscher murine leukemia virus (RLV) and human immunodeficiency virus (HIV). The inhibition by baicalein of reverse transcriptase was highly specific, whereas quercetin and quercetagetin were also strong inhibitors of DNA polymerase beta and DNA polymerase I, respectively. Myricetin was a potent inhibitor of both DNA polymerase alpha and DNA polymerase I (Ono *et al*., 1990). Quercetin also possessed direct inhibitory effect on hepatitis C virus (HCV) NS3. Quercetin, kaempferol, taxifolin and apigenin were able to reduce HCV replication efficiency at very low concentrations. However, quercetin appears to be the most effective modulator of HCV replication capacity in replicon-containing cells. Furthermore, quercetin also showed antiviral activity and decreases HCV particle production in cell culture. NS5A protein expression, which was essential for HCV replication, was also reduced by quercetin. The combination of quercetin and IFNα exerted profound inhibitory effects on NS5A protein levels and HCV replication. Accordingly, quercetin may increase the antiviral gene expression regulated by the IFN-activated JAK-STAT pathway. Quercetin decreased HCV-induced reactive oxygen and nitrogen species (ROS/RNS) generation and lipoperoxidation in replicating cells. It also inhibited liver X receptor (LXR) α-induced lipid accumulation in LXRα-overexpressing and replicon-containing Huh7 cells. The mechanism underlying the LXRα-dependent lipogenesis modulatory effect of quercetin in HCV-replicating cells seemed to involve phosphatidy linositol 3-kinase (PI3K)/AKT pathway inactivation. Thus, inhibition of the PI3K pathway by LY294002 attenuated LXRα upregulation and HCV replication mediated by lipid accumulation, showing an additive effect when combined with quercetin. Inactivation of the PI3K pathway by quercetin contributed to the repression of LXRα-dependent lipogenesis and to the inhibition of viral replication (Pisonero-Vaquero *et al*., 2014; Gonzalez *et al*., 2009; Kim *et al*., 2010; Feld and Hoofnagle 2005; Schindler *et al*., 2007).

The amount of influenza A proteins was significantly decreased and the titer of virus was greatly reduced in Madin-Darby canine kidney treated with flavopiridol. The phosphorylation of Ser-2 in the heptad repeat of the CTD domain in RNA polymerase II was decreased in falvopiridol treated cell which indicated that the transcription elongation activity of RNA pol II was impaired upon treatment. The amount of viral vRNA was also significantly decreased in flavopiridol treated cells while only moderate decrease of mRNA was observed and almost no reduction of cRNA was detected (Wang *et al.*, 2012).

Apigenin and luteolin inhibited EV71-mediated cytopathogenic effect CPE) and EV71 replication. Both molecules also showed inhibitory effect on the viral polyprotein expression. They prevented EV71-induced cell apoptosis, intracellular reactive oxygen species (ROS) generation and cytokines up-regulation. Time-of-drug addition study demonstrated that apigenin and luteolin acted after viral entry. The examining of the effect of apigenin and luteolin on 2A (pro) and 3C (pro) activity, the viral proteases responsible for viral polyprotein processing, showed that they possessed less inhibitory activity on 2A (pro) and 3C (pro). Furthermore, apigenin, but not luteolin interfered with viral IRES activity and inhibited EV71-induced c-Jun N-terminal kinase (JNK) activation which was critical for viral replication. It appeared that one hydroxyl group difference in the B ring between apigenin and luteolin resulted in the distinct antiviral mechanisms (Lv *et al.*, 2014).

Chrysin, acacetin, and apigenin inhibited HIV expression in TNF-alpha-treated OM-10.1 cultures. The three compounds had favorable potencies against HIV activation in relation to their growth inhibitory effects. The inhibition of HIV activation was not dependent on preincubation with flavonoids relative to TNF, and was characterized by a lack of HIV RNA accumulation. NF-kappa B activation after TNF-alpha treatment was not inhibited by these agents, suggesting that some other critical factor(s) are needed for interfering with the viral transcription (Critchfield *et al.*, 1996).

The viral protease is comprised of two viral proteins NS2B and NS3 that were associated with each other to form a heterocomplex. The N-terminal region of the non-structural 3 (NS3) protease formed complex with NS2B cofactor which was essential for viral replication. Quercetin from *Carica papaya* showed highest binding energy against Dengue virus NS2B-NS3 protease which was evident by the formation of six hydrogen bonds with the amino acid residues at the binding site of the receptor (Senthilvel *et al.*, 2013). Quercetin inhibited NS3 activity in a specific dose-dependent manner in an *in vitro* catalysis assay, and also HCV replication in subgenomic HCV RNA replicon cell systems and blocked HCV viral production almost completely. The more dramatic effect of quercetin was related to its ability to cause a global reduction in most of the HSP family members, not only the two (HSP 70 and 40) that were knocked down by

RNA. It also inhibited the cleavage of the engineered NS3 two-coloured cleavable substrate introduced in Huh-7 stably expressing scNS3, and inhibited NS3 cleavage in the Tet-inducible NS3 expression system (Bachmetov *et al.*, 2012). However, antiviral activity of quercetin against hepatitis C virus, enterovirus A71, Dengue virus 2 was mediated by protease inhibition (Zeyu *et al.*, 2016; Bachmetov *et al.*, 2012; Lin *et al.*, 2012). Many other flavonoids inhibited protease in many types of viruses (Lin *et al.*, 2012; Senthilvel *et al.*, 2013; Zeyu *et al.*, 2016).

Baicalin showed inhibitory activity on enterovirus (EV71) infection and was independent of direct virucidal or prophylactic effect and inhibitory viral absorption. The expressions of EV71/3D mRNA and polymerase were significantly blocked by baicalin treatment at early stages of EV71 infection. In addition, baicalin decreased the expressions of FasL and caspase-3, as well as inhibited the apoptosis of EV71-infected human embryonal rhabdomyosarcoma (RD) cells (Li *et al.*, 2015). Many flavonoids exhibited antiviral activity by either preventing the entry of viruses into cells or inhibiting the intracellular replication of virus. Flavonoids with a 5,7-dihydroxyflavone structure such as apigenin, chrysin, silybin and naringenin inhibited replication of rhino viruses, picorno viruses, chikungunya virus (CHIKV), HIV and enterovirus-71 (Pohjala *et al.*, 2011; Jassim and Naji 2003; Zhang *et al.*, 2014). The qRT-PCR, immunofluorescence assay, and Western blot analyses indicated that baicalein, fisetin and quercetagetin affected chikungunya virus RNA production and viral protein expression (Lani *et al.*, 2016).7, 3'-dimetoxyquercetin and 5,7,3',4'- tetramethoxyquercetin from *Deschampsia caespitosa* and *Calamagrostis* blocked the enzymatic systems of the RNA and DNA synthesis in influenza l and herpes simplex virus (Palchykovska *et al.*, 2013).

4.4. Inhibition of Viral Infectivity

Control of viral infections is generally designed as a prophylactic (protective) or therapeutic strategy. Unlike bacterial, fungal and parasitic infections, viruses were not autonomous organisms and therefore, require living cells to replicate. Consequently, most of the steps in their replication involve normal cellular metabolic pathways (Wagner and Hewlett, 1999). Some flavonoids exhibit their antiviral effects *via* inhibition of viral infectivity. Isorhamnetin-3-0-B glucopyranosy l-7-0 -L-rhamnopyranoside and quercetin -3-0-B – glucopyranosly-7-0-L rhamnopyranoside isolated from *Cleome droserifolia* caused inhibition of influenza virus activity and infectivity (El-kosy *et al.*, 2005). Apigenin interacted with heterogeneous nuclear ribonucleoproteins (hnRNPs) and interfered with their RNA editing activity. It selectively blocked EV71 infection by disrupting viral RNA association with hnRNP A1 and A2 proteins (Zhang *et al.*, 2014). Epicatechin-3-O-gallate-(4β!8)-epicatechin-3'-O-gallate blocked attachment of influenza A virus (IAV) and interfered with viral penetration at higher concentrations. Galloylation of the compound core structure was shown to be a prerequisite for anti-IAV activity; o-trihydroxylation in the B-ring increased the anti-IAV activity, it interacted with the receptor binding site of IAV (H1N1) (Derksen *et al.*, 2014).

(-)-Epigallocatechin-3-gallate isolated from green teainhibited the entry ofhepatitis B virus into hepatocytes. At a concentration of 50 μM, itinhibited HBV entry into immortalized human primary hepatocytes by more than 80% (Huang *et al.*, 2014). (")-Epigallocatechin-3-gallate (EGCG) exposure during infection of Huh-7 cells with HCVcc resulted in dose-dependent inhibition of infection. EGCG does not change the expression levels of cellular entry factors (CD81, CLDN1, OCLN, SR-BI). It acted directly on the viral particle and inhibited the binding of the virus to the cell surface. EGCG also inhibited cell-to-cell transmission, which represented the major route of spreading of HCV in the liver of infected patients (Ciesek *et al.*, 2011; Calland *et al.*, 2012; Chen *et al.*, 2012).

Inhibition of virus penetration into host cells was one mechanism whereby flavonoids inhibited respiratory syncytial virus replication (Barnard *et al.*, 1993). The purified flavonoid from *Polygonum perfoliatum* strongly inhibited viral replication and cell-to-cell spread which was vital for the virus's propagation (Zhang *et al.*, 2014). Ladanein inhibited a later step of HCV entry and when it was used in combination with cyclosporin A, a known inhibitor of HCV replication, ladanein synergistically inhibited HCV replication (Haid *et al.*, 2012). When 4',6-dicyanoflavan was present from the beginning of infection or was added no later than the first hour of infection, the compound completely prevented viral RNA and protein synthesis and the virus-induced shutoff of host translation. 4',6-dicyanoflavan had no effect either on virus binding to the cell membrane or on virus penetration into cells, it delayed the uncoating kinetics of neutral red encapsidated rhinovirus. The stabilizing effect of 4',6-dicyanoflavan on virion capsid conformation is responsible for uncoating inhibition (Conti *et al.*, 1992).

Flavonoids also inhibited the fusion of the viral membrane with that of the lysosome. It seemed that prostaglandins participate in the fusion of cell membranes. Since flavonoids inhibited their formation, therefore, they can used asprotective drugs against viral diseases (Nagai *et al.*, 1995a; Nagai *et al.*, 1995b; Carpenedo *et al.*, 1965). Baicalein, fisetin and quercetagetin inhibited chikungunya virus binding to the Vero cells and displayed potent activity against extracellular CHIKV particles (Lani *et al.*, 2016). Naringenin inhibited secretion of HCV particles. A concomitant dose-dependent decrease of core protein, HCV-positive strand RNA and infectious particles were observed in the supernatant of infected Huh-7 cells after naringenin treatment. The inhibitory activity of naringenin was also observed in primary hepatocytes in culture. Naringenin blocked the assembly of intracellular infectious viral particles without affecting intracellular levels of the viral RNA or protein. The maximal inhibition (74% of inhibition) of secretion of HCV RNA was observed at 200 μM naringenin with an IC_{50} of 109 μM (Nahmias *et al.*, 2008; Goldwasser *et al.*, 2011).

Baicalein and genistein significantly reduced the levels of human cytomegalovirus (HCMV) early and late proteins, as well as viral DNA synthesis. Baicalein reduced the levels of HCMV immediate-early proteins to nearly background levels while genistein did not. Pre-incubation of concentrated virus stocks with either of the flavonoids did not inhibit HCMV replication, suggesting that baicalein did not directly inactivate virus particles. Baicalein functionally blocked epidermal growth factor receptor tyrosine kinase activity and HCMV nuclear translocation, while genistein did not. At 24h post infection HCMV-infected cells treated with genistein continued to express immediate-early proteins and efficiently phosphorylate IE1-72. However, HCMV induction of NF-kappaB and increase in the levels of cell cycle regulatory proteins (events that were associated with immediate-early protein functioning) were absent. It seemed that the action of baicalein was mediated by blocking HCMV infection at entry while, the primary mechanism of action of genistein was due to blocking of HCMV immediate-early protein (Evers *et al.*, 2005). Baicalein, exhibited significant direct virucidal activity (SI = 33.4) as well as intracellular anti- Japanese encephalitis virus activity (SI = 15.8) and anti-adsorption activity (SI = 15.8) that lead to the inhibition of virus entry to the cells. Baicalein also interacted with viral structural and/or non-structural protein(s). It inhibited Sendai virus replication through inhibition of virus neuraminidase activity. Baicalein also binds to HIV-1 integrase and reverse transcriptase enzymes (Johari *et al.*, 2012; Dou *et al.*, 2011; Ahn *et al.*, 2001; Kitamura *et al.*, 1998). Flavone *O*-glycoside inhibited HIV-1 entry into cells expressing CD4 and chemokine coreceptors and antagonism of HIV-1 reverse transcriptase (Li *et al.*, 2000).

Neuraminidase (NA) is a key viral protein that is responsible for the release of new virus particles via the recognition and cleavage of the N-acetylneuraminic acid (sialic acid moiety) receptor on the host cell membrane. Neuraminidase activity was decreased after treatment with many flavonoids in comparison with the positive control (Dayem *et al.*, Mercader *et al.*, 2010; 2015; Kirchmair *et al.*, 2012; Dou *et al.*, 2004; Li *et al.*, 2008; Li *et al.*, 2006; Mikki *et al.*, 2008; Mikki *et al.*, 2007). The flavonoids markedly decreased the expression of HA and NA, therefore flavonoids produced additional inhibitory effects on virus release through inhibition of neuraminidase (Dayem *et al.*, 2015). Many flavonoids inhibited the cytopathic effects of wide range of viral infections. For example, EC, ECG, genistein, naringenin, and quercetin showed a high level of cytopathic inhibitory activity against simplex virus type 1 (HSV-1) and type 2 (HSV-

2) (Lyn *et al.*, 2005). ECG inhibited the CPE of hepatitis C virus (Fukazawa *et al.*, 2005). Fisetin and rutin inhibited the CPE of enterovirus A71 (EV-A71) (Lin *et al.*, 2012). 7-O-galloyltricetifavan and 7,4'-di-O-galloyltricetifavan isolated from *Pithecellobium clypearia* inhibited the CPE of respiratory syncytial virus (RSV) (Li *et al.*, 2006). Many flavonoids, including demethylated gardenin A and 3, 2-dihydroxyflavone, inhibit HIV-1 proteinase. Robinetin, myricetin, baicalein, quercetagetin and quercetin 3-*O*-(2-galloyl)-α-l-arabinopyranoside inhibit HIV-1 integrase which enables the viral genetic material to be integrated into the DNA of the infected cell, a step that is essential for HIV replication and infectivity (Brinkworth *et al.*, 1992; Fesen *et al.*, 1994; Kim *et al.*, 1998).

5. FUTURE PERSPECTIVES

Infectious diseases remain one of the most important causes of morbidity and mortality around the world. Due to indiscriminate use of antimicrobial drugs, the microorganisms have developed resistance to many antibiotics. It has created immense clinical problems in the treatment of infectious diseases. Flavonoids showed promising antibacterial, antifungal and antiviral effects, however, there are limited pharmacological and pharmacokinetic human trials. Hence flavonoids should be subjected to animal and human studies to determine their effectiveness in whole-organism systems, their pharmacokinetics, their acute, subacute and chronic toxicity, as well as an examination of their effects on beneficial normal microbiota. Chemical modification to enhance the effects and/or improve kinetics also should be performed. Structure–activity studies revealed that it might be possible to prepare a potent antibacterial flavanone by synthesising a compound with halogenation of the B ring as well as lavandulyl or geranyl substitution of the A ring. Enhancing of natural biosynthetic pathways and production of structural analogues of active flavonoids through biotechnology also should be carried out. Finally, according to the preliminary studies, it appeared that natural, hemisynthetic and synthetic flavonoids alone or in combination with other preventive and/or therapeutic strategies will become effective future drugs against the most common infections.

6. CONCLUSIONS

Flavonoids are a group of polyphenolic compounds, which are widely distributed throughout the plant kingdom. Flavonoids showed broad spectrum antiviral antibacterial and antifungal activity. This article highlights the antiviral, antibacterial and antifungal effects of various flavonoids and the mechanism of action of flavonoids against different pathogens.

REFERENCES

Abdal Dayem, A., Choi, H.Y., Kim, Y.B. and Cho, S.G. (2015). Antiviral effect of methylated flavonol isorhamnetin against influenza. *PLoS ONE*, 10(3): e0121610. doi:10.1371/ journal. pone.0121610

Afifi, F.U., Al-Khalil, S., Abdul-Haq, B.K., Al-Eisawi, D.M., Sharaf, M. and Wong, L.K. (1991). Antifungal flavonoids from *Varthemia iphionoides*. *Phytotherapy Res.*, 5(4): 173–175.

Ahmad, A., Kaleem, M., Ahmed, Z. and Shafiq, H. (2015). Therapeutic potential of flavonoids and their mechanism of action against microbial and viral infections-A review. *Food Research International*, http://dx.doi.org/10.1016/j.foodres.2015.06. 021.

Ahmadu, A.A., Onanuga, A. and Ebeshi, B.U. (2011). Isolation of antibacterial flavonoids from the aerial parts of *Indigofera secundiflora*. *Pharmacognosy Journal*, 3(19): 25–28.

Ahn, H.C., Lee, S.Y., Kim, J.W., Son, W.S., Shin, C.G. and Lee, B.J. (2001). Binding aspects of baicalein to HIV-1 integrase. *Mol. Cells*, 31: 127–130.

Akroum, S., Bendjeddou, D., Satta, D. and Lalaoui, K. (2009). Antibacterial activity and acute toxicity effect of flavonoids extracted from *Mentha longifolia*. *American-Eurasian Journal of Scientific Research*, 4(2): 93–96.

Alcaraz, L.E., Blanco, S.E., Puig, O.N., Tomas, F. and Ferretti, F.N. (2000). Antibacterial activity of flavonoids against methicillin resistant *Staphylococcus aureus* strains. *Journal of Theoretical Biology*, 205(2): 231–240.

Alvarez, M., Debattista, N. and Pappano, N. (2006). Synergism of flavonoids with bacteriostatic action against *Staphylococcus aureus* ATCC 25 923 and *Escherichia coli* ATCC 25 922. *Biocell*, 30: 39–42.

Alves LA, Freires IA, Pereira TM, Souza A, Lima EO, Castro RD (2013). Effect of *Schinus terebinthifolius* on *Candida albicans* growth kinetics, cell wall formation and micromorphology. *Acta Odontol Scand.*, 71: 965–971.

Alves, C.T., Ferreira, I.C.F.R., Barros, L., Silva, S., Azeredo, J. and Henriques, M. (2014). Antifungal activity of phenolic compounds identified in flowers from North Eastern Portugal against *Candida* species. *Future Microbiol.*, 9(2): 139–146.

Amin, M.U., Khurram, M., Khattak, B. and Khan, J. (2015). Antibiotic additive and synergistic action of rutin, morin and quercetin against methicillin resistant *Staphylococcus aureus*. *BMC Complementary and Alternative Medicine*, 15: 59. doi: 10.1186/s12906-015-0580-0.

An, J., Zuo, G.Y., Hao, X.Y., Wang, G.C. and Li, Z.S. (2011). Antibacterial and synergy of a flavanonol rhamnoside with antibiotics against clinical isolates of methicillin-resistant *Staphylococcus aureus* (MRSA). *Phytomedicine*, 18(11): 990–993.

Anandhi, D., Srinivasan, P.T., Praveen Kumar, G. and Jagatheesh, S. (2014) DNA fragmentation induced by the glycosides and flavonoids from *C. coriaria*. *Int. J. Curr. Microbiol. App. Sci.*, 3(12): 666–673.

Antonelli, G. and Turriziani, O. (2010). Antiviral therapy: Old and current issues. *Int. J. Antimicrob. Agents*, 40(2): 95–102.

Anusuya, S. and Gromiha, M.M. (2016). Quercetin derivatives as non-nucleoside inhibitors for dengue polymerase: Molecular docking, molecular dynamics simulation, and binding free energy calculation. *J. Biomol. Struct. Dyn.*, 29: 1–15.

Ashfaq, U.A. and Idrees, S. (2014). Medicinal plants against Hepatitis C virus. *World Journal of Gastroenterology*, 20(11): 2941–2947.

Bachmetov, L., Gal-Tanamy, M., Shapira, A., Vorobeychik, M., Giterman-Galam, T., Sathiyamoorthy, P., Golan-Goldhirsh, A., Benhar, I., Tur-Kaspa, R. and Zemel, R. (2012). Suppression of hepatitis C virus by the flavonoid quercetin is mediated by inhibition of NS3 protease activity. *J. Viral Hepatitis*, 19: e81–88.

Bae, E.A., Han, M.J., Lee, M. and Kim, D.H. (2000). *In vitro* inhibitory effect of some flavonoids on rotavirus infectivity. *Biol. Pharm. Bull.*, 23(9): 1122–1124.

Barnard, D.L., Huffman, J.H., Meyerson, L.R. and Sidwell, R.W. (1993). Mode of inhibition of respiratory syncytial virus by a plant flavonoid, SP-303. *Chemotherapy*, 39(3): 212–217.

Bashir, H.S., Mohammed, A.M., Magsoud, A.S. and Shaoub, A.M. (2013). Isolation of three flavonoids from *Withania somnifera* leaves (*Solanaceae*) and their antimicrobial activities. *J. of Forest Products and Industries*, 2(5): 39–45.

Basile, A., Giordano, S., Lopez-Sae, J.A. and Cobianchi, R.C. (1999). Antibacterial activity of pure flavonoids isolated from mosses. *Phytochemistry*, 52: 1479–1482.

Bernard, F.X., Sablé, S., Cameron, B., Provost, J., Desnottes, J.F., Crouzet, J., Blanche, F. (1997). Glycosylated flavones as selective inhibitors of topoisomerase IV. *Antimicrob. Agents Chemother.*, 41: 992–998.

Bitencourt, T.A., Komoto, T.T., Massaroto, B.G., Miranda, C.E., Beleboni, R.O., Marins, M. and Fachin, A.L. (2013). Trans-chalcone and quercetin down-regulate fatty acid synthase gene expression and reduce ergosterol content in the human pathogenic dermatophyte *Trichophyton rubrum*. *BMC Complement Altern. Med.*, 13: 229. doi: 10.1186/1472-6882-13-229.

Blanco, A.R., Sudano-Roccaro, A., Spoto, G.C., Nostro, A. and Rusciano, D. (2005) Epigallocatechin gallate inhibits biofilm formation by ocular staphylococcal isolates. *Antimicrob Agents Chemother*, 49(10): 4339–4343.

Bolintineanu, D., Hazrati, E., Davis, H.T., Lehrer, R.I. and Kaznessis, Y.N. (2010) Antimicrobial mechanism of pore-forming protegrin peptides: 100 Pores to kill *E coli*. *Peptides*, 31: 1–8.

Borges, A., Serra, S., Cristina Abreu, A., Saavedra, M.J., Salgado, A. and SimO—es, M. (2014). Evaluation of the effects of selected phytochemicals on quorum sensing inhibition and *in vitro* cytotoxicity. *Biofouling*, 30: 183–195.

Braun, P.C. (2009). The effects of tea polyphenols on *Candida albicans*: Inhibition of biofilm formation and proteasome inactivation. *Canadian Journal of Microbiology*, 55(9): 1033–1039.

Brinkworth, R.I., Stoermer, M.J. and Fairlie, D.P. (1992). Flavones are inhibitors of HIV-1 proteinase. *Biochem. Biophys. Res. Commun.*, 188: 631–637.

Bylka, W., Szaufer, M., Matlawska, J. and Goslinska, O. (2004). Antimicrobial activity of isocytisoside and extracts of *Aquilegia vulgaris* L. *Lett. Appl. Microbiol.*, 39: 93–97.

Calland, N., Albecka, A., Belouzard, S., Wychowski, C., Duverlie, G., Descamps, V., Hober, D., Dubuisson, J., Rouillé, Y. and Séron, K. (2012). (")-Epigallocatechin-3-gallate is a new inhibitor of hepatitis C virus entry. *Hepatology*, 55: 720–729.

Carpenedo, F., Bortignon, C., Bruni, A. and Santi, R. (1969). Effect of quercetin on membrane-linked activities. *Biochem Pharmacol.*, 18: 1495–1500.

Chacha, M., Bojase-Moleta, G. and Majinda, R.R.T. (2005). Antimicrobial and radical scavenging flavonoids from the stem wood of *Erythrina latissima*. *Phytochemistry*, 66(1): 99–104.

Chan, B.C., Ip, M., Gong, H., Lui, S.L., See, R.H., Jolivalt, C., Fung, K.P., Leung, P.C., Reiner, N.E. and Lau, C.B. (2013). Synergistic effects of diosmetin with erythromycin against ABC transporter over-expressed methicillin-resistant *Staphylococcus aureus* (MRSA) RN4220/pUL5054 and inhibition of MRSA pyruvate kinase. *Phytomedicine*, 20(7): 611–614.

Chan, B.C., Ip, M., Lau, C.B., Lui, S.L., Jolivalt, C., Ganem-Elbaz, C., Litaudon, M., Reiner, N.E., Gong, H., See, R.H., Fung, K.P. and Leung, P.C. (2011). Synergistic effects of baicalein with ciprofloxacin against NorA over-expressed methicillin-resistant *Staphylococcus aureus* (MRSA) and inhibition of MRSA pyruvate kinase. *J. Ethnopharmacol.*, 137(1): 767–773.

Chang, P.C., Li, H.Y., Tang, H.J., Liu, J.W., Wang, J.J. and Chuang, Y.C. (2007). *In vitro* synergy of baicalein and gentamicin against vancomycin-resistant *Enterococcus*. *J. Microbiol Immunol Infect*, 40(1): 56–61.

Chen, C., Qiu, H., Gong, J., Liu, Q., Xiao, H., Chen, X.W., Sun, B.L. and Yang, R.G. (2012). (-)-Epigallocatechin-3-gallate inhibits the replication cycle of hepatitis C virus. *Arch. Virol.*, 157: 1301–1312.

Chinnam, N., Dadi, P.K., Sabri SA, Ahmad, M., Kabir, M.A. and Ahmad, Z. (2010). Dietary bioflavonoids inhibit *Escherichia coli* ATP synthase in a differential manner. *Int. J. Biol. Macromol.*, 46(5): 478–486.

Cho, Y.S., Oh, J.J. and Oh, K.H. (2011). Synergistic anti-bacterial and proteomic effects of epigallocatechin gallate on clinical isolates of imipenem-resistant *Klebsiella pneumoniae*. *Phytomedicine*, 18(11): 941–946.

Christopher, R., Nyandoro, S.S., Chacha, M. and de Koning, C.B. (2014). A new cinnamoylglycoflavonoid, antimycobacterial and antioxidant constituents from *Heritiera littoralis* leaf extracts. *Nat. Prod. Res.*, 28: 351–358.

Ciesek, S., von Hahn, T., Colpitts, C.C., Schang, L.M., Friesland, M., Steinmann, J., Manns, M.P., Ott, M., Wedemeyer, H., Meuleman, P., Pietschmann, T. and Steinmann, E. (2011). The green tea polyphenol, epigallocatechin-3-gallate, inhibits hepatitis C virus entry. *Hepatology*, 54: 1947–1955.

Citoglu, G.S., Sever, B., Antus, S., Baitz-Gacs, E. and Altanlar, N. (2005). Antifungal diterpenoids and flavonoids from *Ballota inaequidens*. *Pharmaceutical Biolog*, 42(8): *http://dx.doi.org/10.1080/13880200490902626*

Clara, C., Matasyoh, J.C., Wagara, I.N., Nakavuma, J. (2014). Antifungal activity of flavonoids isolated from *Monanthotaxis littoralis* against mycotoxigenic fungi from maize. *American Journal of Chemistry and Application Chemistry and Application*, 1(4): 54–60.

Collin, F., Karkare, S. and Maxwell, A. (2011). Exploiting bacterial DNA gyrase as a drug target: Current state and perspectives. *Appl Microbiol Biotechnol.*, 92(3): 479–497.

Constantinou, A., Mehta, R., Runyan, C., Rao, K., Vaughan, A. and Moon, R. (1995). Flavonoids as DNA topoisomerase antagonists and poisons: Structure–activity relationships. *J. Nat. Prod.*, 58: 217–225.

Conti, C., Tomao, P., Genovese, D., Desideri, N., Stein, M.L. and Orsi, N. (1992). Mechanism of action of the antirhinovirus flavanoid 4',6-dicyanoflavan. *Antimicrob. Agents Chemother.*, 36(1): 95–99.

Costanzo, C.D.G., Fernandes, V.C., Zingaretti, C., Beleboni, R.O., Pereira, A.M.S., Marins, M., Taleb-Contini, S.T.H., Pereira, P.S. and Fachin, A.L. (2013). Isolation of flavonoids from *Anemopaegma arvense* (Vell) Stellf. ex de Souza and their antifungal activity against *Trichophyton rubrum*. *Brazilian Journal of Pharmaceutical Sciences*, 49(3): 559–565.

Coulerie, P., Maciuk, A., Eydoux, C., Hnawia, E., Lebouvier, N., Figadère, B., Guillemot, J., Nour, M. (2014). New inhibitors of the DENV-NS5 RdRp from *Carpolepis laurifolia* as potential antiviral drugs for dengue treatment. *Rec. Nat. Prod.*, 8(3): 286–289.

Critchfield, J.W., Butera, S.T. and Folks, T.M. (1996). Inhibition of HIV activation in latently infected cells by flavonoid compounds. *AIDS Res. Hum. Retroviruses*, 12(1): 39–46.

Cushnie, T.P. and Lamb, A.J. (2011). Recent advances in understanding the antibacterial properties of flavonoids. *Int. J. Antimicrob. Agents*, 38: 99–107.

Cushnie, T.P.T. and Lamb, A.J. (2005). Antimicrobial activity of flavonoids. *International Journal of Antimicrobial Agents*, 26(5): 343–356.

Da Silva, C.R., de Andrade Neto, J.B., de Sousa Campos, R., Figueiredo, N.S., Sampaio, L.S., MagalhE—es, H.I. *et al.* (2014). Synergistic effect of the flavonoid catechin, quercetin, or epigallocatechin gallate with fluconazole induces apoptosis in *Candida tropicalis* resistant to fluconazole. *Antimicrob Agents Chemother.*, 58(3): 1468–1478.

De Meyer, N., Haemers, A., Mishra, L., Pandey, H.K., Pieters, L.A., Vanden Berghe, D.A. *et al.* (1991). 4-Hydroxy-3-methoxyflavones with potent antipicornavirus activity. *J. Med. Chem.*, 34: 736–746.

Derksen, A., Hensel, A., Hafezi, W., Herrmann, F., Schmidt, T.J., Ehrhardt, C., Ludwig, S. *et al.* (2014). 3-O-galloylated procyanidins from *Rumex acetosa* L inhibit the attachment of influenza A virus. *PLoS ONE*, 9(10): e110089. doi: 10.1371/ journal. pone. 0110089.

Dixit, A., Rohilla, A. and Singh, V. (2012). *Alpinia officinarum*: Phytochemistry and Pleitropism. *Int. J. Pharm. Phytopharmacol. Res.*, 2(2): 122–125.

Djouossi, M.G., Tamokou, J.D., Ngnokam, D., Kuiate, H.R., Tapondjou, L.A., Harakat, D. and Voutquenne-Nazabadioko, L. (2015). Antimicrobial and antioxidant flavonoids from the leaves of *Oncoba spinosa* Forssk (Salicaceae). *BMC Complementary and Alternative Medicine*, 15: 134. doi: 10.1186/s12906-015-0660-1

Dll'Aica, I., Dona, M., Tonello, F., Piris, A., Mock, M., Montecucco, C. and Garbisa, S. (2004). Potent inhibitors of anthrax lethal factor from green tea. *EMBO Reports*, 5(4): 418–422.

Dos Santos, A.E., Kuster, R.M., Yamamoto, K.A., Salles, T.S., Campos, R., de Meneses, M.D., Soares, M.R., Ferreira, D. (2014). Quercetin and quercetin 3-O-glycosides from *Bauhinia longifolia* (Bong.) Steud show anti-Mayaro virus activity. *Parasit Vectors*, 7: 130. doi: 10.1186/1756-3305-7-130.

Dou, J., Chen, L., Xu, G., Zhang, L., Zhou, H., Wang, H., Su, Z., Ke, M., Guo, Q. and Zhou, C. (2011). Effects of baicalein on Sendai virus *in vivo* are linked to serum baicalin and its inhibition of hemagglutinin-neuraminidase. *Arch. Virol*, 156: 793–801.

Du, J., He, Z.D., Jiang, R.W., Ye, W.C., Xu, H.X. and But, P.P.H. (2003). Antiviral flavonoids from the root bark of *Morus alba* L. Phytochemistry, 62(8): 1235–1238.

Dzoyem, J.P., Hamamoto, H., Ngameni, B., Ngadjui, B.T. and Sekimizu, K. (2013). Antimicrobial action mechanism of flavonoids from *Dorstenia* species. *Drug Discoveries & Therapeutics*, 7(2): 66–72.

Edziri, H., Mastouri, M., Mahjoub, M.A., Mighri, Z., Mahjoub, A. and Verschaeve, L. (2012). Antibacterial, antifungal and cytotoxic activities of two flavonoids from *Retama raetam* flowers. *Molecules*, 17: 7284–7293.

Eggimann, P., Garbino, J. and Pittet, D. (2003). Epidemiology of Candida species infections in critically ill non-immunosuppressed patients. *Lancet Infect. Dis.*, 3: 685–702.

El-kosy, R.H., Ismail, L.D., El-Gendy, O.D., Said, Z.N. and Abdel-Wahab, K.S. (2005). Phytomedicine: Anti Influenza A virus activity of three herbal extracts. *Egyptian Journal of Virology*, 2(1): 21–39.

Eumkeb, G., Chukrathok, S. (2013) Synergistic activity and mechanism of action of ceftazidime and apigenin combination against ceftazidime-resistant *Enterobacter cloacae*. *Phytomedicine*, 20(3–4): 262–269.

Eumkeb, G., Siriwong, S. and Thumanu, K (2012). Synergistic activity of luteolin and amoxicillin combination against amoxicillin-resistant *Escherichia coli* and mode of action. *J. Photochem. Photobiol B.*, 117: 247–253.

Eumkeb, G., Siriwong, S., Phitaktim, S., Rojtinnakorn, N. and Sakdarat, S. (2012). Synergistic activity and mode of action of flavonoids isolated from smaller galangal and amoxicillin combinations against amoxicillin-resistant *Escherichia coli*. *J. Appl. Microbiol.*, 112(1): 55–64.

Evensen, N.A. and Braun, P.C. (2009). The effects of tea polyphenols on *Candida albicans*: Inhibition of biofilm formation and proteasome inactivation. *Can. J. Microbiol.*, 55: 1033–1039.

Evers, D.L., Chao, C.F., Wang, X., Zhang, Z., Huong, S.M. and Huang, E.S. (2005). Human cytomegalovirus-inhibitory flavonoids: Studies on antiviral activity and mechanism of action. *Antiviral Res.*, 68(3): 124–134.

Fan, D., Zhou, X., Zhao, C., Chen, H., Zhao, Y. and Gong, X. (2012). Antiinflammatory, antiviral and quantitative study of quercetin-3-O-beta-D-glucuronide in *Polygonum perfoliatum* L. *Fitoterapia*, 82: 805–810.

Faria, N.C., Kim, J.H., Goncalves, L.A., Martins, M.L., Chan, K.L., Campbell, B.C. (2012). Enhanced activity of antifungal drugs using natural phenolics against yeast strains of *Candida* and *Cryptococcus*. *Letters in Applied Microbiology*, 52(5): 506–513.

Fassina, G., Buffa, A., Benelli, R., Varnier, O.E., Noonan, D.M. and Albini, A. (2002). Polyphenolic antioxidant (-)-epigallocatechin-3-gallate from green tea as a candidate anti-HIV agent. *AIDS*, 16: 939–941.

Fathima, A. and Rao, J.R. (2016). Selective toxicity of catechin-a natural flavonoid towards bacteria. *Appl. Microbiol. Biotechnol.*, doi 10.1007/s00253-016-7492-x

Feld, J.J. and Hoofnagle, J.H. (2005). Mechanism of action of interferon and ribavirin in treatment of hepatitis C. *Nature,* 436: 967–972.

Fesen, M.R., Pommier, Y., Leteurtre, F., Hiroguchi, S., Yung, J. and Kohn, K.W. (1994). Inhibition of HIV-1 integrase by flavones, caffeic acid phenethyl ester (CAPE) and related compounds. *Biochem. Pharmacol.*, 48: 595–608.

Filho, A.A.O., de Oliveira, H.M.B., de Sousa, J.P., Meireles, D.R.P., Maia, G.L., Filho, J.M.B., JR—nior, J.P. and Lima, E.O. (2016). *In vitro* anti-candida activity and mechanism of action of the flavonoid isolated from *Praxelis clematidea* against *Candida albicans* species. *Journal of Applied Pharmaceutical Science*, 6(01): 066–069.

Filho, A.A.O., Fernandes, H.M.B., Sousa, J.P., Maia, G.L.A., Barbosa-Filho, J.M. *et al.* (2013). Anti bacterial activity of flavonoid 5.7.4'-trimethoxyflavone isolated from *Praxelis clematides* RM King & Robinson. *BoletJ—n Latinoamericano y del Caribe de Plantas Medicinales y AromD—ticas*, 12(4): 400–404.

Frost, D.J., Brandt, K.D., Cugier, D. and Goldman, R. (1995). A whole-cell *Candida albicans* assay for the detection of inhibitors towards fungal cell wall synthesis and assembly. *J. Antibiotics.*, 48(4): 306–310.

Fukazawa, H., Suzuki, T., Wakita, T. and Murakami, Y. (2012) A cell-based, microplate colorimetric screen identifies 7,8-benzoflavone and green tea gallate catechins as inhibitors of the hepatitis C virus. *Biol. Pharm. Bull.*, 35(8): 1320–1327.

Galochkina, A.V., Anikin, V.B., Babkin, V.A., Ostrouhova, L.A. and Zarubaev, V.V. (2016). Virus-inhibiting activity of dihydroquercetin, a flavonoid from *Larix sibirica*, against coxsackievirus B4 in a model of viral pancreatitis. *Arch. Virol.*, 161(4): 929–938.

Garrett, R., Romanos, M.T.V., Borges, R.M., Santos, M.G., Rocha, L., Jorge, A. and da Silva, R. (2012). Antiherpetic activity of a flavonoid fraction from *Ocotea notata* leaves. *Revista Brasileira de Farmacognosia Brazilian Journal of Pharmacognosy*, 22(2): 306–313.

Gerdin, B. and Srensso, E. (1983). Inhibitory effect of flavonoids on increased microvascular permeability induced by various agents in rat skin. *Int. J. Micro. Cir. Clin. Exp.*, 2: 39–46.

Ghazal, S.A., Abuzarqa, M. and Maasneh, A.M. (1992). Antimicrobial activity of *Polygonum equisetiforme* extracts and flavonoids. *Phytotherapy Res.*, 6(5): 265–269.

Goldwasser, J., Cohen, P.Y., Lin, W., Kitsberg, D., Balaguer, P., Polyak, S.J., Chung, R.T., Yarmush, M.L. and Nahmias, Y. (2011). Naringenin inhibits the assembly and long-term production of infectious hepatitis C virus particles through a PPAR-mediated mechanism. *J. Hepatol.*, 55: 963–971.

Gonzalez, O., Fontanes, V., Raychaudhuri, S., Loo, R., Loo, J., Arumugaswami, V., Sun, R., Dasgupta, A. and French, S.W. (2009). The heat shock protein inhibitor Quercetin attenuates hepatitis C virus production. *Hepatology*, 50: 1756–1764.

Gordon, N.C. and Wareham, D.W. (2010). Antimicrobial activity of the green tea polyphenol (")-epigallocatechin-3-gallate (EGCG) against clinical isolates of *Stenotrophomonas maltophilia*. *Int. J. Antimicrob. Agents.*, 36: 129–131.

Gradisar, H., Pristovsek, P., Plaper, A. and Jerala, R. (2007). Green tea catechins inhibit bacterial DNA gyrase by interaction with its ATP binding site. *J. Med. Chem.*, 50(2): 264–271.

Haid, S., NovodomskD—, A., Gentzsch, J., Grethe, C., Geuenich, S., Bankwitz, D. *et al.* (2012). A plant-derived flavonoid inhibits entry of all HCV genotypes into human hepatocytes. *Gastroenterology*, 143: 213–222.

Haraguchi, H., Tanimoto, K., Tamura, Y., Mizutani, K. and Kinoshita, T. (1998). Mode of antibacterial action of retrochalcones from *Glycyrrhiza inflate*. *Phytochemistry*, 48(1): 125–129.

Hazra, K.M., Roy, R.N., Sen, S.K. and Laskar, S. (2007). Isolation of antibacterial pentahydroxy flavones from the seeds of *Mimusops elengi* Linn. *African Journal of Biotechnology*, 6(12): 1446–1449.

Hirasawa, M. and Takada, K. (2004). Multiple effects of green tea catechin on the antifungal activity of antimycotics against *Candida albicans*. *J. Antimicrob. Chemother.*, 53: 225–229.

Ho, K. and Cheng, T. (2010). Common superficial fungal infections – a short review. *Medical. Bull.*, 15(11): 23–27.

Hossion, A.M., Zamami, Y., Kandahary, R.K., Tsuchiya, T., Ogawa, W., Iwado, A., Sasaki, K. (2011). Quercetin diacylglycoside analogues showing dual inhibition of DNA gyrase and topoisomerase IV as novel antibacterial agents. *J. Med. Chem.*, 54(11): 3686–3703.

Huang, H.C., Tao, M.H., Hung, T.M., Chen, J.C., Lin, Z.J. and Huang, C. (2014). (-)-Epigallocatechin-3-gallate inhibits entry of hepatitis B virus into hepatocytes. *Antiviral. Res.*, 111: 100–111.

Huang, W.H., Zhou, G.X., Wang, G.C., Chung, H.Y., Ye, W.C. and Li, Y.L. (2012). A new biflavonoid with antiviral activity from the roots of *Wikstroemia indica*. *J. Asian. Nat. Prod. Res.*, 14(4): 401–406.

Huber, B., Eberl, L., Feucht, W. and Polster, J. (2003). Influence of polyphenols on bacterial biofilm formation and quorum-sensing. *Z Naturforsch C*, 58: 879–884.

Hufford, C.D., Jia, Y., Croom, E.M., Muhammed, I., Okunade, A.I., Clark, A.M. and Rogers, R.D. (1993). Antimicrobial compounds from *Petalostemum purpureum*. *J. Nat. Product.*, 56: 1878–1889.

Hwang, I.S., Lee, J., Jin, H.G., Woo, E.R. and Lee, D.G. (2012). Amentoflavone stimulates mitochondrial dysfunction and induces apoptotic cell death in *Candida albicans*. *Mycopathologia*, 173(4): 207–218.

Ikigai, H., Nakae, T., Hara, Y. and Shimamura, T. (1993). Bactericidal catechins damage the lipid bilayer. *Biochim. Biophys. Acta*, 1147: 132–136.

Jamil, S., Abdul Lathiff, S.M., Abdullah, S.A., Jemaon, N. and Sirat, H.M. (2014). Antimicrobial flavonoids from *Artocarpus anisophyllus* Miq. and *Artocarpus lowii* King. *J. Teknology.*, 71(1): 95–99.

Jassim, S.A. and Naji, M.A. (2003). Novel antiviral agents: A medicinal plant perspective. *J. Appl. Microbiol.*, 95(3): 412–427.

Jayasinghe, L., Balasooriya, B.A., Padmini, W.C., Hara, N. and Fujimoto, Y. (2004). Geranyl chalcone derivatives with antifungal and radical scavenging properties from the leaves of *Artocarpus nobilis*. *Phytochemistry*, 65(9): 1287–1290.

Ji, P., Chen, C., Hu, Y., Zhan, Z., Pan, W., Li, R., Li, E., Ge, H.M. and Yang, G. (2015). Antiviral activity of *Paulownia tomentosa* against enterovirus 71 of hand, foot, and mouth disease. *Biol. Pharm. Bull.*, 38(1): 1–6.

Jiang, L., Li, H., Wang, L., Song, Z., Shi, L., Li, W., Deng, X. and Wang, J. (2016). Isorhamnetin attenuates *Staphylococcus aureus* induced lung cell injury by inhibiting alpha-hemolysin expression. *J. Microbiol Biotechnol.*, 26(3): 596–602.

Johari, J., Kianmehr, A., Mustafa, M.R., Abubakar, S. and Zandi, K. (2012). Antiviral activity of baicalein and quercetin against the Japanese encephalitis virus. *Int. J. Mol. Sci.*, 13: 16785–16795.

Jonathan, G. (2010). The grapefruit flavonoid naringenin as a Hepatitis C virus therapy: Efficacy, mechanism and delivery. PhD. thesis, Harvard-MIT Division of Health Sciences and Technology.

Jung, H.J., Park, K., Lee, I.S., Kim, H.S., Yeo, S.H., Woo, E.R. and Lee, D.G. (2007). S-phase accumulation of *Candida albicans* by anticandidal effect of amentoflavone isolated from *Selaginella tamariscina*. *Biol. Pharm. Bull.*, 30(10): 1969–1971.

Kanwal, Q., Hussain, I., Latif Siddiqui, H. and Javaid, A. (2010). Antifungal activity of flavonoids isolated from mango (*Mangifera indica* L.) leaves. *Nat. Prod. Res.*, 24(20): 1907–1914.

Kanwal, Q., Hussain, I., Siddiqui, H.L. and Javaid, A. (2009). Antifungal activity of flavonoids isolated from mango (*Mangifera indica* L.) leaves. *Journal of the Serbian Chemical Society*, 74(12): 1389–1399.

Kaul, T.N., Middleton, E. and Jr Ogra, P.L. (1985). Antiviral effect of flavonoids on human viruses. *J. Med. Virol.*, 15(1): 71–79.

Kaur, R.T., Gupte, S. and Kaur, M. (2015). A review on emerging fungal infections and their significance. *Journal of Bacteriology & Mycology*, 1(2): doi: 10.15406/ jbmoa.2015.01.00009

Kemertelidze, E.P., Shalashvili, K.G., Korsantiya, B.M., Nizharadze, N.O. and Chipashvili, N.S. (2007). Therapeutic effect of phenolic compounds isolated from *Rhododendron ungernii* leaves. *Pharm. Chem. J-USSR*, 41: 10–13.

Kim, H.J., Woo, E.R., Shin, C.G. and Park, H. (1998). A new flavonol glycoside gallate ester from *Acer okamotoanum* and its inhibitory activity against human immunodeficiency virus-1 (HIV-1) integrase. J. Nat. Prod., 61: 145–148.

Kim, K., Kim, K.H., Kim, H.Y., Cho, H.K., Sakamoto, N. and Cheong, J. (2010). Curcumin inhibits hepatitis C virus replication *via* suppressing the Akt-SREBP-1 pathway. *FEBS Lett.*, 584: 707–712.

Kirchmair, J., Liedl, K.R. and Rollinger, J.M. (2012). Influenza neuraminidase: A drug gable target for natural products. Natural Product Reports, 29(1): 11–36.

Kitamura, K., Honda, M., Yoshizaki, H., Yamamoto, S., Nakane, H., Fukushima, M., Ono, K. and Tokunaga, T. (1998). Baicalin, an inhibitor of HIV-1 production *in vitro*. *Antiviral Res.*, 37: 131–140.

Kobric, D.J., Syed, A., Tenenbaum, H.C. and Levesque, C.M. (2012). Antifungal efficacy of Citrus fruit flavonoids against *Candida albicans* biofilms. Conference: AADR Annual Meeting 2012, *https://www.researchgate.net/publication 266778789_ Antifungal_ Efficacy* _of_Citrus_Fruit_Flavonoids_ Against_Candida_ albicans_ Biofilms

Kuete, V., Ngameni, B., Mbaveng, A.T., Ngadjui, B., Meyer, J.J. and Lall, N. (2010). Evaluation of flavonoids from *Dorstenia barteri* for their antimycobacterial, antigonorrheal and anti-reverse transcriptase activities. *Actatropica*, 116: 100–104.

Kumar, S. and Pandey, A.K. (2013). Chemistry and biological activities of flavonoids: An overview. Hindawi Publishing Corporation the Scientific World Journal, Article ID 162750.

Lani, R., Hassandarvish, P., Shu, M.H., Phoon, W.H., Chu, J.J., Higgs, S., Vanlandingham, D., Abu Bakar, S. and Zandi, K. (2016). Antiviral activity of selected flavonoids against chikungunya virus. *Antiviral Res.*, 133: 50–61.

Lee, J., Choi, Y., Woo, E.R. and Lee, D.G. (2009). Isocryptomerin, a novel membrane-active antifungal compound from *Selaginella tamariscina*. *Biochem. Biophys. Res. Commun.*, 379(3): 676–680.

Lee, J., Park, J., Cho, H.S., Joo, S.W., Cho, M.H. and Lee, J. (2013). Anti-biofilm activities of quercetin and tannic acid against *Staphylococcus aureus*. *Biofouling*, 29: 491–499.

Lee, J.S., Kim, H.J. and Lee, Y.S. (2003). A new anti HIV flavonoid glucoronide from *Chrysanthemum morifolium*. *Planta Medica*, 69: 859–861.

Lee, K.A., Moon, S.H., Lee, J.Y., Kim, K.T., Park, Y.S. and Paik, H.D. (2013). Antibacterial activity of a novel flavonoid, 7-O-butyl naringenin, against methicillin-resistant *Staphylococcus aureus* (MRSA). *Food Sci. Biotechnol.*, 22(6): 1725–1728.

Lee, M.H., Han, D.W., Hyon, S.H. and Park, J.C. (2011). Apoptosis of human fibrosarcoma HT-1080 cells by epigallocatechin-3-O-gallate *via* induction of p53 and caspases as well as suppression of Bcl-2 and phosphorylated nuclear factor-κB. *Apoptosis,* 16: 75–85.

Lee, W.J., Moon, J.S., Kim, Y.T., Bach, T.T., Hai, D.V. and Kim, S.U. (2016). Inhibition of the calcineurin pathway by two favonoids isolated from *Miliusa sinensis* Finet & Gagnep. *J. Microbiol. Biotechnol.*, 26(10): 1696–1700.

Li, B.H., Zhang, R., Du, Y.T., Sun, Y.H. and Tian, W.X. (2006). Inactivation mechanism of the beta-ketoacyl-[acyl carrier protein] reductase of bacterial type-II fatty acid synthase by epigallocatechin gallate. *Biochem. Cell. Biol.*, 84(5): 755–762.

Li, B.Q., Fu, T., Dongyan, Y., Mikovits, J.A., Ruscetti, F.W. and Wang, J.M. (2000). Flavonoid baicalin inhibits HIV-1 infection at the level of viral entry. *Biochem. Biophys. Res. Commun.*, 276: 534–538.

Li, B.Q., Fu, T., Yan, Y.D., Baylor, N.W., Ruscetti, F.W. and Kung, H.F. (1993). Inhibition of HIV infection by baicalin-a flavonoid compound purified from Chinese herbal medicine. *Cell Mol. Biol. Res.*, 39(2): 119–124.

Li, S., Zhang, Z., Cain, A., Wang, B., Long, M. and Taylor, J. (2005). Antifungal activity of camptothecin, trifolin, and hyperoside isolated from *Camptotheca acuminata. J. Agric. Food Chem.*, 53(1): 32–37.

Li, X., Liu, Y., Wu, T., Hin, Y., Cheng, H., Wan, C., Qian, W., Xing, F. and Shi, W. (2015). The antiviral effect of baicalin on enterovirus 71 *in vitro*. *Viruses*, 7(8): 4756–4771.

Li, Y., Leung, K.T., Yao, F., Ooi, L.S.M. and Ooi, V.E.C. (2006). Antiviral flavans from the leaves of *Pithecellobium clypearia. J. Nat. Prod.*, 69: 833–835.

Lim, Y.H., Kim, I.H., Seo, J.J. (2007). *In vitro* activity of kaempferol isolated from the *Impatiens balsamina* alone and in combination with erythromycin or clindamycin against *Propionibacterium acnes. J. Microbiol.*, 45(5): 473–477.

Lin, Y.J., Chang, Y.C., Hsiao, N.W., Hsieh, J.L., Wang, C.Y., Kung, S.H., Tsai, F.J., Lan, Y.C. and Lin, C.W. (2012). Fisetin and rutin as 3C protease inhibitors of enterovirus A 71. *J. Virol. Methods.*, 182(1–2): 93–98.

Lin, Y.M., Anderson, H., Flavin, M.T., Pai, Y.H., Mata-Greenwood, E., Pengsuparp, T., Pezzuto, J.M., Schinazi, R.F., Hughes, S.H. and Chen, F.C. (1997). *In vitro* anti-HIV activity of biflavonoids isolated from *Rhus succedanea* and *Garcinia multiflora. J. Nat. Prod.*, 60(9): 884–888.

Lipson, S.M. (2013). Flavonoid-associated direct loss of rotavirus antigen/antigen activity in cell-free suspension. *Journal of Medicinally Active Plants*, 2(1): 10–24.

Liu, A.L., Wang, H.D., Lee, S.M., Wang, Y.T. and Du, G.H. (2008). Structure–activity relationship of flavonoids as influenza virus neuraminidase inhibitors and their *in vitro* anti-viral activities. *Bioorg. Med. Chem.*, 16: 7141–7147.

Lopez-Lazaro, M. (2009). Distribution and biological activities of the flavonoid luteolin. *Mini Reviews in Medicinal Chemistry*, 9(1): 31–59.

Luo, G., Hamatake, R.K., Mathis, D.M., Racela, J., Rigat, K.L., Lemm, J. and Colonno, R.J. (2000). De novo initiation of RNA synthesis by the RNA-dependent RNA polymerase (NS5B) of hepatitis C virus. *J. Virol.*, 74: 851–863.

Lv, X., Qiu, M., Chen, D., Zheng, N., Jin, Y. and Wu, Z. (2014). Apigenin inhibits enterovirus 71 replication through suppressing viral IRES activity and modulating cellular JNK pathway. *Antiviral Res.*, 109: 30–41.

Lyu, S.Y., Rhim, J.Y. and Park, W.B. (2005).Antiherpetic activities of flavonoids against herpes simplex virus type 1 (HSV-1) and type 2 (HSV-2) *in vitro. Arch. Pharm. Res.*, 28(11): 1293–1301.

Mandalari, G., Bennett, N., Bisignano, G., Trombetta, D., Saija, A., Faulds, C.B., Gasson, M.J., Narbad, A. (2007). Antimicrobial activity of flavonoids extracted from bergamot (*Citrus bergamia* Risso) peel, a byproduct of the essential oil industry. *J. Appl. Microbiol.*, 103(6): 2056–2064.

Mangoyi, R., Midiwo, J. and Mukanganyama, S. (2015). Isolation and characterization of an antifungal compound 5-hydroxy-7,4'-dimethoxyflavone from *Combretum zeyheri*. *BMC Complement Altern Med.*, 15: 405. doi: 10.1186/s12906-015-0934-7. Maritini, N.D., Katerere, D.R. and Eloff, J. (2004). Biological activity of five antibacterial flavonoids from *Combretum erythrophyllum* (Combretaceae). *Journal of Ethnopharmacology*, 93(2–3): 207–212.

Matsunaga, T., Nakahara, A., Minnatul, K.M., Noiri, Y., Ebisu, S., Kato, A. *et al.* (2010). The inhibitory effects of catechins on biofilm formation by the periodontopathogenic bacterium, *Eikenella corrodens*. *Biosci Biotechnol Biochem.*, 74: 2445–2450.

Mercader, A.G. and Pomilio, A.B. (2010). QSAR study of flavonoids and biflavonoids as influenza H1N1 virus neuraminidase inhibitors. *Eur. J. Med. Chem.*, 45: 1724–1730.

Miki, K., Nagai, T., Nakamura, T., Tuji, M., Koyama, K., Kinoshita, K. *et al.* (2008). Synthesis and evaluation of influenza virus sialidase inhibitory activity of hinokiflavone-sialic acid conjugates. *Heterocycles*, 75: 879–885.

Miki, K., Nagai, T., Suzuki, K., Tsujimura, R., Koyama, K., Kinoshita, K. *et al.* (2007). Antiinfluenza virus activity of biflavonoids. *Bioorg Med Chem Lett.*, 17: 772–775.

Min, B.S., Lee, H.K., Lee, S.M., Kim, Y.H., Bae, K.H., Otake, T. *et al.* (2002). Anti-human immunodeficiency virus-type 1 activity of constituents from *Juglans mandshurica*. *Arch. Pharm. Res.*, 25: 441–445.

Mohammed, R.S., El Souda, S.S., Taie, H.A.A., Moharam. M.E., Shaker, K.H. (2015). Antioxidant, antimicrobial activities of flavonoids glycoside from *Leucaena leucocephala* leaves. *Journal of Applied Pharmaceutical Science*, 5(6): 138–147.

Mori, A., Nishino, C., Enoki, N. and Tawata, S. (1987). Antibacterial activity and mode of action of plant flavonoids against *Proteus vulgaris* and *Staphylococcus aureus*. *Phytochemistry*, 26: 2231–2234.

Moskaug, J., Carlsen, H., Myhrstad, M. and Blomhoff, R. (2004). Molecular imaging of the biological effects of quercetin and quercetin-rich foods. *Mechanisms of Ageing and Development*, 125: 315–324.

Mun, S.H., Lee, Y.S., Han, S.H., Lee, S.W., Cha, S.W., Kim, S.B. *et al.* (2015). *In vitro* potential effect of morin in the combination with β-lactam antibiotics against methicillin-resistant *Staphylococcus aureus*. *Foodborne Pathog Dis.*, 12(6): 545–550.

Murali, K.S., Sivasubramanian, S., Vincent, S., Murugan, S.B., Giridaran, B., Dinesh, S. *et al.* (2012). Anti-chikungunya activity of luteolin and apigenin rich fraction from *Cynodon dactylon*. *Asian. Pac. J. Trop. Med.*, 8(5): 352–358.

Mutai, P., Heydenreich, M., Thoithi, G., Mugumbate, G. and Chibale, K. (2013). 3-Hydroxy isoflavanones from the stem bark of *Dalbergia melanoxylon*: Isolation, anti-mycobacterial evaluation and molecular docking studies. *Phytochem Lett.,* 6: 671–675.

Nafisi, S.H., Shadaloi, A., Feizbakhsh, A. and Tajmir-Riahi, H.A. (2009). RNA binding to antioxidant flavonoids. *J. Photochem. Photobiol. B.*, 94: 1–7.

Nagai, T., Miyaichi, Y., Tomimori, T., Suzuki, Y. and Yamada, H. (1992). *In vivo* anti-influenza virus activity of plant flavonoids possessing inhibitory activity for influenza virus sialidase. *Antiviral Res.*, 19: 207–217.

Nagai, T., Suzuki, Y., Tomimori, T. and Yamada, H. (1995b). Antiviral activity of plant flavonoid, 5,7,4-trihydroxy-8-methoxyflavone, from the roots of *Scutellaria baicalensis* against influenza A (H3N2) and B viruses. *Biol. Pharm. Bull.*, 18: 295–299.

Nagai, T., Miyaichi, Y., Tomimori, T., Suzuki, Y. and Yamada, H. (1990). Inhibition of influenza virus sialidase and anti-influenza virus activity by plant flavonoids. *Chem. Pharm. Bull.* (Tokyo), *38(5): 1329–1332.*

Nagai, T., Moriguchi, R., Suzuki, Y., Tomimori, T. and Yamada, H. (1995a). Mode of action of the anti-influenza virus activity of plant flavonoid, 5,7,4'-trihydroxy-8-methoxyflavone, from the roots of *Scutellaria baicalensis*. *Antiviral Res.*, 26(1): 11–25.

Nahmias, Y., Goldwasser, J., Casali, M., van Poll, D., Wakita, T., Chung, R.T. *et al.*, (2008). Apolipoprotein B-dependent hepatitis C virus secretion is inhibited by the grapefruit flavonoid naringenin. *Hepatology*, 47: 1437–1445.

Nakane, H. and Ono, K. (1990). Differential inhibitory effects of some catechin derivatives on the activities of human immunodeficiency virus reverse transcriptase and cellular deoxyribonucleic and ribonucleic acid polymerases. *Biochemistry*, 29(11): 2841–2845.

Nayaka, H.B., Londonkar, R.L., Umesh, M.K. and Tukappa, A. (2014). Antibacterial attributes of apigenin isolated from *Portulaca oleracea* L. *International Journal of Bacteriology*, Article ID 175851.

Nema, R. (2012), Antibacterial activity of a new flavone glycoside from the seeds of *Cassia sophera* Linn. *International Research Journal of Pharmacy*, 3(4): 369–371.

Nessa, F., Ismail, Z. and Mohamed, N. (2012). Antimicrobial activities of extracts and favonoid glycosides of corn silk (*Zea mays* L). *International Journal of Biotechnology for Wellness Industries*, 1: 115–121.

Ng, T.B., Ling, J.M., Wang, Z.T., Cai, J.N. and Xu, G.J. (1996). Examination of coumarins, flavonoids and polysaccharopeptide for antibacterial activity. *Gen. Pharmacol.*, 27(7): 1237–1240.

Novy, P., Rondevaldova, J., Kourimska, L. and Kokoska. L. (2013). Synergistic interactions of epigallocatechin gallate and oxytetracycline against various drug resistant *Staphylococcus aureus* strains *in vitro*. *Phytomedicine*, 20(5): 432–435.

Novy, P., Urban, J., Leuner, O., Vadlejch, J. and Kokoska, L. (2011). *In vitro* synergistic effects of baicalin with oxytetracycline and tetracycline against *Staphylococcus aureus*. *J. Antimicrob. Chemother.*, 66(6): 1298–1300.

Ohemeng, K.A., Schwender, C.F., Fu, K.P. and Barrett, J.F. (1993). DNA gyrase inhibitory and antibacterial activity of some flavones (1). *Bioorganic & Medicinal Chemistry Letters*, 3(2): 225–230.

Olugbuyiro, J.O. and Moody, J.O. (2013). Anti-Tubercular compounds from *Spondias mombin*. *Int. J. Pure. Appl. Sci. Technol.*, 19: 76.

Ono, K., Nakane, H., Fukushima, M., Chermann, J.C. and Barré-Sinoussi, F. (1990). Differential inhibitory effects of various flavonoids on the activities of reverse transcriptase and cellular DNA and RNA polymerases. *Eur. J. Biochem.*, 190(3): 469–476.

Onsare, J.G. and Arora, D.S. (2015). Antibio film potential of flavonoids extracted from *Moringa oleifera* seed coat against *Staphylococcus aureus, Pseudomonas aeruginosa* and *Candida albicans*. *J Appl Microbiol.*, 118(2): 313–325.

Orhan, D.D., Ozçelik, B., Ozgen, S. and Ergun, F. (2010). Antibacterial, antifungal, and antiviral activities of some flavonoids. *Microbiol Res.*, 165(6): 496–504.

Osawa, K., Yasuda, H., Maruyama, T., Morita, H., Takeya, K. and Itokawa, H. (1992). Isoflavanones from the heartwood of *Swartzia polyphylla* and their antibacterial activity against cariogenic bacteria. *Chemical and Pharmaceutical Bulletin*, 40(11): 2970–2974.

Otsuka, N., Liu, M.H., Shiota, S., Ogawa, W., Kuroda, T., Hatano, T. and Tsuchiya, T. (2008). Anti-methicillin resistant *Staphylococcus aureus* (MRSA) compounds isolated from *Laurus nobilis*. *Biol. Pharm. Bull.*, 31: 1794–1797.

6—zçelik, B., Orhan, D.D., 6—zgen, S. and Ergun, F. (2008). Antimicrobial activity of flavonoids against extended-spectrum β-lactamase (ESβL)-producing *Klebsiella pneumonia*. *Trop. J. Pharm. Res.*, 7(4): 1151–1157.

Palchykovska, L.G., Vasylchenko, O.V., Platonov, M.O., Starosyla, D.B., Porva, J.I., Rymar, S.J. *et al.* (2013). Antiviral properties of herbal flavonoids – inhibitors of the DNA and RNA synthesis. *Biopolymers and Cell*, 29(2): 150–156.

Pang, S., Ge, Y., Wang, L.S., Liu, X., Lin, C.W. and Yang, H. (2013). Isolation and purification of orientin and isovitexin from *Thlaspi arvense* Linn. *Advanced Materials Research*, 781: 615–618.

Peralta, M.A., da Silva, M.A., Ortega, M.G., Cabrera, J.L., Paraje, M.G. (2015). Antifungal activity of a prenylated flavonoid from *Dalea elegans* against *Candida albicans* biofilms. *Phytomedicine*, 22(11): 975–980.

Perumal, S., Mahmud, R. and Ramanathan, S. (2015). Anti-infective potential of caffeic acid and epicatechin 3-gallate isolated from methanol extract of *Euphorbia hirta* (L.) against *Pseudomonas aeruginosa. Nat. Prod. Res.*, 29(18): 1766–1769.

Phosrithong, N., Samee, W. and Ungwitayatorn (2012). 3D-QSAR studies of natural flavonoid compounds as reverse transcriptase inhibitors. *J. Med. Chem. Res.*, 21: 559. doi:10.1007/s00044-011-9570-z

Pina-Vaz, C., Gonçalves Rodrigues, A., Pinto, E., Costa-de-Oliveira, S., Tavares, C., Salgueiro, L., Cavaleiro, C., Gonçalves, M.J. and Martinez-de-Oliveira, J. (2004). Antifungal activity of Thymus oils and their major compounds. *J. Eur. Acad. Dermatol. Venereol.*, 18: 73–78.

Pinto, E., Pina-Vaz, C., Salgueiro, L., Gonçalves, M.J., Costa-de-Oliveira, S., Cavaleiro, C. *et al.* (2006). Antifungal activity of the essential oil of *Thymus pulegioides* on Candida, *Aspergillus* and dermatophyte species. *J. Med. Microbiol.*, 55: 1367–1373.

Pisonero-Vaquero, S., GarcJ—a-Mediavilla, M.V., Jorquera, F., Majano, P.L., Benet, M., Jover, R. *et al.* (2014). Modulation of PI3K-LXRα-dependent lipogenesis mediated by oxidative/nitrosative stress contributes to inhibition of HCV replication by quercetin. *Lab Invest.*, 94(3): 262–274.

Plaper, A., Golob, M., Hafner, I., Oblak, M., Solmajer, T. and Jerala, R. (2003). Characterization of quercetin binding site on DNA gyrase. *Biochem Biophys Res Commun.*, 306(2): 530–536.

Plyuta, V., Zaitseva, J., Lobakova, E., Zagoskina, N., Kuznetsov, A. and Khmel, I. (2013). Effect of plant phenolic compounds on biofilm formation by *Pseudomonas aeruginosa. APMIS*, 121: 1073–1081.

Pohjala, L., Utt, A., Varjak, M., Lulla, A., Merits, A., Ahola, T. and Tammela, P. (2011). Inhibitors of alphavirus entry and replication identified with a stable Chikungunya replicon cell line and virus-based assays. *PLoS ONE*, 6(12): e28923.

Qian, M., Tang, S., Wu, C., Wang, Y., He, T., Chen, T. and Xiao, X. (2015). Synergy between baicalein and penicillins against penicillinase-producing *Staphylococcus aureus. Int. J. Med. Microbiol.*, 305(6): 501–504.

Ragasa, C., Cruz, C., Chiong, I. and Rideout, J. (1997). Antifungal flavonoids from *Waltheria americana. Philippine Journal of Science*, 126(3): 243–250.

Ragasa, C.Y., Co, A.L., Rideout, J.A. (2005). Antifungal metabolites from *Blumea balsamifera. Nat. Prod. Res.*, 19(3): 231–237.

Rahman, M.S., Ali, M.Y. and Ali, M.U. (2008). *In vitro* screening of two flavonoid compounds isolated from *Cassia alata* leaves for fungicidal activities. *J. Bio. Sci.*, 16: 139–142.

Rao, M.S., Duddeck, H. and Dembinski, R. (2002). Isolation and structural elucidation of 3,4',5,7-tetraacetyl quercetin from *Adina cordifolia* (Karam ki Gaach). *Fitoterapia*, 73(4): 353–355.

Rashed, K., Calland, N., Deloison, G., Rouillé, Y. and Séron, K. (2014).*In vitro* antiviral activity of *Pistacia chinensis* flavonoids against hepatitis C virus (HCV). *J. App. Pharm.*, 6(1): 8–18.

Rattanachaikunsopon, P. and Phumkhachorn, P. (2010). Contents and antibacterial activity of flavonoids extracted from leaves of *Psidium guajava*. *Journal of Medicinal Plants Research*, 4(5): 393–396.

Rawat, D. and Nair, D. (2010). Extended-spectrum β-lactamases in Gram negative bacteria. *J. Glob. Infect. Dis.*, 2(3): 263–274.

Ray, P.G. and Majumdar, S.K. (1975). New antifungal from *Alpinia officinarum*. *Ind. J. Exp. Biol.*, 1: 489.

Ray, P.G. and Majumdar, S.K. (1976). Antifungal flavonoid from *Alpinia officinarum*. *Ind. J Exp. Biol.*, 14: 712–714.

Rhama, S. and Madhavan, S. (2011). Antibacterial activity of the flavonoid, patulitrin isolated from the flowers of *Tagetes erecta* L. *International Journal of Pharm Tech Research*, 3(3): 1407–1409.

Robin, V., Irurzun, A., Amoros, M., Boustie, J. and Carrasco, L. (2001). Antipoliovirus flavonoids from *Psiadia dentata*. *Antivir. Chem. Chemother.*, 12(5): 283–291.

Rodanant, P., Khetkam, P., Suksamrarn, A. and Kuvatanasuchati, J. (2015). Coumarins and flavonoid from *Murraya paniculata* (L.) Jack: Antibacterial and anti-inflammation activity. *Pak. J. Pharm. Sci.*, 28(6): 1947–1951.

Romanos, M.T. and Costa, S.S. (2016). Anti-HSV-1 and HSV-2 flavonoids and a new kaempferol triglycoside from the medicinal plant *Kalanchoe daigremontiana*. *Chem. Biodivers.*, doi: 10.1002/cbdv.201600127.

Sakanaka, S. and Okada, Y. (2004). Inhibitory effects of green tea polyphenols on the production of a virulence factor of the periodontal-disease-causing anaerobic bacterium *Porphyromonas gingivalis*. *J. Agric. Food Chem.*, 52: 1688–1692.

Salas, M.P., Celiz, G., Geronazzo, H., Daz, M. and Resnik, S.L. (2011). Antifungal activity of natural and enzymatically-modified flavonoids isolated from citrus species. *Food Chemistry*, 124(4): 1411–1415.

Salvatore, M.J., King, A.B., Graham, A.C., Onishi, H.R., Bartizal, K.F., Abruzzo, G.K., Gill, C.J., Ramjit, H.G., Pitzenberger, S.M. and Witherup, K.M. (1998). Antibacterial activity of lonchocarpol A. *J. Nat. Prod.*, 61: 640–642.

Sami, A.J. and Shakoori, A.R. (2011). Cellulase activity inhibition and growth retardation of associated bacterial strains of *Aulacophora foviecollis* by two glycosylated flavonoids isolated from *Mangifera indica* leaves.*Journal of Medicinal Plant Research*, 5(2): 184–190·

Sampath, M. and Vasanthi, M. (2013). Isolation, structural elucidation of flavonoids from *Polyalthia longifolia* (Sonn) thawaites and evaluation of antibacterial, antioxidant, anticancer potential. *Int. J. Pharm. Pharm. Sci.*, 5(1): 336–341.

Sathiamoorthy, B., Gupta, P., Kumar, M., Chaturyedi, A.K. and Maurya, R. (2007). New antifungal flavonoid glycoside from *Vitex negundo*. *Bioorganic and Medicinal Chemistry Letters*, 17(1): 239–242.

Satoh, E., Ishii, T., Shimizu, Y., Sawamura, S. and Nishimura, M. (2002a). A mechanism of the thearubigin fraction of black tea (*Camellia sinensis*) extract protecting against the effect of tetanus toxin. *The Journal of Toxicological Sciences*, 27(5): 441–447.

Satoh, E., Ishii, T., Shimizu, Y., Sawamura, S. and Nishimura, M. (2002b). The mechanism underlying the protective effect of the thearubigin fraction of black tea (*Camellia sinensis*) extract against the neuromuscular blocking action of botulinum neurotoxins. *Pharmacology & Toxicology*, 90(4): 199–202.

Schindler, C., Levy, D.E. and Decker, T. (2007). JAK–STAT signaling: From interferons to cytokines. *J. Biol. Chem.*, 282: 20059–20063.

Selway, J.W.T. (1986). Antiviral activity of flavones and flavans. *In*: Cody, V., Middleton, E. and Harborne, J.B. (*eds.*), Plant flavonoids in biology and medicine: Biochemical, pharmacological and structure activity relationships. New York: Alan R Liss, Inc, pp. 521–536.

Senthilvel, P., Lavanya, P., Kumar, K.M., Swetha, R., Anitha, P., Bag, S., Sarveswari, S., Vijayakumar, V., Ramaiah, S. and Anbarasu, A. (2013). Flavonoid from *Carica papaya* inhibits NS2B-NS3 protease and prevents Dengue 2 viral assembly. *Bioinformation*, 9(18): 889–895.

Serpa, R., França, E.J., Furlaneto-Maia, L., Andrade, C.G., Diniz, A. and Furlaneto, M.C. (2012). *In vitro* antifungal activity of the flavonoid baicalein against *Candida* species. *J. Med. Microbiol.*, 61(Pt 12): 1704–1708.

Shah, S., Stapleton, P.D. and Taylor, P.W. (2008). The polyphenol (-)-epicatechin gallate disrupts the secretion of virulence-related proteins by *Staphylococcus aureus*. *Lett. Appl. Microbiol.*, 46(2): 181–5.

Shao, L.C., Sheng, C.Q. and Zhang, W.N. (2007). Recent advances in the study of antifungal lead compounds with new chemical scaffolds. *Yao Xue Xue Bao*, 42: 1129–1136.

Sharma, A., Gupta, S., Sarethy, I.P., Dang, S., Gabrani, R. (2012). Green tea extract: Possible mechanism and antibacterial activity on skin pathogens. *Food Chem.*, 135(2): 672–5.

Shehadi, M., Awada, F., Oleik, R., Chokr, A., Hamze, K., Abou Hamdan Harb, A. *et al.* (2014). Comparative analysis of the anti-bacterial activity of four plant extract. *Int. J. Curr. Res. Acad. Rev.*, 2(6): 83–94.

Shinozuka, K., Kikuchi, Y., Nishino, C., Mori, A. and Tawata, S. (1988). Inhibitory effect of flavonoids on DNA-dependent DNA and RNA polymerases. *Experientia*, 44: 882–885.

Sichel, G., Corsaro, C., Scalia, M., Di Bilio, A.J. and Bonomo, R.P. (1991). *In vitro* scavenger activity of some flavonoids and melanins against O2-dot. *Free Radic Biol Med.*, 11: 1–8.

Sivasothy, Y., Sulaiman, S.F., Ooi, K.L., Ibrahim, H. and Awang, K. (2013). Antioxidant and antibacterial activities of flavonoids and curcuminoids from *Zingiber spectabile* Griff. *Food Control.*, 30: 714–720.

Sohn, H.Y., Son, K.H., Kwon, C.S., Kwon, G.S. and Kang, S.S. (2004). Antimicrobial and cytotoxic activity of 18 prenylated flavonoids isolated from medicinal plants: *Morus alba* L., *Morus mongolica* Schneider, *Broussnetia papyrifera* (L.) Vent, *Sophora flavescens* Ait and *Echinosophora koreensis* Nakai. *Phytomedicine*, 11(7–8): 666–672.

Song, J.H., Park, K.S., Kwon, D.H. and Choi, H.J. (2013). Anti-human rhinovirus 2 activity and mode of action of quercetin-7-glucoside from *Lagerstroemia speciosa*. *J. Med. Food*, 16(4): 274–279.

Song, M., Gao, M.H., Huang, W.H., Li, M.M., Li, H., Li, Y.L., Zhang, X.Q. and Ye, W.C. (2016). Flavonoids from the seeds of *Hovenia acerba* and their *in vitro* antiviral activity. *J. Pharm. Biomed. Sci.*, 6(6): 401–409.

Stapleton, P.D., Shah, S., Hamilton-Miller, J.M., Hara, Y., Nagaoka, Y., Kumagai, A., Uesato, S. and Taylor, P.W. (2004). Anti *Staphylococcus aureus* activity and oxacillin resistance modulating capacity of 3-*O*-acyl-catechins. *Int. J. Antimicrob. Agents.*, 24: 374–380.

Su, Y., Ma, L., Wen, Y., Wang, H. and Zhang, S. (2014) Studies of the *in vitro* anti-bacterial activities of several polyphenols against clinical isolates of methicillin-resistant *Staphylococcus aureus*. *Molecules*, 19(8): 12630–12639.

Sugita-Konishi, Y., Hara-Kudo, Y., Amano, F., Okubo, T., Aoi, N., Iwaki, M. and Kumagai, S. (1999). Epigallocatechin gallate and gallocatechin gallate in green tea catechins inhibit extracellular release of Vero toxin from enterohemorrhagic *Escherichia coli* O157:H7. *Biochim. Biophys. Acta*, 1472(1–2): 42–50.

Suriyanarayanan, B., Shanmugam, K. and Santhosh, R.S. (2013). Synthetic quercetin inhibits mycobacterial growth possibly by interacting with DNA gyrase. *Romanian Biotechnological Letters*, 18(5): 8587–8593.

Svetaz, L., Agüero, M.B., Alvarez, S., Luna, L., Feresin, G., Derita, M. *et al.*, (2007). Antifungal activity of *Zuccagnia punctata* Cav.: Evidence for the mechanism of action. *Planta Med.*, 73(10): 1074–1080.

Takahashi, T., Kokubo, R. and Sakaino, M. (2004). Antimicrobial activities of eucalyptus leaf extracts and flavonoids from *Eucalyptus maculate*. *Letters in Applied Microbiology*, 39: 60–64.

Talalay, P., Fahey, J.W., Holtzclaw, W.D., Prestera, T. and Zhang, Y. (1995). Chemoprotection against cancer by phase 2 enzyme induction. *Toxicol Lett.*, 82–83: 173–179.

Tang, F., Li, W.H., Zhou, X., Liu, Y.H., Li, Z., Tang, Y.S. *et al.* (2014). Puerarin protects against *Staphylococcus aureus* induced injury of human alveolar epithelial aA49 cells *via* downregulating alpha-hemolysin secretion. *Microb. Drug Resist.*, 20: 357–363.

Teffo, L.S., Aderogba, M.A. and Eloff, J.N. (2010). Antibacterial and antioxidant activities of four kaempferol methyl ethers isolated from *Dodonaea viscose* Jacq. var. *Angustifolia* leaf extracts. *South African Journal of Botany*, 76(1): 25–29.

Toda, M., Okubo, S., Ikigai, H., Suzuki, T., Suzuki, Y. and Shimamura, T. (1991a). The protective activity of tea against infection by *Vibrio cholerae* O1. *Journal of Applied Microbiology*, 70(2): 109–112.

Toda, M., Okubo, S., Ikigai, H., Suzuki, T., Suzuki, Y., Hara, Y., Shimamura, T. (1991b). The protective activity of tea catechins against experimental infection by *Vibrio cholera* O1. *Microbiology and Immunology*, 36(9): 999–1001.

Toyoshima, Y., Okubo, S. and Toda, M. (1994). Effect of catechin on the ultrastructure of *Trichophyton mentagrophytes*. *Kansenshogaku Zasshi*, 68: 295–303.

Tripathi, V.D. and Rastogi, R.P. (1981). *In vitro* anti-HIV activity of flavonoids isolated from *Garcinia multifolia*. *J. Sci. Indian Res.*, 40: 116–121.

Tsuchiya, H. and Iinuma, M. (2000). Reduction of membrane fluidity by antibacterial sophoraflavanone G isolated from *Sophora exigua*. *Phytomedicine*, 7: 161–165.

@—rményi, F.G., Saraiva, G.D., Casanova, L.M., Matos, A.D., de MagalhE—es Camargo, L.M., Valsaraj, R., Pushpangadan, P., Smitt, U.W., Adsersen, A., Christensen, S.B., Sittie, A., Nyman, U., Nielsen, C. and Olsen, C.E. (1997). New anti-HIV-1, antimalarial, and antifungal compounds from *Terminalia bellerica*. *J. Nat. Prod.*, 60: 739–742.

Van Hoof, L., Vanden Berghe, D.A., Hatfield, G.M. and Vlietinck, A.J. (1984). Plant antiviral agents; V. 3-Methoxyflavones as potent inhibitors of viral-induced block of cell synthesis. *Planta Med.*, 50: 513–517.

Vandeputte, O.M., Kiendrebeogo, M., Rajaonson, S., Diallo, B., Mol, A., El Jaziri, M. *et al.* (2010). Identification of catechin as one of the flavonoids from *Combretum albiflorum* bark extract that reduces the production of quorum-sensing-controlled virulence factors in *Pseudomonas aeruginosa* PAO1. *Appl. Environ. Microbiol.*, 76: 243–253.

Vikram, A., Jayaprakasha, G., Jesudhasan, P., Pillai, S. and Patil, B. (2010). Suppression of bacterial cell-cell signalling, biofilm formation and T type III secretion system by citrus flavonoids. *J. Appl. Microbiol.*, 109: 515–527.

Vlietinck, A., De Bruyne, T., Apers, S. and Pieters, L. (1998). Plant-derived leading compounds for chemotherapy of human immunodeficiency virus (HIV) infection. *Planta Medica*, 64(02): 97–109.

Wachter, G.A., Hoffmann, J.J., Furbacher, T., Blake, M.E. and Timmermann, B.N. (1999). Antibacterial and antifungal flavanones from *Eysenhardtia texana*. *Phytochemistry*, 52: 1469–1471.

Wagner, E.K., Hewlett, M.J. (1999). Basic Virology. Malden, MA, USA, Blackwell Science.

Wagoner, J., Negash, A., Kane, O.J., Martinez, L.E., Nahmias, Y., Bourne, N. *et al.* (2010). Multiple effects of silymarin on the hepatitis C virus lifecycle. *Hepatology*, 51: 1912–1921.

Wang, H.K., Xia, Y., Yang, Z.Y., Natschke, S.L. and Lee, K.H. (1998). Recent advances in the discovery and development of flavonoids and their analogues as antitumor and anti-HIV agents. *Adv. Exp. Med. Biol.*, 439: 191–225.

Wang, J., Qiu, J., Dong, J., Li, H., Luo, M., Dai, X. *et al.* (2011). Chrysin protects mice from *Staphylococcus aureus* pneumonia. *J. Appl. Microbiol.*, 111: 1551–1558.

Wang, S., Zhang, J. and Ye, X. (2012). Protein kinase inhibitor flavopiridol inhibits the replication of influenza virus *in vitro*. *Wei Sheng Wu Xue Bao.*, 52(9): 1137–1142.

Wang, S.Y., Sun, Z.L., Liu, T., Gibbons, S., Zhang, W.J. and Qing, M. (2014). Flavonoids from *Sophora moorcroftiana* and their synergistic antibacterial effects on MRSA. *Phytother Res.*, 28(7): 1071–1076.

Wink, M. (2013). Evolution of secondary metabolites froman ecological and molecular phylogenetic perspective. *Phytochemistry*, 64: 3–19.

Wleklik, M., Luczak, M., Panasiak, W., Kobus, M. and Lammer-Zarawska, E. (1988). Structural basis for antiviral activity of flavonoids-naturally occurring compounds. *Acta Virol.*, 32(6): 522–525.

Woz nicka, E., Kuz niar, A., Nowak, D., Nykiel, E., Kopacz, M., Gruszecka, J. *et al.* (2013). Comparative study on the antibacterial activity of some flavonoids and their sulfonic derivatives. *Acta Pol. Pharm.*, 70(3): 567–571.

Wu, D., Kong, Y., Han, C., Chen, J., Hu, L., Jiang, H. and Shen, X. (2008). D-Alanine: D-alanine ligase as a new target for the flavonoids quercetin and apigenin. *Int. J. Antimicrob. Agents*, 32: 421–426.

Wu, Q., Yu, C., Yan, Y., Chen, J., Zhang, C. and Wen, X. (2010). Antiviral flavonoids from *Mosla scabra*. *Fitoterapia*, 81(5): 429–433.

Wu, T., He, M., Zang, X., Zhou, Y., Qiu, T., Pan, S. and Xu, X. (2013). A structure–activity relationship study of flavonoids as inhibitors of *E. coli* by membrane interaction effect. *Biochimica et Biophysica Acta (BBA) - Biomembranes*, 1828(11): 2751–2756.

Wu, T., Zang, X., He, M., Pan, S. and Xu, X. (2013). Structure–activity relationship of flavonoids on their anti *Escherichia coli* activity and inhibition of DNA gyrase. *J. Agric. Food Chem.,* 61(34): 8185–8190.

Xu, H. and Lee, S.F. (2001). Activity of plant flavonoids against antibiotic resistant bacteria. *Phytother Res.*, 15: 39–43.

Xu, J.J., Wu, X., Li, M.M., Li, G.Q., Yang, Y.T., Luo, H.J. *et al.* (2014). Antiviral activity of polymethoxylated flavones from Guangchenpi, the edible and medicinal pericarps of *Citrus reticulata* 'Chachi'. *J. Agric. Food Chem.*, 62(10): 2182–2189.

Yahiro, K., Shirasaka, D., Tagashira, M., Wada, A., Morinaga, N. and Kuroda, F. (2005). Inhibitory effects of polyphenols on gastric injury by *Helicobacter pylori* VacA toxin. *Helicobacter,* 10(3): 231–239.

Yarmolinsky, L., Huleihel, M., Zaccai, M. and Ben-Shabat, S. (2012). Potent antiviral flavone glycosides from *Ficus benjamina* leaves. *Fitoterapia*, 83(2): 362–367.

Yenjai, C., Prasanphen, K., Daodee, S., Wongpanich, V. and Kittakoop, P. (2004). Bioactive flavonoids from *Kaempferia parviflora*. *Fitoterapia*, 75(1): 89–92.

Yun, J.E., Lee, H., Ko, H.J., Woo, E.R. and Lee, D.G. (2015). Fungicidal effect of isoquercitrin *via* inducing membrane disturbance. *Biochimica et Biophysica Acta*, 1848: 695–701.

Zandi, K., Teoh, B.T., Sam, S.S., Wong, P.F., Mustafa, M.R. and AbuBakar, S. (2011). Antiviral activity of four types of bioflavonoid against dengue virus type-2. *Virology Journal*, 8: 560.

Zeyu, C., Yue, D., Zhipeng, K., Liang, C., Na, L., Gang, D., Zhenzhong, W. and Wei, X. (2016). Luteoloside acts as 3C protease inhibitor of enterovirus 71 *in vitro*. *PLOS ONE*, 11(2): e0148693. doi: 10.1371/journal.pone.0148693

Zhang, Q.G., Wei, F., Liu, Q., Chen, L.J., Liu, Y.Y., Luo, F. *et al.* (2014). The flavonoid from *Polygonum perfoliatum* L. inhibits herpes simplex virus 1 infection. *Acta Virol.*, 58(4): 368–373.

Zhang, W., Qiao, H., Lv, Y., Wang, J., Chen, X., Hou, Y. *et al.* (2014). Apigenin inhibits enterovirus-71 infection by disrupting viral RNA association with trans-acting factors. *PLoS ONE*, 9(10): e110429. doi: 10.1371/journal.pone.0110429.

Zhang, Y., Wang, J.F., Dong, J., Wei, J.Y., Wang, Y.N., Dai, X.H. *et al.* (2013). Inhibition of alpha-toxin production by subinhibitory concentrations of naringenin controls *Staphylococcus aureus* pneumonia. *Fitoterapia*, 86: 92–99.

Zhang, Y.M. and Rock, C.O. (2004). Evaluation of epigallocatechin gallate and related plant polyphenols as inhibitors of the FabG and FabI reductases of bacterial type II fatty-acid synthase. *J. Biol. Chem.*, 279(30): 30994–31001.

Zheng, W.F., Tan, R.X., Yang, L. and Liu, Z.L. (1996). Two flavones from *Artemisia giraldii* and their antimicrobial activity. *Planta Med.*, 62: 160–162.

Zhou, Z.L., Yin, W.Q., Zou, X.P., Huang, D.Y., Zhou, C.L., LI, L.M. *et al.* (2014). Flavonoid glycosides and potential antivirus activity of isolated compounds from the leaves of *Eucalyptus citriodora. Journal of the Korean Society for Applied Biological Chemistry*, 57(6): 813–817.

Zhu, Q.C., Wang, Y., Liu, Y.P., Zhang, R.Q., Li, X., Su, W.H. *et al.* (2011). Inhibition of enterovirus 71 replication by chrysosplenetin and penduletin. *Eur. J. Pharm. Sci.*, 44: 392–398.

3

Beneficial Effects and Molecular Mechanisms of Flavonoids Against Gastrointestinal Diseases and Disorders

Periyanaina Kesika[1] and Bhagavathi Sundaram Sivamaruthi[1*]

ABSTRACT

Flavonoids are one of the major ubiquitous groups of secondary metabolites of dietary phytochemicals. Flavonoids are sub-grouped as anthocyanidins, flavan-3-ols, flavanones, flavones, flavonols, and isoflavonoid. These low molecular weight polyphenolic compounds contribute the nutrition, taste, and color of the fruits, flowers, legumes and vegetables. Oxidative stress is one of the primary factors that is associated with many intestinal diseases mainly inflammatory bowel disease, intestinal neoplasia, etc., Consumption of natural source of flavonoids as a food supplement provides several beneficial effects that promote the human health. Flavonoids exhibit numerous pharmacological activities like anti-inflammatory, antioxidant, anti-cancer (cytotoxicity and antiproliferative activity), and anti-mutagenic ability against the gastrointestinal diseases. This chapter focuses on the beneficial effects and mechanism of flavonoids against the gastrointestinal (GI) diseases mainly inflammatory bowel diseases (Crohn's disease and ulcerative colitis), intestinal neoplasia (colorectal cancer), and GI disorders especially irritable bowel syndrome and functional dyspepsia.

Key words: Colorectal cancer, Flavonoids, Inflammatory bowel diseases, Oxidative stress.

1. INTRODUCTION

Gastrointestinal (GI) diseases impose a major burden on human health and the patients with GI disease exhibit symptoms with structural

[1] Department of Pharmaceutical Sciences, Faculty of Pharmacy, Chiang Mai University, Chiang Mai-50200, Thailand.

**Corresponding author*: E-mail: sivasgene@gmail.com

changes. The most commonly occurring and most studied GI diseases include inflammatory bowel disease (IBD) and intestinal neoplasia (IN) (Knutsson and Bøggild, 2010). The most common IBD are ulcerative colitis (UC) and Crohn's disease (CD), which is characterized by chronic or acute inflammation that requires a prolonged treatment to overcome the clinical relapse and remission that occurs alternatively (Baumgart and Carding, 2007; Calder *et al.,* 2009; Ordás *et al.,* 2012; Vezza *et al.,* 2016). Prevalence of UC is higher than that of Crohn's disease, and the incidence of UC is higher in developed countries than that of the developing countries. Both prevalence and incidence rates of UC and CD are higher in UK, Northern Europe and North America (Loftus, 2004; Baumgart and Carding, 2007; Ordás *et al.,* 2012). IN is the most common leading cause of death in many countries than that of the other cancers. Colorectal cancer (CRC) is the third most common cause of morbidity and fourth most common cause of mortality, thereby causing worldwide health burden (World Cancer Research Fund and American Institute for Cancer Research, 2007; Haggar and Boushey, 2009; Siegel *et al.,* 2014; Torre *et al.,* 2015).

GI disorders (GID) are functional disorders of the GI tract which impacts the public health that leads to a significant social and economic burden (Talley, 2008). The patients with GID exhibit chronic symptoms without any evidence of structural or metabolic abnormalities (Talley, 2008; Knutsson and Bøggild, 2010). GID includes irritable bowel syndrome (IBS), functional dyspepsia (FD), functional constipation, functional diarrhea, and functional bloating, among which, IBS and FD are the most common FGIDs (Drossman, 2006; Tack *et al.,* 2006; Suzuki *et al.,* 2009). The Rome IV diagnostic criteria provide a symptom-based classification of functional gastrointestinal disorders (FGIDs), which is termed as disorders of gut-brain interaction (Aziz *et al.,* 2016; Benninga *et al.,* 2016; Cotton *et al.,* 2016; Drossman, 2016; Hyams *et al.,* 2016; Keefer *et al.,* 2016; Lacy *et al.,* 2016; Rao *et al.,* 2016; Sood and Ford, 2016; Stanghellini *et al.,* 2016; Schmulson and Drossman, 2017; Zeevenhooven *et al.,* 2017) (Table 1). The prevalence of IBS is approximately 9-23% of the world population (Grundmann and Yoon, 2010; Canavan *et al.,* 2014; Oswiecimska *et al.,* 2017) and FD is prevalent throughout the world (Mahadeva and Goh 2006; Kumar *et al.,* 2012).

Consumption of foods and beverages that are rich in naturally occurring antioxidants like flavonoids and other phytochemicals are believed to maintain the health and to reduce the risk of developing disorders and diseases in human. Scientifically, flavonoids are considered to be the most active nutraceutical compound that exhibits much health promoting beneficial properties (Tapas *et al.,* 2008; Devi *et al.,* 2015), and consumption of foods that are rich in flavonoids are considered to be safe for humans (Kozłowska and Szostak-Wegierek, 2014).

Table 1: Classification of FGID according to the Rome IV diagnostic criteria

Reference	*Functional Disorders*	*Gastrointestinal Disorders (FGID)* *Catagories*	*Subcatagories*
Aziz *et al.*, 2016	Functional esophageal disorders	Functional heartburn Functional chest pain Functional dysphagia Globus Reflux hypersensitivity	
Stanghellini *et al.*, 2016	Functional gastroduodenal disorders	Functional dyspepsia	Postprandial distress syndrome Epigastric pain syndrome
		Belching disorders	Gastric belching Supragastric belching
		Nausea and vomiting disorders	Chronic nausea and vomiting syndrome Cannabinoid hyperemesis syndrome Cyclic vomiting syndrome
		Rumination syndrome	
Lacy *et al.*, 2016	Functional bowel disorders	Irritable bowel syndrome (IBS)	IBS-C (IBS with predominant constipation) IBS-D (IBS with predominant diarrhea) IBS-M (IBS with diarrhea and constipation) IBS-U (Unclassified IBS)
		Functional constipation Functional diarrhea Functional abdominal bloating Unspecified functional bowel disorder Opioid-induced constipation	
Keefer *et al.*, 2016	Centrally mediated disorders of GI pain	Narcotic bowel syndrome/ opioid-induced gastrointestinal hyperalgesia Centrally mediated abdominal pain syndrome	
Cotton *et al.*, 2016	Functional gallbladder and sphincter of Oddi disorders	Biliary pain	Functional gallbladder disorder Functional biliary sphincter of Oddi disorder
		Functional pancreatic sphincter of Oddi disorder	
Rao *et al.*, 2016	Functional anorectal	Functional fecal incontinence	

Table 1: *(Contd...)*

Table 1: *(Contd...)*

Reference	*Functional Disorders*	*Gastrointestinal Disorders (FGID) Catagories*	*Subcatagories*
	disorders	Functional anorectal pain	Proctalgia fugax Levator ani syndrome Unspecified functional anorectal pain
		Functional defecation disorders	Dyssynergic defecation Inadequate defecatory propulsion
Benninga *et al.*, 2016; Zeevenhooven *et al.*, 2017	Childhood functional GI disorders in infant/toddler	Infant regurgitation Infant rumination syndrome Cyclic vomiting syndrome Infant colic Functional diarrhea Infant dyschezia Functional constipation	
Hyams *et al.*, 2016	Childhood functional GI disorders in child/adolescent	Functional nausea and vomiting disorders	Functional nausea and functional vomiting Rumination syndrome Cyclic vomiting syndrome Aerophagia
		Functional abdominal pain disorders	Functional dyspepsia Irritable bowel syndrome Abdominal migraine Functional abdominal pain-not otherwise specified
		Functional defecation disorders	Functional constipation Nonretentive fecal incontinence

Since natural products have a great demand among most of the people for the prevention and treatment of diseases such as GI disease and disorders, many researchers have focused on studying the biological activities of natural phenolic products to consider and justify as an effective and potential therapeutic products. This chapter describes the therapeutic effects and molecular mechanism of flavonoids against the GI diseases (IBD and IN) and disorders (IBS and FD).

2. MOLECULAR MECHANISMS INVOLVED IN THE THERAPEUTIC EFFECT OF FLAVONOIDS AGAINST GASTROINTESTINAL DISEASES AND DISORDERS

2.1. Gastrointestinal Diseases

Inflammation is either an acute or chronic biological response caused by infection or injuries in tissue (Medzhitov, 2008). Inflammation and imbalance in immune homeostasis lead to the gastrointestinal diseases that include inflammatory bowel disease (IBD), and intestinal neoplasia (IN).

2.1.1. *Inflammatory bowel disease*

Even though multiple factors including environmental factors, genetic factors, and immune factors are involved in the cause of IBD including UC and CD, the specific etiology of the disease is unknown (Baumgart and Carding, 2007; Calder *et al.,* 2009; Ordás *et al.,* 2012; Vezza *et al.,* 2016). UC affects the large intestine of the GI tract. UC is characterized by mucosal and non-transmural inflammation, crypt abscess, edema, ulcers, and fibrosis. The symptoms of UC includes bloody diarrhea, abdominal cramping, and passage of mucous or pus or both during the bowel movements (Baumgart and Sandborn, 2007; Xavier and Podolsky, 2007; Ordás *et al.,* 2012). CD causes chronic inflammation at any part or the entire part of the GI tract. CD is characterized by segmental, patchy, transmural inflammation, edema, granuloma, and fitulas. The symptoms mostly depend on the location of the disease and also includes fever, abdominal pain, and passage of mucous or blood or both during the bowel obstruction or diarrhea (Baumgart and Sandborn, 2007; Xavier and Podolsky, 2007; Baumgart and Sandborn, 2012).

Numerous experimental models of intestinal inflammation were used to study the pathogenesis of IBD, and to test new approaches for therapy (Elson *et al.,* 1995; Mizoguchi 2012; Neurath, 2012; Kolios, 2016). Due to the altered function and microbiota of the GI tract, an abnormal interaction between the host and commensal microbes, and enhanced intestinal permeability occur in the host with IBD. Chronic intestinal injuries are caused due to the activation of host immune response to the continuous stimulation of microbes including pathogenic bacteria and commensal enteric bacteria mainly *Escherichia coli* that become pathogenic to host. Therefore, it is considered to identify natural products that protect the intestinal epithelial barrier, ameliorate the intestinal inflammation and modulate the mucosal immune response for the therapy of IBD (Sartor, 2008).

2.1.1.1. *Therapeutic effect and molecular mechanism of flavonoids targeting the intestinal inflammation*

The subgroups of flavonoids include flavanones, isoflavones, flavones, flavonols, flavan-3-ols, and anthocyanidins. Several reports revealed that flavonoids possesses many pharmacological properties such as antioxidant, antibacterial, anti-diabetic, anti-inflammatory, anti-ulcer, anti-cancer, anti-depressant, antiviral, antihypertensive, anti-allergic, anti-parasitic, immunomodulatory, cardioprotective, and neuroprotective properties (Mota *et al.,* 2009; Jan *et al.,* 2010; Calderon-Montano *et al.,* 2011; Nishitani *et al.,* 2013; Romano *et al.,* 2013; Somani *et al.,* 2015). Flavonoids are considered as anti-inflammatory compound due to its ability to exhibit free radical scavenging property, inhibition of the enzymatic activities induced during the inflammation process, and inhibition or immunomodulation of signaling pathway (Comalada *et al.,* 2005; Tuñón *et al.,* 2009).

Oxidative stress plays a significant role in the pathophysiology of many intestinal diseases mainly IBD, intestinal neoplasia, etc., Imbalance between the production of free radicals such as reactive oxygen species (ROS) and reactive nitrogen species (RNS), and insufficient amount of antioxidants to scavenge the increased amount of oxidants and nitrosants results in oxidative stress and nitrosative stress, which are associated with the chronic intestinal inflammation (Rezaie *et al.,* 2007; Zhu and Li, 2012; Piechota-Polanczyk and Fichna, 2014; Balmus *et al.,* 2016). Free radicals are scavenged by the antioxidant enzymes including catalase (CAT), superoxide dismutase (SOD), and glutathione peroxidase (GPX), and non-enzymatic antioxidant including reduced glutathione (GSH) to prevent the free radical induced damages like DNA damage, lipid peroxidation, apoptosis, and protein damage (Krinsky, 1992; Lü *et al.,* 2010; Nimse and Pal, 2015).

In normal physiological condition, Nitric oxide (NO) is produced in low levels by the consecutive nitric oxide synthase (NOS) enzymes (endothelial NOS and neuronal NOS) and exhibits a protective effect. Whereas, in the abnormal conditions, NO is produced in large amounts by inducible isoform of nitric oxide synthase (iNOS) and induce inflammation (Bogdan, 2001; Korhonen *et al.,* 2005; Sharma *et al.,* 2007). Pathogen-associated molecular patterns (PAMPs) such as bacterial lipopolysaccharides (LPS), and the pro-inflammatory cytokines namely, interleukin-1 beta (IL-1β), interleukin-6 (IL-6), interferon gamma (IFN-γ), and tumor necrosis factor-alpha (TNF-α) stimulates the overexpression of iNOS in macrophages. The inflammatory transcription factors namely, signal transducer and activator of transcription 1 (STAT-1), and nuclear factor-κB (NF-κB) plays an important role in the induction of NOS (Xie *et al.,* 1994; Gao *et al.,* 1997).

Recruitment of blood polymorphonuclear leukocytes and macrophages at the affected site are regulated by the activation of NF-κB signaling pathway through the enhanced expression of pro-inflammatory cytokines (IL-1β, IL-6, IFN-γ, and TNF-α), and pro-inflammatory chemokines namely, macrophage inflammatory proteins (MIP), monocyte chemoattractant protein (MCP)-1, MCP-3, and IL-8. During the recruitment of immune cells, the adhesion molecules namely, E-selectins, P-selectins, macrophage 1 antigen (Mac-1), the lymphocyte function-associated antigen 1 (LFA-1), intercellular adhesion molecule 1 (ICAM-1) are released in enormous amount (Fournier and Parkos, 2012; Leick *et al.,* 2014). Infiltration of leukocytes on the mucosal tissues is a significant pathological characteristic in IBD. During inflammation, neutrophils generate an enormous amount of ROS, myeloperoxidase (MPO), through nicotinamide adenine dinucleotide phosphate (NADPH) oxidase system causing cytotoxicity by means of oxidative burst that leads to induction of enhanced expression of pro-inflammatory mediators (Fournier and Parkos, 2012).

Increased expressions of eicosanoids are found to be associated with the pathogenesis of IBD. Eicosanoids namely, prostaglandins, and leukotrienes are synthesized by the metabolism of arachidonic acid through cyclooxygenase (COX including COX-1, and COX-2), and lipoxygenase (LOX), respectively. COX-1 is responsible for the synthesis of thromboxanes and anti-inflammatory prostaglandins. COX-2 is responsible for the synthesis of inflammatory prostaglandins, which is involved in the intestinal inflammation (Willoughby *et al.,* 2000).

PAMPs are recognized by host pattern recognition receptors (PRRs). Toll-like receptors (TLRs) are the PRRs of the host innate immune system and TLRs also associated with the pathogenesis of inflammatory diseases. LPS is recognized by the TLR-4, which induces the activation of NF-κB *via* Toll/interleukin 1 receptor domain-containing adaptor protein inducing IFN-β (TRIF) and myeloid differentiation primary response gene 88 (MyD88) signaling pathway, and interferon-regulatory factor 3 *via* TRIF signaling pathway, thereby NF-κB activation results in the expression of pro-inflammatory cytokines and mediators (Kawai and Akira, 2010; Kawai and Akira, 2011; Płóciennikowska *et al.,* 2015). Flavonoids targeting the cellular and molecular mechanism involved in the inflammatory intestinal disease were illustrated in Fig. 1.

2.1.1.1.1. *Chalcones*

Lee group investigated the anti-inflammatory property of flavonoid phloretin (dihydrochalcone) using an *in vitro* and *in vivo* models of intestinal inflammation. Pretreatment of phloretin inhibited the inflammatory response in the HT-29 cells by suppressing the expression of inflammatory cytokine TNF-α. Oral administration of phloretin (20 mg/kg per day for 5 days) was more effective in the reduction of myeloperoxidase (MPO) activity, which is an inflammatory marker (leukocyte infiltration marker) in the trinitrobenzene sulfonic acid (TNBS) induced experimental colitis in rat model when compared to that of the conventionally used drug 5-ASA (100 mg/kg per day for 5 days) for IBD treatment. Phloretin also inhibited the formation of *E. coli* O157:H7 biofilm and suppressed the expression of its virulence genes (Lee *et al.,* 2011).

2.1.1.1.2. *Flavanones*

Naringenin exhibits anti-inflammatory property (Fig. 1) by inhibiting the expression (mRNA and protein) of iNOS and suppressing the activation of

NF-κB in the *in vitro* model, LPS induced inflammation in macrophage cells (Hämäläinen *et al.,* 2007). Wang group revealed the protective role of naringenin that inhibits the TLR-4 mediated NF-κB signaling in the experimental colitis in a mouse model. Pre-treatment of naringenin (oral dose: 50 mg/kg of body weight) was effective in the suppression of mRNA levels of pro-inflammatory mediators (monocyte chemoattractant protein-1 (MCP-1), intercellular adhesion molecule-1 (ICAM-1), cyclooxygenase (COX-2), and iNOS), pro-inflammatory cytokines (IL-6, and TNF-α), expression (mRNA and protein) of TLR4 in the dextran sulfate sodium (DSS) induced experimental colitis model. Naringenin reduced the activation of NF-κB by the inhibition of phosphorylation of IκBα, and NF-κB (p56), and suppression of the nuclear translocation of NF-κB (p56) in the colonic mucosa and activated macrophages (RAW264.7) (Dou *et al.,* 2013). Al-Rejaie group investigated the protective effect of naringenin against the acetic acid induced experimental UC in a rat model and evidenced the antioxidant and anti-inflammatory property effect of naringenin (Al-Rejaie *et al.,* 2013).

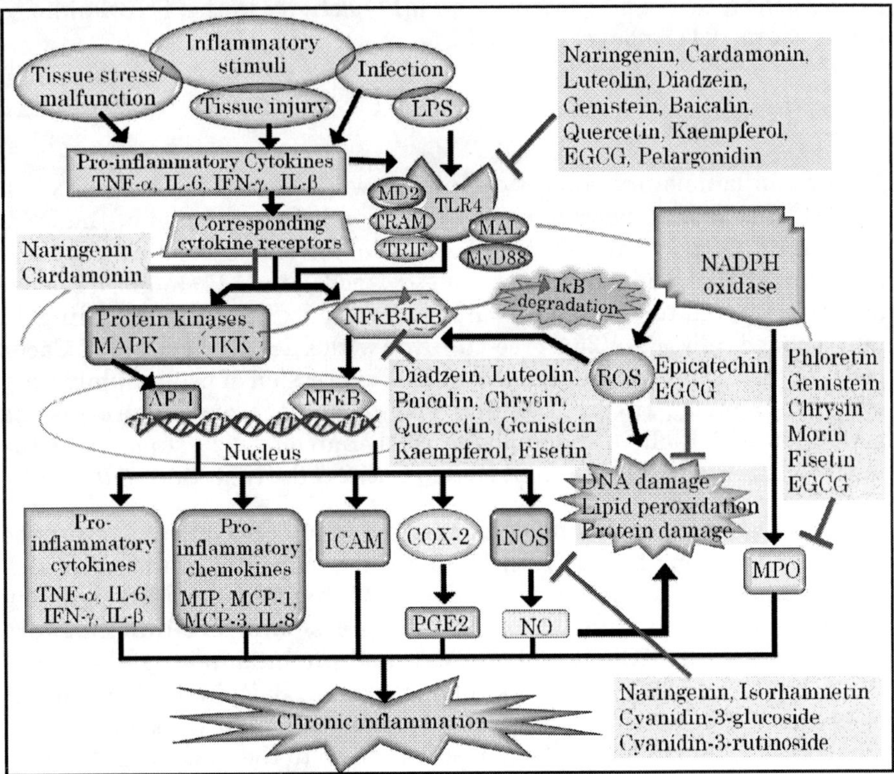

Fig. 1: Flavonoids targeting the cellular and molecular mechanism involved in the inflammatory intestinal disease.

Cardamonin effectively improved the physiological conditions in the DSS-induced experimental colitis in a mouse model. Cardomonin was found to suppress the MPO activity, NO, IL-6, and TNF-α in the colon, blocked the activation of NF-κB and MAPK pathway by inhibiting the phosphorylation of IκBα, NF-κB p65, nuclear translocation of NF-κB p65 in the colon tissues and RAW264.7 cells, reduction of inflammatory mediators, and suppression of TLR4, MyD88, mitogen-activated protein kinase (MAPK) of extracellular signal-regulated kinase (ERK1/2) and c-Jun NH -terminal kinase (JNK) in *in vitro* and *in vivo* models of inflammatory response (Ren *et al.,* 2015).

2.1.1.1.3. *Isoflavones*

Daidzein and genistein inhibited the mRNA and protein expression of iNOS and suppressed the activation of inflammatory transcription factors (STAT-1 and NF-κB) in the LPS induced inflammation in macrophage cells, which evidenced the anti-inflammatory property of these isoflavones (Hämäläinen *et al.,* 2007). Another study by Seibel *et al.* revealed the effective role of genistein against the inflammatory response *via* suppression of COX-2 expression (mRNA and protein), and MPO activity in the TNBS induced colitis rat model (Seibel *et al.,* 2009).

2.1.1.1.4. *Flavones*

The anti-inflammatory property of luteolin was evidenced by the reduction of $CD4^+$ T cells and macrophages infiltration in colon region of the DSS-induced colitis mouse model, and the effect of flavonoid luteolin on the NF-κB pathway was studied using the *in vitro* model, the LPS induced release of pro-inflammatory cytokine and activation of NF-κB signaling in macrophage cells (RAW264.7) co-cultured with intestinal epithelial Caco2 cells. Luteolin down-regulated the mRNA expression of pro-inflammatory cytokines namely, IL-1β, IL-6, and TNF-α, and thereby suppresses the activation of NF-κB in macrophage cells. Luteolin also suppressed the mRNA expression of TNF-α and IL-8 in Caco2 cells (Nishitani *et al.,* 2013).

Cui *et al.* showed that baicalin exerts its protective effect against the intestinal inflammation in TNBS induced experimental colitis rat model. Administration of baicalin exhibited potent inhibition of NF-κB signaling pathway by suppressing the protein expression of pro-inflammatory mediators (Cox-2, MCP-1, and ICAM-1) and pro-inflammatory cytokines (IL-6, IL-1 β, and TNF- α) in the colonic mucosa. Baicalin is also found to block the TLR4 protein expression, phosphorylation of NF- κB p65, I κB, and translocation of NF-κB from the cytoplasm to the nucleus in the LPS stimulated RAW264.7 cells (Cui *et al.,* 2014).

The flavonoid chrysin has been shown to exhibit a protective effect in attenuating the murine IBD by restoration of physiological conditions. Reduction of MPO activity, inflammatory mediators (prostaglandin (PGE2), and NO), pro-inflammatory cytokines (IL-6, and IL-1 β) in colonic mucosa, and inhibition of NF-κB pathway in intestinal epithelial cells (IEC-6) by chrysin have been reported (Shin *et al.,* 2009). Chrysin was found to exhibit protective effects against the intestinal inflammation (Dou *et al.,* 2013) similar to that of the baicalin studied by Cui *et al.* The role of chrysin in preventing the chemically (DSS, TNBS) induced experimental colitis mice model by the activation of pregnane x receptor (PXR) mediated inhibition of NF- κB signaling pathway have been reported by Mani group (Dou *et al.,* 2013).

2.1.1.1.5. *Flavonols*

Zarzuelo group evidenced the anti-inflammatory property of morin (2',3,4',5,7-pentahydroxyflavone) using the TNBS induced colitis in a rat model. Morin reduced the mucosal damage and MPO activity in the colon of the experimental colitis model (Ocete *et al.,* 1998). A preliminary study revealed the anti-inflammatory capacity of quercitrin in an experimental enterocolitis in a rat model (Galsanov *et al.,* 1976). Isorhamnetin suppressed the mRNA and protein expression of iNOS. Quercetin and Kaempferol exhibited anti-inflammatory property, which was evidenced by the inhibition of the of iNOS expression and suppressed the activation of NF-κB, and STAT-1 in the activated macrophage cells (Hämäläinen *et al.,* 2007).

Anderson group revealed that quercetin (250 μM) reduced the hydrogen peroxide (H_2O_2) induced DNA damage in lymphocytes isolated from the healthy volunteers, CD, and UC patients. Quercetin was more efficient in reducing the oxidative stress in the lymphocytes from the UC patients than that of the CD patients (Najafzadeh *et al.,* 2009). Manconi group developed a chitosan/nutriose coated nanovesicles as a quercetin delivery tool for the treatment of GI inflammatory diseases. Chitosan is a polymer, and nutriose is a starch derivative that possesses prebiotic property, which in combination with quercetin provides a synergic effect. Oral administration of nanovesicles containing quercetin (9 mg/kg per day for 3 days (intense inflammation period)) restored the physiological conditions in TNBS induced colitis rat model (Castangia *et al.,* 2015).

A recent study reported the GI protective effect of quercetrin against oxidative stress induced by indomethacin in rat model. Indomethacin is a nonsteroidal anti-inflammatory drug (NSAID), which causes many adverse effects, that damages the GI mucosa. This drug increases the NADPH oxidase and xanthine oxidase (XOD) activity, superoxide ($O^{2\circ-}$) production, and suppresses the activity of SOD, GPX, and Nrf2 by inhibiting the nuclear translocation of Nrf2. Pretreatment with quercetrin (single oral dose of 50, and 100-mg/kg) prevented these adverse effects caused by indomethacin (Carrasco-Pozo *et al.,* 2016). Therefore, quercetrin might be used during the treatments with NSAID to prevent its adverse effects.

The activity of fisetin against the intestinal inflammation was investigated using the DSS-induced colitis mouse model and evidenced that fisetin (5, 10 mg/kg of body weight) was effective in the inhibition of lipid peroxidation, restoration of reduced glutathione (GSH), suppression of myeloperoxidase activity, nitrite levels, pro-inflammatory cytokines (IL-1β, IL-6, and TNF-α), and protein expression of iNOS and COX-2 in the colonic mucosa. Fisetin also attenuated the translocation of NF-κB (p56) from cytoplasm to nucleus, inhibited the phosphorylation of IκBα, Akt, p38 MAPK, and suppressed the NF-κB (p65)-DNA binding activity thereby inhibited the activation of NF-κB (p56), Akt, and p38 MAPK signaling in the experimental colitis (Sahu *et al.,* 2016).

2.1.1.1.6. *Flavan-3-ols*

An *in vitro* study revealed that epicatechin (100 μM) was effective in the reduction of DNA damage induced by 2-amino-3-methylimadazo[4,5-f]-quinoline (IQ), a food mutagen in lymphocytes isolated from IBD (CD and UC) patients and healthy volunteers. Epicatechin was more effective in the lymphocytes isolated from the UC patients compared to that of the CD patients (Najafzadeh *et al.,* 2009).

Epigallocatechin-3-gallate (EGCG) is a well-known flavonoid for its protective effect against inflammation. EGCG showed inhibition of NO production, iNOS activity, iNOS protein expression and suppressed the activation of NF-kB in LPS induced murine peritoneal macrophages (Lin and Lin, 1997). Lügering group reported the antioxidant property and anti-inflammatory property of EGCG in combination with piperine and revealed that it reduced the lipid peroxidation and myeloperoxidase (MPO) activity, increased the SOD and GPX activity in the colonic mucosa of the DSS-induced experimental colitis murine model. EGCG in combination with piperine down-regulated the expression of inflammatory cytokine, IL-8 in the *in vitro* model LPS induced HT29 cells (Brückner *et al.,* 2012).

2.1.1.1.7. *Anthocyanins*

The anthocyanin pelargonidin exhibited a protective effect against inflammatory response by the inhibition of mRNA and protein expression of iNOS in the LPS induced inflammation in macrophage cells (Hämäläinen *et al.,* 2007). Another study by Jung *et al.* reported the anti-inflammatory property of Rubus fruit (Korean raspberries, black raspberries, and blackberries) anthocyanin fractions, cyanidin-3-glucoside and cyanidin-3-rutinoside that showed inhibition of NO activity, iNOS, and suppressed the NF-κB activation in Caco-2 cell lines stimulated with the conditioned medium of LPS activated macrophage cells (Jung *et al.,* 2015).

Recently, Scharl group performed open-label clinical trial and evidenced the protective effect of anthocyanin-rich bilberry extract (ABE) in the intestine of the UC patients. The study revealed that ABE treatment exhibited inhibition of NF-κB (p65) phosphorylation, and pro-inflammatory cytokines (TNF-α, and IFN-γ) in colon tissues, and reduction of pro-inflammatory cytokine and mediator (TNF-α and MCP-1), elevation of Th17 cytokine (IL-22), and anti-inflammatory cytokine (IL-10 which is a key immune regulator) in the serum of UC patients. ARBE also blocked the IFN-γ receptor 2 expressions in human monocytic (THP-1) cells. Both *in vitro* and *in vivo* study revealed the therapeutic use of anthocyanin-rich bilberry extract in UC patients by modulating the expression of cytokines and inhibition of IFN-γ signaling (Roth *et al.,* 2016).

2.1.2. *Intestinal neoplasia*

2.1.2.1. *Colorectal cancer*

CRC is also a multifactorial disease, and the major risk factors include IBD, hereditary and procarcinogens (Balkwill and Mantovani, 2001; Benson, 2007; Pan *et al.,* 2011). The progression of colitis-associated CRC (CACRC) is the second most common cause of mortality in developed countries (Sobczak *et al.,* 2014).

2.1.2.2. *Therapeutic effect and molecular mechanism of flavonoids targeting CRC*

The tumor suppressor gene p53 is referred as "the guardian angels of the genome," and this efficient effector molecule regulates the cell cycle by inhibiting the progression of cell cycle in G1 phase or inducing apoptosis in the prevention of cancer (Lane, 1992; Ryan, 2011). The mutation in p53 leads to induction of increased proliferation of cells and progression of the tumor. p53 also plays a major role in the cause of colon cancer (Bedeir and Krasinskas, 2011). Cancer stem cells (CSCs) have been reported to be the core cells that are capable of initiating the tumor and progression of adenoma. The markers of colon CSCs include CD166, CD44, CD24, CD133, and ALDH1b1 (Todaro *et al.,* 2010).

Wnt, Shh, and BMP signaling pathways are involved in the pathogenesis of CRC, while constitutive stimulation of Wnt signaling pathway is associated with the primary cause of CRC (Todaro *et al.,* 2010). β-catenin mediated Wnt signaling pathway is found to be involved in the intestinal homeostasis. β-catenin is a signal transducer, which plays a significant role in Wnt signaling pathway in regulating the proliferation of intestinal stem cells (Fevr *et al.,* 2007). Cytoplasmic β-catenin is controlled by the multiprotein destruction complex comprised of adenomatous polyposis coli

(APC), axin, Glycogen synthase kinase 3β (GSK 3β), and casein kinase 1α/ε, which promotes the β-catenin phosphorylation for inducing the β-catenin ubiquitination followed by degradation of β-catenin in the absence of Wnt signaling. Stabilized cytoplasmic β-catenin is translocated from cytoplasm to nucleus, and it interacts with the T-cell factor (Tcf)/lymphoid enhancer factor 1 (LEF-1), which modulates the expression of specific developmental genes, cell cycle genes, and oncogenes. Mutations in CRC are largely activated in the axin, APC (tumor suppressor gene), and in the Tcf/LEF-1. Therefore, the mutation blocks the degradation of β-catenin and results in translocation of enormous amount of β-catenin from cytoplasm to nucleus, which leads to the constitutive stimulation of canonical (β-catenin mediated Wnt signaling) pathway (Behrens and Lustig, 2004; Clevers, 2006; Yang, 2012; Amado *et al.,* 2014).

Nuclear factor erythroid 2-related factor 2 (Nrf2) is a transcription factor that plays a significant role in regulating the expression of antioxidant response element (ARE) mediated genes that encode enzymatic antioxidants, detoxifying enzymes, and proteasomes. Nrf2 is highly sensitive to oxidative stress. Therefore it translocates into the nucleus and binds to ARE genes and promotes the elevated expression of phase II enzymes and antioxidants (Zhang, 2006; Li and Kong, 2009; Chen *et al.,* 2015). Nrf-2 is reported to be a significant factor that is associated with inflammation and cancer (Kou *et al.,* 2013; Niture *et al.,* 2014; Chen *et al.,* 2015).

NF-κB activation is found to play a key role in promoting inflammation-induced growth and progression of premalignant cells in the intestine (Karin and Greten, 2005; Mariani *et al.,* 2014). The NF-κB regulated pro-inflammatory cytokine IL-6 has been reported for its role in Stat-3 mediated enhancement of colitis-associated CRC cell proliferation (Becker *et al.,* 2005; Grivennikov *et al.,* 2009).

Flavonoids targeting the cellular and molecular mechanism involved in the intestinal neoplasia were illustrated in Fig. 2. A recent study by Huo *et al.* reported the protective effect of licorice flavonoids (LF) against colitis-associated carcinogenesis in AOM/DSS-induced intestinal inflammation in mouse model. LF extract contains echinatin, enoxolone, kanzonol E, licochalcone, licoflavone, pinocembrinchalcone, tetrahydroxychalcone and isoflavones namely, formononetin and glabrone. Administration of LFs (single daily dose for 10 weeks) suppressed the tumorigenesis in AOM/DSS-induced mouse model. LF showed the anti-inflammatory and immunomodulating property by inhibition of NFκ-B and p53 activation, Jak 2 and Stat 3 phosphorylation, and down-regulation of pro-inflammatory mediators (Cox-2, and iNOS) and pro-inflammatory cytokines (IL-6, IL-1β, and TNF-α) expression in the colon tissues of experimental CACRC mouse model (Huo *et al.,* 2016).

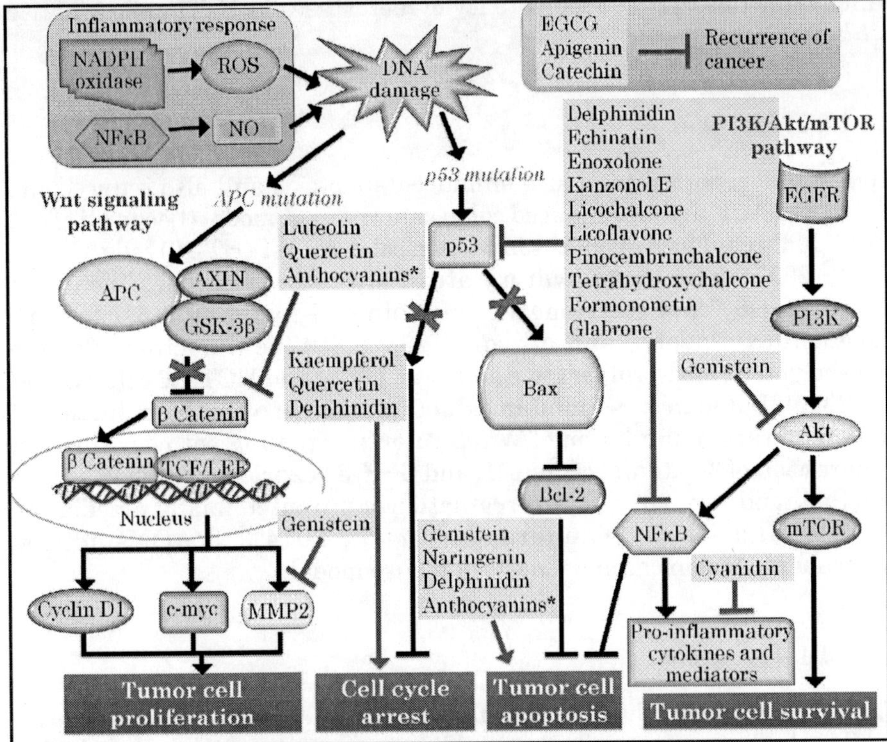

Fig. 2: Flavonoids targeting the cellular and molecular mechanism involved in the intestinal neoplasia. Anthocyanins* represents Pet-3-rut-5-glc, Mal-3-rut-5-glc, Cya-3-O(6-O-malonyl-β-D-glc), Peo-3-(p-coum)-isophoro-5-glc, Peo-3-rut-5-glc, Pet-3-(p-coum)-rut-5-glc, Peo-3-caffeyl-rut-5-glc, Pel-3-(p-coum)-rut-5-glc, Pel-3-(4-ferul-rut)-5-glc, Peo-3-(p-coum)-rut-5-glc, and Mal-3-(p-coum)-rut-5-glc.

2.1.2.2.1. *Flavanones*

Naringenin exhibited anti-proliferative property, reduced the number of aberrant crypt foci (ACF), and induced increased apoptosis in AOM induced colon cancer in a rat model (Leonardi *et al.*, 2010).

2.1.2.2.2. *Isoflavones*

Genistein was found to show anti-proliferative property, induction of apoptosis, suppression of Akt phosphorylation and the expression of miR-95, SGK1 and Akt mRNA in human colon cancer (HCT-116) cells (Qin *et al.*, 2015). Shafiee *et al.* reported the anti-proliferative activity of genistein through inhibition of p38 MAPK expression and its phosphorylation in human colon cancer (HT29) cells. It also induced increased apoptosis through activating the caspase-3 and suppressed the activity of MMP2, which indicates the reduced potency of metastases in HT29 cells (Shafiee *et al.,* 2016).

2.1.2.2.3. *Flavones*

Apigenin is reported to induce enhanced apoptosis and also reduced the number of ACF in AOM induced colon cancer in rat model (Leonardi *et al.,* 2010). It also induced apoptosis in human colon cancer (HT-29) cells (Chung *et al.,* 2007). The novel hydroxylated polymethoxyflavones including 5-hydroxy-6,7,8,4'-tetramethoxyflavone, 5-hydroxy-3,6,7,8,3',4'-hexamethoxyflavone, and 5-hydroxy-6,7,8,3',4'-pentamethoxyflavone showed potent anti-proliferative ability in HT29 and HCT116 cells (Qiu *et al.,* 2010). Luteolin was found to exhibit protective effect by reduction of cell proliferation, inhibition of Wnt/β-catenin signaling pathway through suppression of β-catenin, cyclin D1, and GSK-3β expression (Ashok kumar and Sudhandiran, 2011), down-regulation of pro-inflammatory mediators (COX-2, and iNOS) (Pandurangan *et al.,* 2014), in AOM-induced experimental colon carcinogenesis in mouse model.

2.1.2.2.4. *Flavonols*

The synergic protective effect of flavonoids (kaempferol and quercetin) exhibited strong cytotoxicity, anti-proliferative property through inducing cell cycle arrest in G2/M phase in human colon CRC (HT-116) cells (Jaramillo-Carmona *et al.,* 2014). Shan et al. reported the protective effect of quercetin in an *in vitro* model, human colon cancer (SW480) cell and revealed that quercetin exhibited dose-dependent (20, 40, 60, 80 µmol/L) by suppression of mRNA and protein expression of cyclin D1, and survivin, and stimulation of increased apoptosis in SW480 cells. Quercetin (160 µmol/L) was found to inhibit canonical (Wnt/β-catenin) signaling pathway by suppression of β-catenin/Tcf mRNA expression, in SW480 cells which were transiently transfected with TCF-4 reporter gene (Shan *et al.,* 2009). Quercetin has been found to show dose-dependent inhibition of cell proliferation, and induction of increased cell cycle arrest in G1 phase. It also exhibited apoptotic effect by inducing the elevated expression of p21, p53, and AMPK in colon cancer (HT-29) cells (Kim *et al.,* 2010).

2.1.2.2.5. *Flavan-3-ols*

Hoensch group investigated the preventive effect of flavonoids (EGCG and apigenin) against the risk of CRC recurrence in post-surgical patients who had resected CRC, and in patients who undergone adenoma polypectomy. Daily supplementation (2-5 years) of flavan-3-ol (EGCG 20 mg) and flavones (apigenin 20 mg) reduced the rate of cancer recurrence in patients with resected CRC (Hoensch *et al.,* 2008). Similarly, a randomized clinical trial was performed by Lee group, and they studied the preventive effect of green tea extract (GTE) in patients who underwent removal of CRC by endoscopy. Daily supplementation (1 year) of GTE (0.9 g of GTE containing 0.2 g of EGCG and 0.6 g of catechin) reduced the metachronous colorectal adenoma in Korean patients who had removed the CRC (Shin *et al.,* 2017). These studies evidenced that EGCG, catechin, and apigenin might be effective when used for preventive measure of recurrence risk and during the treatment of CRC.

2.1.2.2.6. *Anthocyanins*

The aglycone forms of anthocyanins are termed as anthocyanidin. The anthocyanidins namely, cyanidin, and delphinidin showed potent anti-proliferative property, and anti-inflammatory property by inhibiting the mRNA expression of pro-inflammatory mediators (iNOS and COX-2) in HT29 cells (Kim *et al.,* 2008). Delphinidin exhibited anti-proliferative property, inhibited NFκ-B signaling pathway, induced apoptosis and cell cycle arrest in HCT116 cells (Yun *et al.,* 2009).

A study by Vanamala group demonstrated the protective effect of anthocyanin-containing extract of baked purple potato (PP) in human colon cancer cell lines and revealed that the extract inhibited the proliferation of HCT-116 and HT-29, and induced apoptosis (Madiwale *et al.,* 2012). This research group further investigated the anti-cancer property of the PP anthocyanin extract (PPAE) using the *in vitro* model, colon CSCs that are positive for ALDH1b1, CD133, and CD44 markers with the presence and absence of p53 function, and *in vivo* model, azoxymethane (AOM) induced experimental colon cancer in the mouse. Anthocyanins present in PPAE includes Pet-3-rut-5-glc, Mal-3-rut-5-glc, Cya-3-O(6-O-malonyl-β-D-glc), Peo-3-(p-coum)-isophoro-5-glc, Peo-3-rut-5-glc, Pet-3-(p-coum)-rut-5-glc, Peo-3-caffeyl-rut-5-glc, Pel-3-(p-coum)-rut-5-glc, Pel-3-(4-ferul-rut)-5-glc, Peo-3-(p-coum)-rut-5-glc, and Mal-3-(p-coum)-rut-5-glc. The *in vitro* study revealed that PPAE exhibited p53 independent inhibition of Wnt pathway by reducing the β-catenin, cMyc, and cyclin D1 protein expression in terms of inhibiting proliferation, and induction of mitochondrial apoptosis by upregulating Bax and cytochrome c in colon CSCs. The *in vivo* study revealed that PPAE was found to induce apoptosis and reduced the tumor incidence rate in a colon cancer mouse model, which overall evidenced the anti-cancer property of PPAE (Charepalli *et al.,* 2015).

Another study reported the chemopreventive effect of anthocyanin-rich black soybean (ABS) extract in the intestinal polyposis mouse ($Apc^{\mathrm{Min/+}}$) model. Supplementation of ABS (0.5 %) extract showed a reduction in intestinal tumor development by inhibiting the expression of cytosolic β-catenin, COX-2, and cytosolic phospholipase A2 (PLA2) in the intestinal polyposis mouse model (Park *et al.,* 2015).

2.2. Functional Gastrointestinal Disorder

FGID are caused by many factors mainly improper dietary hygiene, also includes stress, environmental factors, infections, and side effects of some antibiotics, and nonsteroidal anti-inflammatory drugs (Drossman, 2006; Knutsson and Bøggild, 2010; Villarreal *et al.,* 2012; De Palma *et al.,* 2014). Both IBS and FD patients have been reported for their reduced quality of life.

2.2.1. *Irritable bowel syndrome*

IBS is also caused by multiple risk factors, and the most common factors include young age, infections in GI tract, and female sex, and the etiology is largely unknown. The symptoms of IBS include recurrent abdominal discomfort or pain, irregularities in defecation, change in appearance of stool, and also associated with some other conditions like visceral, somatic (migraine, and pain syndromes) and psychiatric (depression, and anxiety) conditions (Soares, 2014; Enck *et al.,* 2016; Oswiecimska *et al.,* 2017).

2.2.1.1. *Therapeutic effect and molecular mechanism of flavonoids targeting IBD*

A study reported that the flavanones namely, naringin, neohesperidin, and hesperidin present in Zhi-Shao-San (Chinese traditional medicine used for IBS treatment) are absorbed effectively in the acetic acid and restraint stress induced experimental IBS rat model (Chen, 2014). Hekmatdoost group investigated the protective effect of soy isoflavones namely, glycetin, genistein, and diadzein in IBS patients in randomized, double-blind, placebo-controlled study. Daily supplementation (6 weeks) of soy isoflavones (glycetin (3 mg), genistein (17 mg), and diadzein (20 mg)) improved the quality of the IBS patients' life (Jalili *et al.,* 2015).

2.2.2. *Functional dyspepsia*

Dyspepsia that lacks structural symptoms and metabolic evidence are referred as FD or non-ulcer dyspepsia (Adam *et al.,* 2005; Holtmann *et al.,* 2006; Knutsson and Bøggild, 2010). The symptoms of FD include epigastric pain, nausea, bloating, epigastric burning, belching, discomfort postprandial fullness, and early satiation (Adam *et al.,* 2005; Mahadeva and Goh, 2006; Knutsson and Bøggild, 2010; Kumar *et al.,* 2012; Jalili *et al.,* 2015).

2.2.2.1. *Therapeutic effect and molecular mechanism of flavonoids targeting FD*

Allan group reported the health-protective effect of *Glycyrrhiza glabra* root extract (GutGard), which is rich in flavonoids (13.2%) including glabridin (3.6%) in FD patients in randomized, double-blind, placebo-controlled study. Supplementation of flavonoid-rich *G. glabra* root extract capsule was effective in exhibiting a significant reduction in FD symptoms (Raveendra *et al.,* 2012). A recent study reported that flavonoid-rich *G. glabra* root extract was compatible with few commercial probiotic drinks, probiotic strains (*Streptococcus thermophilus, Lactobacillus casei, L. plantarum*, and *L. fermentum*), and digestive enzymes (pancreatic α-amylase, pancreatic lipase, phytase, xylanase, and α-glucosidase) indicating the use of this extract in combination with probiotic supplementation (Asha *et al.,* 2017).

3. FUTURE PERSPECTIVES

Further, few or several clinical studies should be performed to evidence the preventive or protective effect, and safety of active flavonoids to consider and justify as an effective and potential therapeutic products for the treatment intestinal inflammatory disease including IBD, and CRC. There are only a few reports evidencing the health promoting effect of flavonoids against IBS and FD. So, further clinical studies should be conducted to investigate the health promoting role of flavonoids against the IBS and FD.

4. CONCLUSIONS

Many flavonoids have been reported for its efficiency and safety in preventing or health-promoting property against intestinal diseases including inflammatory bowel disease including ulcerative colitis and Crohn's disease, and colorectal cancer *in vitro*, *in vivo* and few clinical studies. Further clinical studies with molecular evidence are required to consider flavonoids as a safe therapeutic agent for intestinal diseases.

5. ACKNOWLEDGEMENT

All authors acknowledge the Faculty of Pharmacy and Chiang Mai University, Chiang Mai, Thailand.

REFERENCES

Adam, B., Liebregts, T., Saadat-Gilani, K., Vinson, B. and Holtmann, G. (2005). Validation of the gastrointestinal symptom score for the assessment of symptoms in patients with functional dyspepsia. *Aliment. Pharmacol. Ther.*, 22(4): 357–363.

Al-Rejaie, S.S., Abuohashish, H.M., Al-Enazi, M.M., Al-Assaf, A.H., Parmar, M.Y., Ahmed, M.M. (2013). Protective effect of naringenin on acetic acid-induced ulcerative colitis in rats. *World J. Gastroenterol.*, 19(34): 5633–5644. doi: 10.3748/wjg.v19.i34.5633.

Amado, N.G., Predes, D., Moreno, M.M., Carvalho, I.O., Mendes, F.A. and Abreu, J.G. (2014). Flavonoids and Wnt/β-catenin signaling: Potential role in colorectal cancer therapies. *Int. J. Mol. Sci.*, 15(7): 12094–12106. doi: 10.3390/ijms150712094.

Asha, M.K., Debraj, D., Dethe, S., Bhaskar, A., Muruganantham, N. and Deepak, M. (2017). Effect of flavonoid-rich extract of *Glycyrrhiza glabra* on gut-friendly microorganisms, commercial probiotic preparations, and digestive enzymes. *J. Diet. Suppl.*, 14(3): 323–333.

Ashokkumar, P. and Sudhandiran, G. (2011). Luteolin inhibits cell proliferation during azoxymethane-induced experimental colon carcinogenesis *via* Wnt/β-catenin pathway. *Invest New Drugs*, 29(2): 273–284. doi: 10.1007/s10637-009-9359-9.

Aziz, Q., Fass, R., Gyawali, C.P., Miwa, H., Pandolfino, J.E. and Zerbib, F. (2016). Esophageal disorders. *Gastroenterology*, 150(6): 1368–1379.

Balkwill, F. and Mantovani, A. (2001). Inflammation and cancer: Back to Virchow? *Lancet*, 357(9255): 539–545.

Balmus, I.M., Ciobica, A., Trifan, A. and Stanciu, C. (2016). The implications of oxidative stress and antioxidant therapies in Inflammatory Bowel Disease: Clinical aspects and animal models. *Saudi J Gastroenterol.*, 22(1): 3–17. doi: 10.4103/1319-3767.173753.

Baumgart, D.C. and Carding, S.R. (2007). Inflammatory bowel disease: Cause and immunobiology. *Lancet.*, 369(9573): 1627–1640.

Baumgart, D.C. and Sandborn, W.J. (2007). Inflammatory bowel disease: Clinical aspects and established and evolving therapies. *Lancet*, 369: 1641–1657.

Baumgart, D.C. and Sandborn, W.J. (2012). Crohn's disease. *Lancet*, 380: 1590–1605.

Becker, C., Fantini, M.C., Wirtz, S., Nikolaev, A., Lehr, H.A., Galle, P.R., Rose-John, S. and Neurath, M.F. (2005). IL-6 signaling promotes tumor growth in colorectal cancer. *Cell Cycle*, 4(2): 217–220.

Bedeir, A. and Krasinskas, A.M. (2011). Molecular diagnostics of colorectal cancer. *Arch. Pathol. Lab. Med.*, 135(5): 578–587. doi: 10.1043/2010-0613-RAIR.1.

Behrens, J. and Lustig, B. (2004). The Wnt connection to tumorigenesis. *Int. J. Dev. Biol.*, 48(5–6): 477–487.

Benninga, M.A., Nurko, S., Faure, C., Hyman, P.E., Roberts, lan St. J. and Schechter, N.L. (2016). Childhood functional gastrointestinal disorders: Neonate/Toddler. *Gastroenterology*, 150(6): 1443–1455.e2.

Benson, A.B. 3rd (2007). Epidemiology, disease progression, and economic burden of colorectal cancer. *J. Manag. Care Pharm.*, 13(6 Suppl C): S5–18.

Bogdan, C. (2001). Nitric oxide and the immune response. *Nat. Immunol.*, 2(10): 907–916.

Brückner, M., Westphal, S., Domschke, W., Kucharzik, T. and Lügering, A. (2012). Green tea polyphenol epigallocatechin-3-gallate shows therapeutic antioxidative effects in a murine model of colitis. *J. Crohns. Colitis.*, 6(2): 226–235. doi: 10.1016/j.crohns.2011.08.012.

Calder, P.C., Albers, R., Antoine, J.M., Blum, S., Bourdet-Sicard, R., Ferns, G.A., Folkerts, G., Friedmann, P.S., Frost, G.S., Guarner, F., Løvik, M., Macfarlane, S., Meyer, P.D., M'Rabet, L., Serafini, M., van Eden, W., van Loo, J., Vas Dias, W., Vidry, S., Winklhofer-Roob, B.M. and Zhao, J. (2009). Inflammatory disease processes and interactions with nutrition. *Br. J. Nutr.*, 101(Suppl 1): S1–S45.

Calderon-Montano, J.M., Burgos-Moron, E., Perez-Guerrero, C. and Lopez Lazaro, M. (2011). A review on the dietary flavonoid kaempferol. *Mini. Rev. Med. Chem.*, 11: 298–344.

Canavan, C., West, J. and Card, T. (2014). The epidemiology of irritable bowel syndrome. *Clinical Epidemiology,* 6: 71–80.

Carrasco-Pozo, C., Castillo, R.L., Beltrán, C., Miranda, A., Fuentes, J. and Gotteland, M. (2016). Molecular mechanisms of gastrointestinal protection by quercetin against indomethacin-induced damage: Role of NF-κB and Nrf2. *J. Nutr. Biochem.*, 27: 289–298. doi: 10.1016/j.jnutbio.2015.09.016.

Castangia, I., Nácher, A., Caddeo, C., Merino, V., Díez-Sales, O., Catalán-Latorre, A., Fernàndez-Busquets, X., Fadda, A.M. and Manconi, M. (2015). Therapeutic efficacy of quercetin enzyme-responsive nanovesicles for the treatment of experimental colitis in rats. *Acta Biomater.*, 13: 216–227. doi: 10.1016/j.actbio.2014.11.017.

Charepalli, V., Reddivari, L., Radhakrishnan, S., Vadde, R., Agarwal, R. and Vanamala, J.K. (2015). Anthocyanin-containing purple-fleshed potatoes suppress colon tumorigenesis *via* elimination of colon cancer stem cells. *J. Nutr. Biochem.*, 26(12): 1641–1649. doi: 10.1016/j.jnutbio.2015.08.005.

Chen, B., Lu, Y., Chen, Y. and Cheng, J. (2015). The role of Nrf2 in oxidative stress-induced endothelial injuries. *J. Endocrinol.*, 225(3): R83–R99. doi: 10.1530/JOE-14-0662.

Chen, J., Chen, Z., Ma, L., Liang, Q., Jia, W., Pan, Z., Zeng, Y. and Jiang, B. (2014). Development of determination of four analytes of Zhi-Shao-San decoction using LC-MS/MS and its application to comparative pharmacokinetics in normal and irritable bowel syndrome rat plasma. *Biomed. Chromatogr.*, 28: 1384–1392. doi: 10.1002/bmc.3180.

Chung, C.S., Jiang, Y., Cheng, D. and Birt, D.F. (2007). Impact of adenomatous polyposis coli (APC) tumor supressor gene in human colon cancer cell lines on cell cycle arrest by apigenin. *Mol. Carcinog.*, 46(9): 773–782. doi: 10.1002/mc.20306.

Clevers, H. (2006). Wnt/beta-catenin signaling in development and disease. *Cell*, 127(3): 469–480.

Comalada, M., Camuesco, D., Sierra, S., Ballester, I., Xaus, J., Galvez, J. and Zarzuelo, A. (2005). *In vivo* quercitrin anti-inflammatory effect involves release of quercetin, which inhibits inflammation through downregulation of the NF-kappaB pathway. *Eur. J. Immunol.*, 35: 584–592.

Cotton, P.B., Elta, G.H., Carter, C.R., Pasricha, P.J. and Corazziari, E.S. (2016). Gallbladder and sphincter of oddi disorders. *Gastroenterology*, 150(6): 1420–1429.e2.

Cui, L., Feng, L., Zhang, Z.H. and Jia, X.B. (2014). The anti-inflammation effect of baicalin on experimental colitis through inhibiting TLR4/NF-κB pathway activation. *Int. Immunopharmacol.*, 23(1): 294–303. doi: 10.1016/j.intimp.2014.09.005.

De Palma, G., Collins, S.M. and Bercik, P. (2014). The microbiota gut-brain axis in functional gastrointestinal disorders. *Gut Microbes.*, 5(3): 419–429.

Devi, K.P., Malar, D.S., Nabavi, S.F., Sureda, A., Xiao, J., Nabavi, S.M. and Daglia, M. (2015). Kaempferol and inflammation: From chemistry to medicine. *Pharmacol Res.*, 99: 1–10.

Dou, W., Zhang, J., Sun, A., Zhang, E., Ding, L., Mukherjee, S., Wei, X., Chou, G., Wang, Z.T. and Mani, S. (2013). Protective effect of naringenin against experimental colitis *via* suppression of Toll-like receptor 4/NF-κB signalling. *Br. J. Nutr.*, 110(4): 599–608. doi: 10.1017/S0007114512005594.

Dou, W., Zhang, J., Zhang, E., Sun, A., Ding, L., Chou, G., Wang, Z. and Mani, S. (2013). Chrysin ameliorates chemically induced colitis in the mouse through modulation of a PXR/NF-κB signaling pathway. *J. Pharmacol. Exp. Ther.*, 345(3): 473–482. doi: 10.1124/jpet.112.201863.

Drossman, D.A. (2006). The functional gastrointestinal disorders and the Rome III process. *Gastroenterology*, 130: 1377–1390.

Drossman, D.A. (2016). Functional gastrointestinal disorders: What's new for Rome IV? *Lancet Gastroenterol Hepatol*, 1(1): 6"8.

Elson, C.O., Sartor, R.B., Tennyson, G.S. and Riddell, R.H. (1995). Experimental models of inflammatory bowel disease. *Gastroenterology*, 109(4): 1344–1367.

Enck, P., Aziz, Q., Barbara, G., Farmer, A.D., Fukudo, S., Mayer, E.A., Niesler, B., Quigley, E.M., Rajili -Stojanovi , M., Schemann, M., Schwille-Kiuntke, J., Simren, M., Zipfel, S. and Spiller, R.C. (2016). Irritable bowel syndrome. *Nat. Rev. Dis. Primers.*, 2: 16014. doi: 10.1038/nrdp.2016.14.

Fevr, T., Robine, S., Louvard, D. and Huelsken, J. (2007). Wnt/beta-catenin is essential for intestinal homeostasis and maintenance of intestinal stem cells. *Mol. Cell. Biol.*, 27(21): 7551–7559.

Fournier, B.M. and Parkos, C.A. (2012). The role of neutrophils during intestinal inflammation. *Mucosal Immunol.*, 5(4): 354–366. doi: 10.1038/mi.2012.24.

Galsanov, S.H.B., Tourova, A.D. and Klimenko, E.D. (1976). Effect of quercitrin on structural changes in the large and small intestines in experimental enterocolitis. *Biull. Eksp. Biol. Med.*, 81(5): 623–625.

Gao, J., Morrison, D.C., Parmely, T.J., Russell, S.W. and Murphy, W.J. (1997). An interferon-gamma-activated site (GAS) is necessary for full expression of the mouse iNOS gene in response to interferon-gamma and lipopolysaccharide. *J. Biol. Chem.*, 272(2): 1226–1230.

Grivennikov, S., Karin, E., Terzic, J., Mucida, D., Yu, G.Y., Vallabhapurapu, S., Scheller, J., Rose-John, S., Cheroutre, H., Eckmann, L. and Karin, M. (2009). IL-6 and Stat3 are required for survival of intestinal epithelial cells and development of colitis-associated cancer. *Cancer Cell*, 15(2): 103–113. doi: 10.1016/j.ccr.2009.01.001.

Grundmann, O. and Yoon, S.L. (2010). Irritable bowel syndrome: Epidemiology, diagnosis and treatment: An update for health-care practitioners. *J. Gastroenterol Hepatol.*, 25(4): 691–699.

Haggar, F.A. and Boushey, R.P. (2009). Colorectal cancer epidemiology: Incidence, mortality, survival, and risk factors. *Clin. Colon. Rectal. Surg.*, 22(4): 191–197. doi: 10.1055/s-0029-1242458.

Hämäläinen, M., Nieminen, R., Vuorela, P., Heinonen, M. and Moilanen, E. (2007). Anti-inflammatory effects of flavonoids: Genistein, kaempferol, quercetin, and daidzein inhibit STAT-1 and NF-kappaB activations, whereas flavone, isorhamnetin, naringenin, and pelargonidin inhibit only NF-kappaB activation along with their inhibitory effect on iNOS expression and NO production in activated macrophages. *Mediators Inflamm.*, 2007: 45673. doi: 10.1155/2007/45673.

Hoensch, H., Groh, B., Edler, L. and Kirch, W. (2008). Prospective cohort comparison of flavonoid treatment in patients with resected colorectal cancer to prevent recurrence. *World J. Gastroenterol.*, 14(14): 2187–2193. doi: 10.3748/wjg.14.2187.

Holtmann, G., Talley, N.J., Liebregts, T., Adam, B. and Parow, C. (2006). A placebo-controlled trial of itopride in functional dyspepsia. *N. Engl. J. Med.*, 354(8): 832–840.

Huo, X., Liu, D., Gao, L., Li, L. and Cao, L. (2016). Flavonoids extracted from licorice prevents colitis-associated carcinogenesis in AOM/DSS mouse model. *Int. J. Mol. Sci.*, 17(9). pii: E1343. doi: 10.3390/ijms17091343.

Hyams, J.S., Lorenzo, C.D., Saps, M., Shulman, R.J., Staiano, A. and van Tilburg, M. (2016). Childhood functional gastrointestinal disorders: Child/Adolescent. *Gastroenterology*, 150(6): 1456–1468.e2.

Jalili, M., Vahedi, H., Janani, L., Poustchi, H., Malekzadeh, R. and Hekmatdoost, A. (2015). Soy isoflavones supplementation for patients with irritable bowel syndrome: A randomized double blind clinical trial. *Middle East J. Dig. Dis.*, 7: 170–176.

Jan, A.T., Kamli, M.R., Murtaza, I., Singh, J.B., Ali, A. and Haq, Q. (2010). Dietary flavonoid quercetin and associated health benefits-an overview. *Food Rev. Int.*, 26: 302–317.

Jaramillo-Carmona, S., Lopez, S., Abia, R., Rodriguez-Arcos, R., Jimenez, A., Guillen, R. and Muriana, F.J.G. (2014). Combination of quercetin and kaempferol enhances *in vitro* cytotoxicity on human colon cancer (HCT-116) cells. *Rec. Nat. Prod.*, 8(3): 262–271.

Jung, H., Lee, H.J., Cho, H. and Hwang, K.T. (2015). Anti-inflammatory activities of *Rubus* fruit anthocyanins in inflamed human intestinal epithelial cells. *Journal of Food Biochemistry*, 39: 300–309. doi:10.1111/jfbc.12130

Karin, M. and Greten, F.R. (2005). NF-kappaB: Linking inflammation and immunity to cancer development and progression. *Nat. Rev. Immunol.*, 5(10): 749–759.

Kawai, T. and Akira, S. (2010). The role of pattern-recognition receptors in innate immunity: Update on Toll-like receptors. *Nat. Immunol.*, 11(5): 373–384. doi: 10.1038/ni.1863.

Kawai, T. and Akira, S. (2011). Toll-like receptors and their crosstalk with other innate receptors in infection and immunity. *Immunity*, 34(5): 637–650. doi: 10.1016/j.immuni.2011.05.006.

Keefer, L., Drossman, D.A., Guthrie, E., Simrén, M., Tillisch, K., Olden, K. and Whorwell, P.J. (2016). Centrally mediated disorders of gastrointestinal pain. *Gastroenterology*, 150(6): 1408–1419.

Kim, H.J., Kim, S.K., Kim, B.S., Lee, S.H., Park, Y.S., Park, B.K., Kim, S.J., Kim, J., Choi, C., Kim, J.S., Cho, S.D., Jung, J.W., Roh, K.H., Kang, K.S. and Jung, J.Y. (2010). Apoptotic effect of quercetin on HT-29 colon cancer cells *via* the AMPK signaling pathway. *J. Agric. Food Chem.*, 58(15): 8643–8650. doi: 10.1021/jf101510z.

Kim, J.M., Kim, J.S., Yoo, H., Choung, M.G. and Sung, M.K. (2008). Effects of black soybean [*Glycine max* (L.) Merr.] seed coats and its anthocyanidins on colonic inflammation and cell proliferation *in vitro* and *in vivo*. *J. Agric. Food Chem.*, 56(18): 8427–8433. doi: 10.1021/jf801342p.

Knutsson, A. and Bøggild, H. (2010). Gastrointestinal disorders among shift workers. *Scand. J. Work Environ. Health*, 36(2): 85–95.

Kolios, G. (2016). Animal models of inflammatory bowel disease: How useful are they really? *Curr. Opin. Gastroenterol.*, 32(4): 251–257.

Korhonen, R., Lahti, A., Kankaanranta, H. and Moilanen, E. (2005). Nitric oxide production and signaling in inflammation. *Curr. Drug Targets Inflamm. Allergy*, 4(4): 471–479.

Kou, X., Kirberger, M., Yang, Y. and Chen, N. (2013). Natural products for cancer prevention associated with Nrf2–ARE pathway. *Food Science and Human Wellness*, 2(1): 22–28.

Kozlowska, A. and Szostak-Wegierek, D. (2014). Flavonoids–food sources and health benefits. *Rocz Panstw Zakl Hig.*, 65(2): 79–85.

Krinsky, N.I. (1992). Mechanism of action of biological antioxidants. *Proc. Soc. Exp. Biol. Med.*, 200(2): 248–254.

Kumar, A., Pate, J. and Sawant, P. (2012). Epidemiology of functional dyspepsia. *J. Assoc. Physicians. India*, 60(Suppl): 9–12.

Lacy, B.E., Mearin, F., Chang, L., Chey, W.D., Lembo, A.J., Simren, M. and Spiller, R. (2016). Bowel disorders. *Gastroenterology*, 150(6): 1393–1407.e5.

Lane, D.P. (1992). Cancer. p53, guardian of the genome. *Nature*, 358(6381): 15–16.

Lee, J.H., Regmi, S.C., Kim, J.A., Cho, M.H., Yun, H., Lee, C.S. and Lee, J. (2011). Apple flavonoid phloretin inhibits *Escherichia coli* O157: H7 biofilm formation and ameliorates colon inflammation in rats. *Infect Immun.*, 79(12): 4819–4827. doi: 10.1128/IAI.05580-11.

Leick, M., Azcutia, V., Newton, G. and Luscinskas, F.W. (2014). Leukocyte recruitment in inflammation: Basic concepts and new mechanistic insights based on new models and microscopic imaging technologies. *Cell Tissue Res.*, 355(3): 647–656. doi:10.1007/s00441-014-1809-9.

Leonardi, T., Vanamala, J., Taddeo, S.S., Davidson, L.A., Murphy, M.E., Patil, B.S., Wang, N., Carroll, R.J., Chapkin, R.S., Lupton, J.R. and Turner, N.D. (2010). Apigenin and naringenin suppress colon carcinogenesis through the aberrant crypt stage in azoxymethane-treated rats. *Exp. Biol. Med.* (Maywood), 235(6): 710–717. doi: 10.1258/ebm.2010.009359.

Li, W. and Kong, A.N. (2009). Molecular mechanisms of Nrf2-mediated antioxidant response. *Mol. Carcinog.*, 48(2): 91–104. doi:10.1002/mc.20465.

Lin, Y.L. and Lin, J.K. (1997). (-)-Epigallocatechin-3-gallate blocks the induction of nitric oxide synthase by down-regulating lipopolysaccharide-induced activity of transcription factor nuclear factor-kappaB. *Mol. Pharmacol.*, 52(3): 465–472.

Loftus, Jr. E.V. (2004). Clinical epidemiology of inflammatory bowel disease: Incidence, prevalence, and environmental influences. *Gastroenterology*, 126: 1504–1517.

Lü, J-M., Lin, P.H., Yao, Q. and Chen, C. (2010). Chemical and molecular mechanisms of antioxidants: Experimental approaches and model systems. *Journal of Cellular and Molecular Medicine*, 14(4): 840–860. doi:10.1111/j.1582-4934.2009.00897.x.

Madiwale, G.P., Reddivari, L., Stone, M., Holm, D.G. and Vanamala, J. (2012). Combined effects of storage and processing on the bioactive compounds and pro-apoptotic properties of color-fleshed potatoes in human colon cancer cells. *J. Agric. Food Chem.*, 60(44): 11088–11096. doi: 10.1021/jf303528p.

Mahadeva, S. and Goh, K.L. (2006). Epidemiology of functional dyspepsia: A global perspective. *World J. Gastroenterol.*, 12(17): 2661–2666.

Mariani, F., Sena, P. and Roncucci, L. (2014) Inflammatory pathways in the early steps of colorectal cancer development. *World J. Gastroenterol.*, 20(29): 971631. doi: 10.3748/wjg.v20.i29.9716.

Medzhitov, R. (2008). Origin and physiological roles of inflammation. *Nature*, 454(7203): 428–435.

Mizoguchi, A. (2012). Animal models of inflammatory bowel disease. *Prog. Mol. Biol. Transl. Sci.*, 105: 263–320.

Mota, K.S., Dias, G.E., Pinto, M.E., Luiz-Ferreira, A., Souza-Brito, A.R., Hiruma-Lima, C.A., Barbosa-Filho, J.M. and Batista, L.M. (2009). Flavonoids with gastroprotective activity. *Molecules*, 14(3): 979–1012.

Najafzadeh, M., Reynolds, P.D., Baumgartner, A. and Anderson, D. (2009). Flavonoids inhibit the genotoxicity of hydrogen peroxide (H_2O_2) and of the food mutagen 2-amino-3-methylimadazo[4,5-f]-quinoline (IQ) in lymphocytes from patients with inflammatory bowel disease (IBD). *Mutagenesis*, 24(5): 405–411. doi: 10.1093/mutage/gep016.

Neurath, M.F. (2012). Animal models of inflammatory bowel diseases: Illuminating the pathogenesis of colitis, ileitis and cancer. *Dig. Dis.*, 30 (Suppl 1): 91–94.

Nimse, S.B. and Pal, D. (2015). Free radicals, natural antioxidants, and their reaction mechanisms. *RSC Adv.*, 5: 27986–28006.

Nishitani, Y., Yamamoto, K., Yoshida, M., Azuma, T., Kanazawa, K., Hashimoto, T. and Mizuno, M. (2013). Intestinal anti-inflammatory activity of luteolin: Role of the aglycone in NF-kappaB inactivation in macrophages co-cultured with intestinal epithelial cells. *Bio-Factors*, 39(5): 522–533.

Nishitani, Y., Yamamoto, K., Yoshida, M., Azuma, T., Kanazawa, K., Hashimoto, T. and Mizuno, M. (2013). Intestinal anti-inflammatory activity of luteolin: Role of the aglycone in NF-κB inactivation in macrophages co-cultured with intestinal epithelial cells. *BioFactors*, 39(5): 522–533. doi: 10.1002/biof.1091.

Niture, S.K., Khatri, R. and Jaiswal, A.K. (2014). Regulation of Nrf2-an update. *Free Radic Biol Med.*, 66: 36–44. doi: 10.1016/j.freeradbiomed.2013.02.008.

Ocete, M.A., Gálvez, J., Crespo, M.E., Cruz, T., González, M., Torres, M.I. and Zarzuelo, A. (1998). Effects of morin on an experimental model of acute colitis in rats. *Pharmacology*, 57(5): 261–270.

Ordás, I., Eckmann, L., Talamini, M., Baumgart, D.C. and Sandborn, W.J. (2012). Ulcerative colitis. *Lancet*, 380: 1606–1619.

Oswiecimska, J., Szymlak, A., Roczniak, W., Girczys-PoB edniok, K. and KwiecieD , J. (2017). New insights into the pathogenesis and treatment of irritable bowel syndrome. *Adv. Med. Sci.*, 62(1): 17–30. doi: 10.1016/j.advms.2016.11.001.

Pan, M.H., Lai, C.S., Wu, J.C. and Ho, C.T. (2011). Molecular mechanisms for chemoprevention of colorectal cancer by natural dietary compounds. *Mol. Nutr. Food Res.*, 55(1): 32–45. doi: 10.1002/mnfr.201000412.

Pandurangan, A.K., Kumar, S.A.S., Dharmalingam, P. and Ganapasam, S. (2014). Luteolin, a bioflavonoid inhibits azoxymethane-induced colon carcinogenesis: Involvement of iNOS and COX-2. *Pharmacogn Mag.*, 10(Suppl 2): S306–S310. doi:10.4103/0973-1296.133285.

Park, M-Y., Kim, J-M., Kim, J-S., Choung, M-G. and Sung, M.K. (2015). Chemopreventive action of anthocyanin-rich black soybean fraction in $APC^{Min/+}$ intestinal polyposis model. *Journal of Cancer Prevention*, 20(3): 193–201. doi:10.15430/JCP.2015.20.3.193.

Piechota-Polanczyk, A. and Fichna, J. (2014). Review article: The role of oxidative stress in pathogenesis and treatment of inflammatory bowel diseases. *Naunyn Schmiedebergs Arch. Pharmacol.*, 387(7): 605–620. doi: 10.1007/s00210-014-0985-1.

Plociennikowska, A., Hromada-Judycka, A., Borz cka, K. and Kwiatkowska, K. (2015). Co-operation of TLR4 and raft proteins in LPS-induced pro-inflammatory signaling. *Cell. Mol. Life Sci.*, 72(3): 557–581. doi: 10.1007/s00018-014-1762-5.

Qin, J., Chen, J.X., Zhu, Z. and Teng, J.A. (2015). Genistein inhibits human colorectal cancer growth and suppresses MiR-95, Akt and SGK1. *Cell Physiol Biochem.*, 35: 2069–2077.

Qiu, P., Dong, P., Guan, H., Li, S., Ho, C.T., Pan, M.H., McClements, D.J. and Xiao, H. (2010). Inhibitory effects of 5-hydroxy polymethoxyflavones on colon cancer cells. *Mol. Nutr. Food Res.*, 54 (Suppl 2): S244–S252. doi: 10.1002/mnfr.200900605.

Rao, S.S.C., Bharucha, A.E., Chiarioni, G., Felt-Bersma, R., Knowles, C., Malcolm, A., Wald, A. (2016). Anorectal disorders. *Gastroenterology,* 150(6): 1430–1442.e4.

Raveendra, K.R., Jayachandra, Srinivasa V., Sushma, K.R., Allan, J.J., Goudar, K.S., Shivaprasad, H.N., Venkateshwarlu, K., Geetharani, P., Sushma, G. and Agarwal, A. (2012). An extract of *Glycyrrhiza glabra* (GutGard) alleviates symptoms of functional dyspepsia: A randomized, double-blind, placebo-controlled study. *Evid. Based Complement Alternat. Med.*, 2012: 216970. doi: 10.1155/2012/216970.

Ren, G., Sun, A., Deng, C., Zhang, J., Wu, X., Wei, X., Mani, S., Dou, W. and Wang, Z. (2015). The anti-inflammatory effect and potential mechanism of cardamonin in DSS-induced colitis. *Am. J. Physiol. Gastrointest. Liver Physiol.*, 309(7): G517–G527. doi: 10.1152/ajpgi.00133.2015.

Rezaie, A., Parker, R.D. and Abdollahi, M. (2007). Oxidative stress and pathogenesis of inflammatory bowel disease: An epiphenomenon or the cause? *Dig. Dis. Sci.*, 52(9): 2015–2021.

Romano, B., Pagano, E., Montanaro, V., Fortunato, A.L., Milic, N. and Borrelli, F. (2013). Novel insights into the pharmacology of flavonoids. *Phytother Res.*, 27: 1588–1596.

Roth, S., Spalinger, M.R., Gottier, C., Biedermann, L., Zeitz, J., Lang, S., Weber, A., Rogler, G. and Scharl, M. (2016). Bilberry-derived anthocyanins modulate cytokine expression in the intestine of patients with ulcerative colitis. *PLoS ONE,* 11(5): e0154817. doi: 10.1371/journal.pone.0154817.

Ryan, K.M. (2011). p53 and autophagy in cancer: Guardian of the genome meets guardian of the proteome. *Eur. J. Cancer*, 47(1): 44–50. doi: 10.1016/j.ejca.2010.10.020.

Sahu, B.D., Kumar, J.M., Sistla, R. (2016). Fisetin, a dietary flavonoid, ameliorates experimental colitis in mice: Relevance of NF-κB signaling. *J. Nutr. Biochem.*, 28: 171–182. doi: 10.1016/j.jnutbio.2015.10.004.

Sartor, R.B. (2008). Microbial influences in inflammatory bowel diseases. *Gastroenterology*, 134(2): 577–594.

Schmulson, M.J. and Drossman, D.A. (2017). What Is New in Rome IV. *J. Neurogastroenterol. Motil.*, 23(2): 151–163. doi:10.5056/jnm16214.

Seibel, J., Molzberger, A.F., Hertrampf, T., Laudenbach-Leschowski, U. and Diel, P. (2009). Oral treatment with genistein reduces the expression of molecular and biochemical markers of inflammation in a rat model of chronic TNBS-induced colitis. *Eur. J. Nutr.*, 48(4): 213–220. doi: 10.1007/s00394-009-0004-3.

Shafiee, G., Saidijam, M., Tavilani, H., Ghasemkhani, N. and Khodadadi, I. (2016). Genistein induces apoptosis and inhibits proliferation of HT29 colon cancer cells. *Int. J. Mol. Cell. Med.*, 5(3): 178–191.

Shan, B.E., Wang, M.X. and Li, R.Q. (2009). Quercetin inhibit human SW480 colon cancer growth in association with inhibition of cyclin D1 and survivin expression through Wnt/beta-catenin signaling pathway. *Cancer Invest.*, 27(6): 604–612. doi: 10.1080/07357900802337191.

Sharma, J.N., Al-Omran, A. and Parvathy, S.S. (2007). Role of nitric oxide in inflammatory diseases. *Inflammopharmacology*, 15(6): 252–259. doi: 10.1007/s10787-007-0013-x.

Shin, C.M., Lee, D.H., Seo, A.Y., Lee, H.J., Kim, S.B., Son, W.C., Kim, Y.K., Lee, S.J., Park, S.H., Kim, N., Park, Y.S. and Yoon, H. (2017). Green tea extracts for the prevention of metachronous colorectal polyps among patients who underwent endoscopic removal of colorectal adenomas: A randomized clinical trial. *Clin. Nutr.*, pii: S0261–5614(17): 30038–9. doi: 10.1016/j.clnu.2017.01.014.

Shin, E.K., Kwon, H.S., Kim, Y.H., Shin, H.K. and Kim, J.K. (2009). Chrysin, a natural flavone, improves murine inflammatory bowel diseases. *Biochem. Biophys Res. Commun.*, 381(4): 502–507. doi: 10.1016/j.bbrc.2009.02.071.

Siegel, R., Desantis, C. and Jemal, A. (2014). Colorectal cancer statistics. *CA Cancer J. Clin.*, 64(2): 104–117. doi: 10.3322/caac.21220.

Soares, R.L. (2014). Irritable bowel syndrome: A clinical review. *World J. Gastroenterol.*, 20(34): 12144–12160. doi: 10.3748/wjg.v20.i34.12144.

Sobczak, M., WlazB owski, M., Zatorski, H., Salaga, M. and Fichna, J. (2014). Current overview of colitis-associated colorectal cancer. *Cent. Eur. J. Biol.*, 9(11): 1022–1029. doi: 10.2478/s11535-014-0345-7.

Somani, S.J., Modi, K.P., Majumdar, A.S. and Sadarani, B.N. (2015). Phytochemicals and their potential usefulness in inflammatory bowel disease. *Phytother. Res.*, 29: 339–350.

Sood, R. and Ford, A.C. (2016). Diagnosis: Rome IV criteria for FGIDs–an improvement or more of the same? *Nat. Rev. Gastroenterol. Hepatol.*, 13: 501–502. doi:10.1038/nrgastro.2016.110

Stanghellini, V., Chan, F.K., Hasler, W.L., Malagelada, J.R., Suzuki, H., Tack, J. and Talley, N.J. (2016). Gastroduodenal disorders. *Gastroenterology*, 150(6): 1380–1392. doi: 10.1053/j.gastro.2016.02.011.

Suzuki, H., Inadomi, J.M. and Hibi, T. (2009). Japanese herbal medicine in functional gastrointestinal disorders. *Neurogastroenterol. Motil.*, 21(7): 688–696.

Tack, J., Talley, N.J., Camilleri, M., Holtmann, G., Hu, P., Malagelada, J.R. and Stanghellini, V. (2006). Functional gastroduodenal disorders. *Gastroenterology*, 130: 1466–1479.

Talley, N.J. (2008). Functional gastrointestinal disorders as a public health problem. *Neurogastroenterol. Motil.* 20(Suppl 1): 121–129.

Tapas, A.R., Sakarkar, D.M. and Kakde, R.B. (2008). Flavonoids as Nutraceuticals: A Review. *Trop. J. Pharm. Res.*, 7(3): 1089–1099.

Todaro, M., Francipane, M.G., Medema, J.P. and Stassi, G. (2010). Colon cancer stem cells: Promise of targeted therapy. *Gastroenterology*, 138(6): 2151–2162. doi: 10.1053/j.gastro.2009.12.063.

Torre, L.A., Bray, F., Siegel, R.L., Ferlay, J., Lortet-Tieulent, J. and Jemal, A. (2015). Global cancer statistics, 2012. *CA. Cancer J. Clin.*, 65(2): 87–108. doi: 10.3322/caac.21262.

Tuñón, M.J., García-Mediavilla, M.V., Sánchez-Campos, S. and González-Gallego, J. (2009). Potential of flavonoids as anti-inflammatory agents: modulation of pro-inflammatory gene expression and signal transduction pathways. *Curr. Drug. Metab.*, 10(3): 256–271.

Vezza, T., Rodríguez-Nogales, A., Algieri, F., Utrilla, M.P., Rodriguez-Cabezas, M.E. and Galvez, J. (2016). Flavonoids in inflammatory bowel disease: A Review. *Nutrients,* 8(4): 211. doi: 10.3390/nu8040211.

Villarreal, A.A., Aberger, F.J., Benrud, R. and Gundrum, J.D. (2012). Use of broad-spectrum antibiotics and the development of irritable bowel syndrome. *W.M.J.*, 111: 17–20.

Willoughby, D.A., Moore, A.R. and Colville-Nash, P.R. (2000). COX-1, COX-2, and COX-3 and the future treatment of chronic inflammatory disease. *Lancet*, 355(9204): 646–648.

World Cancer Research Fund and American Institute for Cancer Research (2007). Food, Nutrition, Physical Activity, and the Prevention of Cancer: A Global Perspective. Washington, DC: American Institute for Cancer Research.

Xavier, R.J. and Podolsky, D.K. (2007). Unravelling the pathogenesis of inflammatory bowel disease. *Nature*, 448: 427–434.

Xie, Q.W., Kashiwabara, Y. and Nathan, C. (1994). Role of transcription factor NF-kappa B/Rel in induction of nitric oxide synthase. *J. Biol. Chem.*, 269(7): 4705–4708.

Yang, Y. (2012). Wnt signaling in development and disease. *Cell & Bioscience*, 2: 14. doi:10.1186/2045-3701-2-14.

Yun, J.M., Afaq, F., Khan, N. and Mukhtar, H. (2009). Delphinidin, an anthocyanidin in pigmented fruits and vegetables, induces apoptosis and cell cycle arrest in human colon cancer HCT116 cells. *Mol. Carcinog.*, 48(3): 260–270. doi: 10.1002/mc.20477.

Zeevenhooven, J., Koppen, I.J.N. and Benninga, M.A. (2017). The new rome IV criteria for functional gastrointestinal disorders in infants and toddlers. *Pediatr Gastroenterol Hepatol Nutr.*, 20(1): 1–13.

Zhang, D.D. (2006). Mechanistic studies of the Nrf2-Keap1 signaling pathway. *Drug Metab Rev.,* 38(4): 769–789.

Zhu, H. and Li, Y.R. (2012). Oxidative stress and redox signaling mechanisms of inflammatory bowel disease: Updated experimental and clinical evidence. *Exp. Biol. Med.* (Maywood)., 237(5): 474–480. doi: 10.1258/ebm.2011.011358.

4

Anti-diabetic Potential of Flavonoids and Their Molecular Mechanisms – A Review

SHIVSHARAN B. DHADDE[1] AND BABURAO N. CHANDAKAVATHE[1]

ABSTRACT

Diabetes mellitus (DM) is one of the major health disasters of the 21st century. The World Health Organization estimates that after hypertension and tobacco use, hyperglycemia is the third highest risk factor for early death. Dietary and plant derived products have been evaluated in numerous preclinical and clinical trials for thier antidiabetic activities. Flavonoids are a large class of phenolic compounds found in many natural products. Flavonoids including flavonol, flavanone, flavone, isoflavone, flavan-3-ols and anthocyanin containing foods play positive roles in sustaining blood glucose levels, glucose uptake, insulin release and adjusting immune functions. In this review, the association between flavonoids and DM is focused on the basis of the latest studies. The anti-diabetic activities of flavonoids found in dietary plants and fruits are summarized to delineate the underlying molecular signalling of flavonoids using in vitro and in vivo models.

***Key words*:** Flavonol, Flavanone, Flavone, Isoflavone, Flavan-3-ols, Anthocyanin

1. INTRODUCTION

Diabetes mellitus (DM) is a heterogeneous group of metabolic disorders characterized by the annihilation of pancreatic β-cells or reduced insulin discharge and its action, which results in abnormal metabolism of

[1] D.S.T.S. Mandal's College of Pharmacy, Solapur-413 004, Maharashtra, India
**Corresponding author*: E-mail: sharanapharma@hotmail.com

carbohydrate, protein and lipid (Michael *et al.*, 2004; Chambers, 2006; IDF Diabetes Atlas, 2015). DM is one of the major health disasters of the 21st century. The World Health Organization estimates that after hypertension and tobacco use, hyperglycemia is the third highest risk factor for early death (WHO, 2009). In 2015, around five million people between the age of 20-79 years died from diabetes, which is equivalent to one death at each six seconds. In 2015, International Diabetes Federation (IDF) estimated that one in 11 adults has diabetes and one in two adults with diabetes is undiagnosed. One in seven births is affected by gestational diabetes and nearly 5,42,000 children are suffering from type 1 diabetes. Presently more than 415 million population is diabetic in the world and by 2040, this number is expected to come close to 642 million (IDF Diabetes Atlas, 2015) (Table 1).

Table 1: Estimated number of people with diabetes worldwide and per region in 2015 and 2040 (20-79 years) (IDF Diabetes Atlas, 2015)

Region	***Diabetics in 2015***	***Projected diabetics in 2040***
Africa	14.2 million	34.2 million
South and Central America	29.6 million	48.8 million
Middle East and North Africa	35.4 million	72.1 million
North America and Caribbean	44.3 million	60.5 million
Europe	59.8 million	71.1 million
South East Asia	78.3 million	140.2 million
Western Pacific	153.2 million	214.8 million
In World	415 million	642 million

2. PATHOPHYSIOLOGY OF DM

2.1. Diagnosis, Types and Etiopathogenesis

The approaches used to diagnose DM are based on statistical methods defining unusual or high blood glucose levels and the risk of symptoms and complications. The American Diabetes Association (ADA) fixed criteria for the diagnosis of DM which comprised of symptoms such as polyuria, polydipsia and unexplained weight loss and a random plasma glucose concentration of greater than 200 mg/dL, a fasting plasma glucose concentration of greater than 126 mg/dL, or a plasma glucose concentration of greater than 200 mg/dL 2 h after the ingestion of an oral glucose load (Expert Committee on the Diagnosis and Treatment of Diabetes Mellitus, 2003, Chambers, 2006).

DM has been conventionally categorized into type 1 DM, also known as insulin-dependent DM (IDDM, formerly called juvenile-onset DM), and type 2 DM, also known as non–insulin-dependent DM (NIDDM, formerly referred as adult-onset DM). Other than type 1 and type 2 DM, gestational diabetes appears during pregnancy. Gestational diabetes can lead to serious health risks and is associated with an increased risk of developing type 2 diabetes later in life for both mother and the child (Fetita *et al.,* 2006).

Autoimmune reactions are responsible for type 1 diabetes, in which the immune system of body attacks the insulin-producing pancreatic β-cells. As a consequence, the body can no longer supply the insulin it needs. The disease can affect at any age, but onset usually occurs in children or youngsters. People with type 1 diabetes need insulin regularly in order to control the levels of glucose in their blood. With no insulin, a person with type 1 diabetes will die (IDF Diabetes Atlas, 2015).

Type 2 diabetes is common, usually seen in adults but is increasingly observed in children and adolescents. In type 2 diabetes, the body is able to produce insulin but develop into resistance so that the insulin is ineffective. Over the period, insulin levels may subsequently become deficient. Both the insulin resistance and deficiency lead to hypoglycemia. The features of type 1 and type 2 DM are shown in Table 2 (IDF Diabetes Atlas, 2015; Michael *et al.,* 2004).

Table 2: Features of Type 1 and Type 2 Diabetes Mellitus

Characteristic	*Type 1 DM*	*Type 2 DM*
Onset (age)	Usually <30 years	Usually >40 years
Type of onset	Abrupt	Gradual
Risk factors	Family history of diabetes, genetics, infections and other environmental influences	Excess body weight, physical inactivity, poor nutrition, genetics, family history of diabetes, past history of gestational diabetes and older age
Nutritional status	Often thin	Often obese
Clinical symptoms	• Abnormal thirst and a dry mouth • Frequent urination • Lack of energy, extreme tiredness • Constant hunger • Sudden weight loss • Blurred vision	• Frequent urination • Excessive thirst • Weight loss • Blurred vision
Ketosis	Present	Usually absent
Endogenous insulin	Absent	Variable
Insulin therapy	Required (Without insulin, a person with type 1 diabetes will die)	Sometimes
Oral hypoglycemics	Usually not effective	Often effective
Diet	Mandatory with insulin	Mandatory with or without drug

2.2. Metabolic Disturbances in DM

Glucose is the main energy source for all the living cells and some tissues (*e.g.*, brain) which require a constant delivery of glucose. Maintenance of blood glucose level within a normal physiological range is critical to the maintenance of normal energy use. It is primarily accomplished by two pancreatic hormones, insulin and glucagon (Michael *et al.*, 2004, IDF Diabetes Atlas, 2015). The biochemical actions of insulin are complex and involve many steps to integrate metabolism of carbohydrate, protein and lipid for glucose (energy) homeostasis. In addition to its effects on stimulating tissue glucose uptake, insulin has other major physiological effects on energy homeostasis which are shown in Fig. 1.

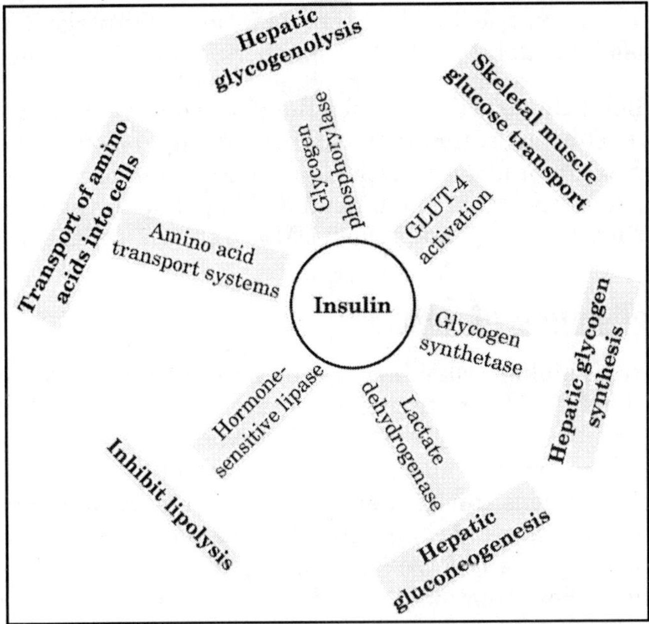

Fig. 1: Biochemical and Pharmacological Actions of Insulin

Exogenous dietary supplement and endogenous hepatic and renal gluconeogenesis and hepatic glycogenolysis are the major sources of blood glucose. In diabetic condition, metabolic process gets affected due to the dearrangement of pancreatic hormones, insulin and glucagon. Carbohydrate metabolism is reduced and on other hand metabolism of proteins and lipids gets increased. Exogenous and endogenous glucose is not used effectively and it accumulates in the blood (hyperglycemia). As blood glucose levels increase, the amount of glucose filtered by the glomeruli eventually exceeds the reabsorption capacity of the proximal tubule cells and glucose appears in the urine (glucosuria). Protein catabolism and the rate of nitrogen excretion are increased when blood insulin falls to low levels; stimulation of hepatic gluconeogenesis converts amino acids to glucose (Michael *et al.*, 2004; Chambers, 2006; IDF Diabetes Atlas).

The breackdown of lipids and fatty acids is also accelerated in the absence of insulin, leading to the formation of ketone bodies, such as acetoacetic acid, β-hydroxybutyric acid and acetone. Renal losses of glucose, nitrogenous substances and ketone bodies promote osmotic diuresis that can result in dehydration, electrolyte abnormalities and acid–base disturbances. Diabetic ketoacidosis is the end result of insulin deficiency in uncontrolled type 1 diabetes (Michael *et al.,* 2004; Chambers, 2006; IDF Diabetes Atlas).

Type 2 diabetics are less prone to develop ketone bodies or diabetic ketoacidosis but may develop a hyperosmolar coma, a condition characterized by severe hyperglycemia and dehydration. The three major metabolic abnormalities that contribute to hyperglycemia in type 2 DM are defective glucose-induced insulin secretion, increased hepatic glucose output and the inability of insulin to stimulate glucose uptake in peripheral target tissues (Michael *et al.,* 2004; Chambers, 2006; IDF Diabetes Atlas).

Even though the exact causes for the development of type 2 diabetes are not clear. The important risk factors are obesity, physical exercise and unhealthy diet. Other factors which play a role are ethnicity, family history of diabetes, past history of gestational diabetes and advancing age. The detailed features of type 1 and type 2 DM are shown in Table 2.

2.3. Complications of DM

Diabetics are at higher risk of developing a number of disabling and life-threatening health problems than non diabetics. Consistently hyperglycemia can lead to serious diseases affecting the cardiovascular system, eyes, kidneys and nerves. Diabetics are also at increased risk of developing infections. Diabetes complications can be prevented or delayed by maintaining blood glucose, blood pressure and cholesterol levels as close to normal as possible. Many complications can be picked up in their early stages by screening programs that allow treatment to prevent them becoming more serious (Michael *et al.,* 2004; Chambers, 2006; IDF Diabetes Atlas).

2.4. Conventional Treatment and Need for New Strategies in the Treatment DM

Taking of a healthy diet, increased physical exercise and maintenance of a normal body weight is the cornerstone of treatment for diabetes, in spite of its type or severity of symptoms. Type 1 diabetics need insulin every day in order to control their blood glucose levels. With no insulin, an individual with type 1 diabetes will die (Michael *et al.,* 2004; Chambers, 2006; IDF Diabetes Atlas).

Unlike type 1 diabetics, most people with type 2 diabetes do not need daily insulin treatment to survive. A number of oral medications are available to control blood glucose levels, which include sulfonylureas (acetohexamide, chlorpropamide, tolazamide, glyburide, glipizide, glimepiride and glibenclamide), meglitinides (repaglinide and nateglinide), biguanides (metformin), thiazolidinediones (pioglitazone and rosiglitazone), α-glucosidase inhibitors (acarbose and miglitol). If blood glucose levels continue to rise, however, people with type 2 diabetes may be prescribed insulin. But oral hypoglycemics are not generally used in the treatment of type 1 diabetes. Moreover, oral hypoglycemic drug therapy results in adverse side effects and limited benefits. In addition, people with all types of diabetes may need access to medications to control blood pressure and cholesterol levels (Michael *et al.,* 2004; Chambers, 2006; IDF Diabetes Atlas).

Heterogeneity of DM, lack of extensive knowledge on pathogenesis of pancreatic β-cell destruction and loss of insulin sensitivity and restricted therapeutic approaches open up new searches for anti-DM candidates that act on the multi-level pathogenesis of DM (Michael *et al.,* 2004; Chambers, 2006; IDF Diabetes Atlas).

Dietary and plant derived products have also been tested in a number of preclinical and clinical trials (Vinayagam and Xu, 2015; Hossain *et al.,* 2016). Since, herbal medicine has been used as monotherapy or as an adjunct to conventional therapeutics, thorough clinical trials and standardized herbal preparations are needed in order to test their efficacy, safety, tolerability and possible clinical recommendations (Michael *et al.,* 2004; Chambers, 2006; IDF Diabetes Atlas).

The use of plant derived products for treating diabetes is not just a seek for safer alternatives to pharmaceuticals, which transiently lower the blood glucose and diabetes-related complications and also enhancing the antioxidant system, insulin secretion and action (Surveswaran *et al.,* 2007).

In this review, the association between flavonoids and DM is focused on the basis of latest studies. The anti-diabetic activities of flavonoids found in dietary plants and fruits summarize the underlying molecular signalling of flavonoids using *in vitro* and *in vivo* models to clarify their anti-diabetic effects.

3. FLAVONOIDS AND THEIR EFFECTS ON DM

Flavonoids are phenolic compounds found in fruits, vegetables, nuts, grains seeds, cocoa, chocolate, tea, soya, red wine, herbs and beverages. Flavonoids including flavonol, flavanone, flavone, isoflavone, flavan-3-ols and anthocyanin containing foods play positive roles in sustaining blood glucose levels, glucose uptake, insulin release and adjusting immune function (Vinayagam and Xu, 2015; Hossain *et al.,* 2016). In current years various approaches have been made to utilize the flavonoids *in vitro* and *in vivo* models by incorporating few novel methods to improve its antidiabetic activity (Table 3).

Table 3: Important anti-diabetic potential and the underlying mechanism of dietary flavonoids

Flavonoid(s)	***Plants/Dietary source***	***Specific mechanism of action***	***Reference***
I. Flavonols			
Quercetin	Apples, berries, red onions, grapes, cherries, broccoli, pepper, coriander, citrus fruits and tea and at high concentrations in capers.	*Stimulation of insulin release:* • Inhibition of transient K_{ATP} channel • Stimulation of whole-cell Ca^{2+} (ICa) current *Inhibition of cell proliferation and induces apoptosis:* • Inhibition of PI3K/Akt signaling	Kittl *et al.*, 2016
		• Strengthening of differentiation of bone marrow mesenchymal stem cells into beta cells. • Increases insulin secretion from the differentiated cells.	Miladpour *et al.*, 2016
		• Inhibition of Toll-like receptor/NF-κB signaling pathway • Improvement in the inflammatory microenvironment. • Inhibition of NF-κβ, IL-1β and IL-6 • Inhibition of oxidized LDL and TNF-α production • Suppression of caspase-3, caspase-9, Blc-2 and Bax	Wang *et al.*, 2016
		• Inhibition of the intestinal glucose transporter GLUT2 • Inhibition of tyrosine kinase	Kwon *et al.*, 2017
		• Stimulation of GLUT4 translocation and expression in skeletal muscle *via* activation of 5' adenosine monophosphate-activated protein kinase (AMPK)	Vinayagam and Xu, 2015

Table 3: *(Contd...)*

Table 3: *(Contd...)*

Flavonoid(s)	***Plants/Dietary source***	***Specific mechanism of action***	***Reference***
Kaempferol 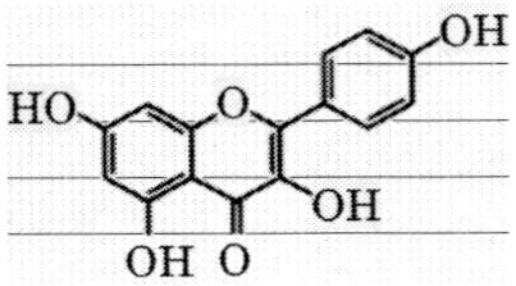	*Ginkgo biloba* L., apple, grape, tomato, tea, potato, broccoli, spinach, and some edible berries.	• Enhancing β-cell survival, improved cAMP signaling	Zhang *et al.*, 2013
		• Decreased PPAR-γ and SREBP-1c expression.	Zhang *et al.*, 2015
		• Enhanced AMPK activity and Glut 4 expression in skeletal muscle	Alkhalidy *et al.*, 2015
		• Inhibition of NF-κB, TNF-α) and IL-6	Luo *et al.*, 2015.
		• Inhibition of lipid peroxidation products, • Restoration of enzymatic antioxidants (superoxide dismutase, catalase, glutathione peroxidase and glutathione-S-transferase) • Restoration of non-enzymatic antioxidants (vitamin C, vitamin E, reduced glutathione)	Al-Numair *et al.*, 2015a
		• Restored deranged activity of membrane-bound ATPases	Al-Numair *et al.*, 2015b
		• Interact with some amino acid residues located within the active site of α-glucosidase	Peng *et al.*, 2016
Isorhamnetin 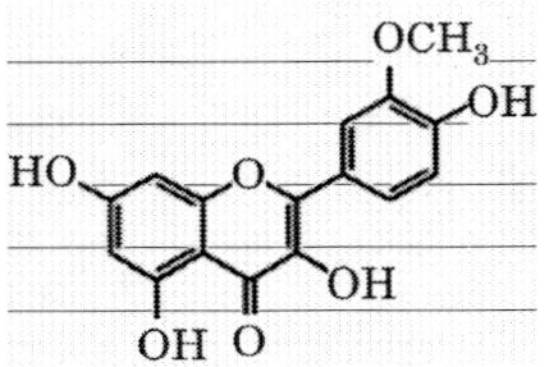	*Ginkgo biloba*, *Hippophae rhamnoides* and *Oenanthe javanica*	• Inhibition of PPARγ, and C/EBPα	Yokozawa *et al.*, 2002
		• Inhibition of aldose reductase and sorbitol accumulation	Lee *et al.*, 2005 and Lim *et al.*, 2006
		• Inhibition of alpha-glucosidase	Shibano *et al.*, 2008
		• GSK-3β inhibition	Middha *et al.*, 2013
		• Decrease the production of inflammatory mediators	Qiu *et al.*, 2016
		• Involvement of the NF-κB signaling pathway	

Table 3: *(Contd...)*

Table 3: *(Contd...)*

Flavonoid(s)	***Plants/Dietary source***	***Specific mechanism of action***	***Reference***
Fisetin 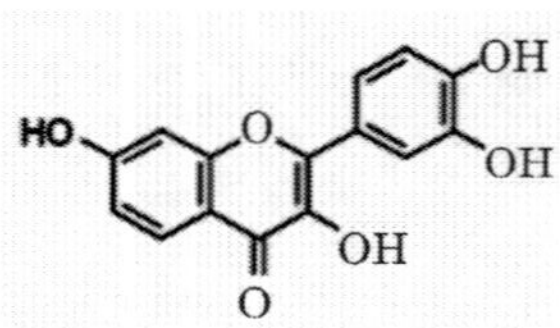	Strawberries, apples, mangoes, persimmons, kiwis, grapes, tomatoes, onions, cucumbers, nuts, and wine.	• Inhibition of pyruvate transport into the mitochondria • Reduction of cytosolic NADH-NAD (+) potential redox	Constantin *et al.*, 2010
		• Inhitition of NF-κB activation • Inhitition IL-6 and TNF-α release • Reduction of CBP/p300 gene expression	Kim *et al.*, 2012
		• Decreased mRNA and protein expression levels of gluconeogenic genes (phosphoenolpyruvate carboxykinase and glucose-6-phosphatase.	Prasath *et al.*, 2014
		• Modulation of hexokinase, pyruvate kinase, lactate dehydrogenase, glucose-6-phosphatase, fructose-1,6-bisphosphatase, glucose-6-phosphate dehydrogenase, glycogen synthase and glycogen phosphorylase	Prasath and Subramanian, 2011
		• Decrease in blood glucose, HbA1c, NF-kB p65 and IL-1β, NO • Elevation of plasma insulin.	Prasath *et al.*, 2013
Myricetin 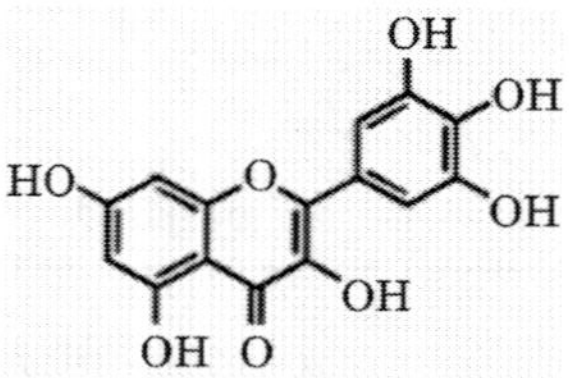	Tea, berries, fruits, wines etc.	• Increased hepatic glycogen • Increased glucose-6-phosphate expression • Increased hepatic glycogen synthase I	Ong and Khoo, 2000
		• Activation of peripheral tissues opioid μ-receptors	Liu *et al.*, 2006
		• Inhibition of α-glucosidase and α-amylase activity	Figueiredo-González *et al.*, 2016

Table 3: *(Contd...)*

Table 3: *(Contd...)*

Flavonoid(s)	***Plants/Dietary source***	***Specific mechanism of action***	***Reference***
Rutin 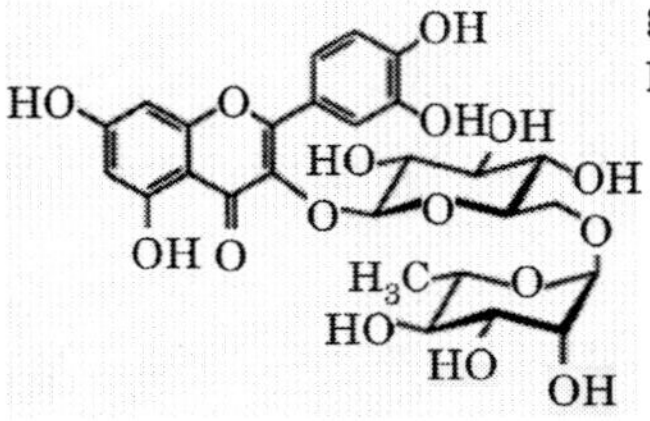	Buckwheat, oranges, grapes, lemons, limes, peaches and berries	• Restoration of glycogen content and the • Restoration of carbohydrate metabolizing enzymes activities • Stimulates mitogen-activated kinase • Protein kinase A activation • Protein kinase II activation • Protein kinase C activation • GLUT-4 the synthesis • Inhibition of inflammatory cytokines • Improvement in antioxidant and plasma lipid profiles • Suppresses human-amylin/hIAPP	Prince and Kamalakkannan, 2006 Kappel *et al.*, 2013a Kappel *et al.*, 2013b. Niture *et al.*, 2014 Aitken *et al.*, 2017
II. Flavanones			
Naringenin 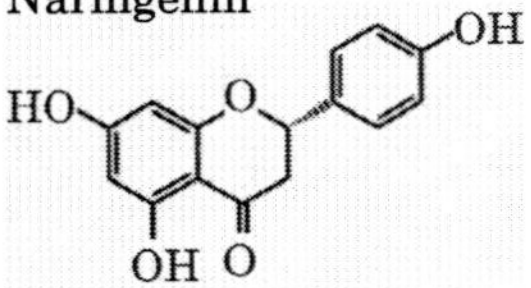	Grapefruit, orange and tomato.	• Decreases poliprotein B secretion in hepatocytes • Inhibition of NF-κB activation • Inhibition of intercellular adhesion molecule-1 (ICAM-1) mRNA expression • Inhibition of intestinal α-glucosidase activity • Downregulation of TGF-β1 and IL-1	Van Acker *et al.*, 2000 Ren *et al.*, 2016 Priscilla *et al.*, 2014 Roy *et al.*, 2016
Hesperidin 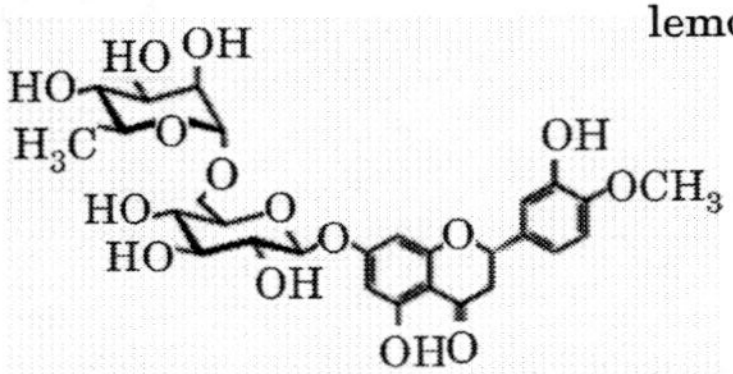	Citrus fruits such as lemons and limes	• Attenuation of oxidative stress • Attenuation proinflammatory cytokine production • Normalisation of SOD, catalase, glutathione • Normalisation of inflammatory cytokines (TNF-α, IL-1β), caspase-3, glial fibrillary acidic protein levels and aquaporin-4 (AQP4) expression in the retina	Mahmoud *et al.*, 2012, Visnagri *et al.*, 2014 Kumar *et al.*, 2013

Table 3: *(Contd...)*

Table 3: *(Contd...)*

Flavonoid(s)	*Plants/Dietary source*	*Specific mechanism of action*	*Reference*
Eriodictyol 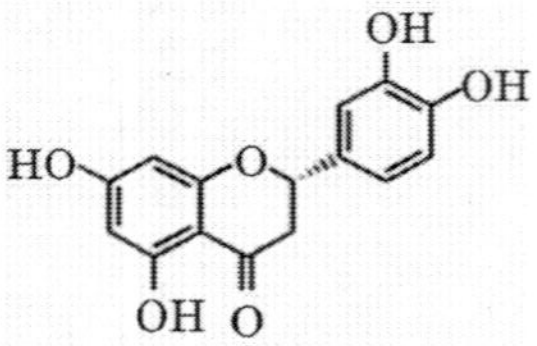	Lemon fruit	• Suppression of oxidative stress • Up-regulation of mRNA expression of PPARγ2 • Inhibition of TNF-α, ICAM-1, VEGF, and eNOS	 Zhang *et al.*, 2012 Bucolo *et al.*, 2012
Naringin 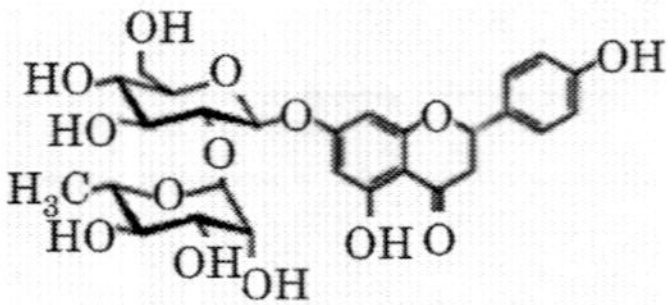	Tomatoes, grapefruits and citrus fruits	• Ameliorates oxidative stress • Increases glucose uptake • Upregulation of PPAR and 5' adenosine monophosphate-activated protein kinase	Dhanya *et al.*, 2015 Pu *et al.*, 2012
III. Flavone			
Apigenin 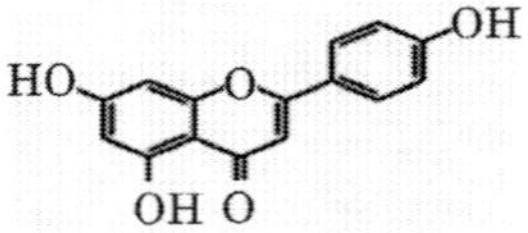	Vegetables, nuts, onion, orange and tea	• Free-radical scavenging activity • Suppression of TNF-α- and IL-1β-induced activation of NF-κB • Improvement in AMPK phosphorylation • Inhibition of NF-κB activation and ICAM-1 mRNA expression • Enhanced GLUT4 translocation • Inhibition of phosphorylation of protein kinase C βII (PKCβII) expression	Panda and Kar, 2007 Zhang *et al.*, 2014 Zang *et al.*, 2006 Ren *et al.*, 2016 Hossain *et al.*, 2014 Qin *et al.*, 2016

Table 3: *(Contd...)*

Table 3: *(Contd...)*

Flavonoid(s)	***Plants/Dietary source***	***Specific mechanism of action***	***Reference***
Luteolin 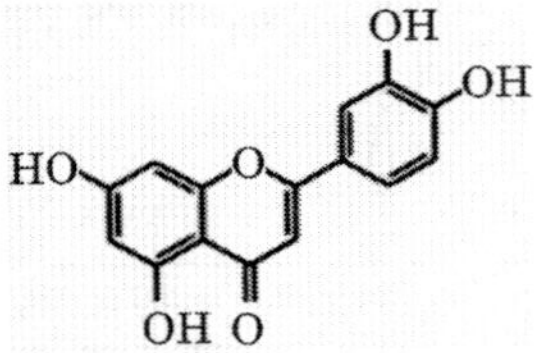	Onion leaves, cabbage, broccoli, parsley, carrots, apple skins, green pepper, perilla leaf and chamomile tea	• Inhibition of proinflammatory cytokine (IL-6 and TNF-α • Inhibition of α-glucosidase activity • Suppression of nuclear factor-κB	Kim *et al.*, 2014 Yan *et al.*, 2014 Nepali *et al.*, 2015
Tangeretin 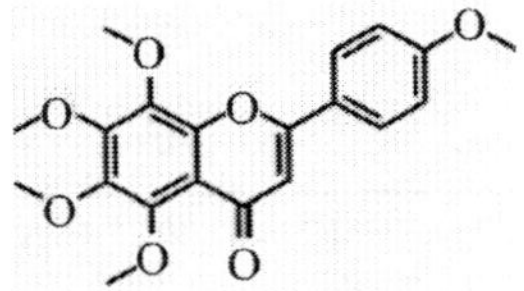	Citrus fruits, including mandarins and oranges	• Inhibition of adiponectin • Inhibition of leptin • Inhibition of resistin • Inhibition of IL-6 • Inhibition of MCP-1 • Modulation of hepatic enzymes (hexokinase, pyruvate kinase, lactate dehydrogenase, glucose -6-phosphatase, fructose-1,6-bisphosphatase, G6PD, glycogen synthase and glycogen phosphorylase) • Increased the secretion of an insulin-sensitizing factor, adiponectin • Stimulates glucose uptake via regulation of AMPK signaling pathways	Kim *et al.*, 2012 Sundaram *et al.*, 2014 Miyata *et al.*, 2011 Kim *et al.*, 2012
IV. Isoflavone			
Daidzein 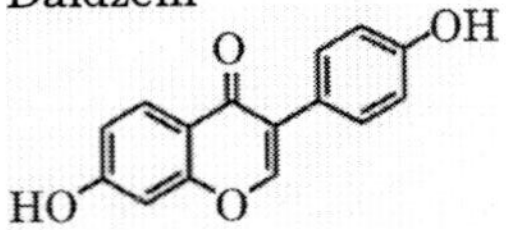	Fruits, nuts, soybeans, and soy-based products	• Decrease in lipid peroxidation, intracellular ROS generation, and indirect nitric oxide levels • Suppression of nitric oxide synthase (iNOS), cyclooxygenase-2 (COX-2), and NF-κB	Park, 2016

Table 3: *(Contd...)*

Table 3: *(Contd...)*

Flavonoid(s)	*Plants/Dietary source*	*Specific mechanism of action*	*Reference*
		• Increased GLUT-4 translocation • AMPK phosphorylation • Down-regulation G6Pase, PEPCK, fatty acid β-oxidation and CPT activities	Park *et al.*, 2013
		• Up-regulation malic enzyme and G6PD activities	Choi *et al.*, 2008
Genistein	legumes and Chinese plants *Genista tinctoria*	• Promoting the cAMP/PKA signaling pathway	Patisaul and Jefferson, 2010
		• Decreased β-cells loss and improved insulin levels • Ameliorates TNFα, iNOS, COX2 and NFκB	El-Kordy *et al.*, 2015
		• Ameliorates Nrf2, HO-1, GPx, and catalase	Eo *et al.*, 2016
V. Flavan-3-ols			
Flavan-3-ol	Fruits, cocoa, and chocolates etc	• Inhibition of secretory sphingomyelinase	Kobayashi *et al.*, 2016
		• Inhibition of MAPK/ERK-VEGF pathway	Zhang *et al.*, 2016
		• Improve insulin sensitivity	Cremonini *et al.*, 2016
		• Decreases NF-κB and TNF-α levels	Cordero-Herrera *et al.*, 2015
VI. Anthocyanins			
Cyanidin	Vegetables, fruits, and red wine	• Inhibition of α-glucosidase activity • Reduction of glucose-dependent insulinotropic polypeptide (GIP) level	Yamane *et al.*, 2016
		• Protection of pancreatic β-cell from apoptosis • Regulation of intrinsic apoptotic pathway-associated proteins, such as proteins belonging to the Bcl-2 family, cytochrome c and caspase-3	Lee *et al.*, 2015a

Table 3: *(Contd...)*

Table 3: *(Contd...)*

Flavonoid(s)	***Plants/Dietary source***	***Specific mechanism of action***	***Reference***
		• Reduction in mRNA levels of MCP-1, TNF-α and IL-6 levels	Moreover Guo *et al.*, 2014
Delphinidin 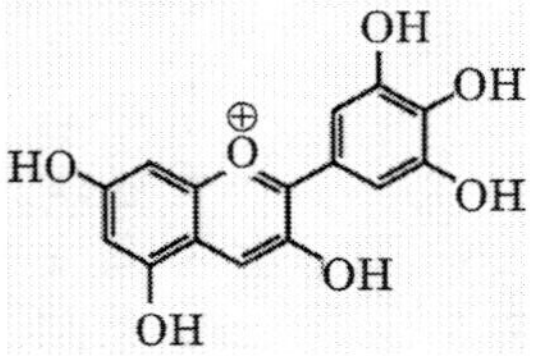	Pomegranate, berries, dark grapes, eggplant, tomato, carrot, purple sweet potato, red cabbage and red onion	• Down regulation of the gluconeogenic enzyme, glucose-6-phosphatase • Increased glucose uptake by cells • Stimulates glucagon-like peptide-1 secretion • increase insulin secretion	Rojo *et al.*, 2012 Gharib *et al.*, 2013 Kato *et al.*, 2015 Johnson and de Mejia, 2016
Malvidin 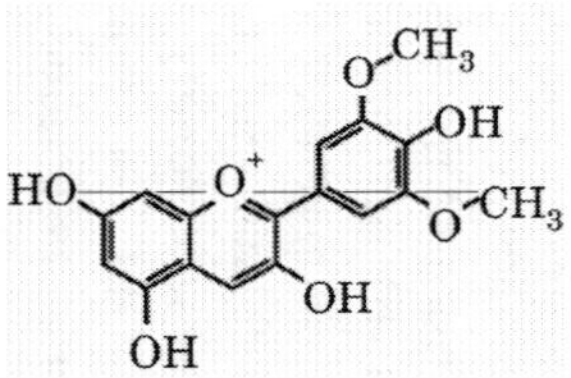	Alcoholic beverages, skins of black grapes, red wine also in other plants.	• Activation of AMPK • Inhibition of pancreatic alpha-amylase	Park *et al.*, 2015 Nickavar and Amin, 2010
Pelargonidin 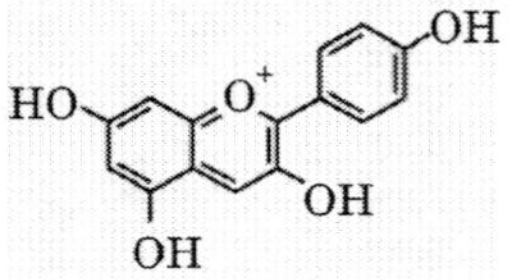	Raspberries, blueberries, blackberries, cranberries and saskatoon berries	• Reduction in TBARS formation • Reduction in nitrite levels • Decrease in oxidative stress	Mirshekar *et al.*, 2010

3.1. Flavonols

Flavonols, a plentiful flavonoids available in nature. Quercetin, kaempferol, isorhamnetin, myricetin and rutin are the main flavonols present in various fruits and vegetables (Vinayagam and Xu, 2015, Hossain *et al.,* 2016).

3.1.1. *Quercetin*

Among the other flavonols, quercetin is the most plentiful flavonoids present in the human diet. Quercetin is found in apples, berries, red onions, grapes, cherries, broccoli, pepper, coriander, citrus fruits and tea and at high concentrations in capers (Vinayagam and Xu, 2015; Hossain *et al.,* 2016).

Quercetin is known for inhibition of nitric oxide (NO) production, antioxidant, anti-hyperglycemic, anti-inflammatory, cytoprotective, hepatoprotective and chemopreventive activities (Vinayagam and Xu, 2015; Hossain *et al.,* 2016).

In vitro studies including pancreatic β-cells and *in vivo* studies in diabetic animals showed that quercetin improves oxidative stress, NF-κβ, pro-inflammatory cytokines (IL-1β and IL-6) and synthesis of oxidized LDL and TNF-α. It also suppresses apoptosis markers (caspase-3, caspase-9, Blc-2 and Bax) in *in vivo* experiments (Kittl *et al.,* 2016; Wang *et al.,* 2016; Zhang *et al.,* 2016; Roslan *et al.,* 2017). Quercetin is also known for its *in vivo* and *in-vitro* insulinotropic actions hence, it may be helpful in metabolic syndrome like DM. Kittl *et al.* (2016), reported that quercetin enhances insulin release and reduces the viability of rat INS-1 β- cells. This study was conducted to better understand short- and long-term effects of quercetin on pancreatic β-cells. Authors conclude that quercetin acutely stimulates insulin release, presumably by transient K_{ATP} channel inhibition and ICa stimulation. Long-term application of quercetin inhibits cell proliferation and induces apoptosis, most likely by inhibition of PI3K/Akt signaling (Kittl *et al.,* 2016). In another *in vitro* study conducted by Miladpour *et al.* (2016), shows that quercetin potentiates transdifferentiation of bone marrow mesenchymal stem cells into the β- cells. This study reveals that quercetin has a strengthening effect on the differentiation of rat bone marrow mesenchymal stem cells into β-cells and increases insulin secretion from the differentiated β-cells. Wang *et al.* (2016), reported that quercetin decreases insulin resistance by improving inflammatory microenvironment in polycystic ovary syndrome rat. The underlying mechanism involves the inhibition of the Toll-like receptor/NF-κB signaling pathway and the improvement in the inflammatory microenvironment. A study conducted on Caco-2E intestinal cells documented that the transport of fructose and glucose by GLUT-2 was strongly inhibited by quercetin. In addition, quercetin stimulates GLUT-4 translocation and expression in skeletal muscle, by mechanisms associated with the activation of AMPK rather than insulin-dependent pathways such as Akt (Vinayagam and Xu, 2015). Inhibition of tyrosine kinase is another mechanism by which quercetin is reported to have effects against diabetes (Vinayagam and Xu, 2015).

3.1.2. *Kaempferol*

Kaempferol is rich in *Ginkgo biloba* L., apple, grape, tomato, tea, potato, broccoli, spinach and some edible berries.

In vitro study in INS-1E cells and human islets results demonstrated that kaempferol treatment promotes viability in palmitate-induced apoptosis and dysfunction. These protective effects of kaempferol are associated with modulation of PDX-1 expression, improved cAMP signaling, anti-apoptotic protein expression and insulin secretion and synthesis in β-cells (Zhang *et al.,* 2013). In hepatocyte, gene expression analysis in high-fat-diet-induced diabetic obese mice showed kaempferol decrease the PPAR-γ and SREBP-1c expression. The anti-obese and anti-diabetic properties of kaempferol were regulated by SREBP-1c and PPAR-γ modulation through AMPK activation (Zhang *et al.,*2015; Hossain *et al.,* 2016).

In vivo study conducted by Alkhalidy *et al.* (2015), showed that long-term dietary supplementation of kaempferol prevents high-fat-diet-induced metabolic disorders in middle-aged obese mice. On cellular and molecular levels, kaempferol improves glycolysis, glucose uptake, glycogen synthesis, AMPK activity and GLUT-4 expression in skeletal muscle. In addition, dietary supplementation of kaempferol significantly ameliorated hyperglycemia and preserved functional islet mass in old adult obese diabetic mice. The action of kaempferol (50 or 150 mg/kg) was evaluated for insulin resistance in 6-week high-fat diet plus streptozotocin (STZ) treated rats. The results showed that kaempferol ameliorated blood lipids and insulin in a dose-dependent manner. Kaempferol effectively restored insulin resistance, it inhibited the phosphorylation of insulin receptor substrate-1 (IRS-1), IkB kinase α (IKKα) and IkB kinase β (IKKβ). These effects were accompanied by a reduction in nucleic and cytosol levels of NF-κB, TNF-α and IL-6 levels (Luo *et al.,* 2015). Al-Numair *et al.* (2015a), evaluate the protective effect of kaempferol against oxidative stress in STZ-induced diabetic rats. Administration of kaempferol to diabetic rats ameliorates plasma glucose, insulin, lipid peroxidation products, enzymatic (superoxide dismutase, catalase, glutathione peroxidase, and glutathione-S-transferase) and non-enzymatic antioxidants (vitamin C, vitamin E, reduced glutathione) levels in liver, kidney, and heart of diabetic rats. Restoration of deranged membrane-bound ATPases in STZ-induced diabetic rats is reported by Al-Numair *et al. (*2015b). Kaempferol also found to show a notable inhibition activity on α-glucosidase in a mixed-type manner with IC_{50} value of $(1.16 \pm 0.04) \times 10^{-5}$ mol/L. Kaempferol bound to α-glucosidase with high affinity and resulted in conformational alteration of α-glucosidase. Authors proposed that kaempferol may interact with some amino acid residues located within the active site of α-glucosidase, occupying the catalytic center of the enzyme to avoid the entrance of p-nitrophenyl-α-D-glucopyranoside and ultimately inhibiting the enzyme activity (Peng *et al.,* 2016).

3.1.3. *Isorhamnetin*

Isorhamnetin, an O-methylated flavonol, is commonly found in medicinal plants such as *Ginkgo biloba*, *Hippophae rhamnoides* and *Oenanthe javanica*. It has several biological properties, including anti-diabetic activities (Vinayagam and Xu, 2015; Hossain *et al.,* 2016). Oral administration of isorhamnetin (10 and 20 mg/kg BW, for 10 days) to STZ-induced diabetes rats ameliorated hyperglycemia and oxidative stress (Yokozawa *et al.,* 2002). Administration of isorhamnetin to diabetic rats caused not only a significant inhibition of serum glucose concentration but also sorbitol accumulation in the lenses, red blood cells, and sciatic nerves (Lee *et al.,* 2005), in addition it also showed aldose reductase inhibitory activity in rat lens (Lim *et al.,* 2006). There is experimental evidence suggesting that isorhamnetin glycosides may possess the antidiabetic effect and their influence on lipid content, endoplasmic reticulum stress markers and the expression of enzymes regulating lipid metabolism (Rodríguez-Rodríguez *et al.*, 2015). Shibano *et al.* (2008), reported that isorhamnetin inhibited the activity of α-glucosidase from rat intestine. Middha *et al.* (2013), conducted silicon–based combinatorial pharmacophore modeling and docking studies, the authors concludes that isorhamnetine could prove to be successful drug candidates for the treatment of diabetes as they are potent, selective, orally bioavailable and nontoxic GSK-3β inhibitors. Isorhamnetin reported for its NF-κB signaling pathway, decrease the production of inflammatory mediators and attenuated oxidative stress in type 2 diabetic rats (Qiu *et al.,* 2016).

3.1.4. *Fisetin*

Fisetin (3,3',4',7-tetrahydroxy flavone) is a dietary flavonoid found in various fruits (strawberries, apples, mangoes, persimmons, kiwis, and grapes), vegetables (tomatoes, onions, and cucumbers), nuts and wine. Fisetin has been reported for its strong anti-inflammatory, anti-oxidant, anti-tumorigenic, anti-invasive, anti-angiogenic, anti-diabetic, neuroprotective and cardioprotective effects in cell culture and in animal models relevant to human diseases (Pal *et al.,* 2016).

Constantin *et al.* (2010), reported that the fisetin inhibition of pyruvate transport into the mitochondria and the reduction of the cytosolic NADH-

NAD $^{(+)}$ potential redox could be the causes of the gluconeogenesis inhibition. A study conducted in human monocytic (THP-1) cells cultured in hyperglycemic condition showed that fisetin (3–10 μM) for 48 h ameliorates NF-κB activation and pro-inflammatory cytokine (IL-6 and TNF-α) release. Fisetin treatment also reduced CBP/p300 gene expression, as well as the levels of acetylation and histone acetyl transferase (HAT) activity of the CBP/p300 protein, which is a known NF-Kb coactivator (Kim *et al.,* 2012). Oral administration of fisetin (10 mg/kg body weight) to diabetic rats for 30 days established a significant decline in blood glucose and glycosylated hemoglobin levels and a significant increase in plasma insulin level. In addition, the mRNA and protein expression levels of gluconeogenic genes, such as phosphoenolpyruvate carboxykinase (PEPCK) and glucose-6-phosphatase, were decreased in diabetic liver tissues (Prasath *et al.,* 2014). Fisetin modulates altered activities of enzymes hexokinase, pyruvate kinase, lactate dehydrogenase, glucose-6-phosphatase, fructose-1,6-bisphosphatase, glucose-6-phosphate dehydrogenase (G6PD), glycogen synthase and glycogen phosphorylase in liver and kidney tissues of diabetic rats (Prasath and Subramanian, 2011). In another study, fisetin treatment showed a significant decline in the levels of blood glucose, glycosylated hemoglobin (HbA1c), NF-kB p65 unit in pancreas and IL-1β in plasma, serum NO with an elevation in plasma insulin. The treatment also improved the antioxidant status in the pancreas as well as a plasma of diabetic rats indicating the antioxidant potential of fisetin (Prasath *et al.,* 2013). Fisetin also showed a protective effect on cataract development in an STZ-induced experimental cataract model (Kan *et al.,* 2014).

3.1.5. *Myricetin*

Myricetin is commonly found in tea, berries, fruits, wines and medicinal plants. It mimics insulin in stimulating lipogenesis and glucose transport in rat adipocytes *in vitro*. It was found that myricetin stimulates lipogenesis in rat adipocytes and enhance the stimulatory effect of insulin. Treatment with myricetin increased hepatic glycogen and glucose-6-phosphate content. It increased hepatic glycogen synthase-I activity and lowered phosphorylase activity in the muscle (Ong and Khoo, 2000). Liu *et al.* (2005), investigated that IV injection of myricetin decreased the plasma glucose concentrations in a dose-dependent manner in STZ-diabetic rats. The increase of glucose utilization by myricetin was further characterized using the enhancement of glycogen synthesis in isolated hepatocytes of STZ-diabetic rats. These results suggest that myricetin has an ability to enhance glucose utilization to lower plasma glucose in diabetic rats lacking insulin. In continuation of above study, the same group of researchers evaluated myricetin for plasma glucose lowering action in STZ-induced diabetic rats and tried to draw its mechanism of action. Findings of this study support that the plasma glucose-lowering action of myricetin in insulin-deficient animals is mediated by activation of opioid μ-receptors of peripheral tissues in response to increased β-endorphin secretion. Opioid μ-receptor activation is held responsible for the enhancement of muscle GLUT-4 gene expression and the attenuation of hepatic PEPCK gene expression observed in these myricetin-treated diabetic animals (Liu *et al.,* 2006). Liu *et al.* continued his research on myricetin and evaluated its action on the improvement of insulin sensitivity in obese Zucker rats. The outcome of findings indicates that myricetin improves insulin sensitivity through increased post-receptor insulin signaling mediated by enhancements in IRS-1-associated PI3-kinase and GLUT-4 activity in muscles of obese Zucker rats (Liu *et al.,* 2007). In another study, myricetin is evaluated on insulin resistance in mice fed a high-fat, high-sucrose diet. Findings of the study suggest that myricetin may have a protective effect against diet-induced obesity and insulin resistance in mice fed HFHS diet and that alleviation of insulin resistance could partly occur by improving obesity and reducing serum proinflammatory cytokine levels (Choi *et al.,* 2014). It is reported that administration of myricetin to STZ-cadmium induced diabetic nephrotoxic rats significantly normalizes the carbohydrate metabolic products like glucose, glycated hemoglobin, glycogen phosphorylase and gluconeogenic enzymes and renal function markers with increased insulin, glycogen, glycogen synthase and expression of GLUT-2, GLUT-4, insulin receptor-1, insulin receptor-2 and protein kinase B (Kandasamy and Ashokkumar, 2014). Myricetin is also evaluated for *in vitro* inhibitory potential against α-glucosidase and α-amylase (Figueiredo-González *et al.,* 2016).

3.1.6. *Rutin*

Rutin is a flavonoid with several pharmacological properties present in buckwheat, oranges, grapes, lemons, limes, peaches and berries (Vinayagam and Xu, 2015). Diabetic mice fed with rutin (100 mg/kg) displayed a significantly lower of plasma glucose and increase in insulin levels along with the restoration of glycogen content and the activities of carbohydrate metabolic enzymes (Prince and Kamalakkannan, 2006). Rutin significantly stimulates the calcium uptake through voltage-dependent calcium channels as well as amitogen-activated kinase (MEK) and protein kinase A (PKA) signaling pathways. In addition, rutin stimulates glucose uptake in the soleus muscle and this effect was mediated by extracellular calcium and calcium-calmodulin-dependent protein kinase II (CaMKII) activation (Kappel *et al.,* 2013). In another study, the author reported that rutin stimulates glucose uptake in the rat soleus muscle *via* the protein kinase C (PI3K) and mitogen-activated protein kinase (MAPK) pathways. Rutin may have an influence on glucose transporter translocation and may directly activate the transporter GLUT-4 the synthesis (Kappel *et al.,* 2013b). This observation is further confirmed by Hsu *et al.* (2014), by conducting the study, rutin potentiates insulin receptor kinase to enhance insulin-dependent GLUT-4 translocation. Niture *et al.* (2014) reported that rutin exhibit significant antidiabetic activity, presumably by inhibiting inflammatory cytokines, improving antioxidant and plasma lipid profiles in high-fat diet and STZ-induced type 2 diabetic rat. More recently, Aitken *et al.* (2017) reported that rutin suppresses human-amylin/hIAPP misfolding and oligomer formation *in-vitro*, and ameliorates diabetes and its impacts in human-amylin/hIAPP transgenic mice.

3.2. Flavanones

Naringenin, hesperidin, eriodictyol and niringin are the major flavanones have been reported to possess antioxidant, antidiabetic, lipid-lowering, anti-atherogenic, and anti-inflammatory activities (Vinayagam and Xu, 2015; Hossain *et al.,* 2016)

3.2.1. *Naringenin*

Naringenin is a weak phytoestrogen found in grapefruit, orange, and tomato. It improves diabetes, inflammation, neuronal diseases, cardiovascular diseases and cancers.

In vitro studies have shown that naringenin had an insulin mimic effect to decrease apolipoprotein B secretion in hepatocytes (Van Acker *et al.,* 2000). Ren *et al.* (2016) reported that naringenin inhibited NF-κB activation and intercellular adhesion molecule-1 (ICAM-1) mRNA expression in palmitic acid-treated endothelial cells and improved nitric oxide production in the presence of insulin. Moreover, oral administration of naringenin exerts significant inhibition of intestinal α-glucosidase activity *in vivo* thereby delaying the absorption of carbohydrates in diabetic rats, thus resulting in significant lowering of postprandial blood glucose levels (Priscilla *et al.,* 2014). Naringenin regulates glucose and lipid metabolism and ameliorates vascular dysfunction in type 2 diabetic rats (Ren *et al.,* 2016). It is reported that naringenin ameliorates renal impairment by downregulation of TGF-β1 and IL-1 *via* modulation of oxidative stress correlates with decreased apoptotic events in the STZ-induced diabetic rat (Roy *et al.,* 2016). In addition, a study conducted by Yan *et al.* (2016), in diabetic nephropathic rats naringenin ameliorated kidney injury through Let-7a/TGFBR1 signaling in diabetic nephropathy. In a recent study, Yoshida and colleague reported that naringenin interferes with the anti-diabetic actions of pioglitazone *via* pharmacodynamic interactions (Yoshida *et al.,* 2016).

3.2.2. *Hesperidin*

Hesperidin is a flavone glycoside abundant in citrus fruits such as lemons and limes that show lipid-lowering and antidiabetic effects. Hesperidin supplementation regulated the activities of glycolytic and gluconeogenesis enzymes of hepatic glucose metabolism and improved hyperglycemia in db/db, C57BL6 mice (Jung *et al.,* 2004; Jung and Choi, 2014). Hesperidin is reported to possess hyperglycemic activity mediated through attenuation of oxidative stress and proinflammatory cytokine production in high fat fed/STZ-induced type 2 diabetic rats (Mahmoud *et al.,* 2012; Visnagri *et al.,* 2014). Hesperidin not only attenuated the diabetic condition but also showed neuromodulatory effects *via* control over hyperglycemia to the down-regulate generation of free radical, release of proinflammatory cytokines in a STZ-induced rodent model (Ashafaq *et al.,* 2014). Treatment with hesperidin (100 mg/kg body weight) for twenty four weeks to STZ-induced diabetic rats, normalised SOD, catalase, glutathione and inflammatory cytokines (TNF-α, IL-1β), caspase-3, glial fibrillary acidic protein levels and aquaporin-4(AQP4) expression in the retina (Kumar *et al.,* 2013).

3.2.3. *Eriodictyol*

Eriodictyol [2-(3,4-dihydroxyphenyl)-5,7-dihydroxy-2,3-dihydrochromen-4-one] is a flavonoid present in lemon fruit. It has reported possessing anti-inflammatory and antioxidant activities. Eriodictyol has been demonstrated (Miyake *et al.,* 1998) that supplementation of lemon flavonoids, such as eriocitrin and hesperidin, significantly suppressed the oxidative stress in diabetic rats. An *in vitro* study conducted by Zhang *et al.* (2012) reported that eriodictyol increased insulin-stimulated glucose uptake in both human hepatocellular liver carcinoma cells (HepG2) and differentiated 3T3-L1 adipocytes under high-glucose conditions. Eriodictyol also up-regulated the mRNA expression of PPAR└2 and adipocyte-specific fatty acid-binding protein (aP2) as well as the protein levels of PPAR└2 in differentiated 3T3-L1 adipocytes. Further more, it reactivated Akt in HepG2 cells with high-glucose-induced insulin resistance. This response was strongly inhibited by pretreatment with the phosphatidylinositol 3-kinase (PI3K) inhibitor LY294002, indicating that eriodictyol increased Akt phosphorylation by activating the PI3K/Akt pathway. Eriodictyol treatment to STZ-induced diabetic rats significantly lowered retinal TNF-α, ICAM-1, VEGF, and eNOS in a dose-dependent manner. Further, treatment with eriodictyol significantly suppressed diabetes-related lipid peroxidation, as well as the BRB breakdown (Bucolo *et al.,* 2012). Administration of citrus flavanones, hesperidin, eriocitrin and eriodictyol increased the serum total antioxidant capacity and restrained the elevation of interleukin-6 (IL-6), macrophage chemoattractant protein-1 (MCP-1), and C-reactive protein (hs-CRP) in C57BL/6J mice fed high-fat diet. In addition, eriocitrin and eriodictyol reduced TBARS levels in the blood serum, and hesperidin and eriodictyol also reduced fat accumulation and liver damage (Ferreira *et al.,* 2016). These reports imply that eriodictyol possess antidiabetic properties and it also improves diabetic related complications.

3.2.4. *Naringin*

Naringin (4',5,7- trihydroxy flavanone-7-rhamnoglucoside) is a major flavanone glycoside obtained from tomatoes, grapefruits and many other citrus fruits. It has been experimentally documented to possess numerous biological properties such as antioxidant, anti-inflammatory, antiapoptotic and antidiabetic activities (Bharti *et al.,* 2014). *In vitro* study conducted in L6 muscle cells report showed that naringin ameliorates oxidative stress and increases glucose uptake (Dhanya *et al.,* 2015). In addition, naringin is effective in protecting against the development of metabolic syndrome through changing the expression of hepatic genes involved in lipid metabolism and gluconeogenesis *via* upregulation of both PPAR and 5' adenosine monophosphate-activated protein kinase (AMPK), involving the activation of multiple types of intracellular signaling in mice exposed to a HFD (Pu *et al.,* 2012). Chen *et al.* (2015) naringin alleviates diabetic kidney disease through inhibiting oxidative stress and inflammatory reaction. Recently, Liu and colleague reported that naringin ameliorates cognitive deficits in STZ-induced diabetic rats (Liu *et al.,* 2016).

3.3. Flavone

Flavones are another class of flavonoids found mainly in celery, parsley, and many different herbs. The major dietary flavones include apigenin, luteolin and tangeritin have been reported to possess antioxidant, anti-inflammatory antidiabetic properties (Jiang *et al.,* 2016).

3.3.1. *Apigenin*

Apigenin is a member of the flavone family and is found in many fruits, vegetables, nuts, onion, orange and tea. Plants containing apigenin, such as passionflower and chamomile, have been used as traditional medicines to treat a variety of diseases (Vinayagam and Xu, 2015, Hossain *et al.,* 2016).

Oral administration of apigenin (0.78 mg/kg body weight) for 10 days was reported to reverse the reduction in hepatic antioxidants in alloxan-induced insulin-dependent diabetic mice, confirming the free-radical scavenging activity (Panda and Kar, 2007). In STZ-induced diabetic rats, intraperitoneal administration of apigenin had a significant anti-hyperglycemic effect (Rauter *et al.,* 2010). In clonal β-cells, apigenin treatment attenuated 2-deoxy-D-ribose-induced apoptosis through its antioxidant effect by controlling the mitochondrial membrane potential (Suh *et al.,* 2012). In human THP-1 monotypic cells, apigenin suppressed TNF-α- and IL-1β-induced activation of NF-κB (Zhang *et al.,* 2014) and, in HepG2 hepatocytes, the flavonoid improved AMPK phosphorylation (Zang *et al.,* 2006). Administration of apigenin 50 or 100 mg/kg once a day for 6 weeks to high-fat diet and STZ induced type 2 diabetic rats ameliorates blood glucose, glycated serum protein, serum lipid, insulin, superoxide dismutase (SOD), malonaldehyde and intercellular adhesion molecule-1 (ICAM-1). In addition, *in vitro*, apigenin inhibited NF-κB activation and ICAM-1 mRNA expression in PA-treated endothelial cells and improved nitric oxide production in the presence of insulin (Ren *et al.,* 2016). Apigenin also preserves the cellular architecture of vital tissues towards normal in STZ-induced diabetic rats and enhanced GLUT4 translocation upon apigenin treatment suggests more glucose lowering as well as β-cell preserving efficacy (Hossain *et al.,* 2014).

In vitro study conducted by Qin *et al.* (2016), showed that apigenin protected against endothelial dysfunction *via* inhibiting phosphorylation of protein kinase C βII (PKCβII) expression and downstream reactive oxygen species (ROS) production in endothelial cells exposed to high glucose. Furthermore, apigenin reduced high glucose-increased apoptosis, Bax expression, caspase-3 activity and phosphorylation of NF-κB in endothelial cells. Moreover, apigenin effectively restored high glucose-reduced Bcl-2 expression and Akt phosphorylation. Importantly, apigenin significantly increased NO production in endothelial cells subjected to high glucose challenge.

3.3.2. *Luteolin*

Luteolin is a flavone obtained from celery, onion leaves, cabbage, broccoli, parsley, carrots, apple skins, green pepper, perilla leaf and chamomile tea. Luteolin has been reported to possess antimutagenic, antitumorigenic, antioxidant, anti-inflammatory and antidiabetic properties (Vinayagam and Xu, 2015, Hossain *et al.,* 2016). Kim *et al.* (2014), reported that luteolin inhibits hyperglycemia-induced proinflammatory cytokine(IL-6 and TNF-α) production and its epigenetic mechanism in human monocytes. The results obtained from molecular docking study indicated that luteolin had a high affinity close to the active site pocket of α-glucosidase and indirectly inhibited the catalytic activity of the enzyme (Yan *et al.,* 2014). Moreover, luteolin prevents uric acid-induced pancreatic β-cell dysfunction (Ding *et al.,* 2014). *In vitro* study conducted in human hepatic cells (HepG2) showed that luteolin induces FOXO1 translocation but inhibit gluconeogenic and lipogenic gene expression (Bumke-Vogt *et al.,* 2014). Luteolin attenuates adipocyte-derived inflammatory responses *via* suppression of nuclear factor-κB/mitogen-activated protein kinases pathway (Nepali *et al.,* 2015). Luteolin also shows anti-diabetic potential in KK-A(y) mice. Treatment with luteolin significantly improved blood glucose, HbA1c, insulin, and HOMR-IR levels (Zang *et al.,* 2016a). Zhang *et al.* (2016b), also reported that luteolin reduces obesity-associated insulin resistance in mice by activating AMPKα1 signalling in adipose tissue macrophages.

3.3.3. *Tangeretin*

Tangeretin, which is prevalent in citrus fruits, including mandarins and oranges. Administration of HFD plus 200 mg/kg bw of tangeretin exhibited a reduction in body weight, total cholesterol (TG), blood glucose and decreased adipocytokines such as adiponectin, leptin, resistin, IL-6, and MCP-1 (Kim *et al.,* 2012). Oral administration of tangeretin (100 mg/kg bw) to STZ-induced diabetic rats for 30 days modulates the activities of hepatic enzymes (hexokinase, pyruvate kinase, lactate dehydrogenase, glucose-6-phosphatase, fructose-1,6-bisphosphatase, G6PD, glycogen synthase and glycogen phosphorylase) *via* enhanced secretion of insulin and decreases the blood glucose by its antioxidant potential (Sundaram *et al.,* 2014). Tangeretin increased the secretion of an insulin-sensitizing factor, adiponectin, but concomitantly decreased the secretion of an insulin-resistance factor, monocyte chemotactic protein-1 (MCP-1), in 3T3-L1 adipocytes (Miyata *et al.,* 2011). Kim *et al.* (2012), reported that tangeretin stimulates glucose uptake *via* regulation of AMPK signaling pathways in C2C12 myotubes and improves glucose tolerance in high-fat diet-induced obese mice.

3.4. Isoflavone

Isoflavones are another class of flavonoids commonly found in leguminous plants, including soyabean and soya products; the major dietary isoflavones are daidzein and genistein, which are present primarily in soy foods. Numerous studies have suggested that isoflavones favorably affect adiposity, glucose homeostasis, insulin secretion and lipid metabolism (Vinayagam and Xu, 2015; Hossain *et al.,* 2016). Ding *et al.* (2016), evaluate the association between soy food and isoflavone consumption and risk of type 2 diabetes in US men and women. The study result revelled that intake of isoflavones was associated with a modestly lower type 2 diabetes risk in US men and women who typically consumed low-to-moderate amounts of soy foods (Vinayagam and Xu, 2015; Hossain *et al.,* 2016).

3.4.1. *Daidzein*

Daidzein belongs to the isoflavone subclass of flavonoids and is found in fruits, nuts, soybeans, and soya-based products (Vinayagam and Xu, 2015; Hossain *et al.,* 2016). Daidzein protects a human umbilical vein endothelial cells (HUVECs) against high-glucose-induced oxidative damage. Treatment with daidzein reduced oxidative stress and significantly increased cell viability. In addition, lipid peroxidation, intracellular ROS generation, and indirect nitric oxide levels induced by the high glucose treatment were significantly reduced in the presence of daidzein (0.02-0.1 mM) in a dose-dependent manner. High glucose levels induced the overexpression of inducible nitric oxide synthase (iNOS), cyclooxygenase-2 (COX-2), and NF-κB proteins in HUVECs, which was suppressed by treatment with 0.04 mM daidzein (Park, 2016). Cheong *et al.* (2014) reported that daidzein promotes glucose uptake through GLUT-4 translocation to the plasma membrane in L6 myocytes and improves glucose homeostasis in type 2 diabetic model mice. In addition, daidzein supplementation markedly improved the AMPK phosphorylation in gastrocnemius muscle of db/db mice. Daidzein showed prominent inhibitory effects against α-glucosidase and α-amylase in STZ-induced diabetic mice (Park *et al.,* 2013). A study conducted by Choi and colleague (2008) suggest that daidzein regulates glucose homeostasis in type 1 diabetic mice by down-regulating G6Pase, PEPCK, fatty acid β-oxidation and CPT activities, while up-regulating malic enzyme and G6PD activities in liver with preservation of pancreatic β-cells.

3.4.2. *Genistein*

Genistein, a naturally occurring soy isoflavone, is a flavonoid presented in legumes and Chinese plants *Genista tinctoria* Linn and *Sophora subprostrala* Chun. Genistein has been reported to improve hyperglycemia caused human vascular endothelial inflammation *ex vivo*, which is at least partially mediated through promoting the cAMP/PKA signaling pathway (Patisaul and Jefferson, 2010). Furthermore, genistein has been shown to protect against oxidative stress and inflammation, neuropathic pain, and neurotrophic and vasculature deficits in the diabetic mouse model (Valsecchi *et al.,* 2011). Indeed, recent findings indicated that genistein administration significantly decreased β-cells loss and improved glucose and insulin levels (El-Kordy *et al.,* 2015). Genistein supplementation improved fasting glucose levels and cutaneous wound closure rate in alloxan induced diabetic mice. Moreover, genistein supplementation restored NLRP3 inflammasome (NLRP3, ASC and caspase-1) at the basal level and ameliorated both inflammation (TNFα, iNOS, COX2 and NFκB) and antioxidant defense system (Nrf2, HO-1, GPx, and catalase) during early stage of wound healing in diabetic mice (Eo *et al.,* 2016).

3.5. Flavan-3-ols

Flavan-3-ols are also referred to as flavanols and are present in various fruits, cocoa, and chocolates (Vinayagam and Xu, 2015; Hossain *et al.,* 2016). In fruits and cocoa, the most common flavan-3-ols are catechin and epicatechin, while in grapes, teas, and seeds of certain leguminous plants, the main flavan-3-ols are epicatechingallate, gallocatechin, epigallocatechin and epigallocatechin gallate.

Sphingomyelinases (SMases) are key enzymes involved in many diseases including diabetes mellitus. Strong inhibition of secretory sphingomyelinase by catechins, particularly by (-)-Epicatechin 3-O-gallate and (-)-3'-O-Methylepigallocatechin 3-O-gallate is reported by Kobayashi *et al.* (2016).

Epigallocatechin-3-gallate is also known for its anti-oxidative and anti-inflammatory effect against various human diseases. It protects retinal vascular endothelial cells from high glucose stress *in vitro* by regulating of inflammatory cytokines and inhibition of the MAPK/ERK-VEGF pathway (Zhang *et al.,* 2016).

Epidemiological studies suggest that moderate consumption of cacao-derived products (*i.e.,* chocolate and cocoa) may reduce the risk of diabetes, myocardial infarction, and cardiovascular disease-associated mortality. Moreover, interventional studies have also suggested that dark chocolate and cocoa consumption is vasculoprotective in normal and type 2 diabetic individuals. (-)-Epicatechin is the main flavanol present in cacao and suggested to be responsible for the beneficial effects observed after dark chocolate/cocoa consumption (Moreno-Ulloa and Moreno-Ulloa, 2016).

Evidence from studies in humans and experimental animals suggest that consumption of the flavan-3-ol (-)-epicatechin and of flavan-3-ol (-)-epicatechin-rich foods may improve insulin sensitivity. In addition, (-)-Epicatechin improves insulin sensitivity in high fat diet-fed mice (Cremonini *et al.,* 2016). Cordero-Herrera *et al.* (2015), reported that (-)-Epicatechin attenuates high-glucose-induced inflammation by epigenetic modulation and decreased NF-κB and TNF-α levels in human monocytes.

3.6. Anthocyanins

Anthocyanidins are another class of flavonoids widely distributed in fruits, vegetables, berries, and red wine. The potential health benefits of anthocyanins include anti-inflammatory, antioxidant, anti-obesity and anti-diabetic effects. More than 600 anthocyanin compounds have been identified; the most prevalent of these compounds include cyanidin, delphinidin, malvidin, peonidin, pelargonidin and petunidin (Vinayagam and Xu, 2015, Hossain *et al.,* 2016). Anthocyanins from fermented berry beverages modulated gene and protein expression to increase insulin secretion from pancreatic β-cells *in vitro* (Johnson and de Mejia, 2016).

3.6.1. *Cyanidin*

Cyanidin and its glycosides belong to anthocyanins and are widely distributed in various human diets through crops, vegetables, fruits, and red wine (Vinayagam and Xu, 2015, Hossain *et al.,* 2016).

The active principle cyanidin 3,5-diglucoside from aronia juice has an inhibitory effect on dipeptidyl peptidase (DPP IV) activity. In addition, it reduces blood glucose levels in diabetes model KK-Ay mice. Furthermore, α-glucosidase activity was inhibited in the upper region of the small intestine KK-Ay diabetic mice. Which induced a reduction of glucose-dependent insulinotropic polypeptide (GIP) level (Yamane *et al.,* 2016).

Cyanidin-3-glucoside (C3G) isolated from mulberry fruits showed cytoprotective actions against pancreatic β-cell apoptosis caused by hydrogen peroxide-induced oxidative stress in MIN6 pancreatic β-cells. C3G inhibited the phosphorylation of ERK and p38 without inducing the phosphorylation of JNK. Furthermore, C3G regulated the intrinsic apoptotic pathway-associated proteins, such as proteins belonging to the Bcl-2 family, cytochrome c and caspase-3 (Lee *et al.,* 2015a). In addition, cyanidin-3-glucoside isolated from mulberry fruits protects pancreatic β-cells against glucotoxicity-induced apoptosis. C3G decreased the generation of intracellular reactive oxygen species, DNA fragmentation and the rate of apoptosis. C3G also prevented pancreatic β–cell apoptosis induced by high glucose conditions by interfering with the intrinsic apoptotic pathways (Lee *et al.,* 2015b).

Moreover Guo *et al.* (2014) showed that C3G significantly reduced macrophage infiltration and the mRNA levels of MCP-1,TNF-α and IL-6 in adipose tissue and phosphorylation of FoxO1 *via* the Akt-dependent pathway, and the extent of phosphorylation represents the FoxO1 transcriptional activity in liver and adipose tissues of HFD and db/db mice.

3.6.2. *Delphinidin*

Delphinidin present in pomegranate, berries, dark grapes, eggplant, tomato, carrot, purple sweet potato, red cabbage and red onion and it possesses strong antioxidant activities (Vinayagam and Nutrition, 2015).

Rojo *et al.* (2012), studied *in vitro* and *in vivo* anti-diabetic effects of delphinidin 3-sambubioside-5-glucoside (D3S5G) isolated from maqui berry . Oral administration of D3S5G improved fasting blood glucose levels and glucose tolerance in hyperglycaemic obese C57BL/6J mice fed a high fat diet. In H4IIE rat liver cells, D3S5G decreased glucose production and enhanced the insulin-stimulated down regulation of the gluconeogenic enzyme, glucose-6-phosphatase. In L6 myotubes D3S5G treatment increased both insulin and non-insulin mediated glucose uptake. In another *in vitro* and *in vivo* study, daily administration of 100 mg/kg delphinidin chloride-loaded liposomes to diabetic mice for eight weeks decreased the rate of albumin and HbA1c glycation (Gharib *et al.,* 2013). Kato *et al.* (2015), reported that delphinidin 3-rutinoside stimulates glucagon-like peptide-1 secretion in murine GLU Tag cell line *via* the Ca^2+/calmodulin-dependent kinase II pathway. Moreover, delphinidin-3-arabinoside, from fermented berry beverages have the potential to modulate DPP-IV and its substrate GLP-1, to increase insulin secretion, and to upregulate expression of mRNA of insulin-receptor associated genes and proteins in pancreatic β-cells (iNS-1E) (Johnson and de Mejia, 2016). A study conducted in double-blind, placebo-controlled, cross-over fashion in ten volunteers with moderate glucose intolerance showed that Delphinol® (standardized maqui berry extract rich with delphinidin as a principal polyphenol) intake prior to rice consumption statistical significantly lowered post prandial blood glucose and insulin as compared to placebo. The researcher identified an inhibition of Na^+-dependant glucose transport by delphinidin. In a diabetic rat model the daily oral application of Delphinol® over a period of four months significantly lowered fasting blood glucose levels and reached values indistinguishable from healthy non-diabetic rats (Hidalgo *et al.*, 2016). In continuation of above study, Alvarado *et al.* (2016) reported that delphinidin-rich maqui berry extract (Delphinol®) lowers fasting and postprandial glycemia and insulinemia in prediabetic individuals during oral glucose tolerance tests.

3.6.3. *Malvidin*

Cyanidin and malvidin in aqueous extracts of black carrots fermented with *Aspergillus oryzae* prevent the impairment of energy, lipid and glucose metabolism in estrogen-deficient rats by AMPK activation (Park *et al.*, 2015). A blueberry extracts rich with malvidin-3-glucoside showed antiproliferative and apoptotic properties in B16-F10 metastatic murine melanoma cells (Bunea *et al.*, 2013). Moreover, malvidin is reported to possess antioxidant and anti-inflammatory effects in RAW264.7 macrophages (Bognar *et al.*, 2013).

Vaccinium arctostaphylos is a traditional medicinal plant in Iran used for the treatment of diabetes mellitus. *V. arctostaphylos* berries extract showed an inhibitory effect on pancreatic α-amylase *in vitro*. The activity-guided purification of extract led to the isolation of malvidin-3-O-beta-glucoside as an a-amylase inhibitor (Nickavar and Amin, 2010).

3.6.4. *Pelargonidin*

Pelargonidin can be found in ripe raspberries, blueberries, blackberries, cranberries and saskatoon berries (Vinayagam and Xu, 2015, Hossain *et al.*, 2016). Pelargonidin treatment counteracts hyperglycemia and relieves the oxidative stress including hemoglobin (Hb) induced iron mediated oxidative reactions by lowering the glycation level and free iron of Hb (Roy *et al.*, 2008). Pelargonidin was also demonstrated to reduce TBARS formation and non-significantly reversed elevation of nitrite level and reduction of antioxidant defensive enzyme superoxide dismutase in diabetic rats (Mirshekar *et al.,* 2010). In addition, chronic oral pelargonidin 10 mg/kg alleviates learning and memory disturbances in STZ-induced diabetic rats (Mirshekar *et al.,* 2011). Pelargonidin-3-galactoside and its aglycone stimulate insulin secretion in rodent pancreatic β-cells *in vitro* in presence of glucose (Jayaprakasam *et al.,* 2005).

4. CONCLUSIONS

The actual antidiabetic potential associated with flavonoids are usually large as a result of their modulatory effects on blood sugar transporter by enhancing insulin secretion, reducing apoptosis and promoting proliferation of pancreatic β-cells, reducing insulin resistance, inflammation and oxidative stress in muscle and promoting translocation of GLUT4 via PI3K/AKT and AMPK pathways. The molecular mechanisms underlying the glucose and lipid metabolism in diabetes would provide new insights in the field of drug development. With the rapidly increasing incidence of diabetes worldwide, there is a greater need for safe and effective functional biomaterials with antidiabetic activity. Hence, meticulously intended human studies are needed to elucidate the molecular mechanism of flavonoids to treat diabetes and its complication.

REFERENCES

Aitken, J.F., Loomes, K.M., Riba-Garcia, I., Unwin, R.D., Prijic, G., Phillips, A.S. *et al.* (2017). Rutin suppresses human-amylin/hIAPP misfolding and oligomer formation *in-vitro*, and ameliorates diabetes and its impacts in human-amylin/hIAPP transgenic mice. *Biochem. Biophys. Res. Commun.*, 482(4): 625–31.

Alkhalidy, H., Moore, W., Zhang, Y., McMillan, R., Wang, A., Ali, M. *et al.* (2015). Small molecule kaempferol promotes insulin sensitivity and preserved pancreatic 5Þ-cell mass in middle-aged obese diabetic mice. *J. Diab. Res.*, 2015: 1–15.

Al-Numair, K.S., Veeramani, C., Alsaif, M.A. and Chandramohan, G. (2015). Influence of kaempferol, a flavonoid compound, on membrane-bound ATPases in streptozotocin-induced diabetic rats. *Pharm. Biol.*, 8: 1–7.

Al-Numair, K.S., Chandramohan, G., Veeramani, C. and Alsaif, M.A. Ameliorative effect of kaempferol, a flavonoid, on oxidative stress in streptozotocin-induced diabetic rats. *Redox Rep.*, 20(5): 198–09.

Alvarado, J.L., Leschot, A., Olivera-Nappa, Á., Salgado, A.M., Rioseco, H., Lyon, C. *et al.*, Delphinidin-Rich Maqui Berry Extract (Delphinol®) Lowers Fasting and Postprandial Glycemia and Insulinemia in Prediabetic Individuals during Oral Glucose Tolerance Tests. *Biomed. Res. Int.*, 2016: 9070537. doi: 10.1155/2016/9070537.

Ashafaq, M., Varshney, L., Khan, M.H., Salman, M., Naseem, M., Wajid, S. and Parvez, S. (2014). Neuromodulatory effects of hesperidin in mitigating oxidative stress in streptozotocin induced diabetes. *Biomed Res Int.*, 2014: 1–9.

Bharti, S., Rani, N., Krishnamurthy, B. and Arya, D.S. (2014). Preclinical evidence for the pharmacological actions of naringin: a review. Planta Med. 2014;80(6):437-51.

Bognar, E., Sarszegi, Z., Szabo, A., Debreceni, B., Kalman, N., Tucsek, Z., *et al.* (2013). Antioxidant and anti-inflammatory effects in RAW264.7 macrophages of malvidin, a major red wine polyphenol. *PLoS One*, 8(6): e65355. doi: 10.1371/journal.pone.0065355.

Bucolo, C., Leggio, G.M., Drago, F., Salomone, S. (2012). Eriodictyol prevents early retinal and plasma abnormalities in streptozotocin-induced diabetic rats. *Biochem Pharmacol.*, 84(1): 88–92.

Bumke-Vogt, C., Osterhoff, M.A., Borchert, A., Guzman-Perez, V., Sarem, Z., Birkenfeld, A.L. *et al.* (2014). The flavones apigenin and luteolin induce FOXO1 translocation but inhibit gluconeogenic and lipogenic gene expression in human cells. *PLoS One, 9(8): e104321.*

Bunea, A., Rugin , D., Sconc a, Z., Pop, R.M., Pintea, A., Socaciu, C. *et al.* (2013). Anthocyanin determination in blueberry extracts from various cultivars and their antiproliferative and apoptotic properties in B16-F10 metastatic murine melanoma cells. *Phytochemistry*, 95: 436–44.

Chen, F., Zhang, N., Ma, X., Huang, T., Shao, Y., Wu, C. and Wang, Q. (2015). Naringin alleviates diabetic kidney disease through inhibiting oxidative stress and inflammatory reaction. *PLoS One*, 10(11): e0143868. doi: 10.1371/journal.pone.0143868.

Cheong, S.H., Furuhashi, K., Ito, K., Nagaoka, M., Yonezawa, T., Miura, Y. *et al.* (2014). Daidzein promotes glucose uptake through glucose transporter 4 translocation to plasma membrane in L6 myocytes and improves glucose homeostasis in Type 2 diabetic model mice. *J. Nutr. Biochem.*, 25(2): 136–43.

Choi, H.N., Kang, M.J., Lee, S.J. and Kim, J.I. (2014). Ameliorative effect of myricetin on insulin resistance in mice fed a high-fat, high-sucrose diet. *Nutr. Res. Pract.*, 8(5): 544–9.

Choi, M.S., Jung, U.J., Yeo, J., Kim, M.J. and Lee, M.K. (2008). Genistein and daidzein prevent diabetes onset by elevating insulin level and altering hepatic gluconeogenic and lipogenic enzyme activities in non-obese diabetic (NOD) mice. *Diabetes Metab Res. Rev.*, 24(1): 74–81.

Constantin, R.P., Constantin, J., Pagadigorria, C.L., Ishii-Iwamoto, E.L., Bracht, A., Ono Mde, K. *et al.* (2010). The actions of fisetin on glucose metabolism in the rat liver. *Cell Biochem Funct.*, 28: 149–58.

Cordero-Herrera, I., Chen, X., Ramos, S. and Devaraj, S. (2015). (-)-Epicatechin attenuates high-glucose-induced inflammation by epigenetic modulation in human monocytes. *Eur. J. Nutr.*, (2015). doi:10.1007/s00394-015-1136-2.

Cremonini, E., Bettaieb, A., Haj, F.G., Fraga, C.G. and Oteiza, P.I. (2016). (-)-Epicatechin improves insulin sensitivity in high fat diet-fed mice. *Arch. Biochem. Biophys.*, 599: 13–21.

Cristina *et al.* (2016). Restoration of density of interstitial cells of Cajal in the jejunum of diabetic rats after quercetin supplementation. *Rev. Esp. Enferm. Dig.*, doi:10.17235/reed.2016.4338/2016.

Davis, S.N. (2006). General principles of antimicrobial therapy, *In*: Brunton, L.L. (*ed.*), Goodman and Gilman's The Pharmacological Basis of Therapeutics. McGraw-Hill., New York, pp. 1200–328.

Dhanya, R., Arun, K.B., Nisha, V.M., Syama, H.P., Nisha, P., Santhosh, Kumar T.R. *et al.* (2015). Preconditioning L6 muscle cells with naringin ameliorates oxidative stress and increases glucose uptake. *PLoS One*, 10(7): e0132429.

Ding, M., Pan, A., Manson, J.E., Willett, W.C., Malik, V., Rosner, B. *et al.* (2016). Consumption of soy foods and isoflavones and risk of type 2 diabetes: A pooled analysis of three US cohorts. *Eur. J. Clin. Nutr.*, 70(12): 1381–7.

Ding, Y., Shi, X., Shuai, X., Xu, Y., Liu, Y., Liang, X. *et al.* (2014). Luteolin prevents uric acid-induced pancreatic β-cell dysfunction. *J. Biomed. Res.*, 28(4): 292–8.

El-Kordy, E.A. and Alshahrani, A.M. (2015). Effect of genistein, a natural soy isoflavone, on pancreatic-cells of streptozotocin-induced diabetic rats: Histological and immunohistochemical study. *J. Microsc. Ultrastruct.*, 3: 108–19.

Eo, H., Lee, H.J. and Lim, Y. (2016). Ameliorative effect of dietary genistein on diabetes induced hyper-inflammation and oxidative stress during early stage of wound healing in alloxan induced diabetic mice. *Biochem Biophys Res. Commun.*, 478(3): 1021–7.

Ferreira, P.S., Spolidorio, L.C., Manthey, J.A. and Cesar, T.B. (2016). Citrus flavanones prevent systemic inflammation and ameliorate oxidative stress in C57BL/6J mice fed high-fat diet. *Food Funct.*, 7(6): 2675–81.

Fetita, L.S., Sobngwi, E., Serradas, P., Calvo, F. and Gautier, J.F. (2006). Consequences of fetal exposure to maternal diabetes in offspring. *J. Clin. Endocrinol. Metab.*, 91: 3718–24.

Figueiredo-González, M., Grosso, C., Valentão, P. and Andrade, P.B. (2016). α-Glucosidase and α-amylase inhibitors from *Myrcia* spp.: A stronger alternative to acarbose? *J. Pharm. Biomed. Anal.*, 118: 322–7.

Gharib, A., Faezizadeh, Z. and Godarzee, M. (2013). Treatment of diabetes in the mouse model by delphinidin and cyanidin hydrochloride in free and liposomal forms. *Planta Med.*, 79(17): 1599–604.

Grzebyk, E. and Piwowar, A. (2016). Inhibitory actions of selected natural substances on formation of advanced glycation endproducts and advanced oxidation protein products. *BMC Complementary and Alternative Medicine,* 16: 381. DOI 10.1186/s12906-016-1353-0.

Guo, H., Xia, M., Zou, T., Ling, W., Zhong, R. and Zhang, W. (2012). Cyanidin 3-glucoside attenuates obesity-associated insulin resistance and hepatic steatosis in high-fat diet-fed and db/db mice *via* the transcription factor FoxO1. *J. Nutr. Biochem.*, 23: 349–60.

Hidalgo, J., Flores, C., Hidalgo, M.A., Perez, M., Yañez, A., Quiñones, L. *et al.* (2014). Delphinol® standardized maqui berry extract reduces postprandial blood glucose increase in individuals with impaired glucose regulation by novel mechanism of sodium glucose cotransporter inhibition. *Panminerva Med.*, 56(2 Suppl 3): 1–7.

Hossain, C.M., Ghosh, M.K., Satapathy, B.S., Dey, N.S. and Mukherjee, B. (2014). Apigenin causes biochemical modulation, GLUT4 and Cd38 alterations to improve diabetes and to protect damages of some vital organs in experimental diabetes. *Am. J. Pharmacol. Toxicol.*, 9: 39–52.

Hossain, M.K., Dayem, A.A., Han, J., Yin, Y., Kim, K., Saha, S.K. *et al.* (2016). Molecular mechanisms of the anti-obesity and anti-diabetic properties of flavonoids. *Int. J. Mol. Sci.*, 17(4): 569.

Hsu, C.Y., Shih, H.Y., Chia, Y.C., Lee, C.H., Ashida, H., Lai, Y.K. and Weng, C.F. (2014). Rutin potentiates insulin receptor kinase to enhance insulin-dependent glucose transporter 4 translocation. *Mol. Nutr. Food. Res.*, 58(6): 1168–76.

International Diabetes Federation (2015). Diabetes Atlas Seventh Edition 2015.

Jayaprakasam, B., Vareed, S.K., Olson, L.K. and Nair, M.G. (2005). Insulin secretion by anthocyanins and anthocyanidins. *J. Agric. Food Chem.*, 53: 2519–23.

Jiang, N. and Doseff, A.I. and Grotewold, E. (2016). Flavones: From Biosynthesis to Health Benefits. *Plants (Basel), 5(2): 27.*

Johnson, M.H. and de Mejia, E.G. (2016). Phenolic compounds from fermented berry beverages modulated gene and protein expression to increase insulin secretion from pancreatic β-cells *in vitro. J. Agric. Food Chem.*, 64(12): 2569–81.

Jung, U.J. and Choi, M.S. (2014). Obesity and its metabolic complications: The role of adipokines and the relationship between obesity, inflammation, insulin resistance, dyslipidemia and nonalcoholic fatty liver disease. *Int. J. Mol. Sci.*, 2014; 15: 6184–223.

Jung, U.J., Lee, M.K., Jeong, K.S. and Choi, M.S. (2004). The hypoglycaemic effects of hesperidin and naringin are partly mediated by hepatic glucose-regulating enzymes in C57BL/KsJ-db/db mice. *J. Nutr.*, 134: 2499–503.

Kan, E., Kiliçkan, E., Ayar, A., Çolak, R. (2015). Effects of two antioxidants; α-lipoic acid and fisetin against diabetic cataract in mice. *Int. Ophthalmol.*, 35(1): 115–20.

Kappel, V.D., Cazarolli, L.H., Pereira, D.F., Postal, B.G., Zamoner, A., Reginatto, F.H. *et al.* (2013b). Involvement of GLUT-4 in the stimulatory effect of rutin on glucose uptake in rat soleus muscle. *J. Pharm. Pharmacol.*, 65(8): 1179–86.

Kappel, V.D., Zanatta, L., Postal, B.G. and Silva, F.R. (2013a). Rutin potentiates calcium uptake *via* voltage-dependent calcium channel associated with stimulation of glucose uptake in skeletal muscle. *Arch. Biochem. Biophys.*, 532(2): 55–60.

Kato, M., Tani, T., Terahara, N. and Tsuda, T. (2015). The anthocyanin delphinidin 3-rutinoside stimulates glucagon-like peptide-1 secretion in murine glutag cell line *via* the Ca^{2+}/calmodulin-dependent kinase II pathway. *PLoS ONE*, 10(5): e0126157. doi: 10.1371/journal.pone.0126157.

Kim, H.J., Kim, S.H. and Yun, J.M. (2012). Fisetin inhibits hyperglycemia-induce-dproinflammatory cytokine production by epigenetic mechanisms. *Evid. Based Complement. Alternat. Med.*, 2012: 1–10.

Kim, H.J., Lee, W. and Yun, J.M. (2014). Luteolin inhibits hyperglycemia-induced proinflammatory cytokine production and its epigenetic mechanism in human monocytes. *Phytother Res.*, 28(9): 1383–91.

Kim, M.S., Hur, H.J., Kwon, D.Y. and Hwang, J.T. (2012). Tangeretin stimulates glucose uptake *via* regulation of AMPK signaling pathways in C2C12 myotubes and improves glucose tolerance in high-fat diet-induced obese mice. *Mol. Cell. Endocrinol.*, 358(1): 127–34.

Kittl, M., Beyreis, M., Tumurkhuu, M., Fürst, J., Helm, K., Pitschmann, A. *et al.* (2016). Quercetin stimulates insulin secretion and reduces the viability of rat INS-1 beta cells. *Cell Physiol Biochem.*, 39: 278–93.

Kobayashi, K., Ishizaki, Y., Kojo, S. and Kikuzaki, H. (). Strong inhibition of secretory sphingomyelinase by catechins, particularly by (-)-Epicatechin 3-O-Gallate and (-)-3'-O-methylepigallocatechin 3-O-gallate. *J. Nutr. Sci. Vitaminol. (Tokyo)*, 62(2): 123–9.

Kumar, B., Gupta, S.K., Srinivasan, B.P., Nag, T.C., Srivastava, S., Saxena, R. and Jha, K.A. (2013). Hesperetin rescues retinal oxidative stress, neuroinflammation and apoptosis in diabetic rats. *Microvasc Res.*, 87: 65–74.

Kwon, O., Eck, P., Chen, S., Corpe, C.P., Lee, J.H., Kruhlak, M. *et al.* (2017). Inhibition of the intestinal glucose transporter GLUT2 by flavonoids. *The FASEB Journal*, 21: 366–77.

Lee, J.S., Kim, Y.R., Park, J.M., Kim, Y.E., Baek, N.I. and Hong, E.K. (2015b). Cyanidin-3-glucoside isolated from mulberry fruits protects pancreatic β-cells against glucotoxicity-induced apoptosis. *Mol. Med. Rep.*, 11(4): 2723–8.

Lee, J.S., Kim, Y.R., Song, I.G., Ha, S.J., Kim, Y.E., Baek, N.I. and Hong, E.K. (2015a). Cyanidin-3-glucoside isolated from mulberry fruit protects pancreatic β-cells against oxidative stress-induced apoptosis. *Int. J. Mol. Med.*, 35(2): 405–12.

Lee, Y.S., Lee, S., Lee, H.S., Kim, B.K., Ohuchi, K. and Shin, K.H. (2005). Inhibitory effects of isorhamnetin-3-O-beta-D-glucoside from *Salicornia herbacea* on rat lens aldose reductase and sorbitol accumulation in streptozotocin-induced diabetic rat tissues. *Biol. Pharm. Bull.*, 28: 916–8.

Lim, S.S., Jung, Y.J., Hyun, S.K., Lee, Y.S. and Choi, J.S. (2006). Rat lens aldose reductase inhibitory constituents of *Nelumbo nucifera* stamens. *Phytother Res.*, 20(10): 825–30.

Liu, I.M., Liou, S.S. and Cheng, J.T. (2006). Mediation of beta-endorphin by myricetin to lower plasma glucose in streptozotocin-induced diabetic rats. *J. Ethnopharmacol.*, 104(1-2): 199–206.

Liu, I.M., Liou, S.S., Lan, T.W., Hsu, F.L. and Cheng, J.T. (2005). Myricetin as the active principle of *Abelmoschus moschatus* to lower plasma glucose in streptozotocin-induced diabetic rats. *Planta Med.*, 71(7): 617–21.

Liu, I.M., Tzeng, T.F., Liou, S.S. and Lan, T.W. (2007). Improvement of insulin sensitivity in obese Zucker rats by myricetin extracted from *Abelmoschus moschatus*. Planta Med., 73(10): 1054–60.

Luo, C., Yang, H., Tang, C., Yao, G., Kong, L., He, H. *et al.* (2015). Kaempferol alleviates insulin resistance *via* hepatic IKK/NF-κB signal in type 2 diabetic rats. *Int. Immunopharmacol.*, 28(1): 744–50.

Mahmoud, A.M., Ashour, M.B., Abdel-Moneim, A. and Ahmed, O.M. (2012). Hesperidin and naringin attenuate hyperglycemia-mediated oxidative stress and proinflammatory cytokine production in high fat fed/streptozotocin-induced type 2 diabetic rats. *J. Diabetes Complications.*, 26(6): 483–90.

Middha, S.K., Goyal, A.K., Faizan, S.A., Sanghamitra, N., Basistha, B. and Usha, T. (2013). Insilico–based combinatorial pharmacophore modelling and docking studies of GSK-3β and GK inhibitors of *Hippophae. J. Biosci.*, 38(4): 805–14.

Miladpour, B., Rasti, M., Owji, A.A., Mostafavipour, Z., Khoshdel, Z., Noorafshan, A. *et al.* Quercetin potentiates transdifferentiation of bone marrow mesenchymal stem cells into the beta cells *in vitro*. *J. Endocrinol. Invest.*, DOI 10.1007/s40618-016-0592-8.

Mirshekar, M., Roghani, M., Khalili, M., Baluchnejadmojarad, T. and Arab, M.S. (2010). Chronic oral pelargonidin alleviates streptozotocin-induced diabetic neuropathic hyperalgesia in rat: Involvement of oxidative stress. *Iran Biomed J.*, 14: 33–9.

Mirshekar, M., Roghani, M., Khalili, M. and Baluchnejadmojarad, T. (2011). Chronic oral pelargonidin alleviates learning and memory disturbances in streptozotocin diabetic rats. *Iran J. Pharm. Res.*, 10(3): 569–75.

Miyake, Y., Yamamoto, K., Tsujihara, N. and Osawa, T. (1998). Protective effects of lemon flavonoids on oxidative stress in diabetic rats. *Lipids.*, 33: 689–95.

Miyata, Y., Tanaka, H., Shimada, A., Sato, T., Ito, A., Yamanouchi, T. *et al.* (2011). Regulation of adipocytokine secretion and adipocyte hypertrophy by polymethoxy flavonoids, nobiletin and tangeretin. *Life Sci.*, 88: 613–18.

Moreno-Ulloa, A. and Moreno-Ulloa, J. (2016). Mortality reduction among persons with type 2 diabetes: (-)-Epicatechin as add-on therapy to metformin? *Med. Hypotheses.*, 91: 86–9.

Nepali, S., Son, J.S., Poudel, B., Lee, J.H., Lee, Y.M., Kim, D.K. (2015). Luteolin is a bioflavonoid that attenuates adipocyte-derived inflammatory responses *via* suppression of nuclear factor-κB/mitogen-activated protein kinases pathway. *Pharmacogn. Mag.*, 11 (43): 627–35.

Nickavar, B. and Amin, G. (2010). Bioassay-guided separation of an alpha-amylase inhibitor anthocyanin from *Vaccinium arctostaphylos* berries. *Z Naturforsch C*, 65(9–10): 567–70.

Niture, N.T., Ansari, A.A. and Naik, S.R. (2014). Anti-hyperglycemic activity of rutin in streptozotocin-induced diabetic rats: An effect mediated through cytokines, antioxidants and lipid biomarkers. *Indian J. Exp. Biol.*, 52(7): 720–7.

Ong, K.C. and Khoo, H.E. (2000). Effects of myricetin on glycemia and glycogen metabolism in diabetic rats. *Life Sci.,* 67(14): 1695–705.

Pal, H.C., Pearlman, R.L. and Afaq, F. (2016). Fisetin and its role in chronic diseases. *Adv. Exp. Med. Biol.*, 928: 213–44.

Panda, S. and Kar, A. (2007). Apigenin (41,5,7-trihydroxyflavone) regulates hyperglycemia, thyroid dysfunction and lipid peroxidation in alloxan-induced diabetic mice. *J. Pharm. Pharmacol.*, 59: 1543–8.

Park, M.H., Ju, J.W., Kim, M. and Han, J.S. (2016). The protective effect of daidzein on high glucose-induced oxidative stress in human umbilical vein endothelial cells. *Z Naturforsch C.,* 71(1–2): 21–8.

Park, M.H., Ju, J.W., Park, M.J. and Han, J.S. (2013). Daidzein inhibits carbohydrate digestive enzymes in vitro and alleviates postprandial hyperglycemia in diabetic mice. *Eur. J. Pharmacol.*, 712(1–3): 48–52.

Park, S., Kang, S., Jeong, D.Y., Jeong, S.Y., Park, J.J. and Yun, H.S. (2015). Cyanidin and malvidin in aqueous extracts of black carrots fermented with *Aspergillus oryzae* prevent the impairment of energy, lipid and glucose metabolism in estrogen-deficient rats by AMPK activation. *Genes Nutr.*, 10(2): 455.

Patisaul, H.B. and Jefferson, W. (2010). The pros and cons of phytoestrogens. *Front Neuroendocrinol,* 31: 400–19.

Peng, X., Zhang, G., Liao, Y. and Gong, D. (2016). Inhibitory kinetics and mechanism of kaempferol on α-glucosidase. *Food Chem.*, 190: 207–15.

Prasath, G.S. and Subramanian, S.P. (2011). Modulatory effects of fisetin, a bioflavonoid, on hyperglycemia by attenuating the key enzymes of carbohydrate metabolism in hepatic and renal tissues in streptozotocin-induced diabetic rats. *Eur. J. Pharmacol.*, 668(3): 492–6.

Prasath, G.S., Pillai, S.I. and Subramanian, S.P. (2014). Fisetin improves glucose homeostasis through the inhibition of gluconeogenic enzymes in hepatic tissues of streptozotocin induced diabetic rats. *Eur. J. Pharmacol.*, 740: 248–54.

Prasath, G.S., Sundaram, C.S. and Subramanian, S.P. (2013). Fisetin averts oxidative stress in pancreatic tissues of streptozotocin-induced diabetic rats. *Endocrine*, 44(2): 359–68.

Prince, P.S.M. and Kamalakkannan, N. (2006). Rutin improves glucose homeostasis in streptozotocin diabetic tissues by altering glycolytic and gluconeogenic enzymes. *J. Biochem. Mol. Toxicol.*, 20: 96–102.

Priscilla, D.H., Roy, D., Suresh, A., Kumar, V. and Thirumurugan, K. (2014). Naringenin inhibits α-glucosidase activity: A promising strategy for the regulation of postprandial hyperglycemia in high fat diet fed streptozotocin induced diabetic rats. *Chem. Biol. Interact.*, 210: 77–85.

Pu, P., Gao, D.M., Mohamed, S., Chen, J., Zhang, J., Zhou, X.Y. *et al.* (2012). Naringin ameliorates metabolic syndrome by activating AMP-activated protein kinase in mice fed a high-fat diet. *Arch Biochem Biophys.*, 518: 61–70.

Qiu, S., Sun, G., Zhang, Y., Li, X. and Wang, R. (2016). Involvement of the NF-κB signaling pathway in the renoprotective effects of isorhamnetin in a type 2 diabetic rat model. *Biomed Reports,* 4: 628–34.

Rauter, A.P., Martins, A., Borges, C., Mota-Filipe, H., Pinto, R., Sepodes, B. *et al.* (2010). Antihyperglycaemic and protective effects of flavonoids on streptozotocin-induced diabetic rats. *Phytother. Res.*, 24: S133–S138.

Ren, B., Qin, W., Wu, F., Wang, S., Pan, C., Wang, L. *et al.* (2016). Apigenin and naringenin regulate glucose and lipid metabolism, and ameliorate vascular dysfunction in type 2 diabetic rats. *Eur. J. Pharmacol.*, 773: 13–23.

Rodríguez-Rodríguez, C., Torres, N., Gutiérrez-Uribe, J.A., Noriega, L.G., Torre-Villalvazo, I., Leal-Díaz, A.M. *et al.* (2015). The effect of isorhamnetin glycosides extracted from *Opuntia ficus-indica* in a mouse model of diet induced obesity. *Food Funct.*, 6: 805–15.

Rojo, L.E., Ribnicky, D., Logendra, S., Poulev, A., Rojas-Silva, P., Kuhn, P. *et al.* (2012). *In vitro* and *in vivo* anti-diabetic effects of anthocyanins from Maqui Berry (*Aristotelia chilensis*). *Food Chem.*, 131(2): 387–96.

Roslan, J., Giribabu, N., Karim, K. and Salleh, N. (2016). Quercetin ameliorates oxidative stress, inflammation and apoptosis in the heart of streptozotocin-nicotinamide-induced adult male diabetic rats. *Biomed Pharmacother.*, 86: 570–82.

Roy, M., Sen, S. and Chakraborti, A.S. (2008). Action of pelargonidin on hyperglycemia and oxidative damage in diabetic rats: Implication for glycation-induced hemoglobin modification. *Life Sci.*, 82: 1102–10.

Roy, S., Ahmed, F., Banerjee, S., Saha, U. (2016). Naringenin ameliorates streptozotocin-induced diabetic rat renal impairment by downregulation of TGF-β1 and IL-1 *via* modulation of oxidative stress correlates with decreased apoptotic events. *Pharm Biol.*, 54(9): 1616–27.

Shibano, M., Kakutani, K., Taniguchi, M., Yasuda, M. and Baba, K. (2008). Antioxidant constituents in the dayflower (*Commelina communis* L.) and their alpha-glucosidase-inhibitory activity. *J. Nat. Med.*, 62(3): 349–53.

Suh, K.S., Oh, S., Woo, J.T., Kim, S.W., Kim, J.W., Kim, Y.S. *et al.* (2012). Apigenin attenuates 2-deoxy-d-ribose-induced oxidative cell damage in HIT-T15 pancreatic. β-cells. *Biol. Pharm. Bull.*, 35: 121–6.

Sundaram, R., Shanthi, P. and Sachdanandam, P. (2014). Effect of tangeretin, a polymethoxylated flavone on glucose metabolism in streptozotocin-induced diabetic rats. *Phytomedicine,* 21(6): 793–9.

Surveswaran, S., Zhong-Cai, Y., Corke, H. and Sun, M. (2007). Systematic evaluation of natural phenolic antioxidants from 133 Indian medicinal plants. *Food Chem.*, 102: 938–53.

Valsecchi, A.E., Franchi, S., Panerai, A.E., Rossi, A., Sacerdote, P. and Colleoni, M. (2011). The soy isoflavone genistein reverses oxidative and inflammatory state, neuropathic pain, neurotrophic and vasculature deficits in diabetes mouse model. *Eur. J. Pharmacol.*, 650: 694–702.

Van Acker, F.A., Schouten, O., Haenen, G.R., van der Vijgh, W.J. and Bast, A. (2000). Flavonoids can replace alpha-tocopherol as an antioxidant. *FEBS Lett.*, 473: 145–8.

Vinayagam, R. and Xu, B. (2015). Antidiabetic properties of dietary flavonoids: A cellular mechanism review. *Nutrition & Metabolism*, 12: 60. DOI 10.1186/s12986-015-0057-7.

Visnagri, A., Kandhare, A.D., Chakravarty, S., Ghosh, P., Bodhankar, S.L. (2014). Hesperidin, a flavanoglycone attenuates experimental diabetic neuropathy *via* modulation of cellular and biochemical marker to improve nerve functions. *Pharm Biol.*, 52(7): 814–28.

Wang, Z., Zhai, D., Zhang, D., Bai, L., Yao, R., Yu, J. *et al.* (2016). Quercetin decreases insulin resistance in a polycystic ovary syndrome rat model by improving inflammatory microenvironment. *Reprod Sci.*, pii: 1933719116667218.

World Health Organization (2009). editor. Global health risks: Mortality and burden of disease attributable to selected major risks. Geneva, Switzerland: World Health Organization.

Yamane, T., Kozuka, M., Konda, D., Nakano, Y., Nakagaki, T., Ohkubo, I. and Ariga, H. (2016). Improvement of blood glucose levels and obesity in mice given aronia juice by inhibition of dipeptidyl peptidase IV and α-glucosidase. *J. Nutr. Biochem.*, 31: 106–12.

Yan, J., Zhang, G., Pan, J. and Wang, Y. (2014). α-Glucosidase inhibition by luteolin: kinetics, interaction and molecular docking. *Int. J. Biol. Macromol.*, 64: 213–23.

Yan, N., Wen, L., Peng, R., Li, H., Liu, H., Peng, H. *et al.* (2016). Naringenin ameliorated kidney injury through Let-7a/TGFBR1 signaling in diabetic nephropathy. *J. Diabetes. Res.*, 2016: 8738760. doi: 10.1155/2016/8738760.

Yokozawa, T., Kim, H.Y., Cho, E.J., Choi, J.S., Chung, H.Y. (2002). Antioxidant effects of isorhamnetin 3,7-di-O-beta-D-glucopyranoside isolated from mustard leaf (*Brassica juncea*) in rats with streptozotocin-induced diabetes. *J. Agric. Food Chem.*, 50: 5490–5.

Yoshida, H., Tsuhako, R., Atsumi, T., Narumi, K., Watanabe, W., Sugita, C. *et al.* (2016). Naringenin interferes with the anti-diabetic actions of pioglitazone *via* pharmacodynamic interactions. *J. Nat. Med.*, 10.1007/s11418-016-1063-4.

Zang, M., Xu, S., Maitland-Toolan, K.A., Zuccollo, A., Hou, X., Jiang, B. *et al.* (2006). Polyphenols stimulate amp-activated protein kinase, lower lipids, and inhibit accelerated atherosclerosis in diabetic ldl receptor-deficient mice. *Diabetes,* 55: 2180–91.

Zang, Y., Zhang, L., Igarashi, K. and Yu, C. (2015). The anti-obesity and anti-diabetic effects of kaempferol glycosides from unripe soybean leaves in high-fat-diet mice. *Food Funct.,* 6: 834–41.

Zang, Y., Igarashi, K. and Li, Y. (2016). Anti-diabetic effects of luteolin and luteolin-7-O-glucoside on KK-A(y) mice. *Biosci Biotechnol Biochem.*, 80(8): 1580–6.

Zhang, L., Han, Y.J., Zhang, X., Wang, X., Bao, B., Qu, W. *et al.* (2016). Luteolin reduces obesity-associated insulin resistance in mice by activating AMPKα1 signalling in adipose tissue macrophages. *Diabetologia, 59(10): 2219–28.*

Zhang, L., Zhang, Z.K. and Liang, S. (2016). Epigallocatechin-3-gallate protects retinal vascular endothelial cells from high glucose stress *in vitro via* the MAPK/ERK-VEGF pathway. *Genet. Mol. Res.,* 15(2). doi: 10.4238/gmr.15027874.

Zhang, W.Y., Lee, J.J., Kim, Y., Kim, I.S., Han, J.H., Lee, S.G. *et al.* (2012). Effect of eriodictyol on glucose uptake and insulin resistance *in vitro*. *J. Agric. Food Chem.*, 60(31): 7652–8.

Zhang, X., Wang, G., Gurley, E.C. and Zhou, H. (2014). Flavonoid apigenin inhibits lipopolysaccharide-induced inflammatory response through multiple mechanisms in macrophages. *PLoS ONE,* 9: e107072.

Zhang, Y., Dong, H., Wang, M. and Zhang, J. Quercetin isolated from toona sinensis leaves attenuates hyperglycemia and protects hepatocytes in high-carbohydrate/high-fat diet and alloxan induced experimental diabetic mice. *Journal of Diabetes Research,* doi.org/10.1155/2016/8492780.

Zhang, Y., Zhen, W., Maechler, P. and Liu, D. (2013). Small molecule kaempferol modulates PDX-1 protein expression and subsequently promotes pancreatic β-cell survival and function *via* CREB. *J. Nutr. Biochem.*, 24(4): 638–46.

5

Molecular Mechanism of Flavonoids for Improvement of Immune System

Om Prakash[1] and Ajeet[2*]

ABSTRACT

Out of the plant's secondary metabolites, flavonoids are one of the eight phytochemical groups which are continuously attracting the attention of drug developers. A variety of experimental observations reported about the flavonoids vs. immunity; which expose the strong evidences for enhancement of immune system. Earlier it was hypothesized, but now has been proved that this ubiquitous dietary chemical impacts significantly on cell homeostasis as well as strengthens the secondary cell systems comprising the inflammatory response. In the present chapter, experimental evidences have been piled-up as well as abstracted into consolidated information explaining the diverse activities of flavonoids in the areas of secretory processes, immunoglobulins, proliferation of immune cells, cytokines, cell-cell interaction, radical scavenging properties, redox activity and so on. These evidences provide a strong base for understanding the mechanism of action of flavonoids for improvement of immune system. This chapter provides an exhaustive coverage of molecular mechanism of flavonoids for improvement of immune system.

Key words: Enhancement, Flavonoids, Immune system, Molecular, Mechanism.

1. INTRODUCTION

Flavonoids belong to a group of plant's secondary metabolites with variable phenolic structures (Romano, 2013). More than 4000 varieties of flavonoids

[1] Department of Biochemistry, University of Lucknow, Uttar Pradesh, India

[2] Department of Pharmacy, Vishveshwarya Group of Institutions, Greater Noida-II, Uttar Pradesh, India

**Corresponding author*: E-mail: ajeet_pharma111@rediffmail.com

are found in roots, stem, bark, leaf, flowers, fruits, wine and so on. Flavonoids are known for acting against many diseases as well as in support of immune system (Peluso, 2015). First evidence of enhancement of immune response by flavonoid came to existence in 1977, when disappearance of Hepatitis-B antigen by Cianidanol was reported. Further, stimulation of immune response by Cianidanol was reported in both normal and diseased human (Salama and Mueller-Eckhardt, 1987). After that, many potential clinical effects of flavonoids were notified, few of them are: anti-atherosclerotic, anti-inflammatory, anti-thrombogenic, anti-osteoporotic, and antiviral effects which were directly correlated with immune system (Kawai, 2011). These effects were also described for their possible mechanism of action for enhancement of immune system, but no consolidated outlook is available till date.

This chapter is organized to expose a basic but multi-directional as well as consolidated molecular mechanism of action of flavonoids for enhancement of immune system. These descriptions are based on experimental information (*in vitro*/ *in vivo*) available in literatures in correlation with structural constituents of flavonoids.

2. COMPONENTS INVOLVED IN IMMUNE-ENHANCEMENT BY FLAVONOIDS

Leukocytes, lymphocyte, mast cells, and immunoglobulin are some of the basic components of immune system, which are observed for evaluation of immune-enhancement (Saleh, 2014). Indications of immune-enhancement by flavonoids are reported in context of lymphocyte proliferation, synthesis of immunoglobulin, anti-oxidant activity by free radical scavenging, impact on nitric oxide synthase, inhibition of enzymes such as: xanthine oxidase, histidine decarboxylase, neutrophil degranulation, induction of thymidine uptake, and inhibition of catabolism of cGMP (Manchope, 2016).

These activities of flavonoids are due to their conjugation behaviour (Cermak and Wolffram, 2006). Which are organised from structural constituents available in flavonoids (Cao, 2014). There are several possible locations for the conjugates on the flavonoid skeleton. The type of conjugate and its location on the flavonoid skeleton establishes enzyme-inhibiting as well as antioxidant activities of the flavonoid (Kandaswami, 2005). Regular intake of flavonoids results in a more predominant formation of several conjugates, which probably results in greater activity (Amponsah, 2012). In addition of these, the functional groups increases the circulatory elimination time and probably also decreases toxicity (Bachmann, 2013). In general the conjugation process for flavonoids (*e.g.* catechins) starts with the interaction of a glucuronide moiety with intestinal cells (Kim, 2009). The flavonoid further binds to albumin and are transported to the liver (Batista, 2012). The liver can extend the conjugation of the flavonoid by adding a sulfate group, a methyl group, or both (D'Andrea, 2015; Toyoda-Hokaiwado, 2011). Among the known mechanism of actions, structural properties of flavonoids have been shown for responsible importance. The immune-enhancing activities of flavonoids are reported due to their specific structural constituents as: planar structure because of a double bond in the central aromatic ring; high reducing power due to phenolic content; stability of oxidized state due to combination of ring and double bond and vicinaldiol component etc. (Brattig, 1984; Cialdella-Kam, 2016; Patel, 2016). [Fig. 1 (a) and 1(b)].

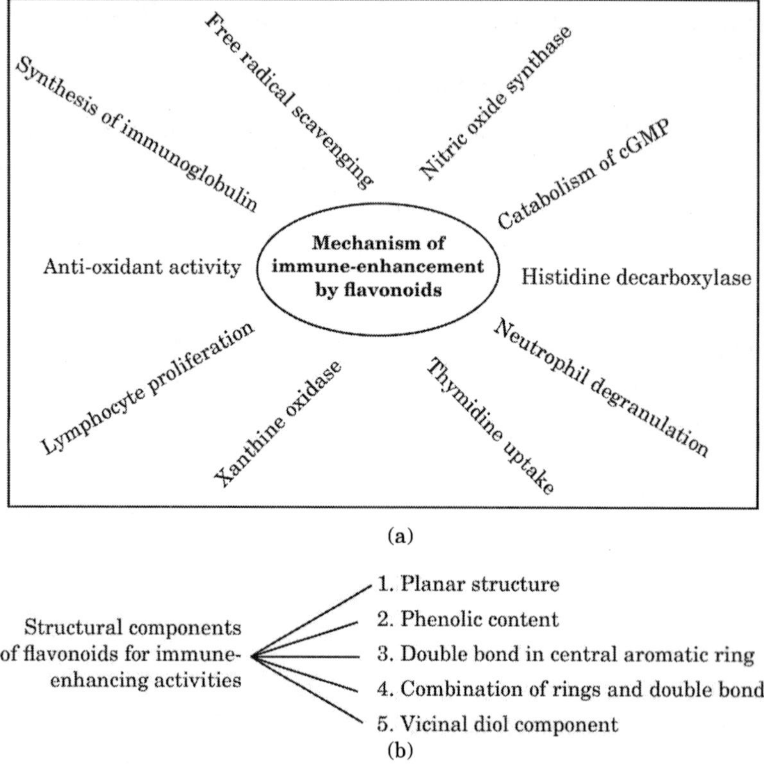

Fig. 1: (a) Major reported mechanism of actions of immune enhancement by flavonoids; (b) Structural components of flavonoids for enhancement of immune activity

3. IMMUNE-ENHANCING EFFECTS OF FLAVONOIDS *VIA* LYMPHOCYTE PROLIFERATION AND SYNTHESIS OF IMMUNOGLOBULIN

The immobilization and firm adhesion of leukocytes to the endothelial wall is the major mechanism responsible for the formation of oxygen-derived free radicals (Manthey, 2000). Flavonoids are lipophilic agents (Li, 2013). They interact with unsaturated fatty acids of membranes of immune cells

(B-cells, macrophases, and mast/leukocytes) and may alter membrane's fluidity and lymphocyte function (Schmitz, 2015).

Immune enhancement properties of flavonoids are well known because of induction of lymphocyte proliferation as well as enhanced synthesis of immunoglobulins in T-cell independent manner (Tanaka and Takahashi, 2013). But these properties are achievable at low concentration of flavonoids. It is notified that requirement of flavonoid's concentration is high for lymphocyte transformation than synthesis of immunoglobulin [Fig. 2]. At higher concentration of flavonoids, lymphocyte responsiveness becomes inhibited (Jennings, 2014; Jeong, 2007).

After first evidence of enhancement of immune response by flavonoid by Cianidanol, stimulation of immune response by Cianidanol was reported in both normal and diseased human (Brattig, 1984). It is reported that, Cianidanol interacts with cell membranes for prevention of lipid peroxidation or reducing the membrane permeability (Brattig, 1984). It is reported that, flavonoids rather stimulate than suppress the immune function.

3.1. Flavonoids and Lymphocyte Proliferation

Lymphocytes include natural killer cells (NK cells) (*i.e.* cytotoxic innate immunity), T cells (*i.e.* cytotoxic adaptive immunity), and B cells (*i.e.* antibody-driven adaptive immunity). Lymphocyte proliferation/ transformation is the process which involves synthesis of DNA after cross-linking of their antigen receptor either following recognition of antigen or stimulation by a polyclonal activator (mitogen) (Baylor, 1992; Lahiri-Chatterjee, 1999). Flavonoid induces uptake of thymidine (*i.e.* deoxythymidine) (Hirano, 1995). This enhances the thymidine pairing with deoxyadenosine in double stranded DNA. These synchronies the cells in G1/early S-phase of cell cycle. Flavonoids also induces DNA synthesis for lymphocyte proliferation, which is evidenced by its ability to orient the cells for inhibition of catabolism of cGMP leading to high level of the nucleotide.

3.2. Enhanced Synthesis of Immunoglobulin

Flavonoid enhances the synthesis of immunoglobulin in T-cell independent manner. This property is different from immune activation during any infection.

3.3. Stabilization of Mast Cells/Leukocytes by Flavonoids

Stabilization of mast cells, followed by inhibition of degranulation of mast cells and inhibition of histamine decarboxylase are reported *via* bioflavonoids (Formica and Regelson, 1995; Saliou, 1998). Since mast cells circulate in blood in an immature form. Stem-cell factor and other cytokines, secreted by endothelial cells and fibroblasts, provide final maturation to mast cells. Therefore stability of mast cells matters for immune enhancement (Landi-Librandi, 2012; Zhang, 2014). Importance of mature mast cells also increases because they participate in early recognition of pathogens at the interface location of tissue and external environment (Sausville, 1999; Wang, 2015). At the instance of pathogen introduction, mature mast cells degranulate to release inflammation mediators (histamine, proteases, and tumour necrosis factor-alpha), which is followed by production of eicosanoids and leukotriene (Altavilla, 2012; Nisar, 2013). Furthermore up-regulation of cytokines and chemokines occurs (Aalinkeel, 2010). In context of innate immunity, flavonoids were found to regulate cytokine release induced by the Toll-like receptor 2 (TLR2) agonist Pam3CSK4 (Lim, 2013). On the other hand, flavonols were found to selectively co-stimulate the IL-1beta secretion but had no impact on the secretion of IL-6 (Lim, 2013).

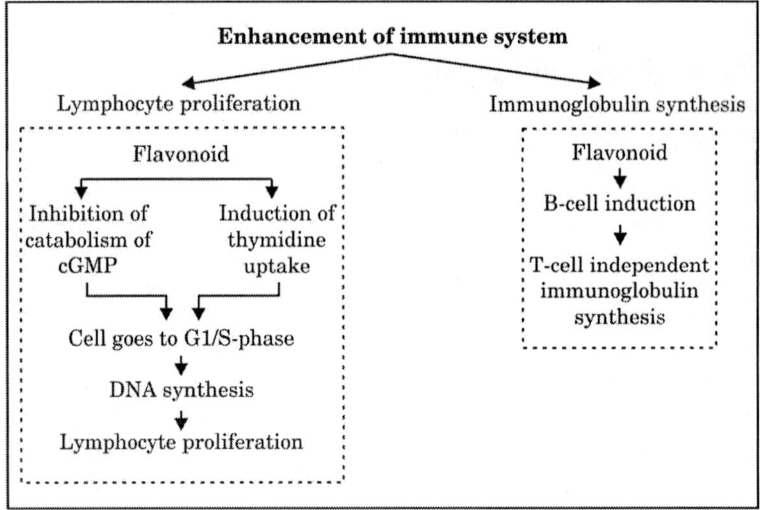

Fig. 2: Possible mechanism of action of immune enhancement by flavonoids *via* lymphocyte proliferation and synthesis of immunoglobulins

4. HIGH REDUCING POWER OF FLAVONOIDS LEADS TO IMMUNE ENHANCEMENT

The cellular damage causes a shift in the net charge of the cell, changing the osmotic pressure, leading to swelling and eventually cell death (Zhan and Yang, 2006). As general inflammatory response, free radicals attract inflammatory mediators towards damaged tissue (Li, 2005). To protect themselves from reactive oxygen species (ROS), living organisms have developed several effective mechanisms (Ablat, 2016; Akram, 2016; Vue,

Chen, 2016; Wang, 2016). The antioxidant-defence mechanisms of the body include enzymes such as superoxide dismutase, catalase, and glutatione peroxidase, but also non-enzymatic counterparts such as glutathione and ascorbic acid (Chandramohan and Parameswari, 2013; Manju, 2005). The increased production of ROS during injury results in consumption and depletion of the endogenous scavenging compounds (Saleem, 2013). Flavonoids also showed additive effect towards endogenous scavenging components (Saleem, 2013). Flavonoids interfere with free radical–producing systems, but they can also increase the function of the endogenous antioxidants. Since flavonoids are phenolic compounds, the availability of high end hydrogen releasing capacity from the hydroxyl groups makes it an anti-oxidant and radical scavenger. Besides this, catechol structure with vicinal diol makes it accessible to proteins (Lopez-Sanchez, 2007; Meng, 2009). Similarly, ringed scaffolds with double bond make it stable even after being oxidized by the free radicals (Lim, 2013; Mercader and Pomilio, 2012).

The flavones and catechins seem to be the most powerful flavonoids for protecting the body against reactive oxygen species (Jeong, 2005). Vitamins A, E and selected flavonoids in the family of catechins are well-defined small molecules that have been proven to possess immunomodulatory properties. Vitamin A or E and a catechin synergize as vaccine adjuvant to enhance immune responses in mice by induction of early interleukin-1 but not interleukin-1beta responses (Patel, 2016).

The mechanisms and the sequence of events by which free radicals interfere with cellular functions are still unclear, but most emphasis comes to lipid peroxidation, which results in cellular membrane damage (Mahapatra, 2009). In a non-animal experiment, increase of ROS production, lipid peroxidation rate and proline concentration have been found to elucidate the innate immunity (Chakraborty, 2016).

4.1. Flavonoids Inhibit Free Radical Generation by Inhibition of Platelets Aggregation

Platelets metabolize the arachidonic acid for its activation and aggregation (Benavente-Garcia and Castillo, 2008). Activated platelets adhere with vascular endothelium to produce lipid peroxides and oxygen free radicals, which further inhibit the generation of prostacyclin and nitrous oxide (Kris-Etherton and Keen, 2002). Flavonoids, as quercetin, kaempferol, and myricetinare effective as inhibitors of platelet aggregation (Formica and Regelson, 1995). They inhibit the thromboxane A2 formation for anti-aggregation (Lee, 2012; Rohdewald, 2002). Flavonoids affect arachidonic acid metabolism in different ways. Some flavonoids specifically block cyclooxygenase or lipoxygenase, whereas others block both the enzymes (Lau, 2010; Li, 2014; Park, 2004).

4.2. Enhanced Antioxidative Effects

Antioxidant activity of flavonoids is well described (Chaphalkar, 2017; Hwang, 2016). It is found to be enhanced after complexation with transient metal cations, which also facilitate the membrane adhesion and fusion, protein-protein and other conjugations (Heim, 2002). Quercetin in particular is known for its iron-chelating and iron-stabilizing properties (Edwin Shackelford, 2005; Shackelford, 2004).

4.3. Nitric Oxide Inhibition by Flavonoids

Nitric oxide is produced by endothelial cells and macrophages (Cho and Kim, 2013). Nitric oxide reacts with free radicals and produces peroxynitrite (McCarty, 2008; Paquay, 2000). Early/low concentration of nitric oxide is important for dilation of blood vessels, while higher concentration creates oxidative damage in macrophages by direct oxidation of LDLs (low density lipopoteins) by peroxynitrite (McCarty, 2008). The release of nitric oxideis controlled by nitric-oxide synthase (Lu, 2009). Flavonoids interfere with nitric-oxide synthase activity to provide free radical scavenging followed by immune enhancement by lowering the production of both nitric oxide and superoxide anions (Sharma, 2016). Silibin is a flavonoid which is known to inhibit nitric oxide in a dose dependent manner (Harasstani, 2010; Lu, 2009).

5. PROTEIN BINDING EFFECT FOR IMMUNE-ENHANCEMENT

Arachidonic acid is the starting point for a general inflammatory response (Alcaraz and Ferrandiz, 1987). Cyclooxygenase and lipoxygenase are involved in release of arachidonic acid (Lau, 2010; Park, 2004; Takahashi, 2006). Therefore these two, play important role as inflammatory mediators. Inhibition of inflammatory mediators is the representation of immune-enhancement. Selected flavonoids (*e.g.* Quercetin) are known to inhibit both cyclooxygenase and lipoxygenase, due to which formation of inflammatory metabolites diminishes (Maioli, 2015). Lipoxygenase of neutrophils generates chemotactic compounds from arachidonic acid as well as provoke release of cytokines (Jean and Bodinier, 1994). Therefore after inhibition of cyclooxygenase and lipoxygenase by flavonoids, inflammatory activities get reduced showing the immune enhancement effect (Vezina, 2012). Secondarily, since eicosanoids are the end products of cyclooxygenase and lipoxygenase pathways, flavonoids show another type of anti-inflammatory feature by inhibiting the eicosanoid biosynthesis (Formica and Regelson, 1995). Besides these, flavonoids also inhibit both cytosolic and membrane tyrosine kinase (Lee, 2012; Tan, 2003). Inhibition of membrane tyrosine kinase reduces uncontrolled cell growth and proliferation (Han, 2007; Li, 2010). It is also involved in variety of signal transduction as well as ATP synthesis (Galati and O'Brien, 2004; Hou, 2015). This property of protein inhibition is extrapolated into inhibition of neutrophil degranulation as well as blockage of release of arachidonic acid by neutrophils and other immune cells (Benavente-Garcia and Castillo, 2008; Park, 2004; Takahashi, 2006). Another target of selected flavonoids, like quercetin, silibin and luteolin, is xanthine oxidase (Ozcelik, 2011), which converts the molecular oxygen into superoxide free radicals (Par and Javor, 1984; Rajendran, 2014). These flavonoids are potential inhibitors of xanthine oxidase (Cao, 2014; Su, 2015), which resulted into free radical exempted injured tissue, showing the enhance immunity by flavonoids. For example, the scavenging ability of rutin may be due to its inhibitory activity on the enzyme xanthine oxidase (Akhlaghi and Bandy, 2009).

6. CONCLUSIONS AND FUTURE PROSPECTS

By this chapter, we can understand that, molecular mechanism of flavonoids for improvement of immune system, are basically linked with specific structural components which are available in a variety of flavonoids. These structural components are motivated for free radical scavenging as well as enzyme binding properties. These properties are observed in various immune enhancing capabilities. Immune enhancing properties of flavonoids can also be utilized for treating avariety of diseases, most importantly *via* improving the innate immunity.

REFERENCES

Aalinkeel, R., Hu, Z., Nair, B.B., Sykes, D.E., Reynolds, J.L., Mahajan, S.D. *et al.* (2010). Genomic analysis highlights the role of the JAK-STAT signaling in the anti-proliferative effects of dietary flavonoid-'Ashwagandha' in prostate cancer cells. *Evidence-Based Complementary and Alternative Medicine: eCAM*, 7(2): 177–87. doi:10.1093/ecam/nem184.

Ablat, N., Lv, D., Ren, R., Xiaokaiti, Y., Ma, X., Zhao, X. *et al.* (2016). Neuroprotective effects of a standardized flavonoid extract from safflower against a rotenone-induced rat model of parkinson's disease. *Molecules,* 21(9). doi:10.3390/molecules21091107.

Akhlaghi, M. and Bandy, B. (2009). Mechanisms of flavonoid protection against myocardial ischemia-reperfusion injury. *Journal of Molecular and Cellular Cardiology*, 46(3): 309–17. doi:10.1016/j.yjmcc.2008.12.003.

Akram, M., Shin, I., Kim, K.A., Noh, D., Baek, S.H., Chang, S.Y. *et al.* (2016). A newly synthesized macakurzin C-derivative attenuates acute and chronic skin inflammation: The Nrf2/heme oxygenase signaling as a potential target. *Toxicology and Applied Pharmacology*, 307: 62–71. doi:10.1016/j.taap.2016.07.013.

Alcaraz, M.J. and Ferrandiz, M.L. (1987). Modification of arachidonic metabolism by flavonoids. *Journal of Ethnopharmacology*, 21(3): 209–29.

Altavilla, D., Minutoli, L., Polito, F., Irrera, N., Arena, S., Magno, C. *et al.* (2012). Effects of flavocoxid, a dual inhibitor of COX and 5-lipoxygenase enzymes, on benign prostatic hyperplasia. *British Journal of Pharmacology*, 167(1): 95–108. doi:10.1111/j.1476-5381.2012.01969.x.

Amponsah, S.K., Bugyei, K.A., Osei-Safo, D., Addai, F.K., Asare, G., Tsegah, E.A. *et al.* (2012). *In vitro* activity of extract and fractions of natural cocoa powder on *Plasmodium falciparum*. *Journal of Medicinal Food*, 15(5): 476–82. doi:10.1089/jmf.2011.0220.

Bachmann, H., Offord-Cavin, E., Phothirath, P., Horcajada, M.N., Romeis, P. and Mathis, G.A. (2013). 1,25-Dihydroxyvitamin D3-glycoside of herbal origin exhibits delayed release pharmacokinetics when compared to its synthetic counterpart. *The Journal of Steroid Biochemistry and Molecular Biology*, 136: 333–6. doi:10.1016/j.jsbmb.2012.09.016.

Batista, L.L., Campesatto, E.A., Assis, M.L., Barbosa, A.P., Grillo, L.A. and Dornelas, C.B. (2012). Comparative study of topical green and red propolis in the repair of wounds induced in rats. *Revista do ColegioBrasileiro de Cirurgioes,* 39(6): 515–20.

Baylor, N.W., Fu, T., Yan, Y.D. and Ruscetti, F.W. (1992). Inhibition of human T cell leukemia virus by the plant flavonoid baicalin (7-glucuronic acid, 5,6-dihydroxyflavone). *The Journal of Infectious Diseases*, 165(3): 433–7.

Benavente-Garcia, O. and Castillo, J. (2008). Update on uses and properties of citrus flavonoids: New findings in anticancer, cardiovascular, and anti-inflammatory activity. *Journal ofAgricultural and Food Chemistry*, 56(15): 6185–205. doi:10.1021/jf8006568.

Brattig, N.W., Diao, G.J. and Berg, P.A. (1984). Immunoenhancing effect of flavonoid compounds on lymphocyte proliferation and immunoglobulin synthesis. *International Journal of Immunopharmacology*, 6(3): 205–15.

Cao, H., Pauff, J.M. and Hille, R. (2014). X-ray crystal structure of a xanthine oxidase complex with the flavonoid inhibitor quercetin. *Journal of Natural Products*, 77(7): 1693–9. doi:10.1021/np500320g.

Cermak, R. and Wolffram, S. (2006). The potential of flavonoids to influence drug metabolism and pharmacokinetics by local gastrointestinal mechanisms. *Current Drug Metabolism,* 7(7): 729–44.

Chakraborty, N., Ghosh, S., Chandra, S., Sengupta, S. and Acharya, K. (2016). Abiotic elicitors mediated elicitation of innate immunity in tomato: An *ex vivo* comparison. *Physiology and Molecular Biology of Plants: An International Journal of Functional Plant Biology,* 22(3): 307–20. doi:10.1007/s12298-016-0373-z.

Chandramohan, Y. and Parameswari, C.S. (2013). Therapeutic efficacy of naringin on cyclosporine (A) induced nephrotoxicity in rats: Involvement of hemeoxygenase-1. *Pharmacological Reports*: *PR*, 65(5): 1336–44.

Chaphalkar, R., Apte, K.G., Talekar, Y., Ojha, S.K. and Nandave, M. (2017). Antioxidants of *Phyllanthus emblica* L. Bark extract provide hepatoprotection against ethanol-induced hepatic damage: A comparison with silymarin. *Oxidative Medicine and Cellular Longevity*, 2017: 3876040. doi:10.1155/2017/3876040.

Cho, Y.J. and Kim, S.J. (2013). Effect of quercetin on the production of nitric oxide in murine macrophages stimulated with lipopolysaccharide from *Prevotella intermedia*. *Journal of Periodontal & Implant Science*, 43(4): 191–7. doi:10.5051/jpis.2013.43.4.191.

Cialdella-Kam, L., Nieman, D.C., Knab, A.M., Shanely, R.A., Meaney, M.P. and Jin, F. *et al.* (2016). A mixed flavonoid-fish oil supplement induces immune-enhancing and anti-inflammatory transcriptomic changes in adult obese and overweight Women-A randomized controlled trial. *Nutrients*, 8(5). doi:10.3390/nu8050277.

D'Andrea, G. (2015). Quercetin: A flavonol with multifaceted therapeutic applications? *Fitoterapia,* 106: 256–71. doi:10.1016/j.fitote.2015.09.018.

Edwin Shackelford, R., Manuszak, R.P., Heard, S.C., Link, C.J. and Wang, S. (2005). Pharmacological manipulation of ataxia-telangiectasia kinase activity as a treatment for Parkinson's disease. *Medical Hypotheses*, 64(4): 736–41. doi:10.1016/j.mehy.2004.08.029.

Formica, J.V. and Regelson, W. (1995). Review of the biology of Quercetin and related bioflavonoids. *Food and Chemical Toxicology: An International Journal Published for the British Industrial Biological Research Association,* 33(12): 1061–80.

Galati, G. And O'Brien, P.J. (2004). Potential toxicity of flavonoids and other dietary phenolics: Significance for their chemopreventive and anticancer properties. *Free Radical Biology & Medicine,* 37(3): 287–303. doi:10.1016/j.freer adbiomed. 2004.04.034.

Han, H.J., Kim, T.J., Jin, Y.R., Hong, S.S., Hwang, J.H., Hwang, B.Y. *et al.* (2007). Cudraflavanone A, a flavonoid isolated from the root bark of *Cudrania tricuspidata*, inhibits vascular smooth muscle cell growth *via* an Akt-dependent pathway. *Plantamedica,* 73(11): 1163–8. doi:10.1055/s-2007-981584.

Harasstani, O.A., Moin, S., Tham, C.L., Liew, C.Y., Ismail, N., Rajajendram, R. *et al.* (2010). Flavonoid combinations cause synergistic inhibition of proinflammatory mediator secretion from lipopolysaccharide-induced RAW 264.7 cells. *Inflammation Research: Official Journal of the European Histamine Research Society* [*et al.*], 59(9): 711–21. doi:10.1007/s00011-010-0182-8.

Heim, K.E., Tagliaferro, A.R. and Bobilya, D.J. (2002). Flavonoid antioxidants: Chemistry, metabolism and structure-activity relationships. *The Journal of Nutritional Biochemistry*, 13(10): 572–84.

Hirano, T., Abe, K., Gotoh, M. and Oka, K. (1995). Citrus flavone tangeretin inhibits leukaemic HL-60 cell growth partially through induction of apoptosis with less cytotoxicity on normal lymphocytes. *British Journal of Cancer*, 72(6): 1380–8.

Hou, X.L., Tong, Q., Wang, W.Q., Shi, C.Y., Xiong, W., Chen, J. *et al.* (2015). Suppression of inflammatory responses by dihydromyricetin, a flavonoid from *Ampelopsis grossedentata, via* Inhibiting the Activation of NF-kappaB and MAPK Signaling Pathways. *Journal of Natural Products,* 78(7): 1689–96. doi:10.1021/acs. jnatprod.5b00275.

Hwang, K.A., Hwang, Y.J. and Song, J. (2016). Antioxidant activities and oxidative stress inhibitory effects of ethanol extracts from *Cornus officinalis* on raw 264.7 cells. *BMC Complementary and Alternative Medicine*, 16: 196. doi:10.1186/s12906-016-1172-3.

Jean, T. and Bodinier, M.C. (1994). Mediators involved in inflammation: Effects of Daflon 500 mg on their release. *Angiology,* 45(6 Pt 2): 554–9.

Jennings, A., Welch, A.A., Spector, T., Macgregor, A. and Cassidy, A. (2014). Intakes of anthocyanins and flavones are associated with biomarkers of insulin resistance and inflammation in women. *The Journal of Nutrition*, 144(2): 202–8. doi:10.3945/ jn.113.184358.

Jeong, J.M., Choi, C.H., Kang, S.K., Lee, I.H., Lee, J.Y. and Jung, H. (2007). Antioxidant and chemosensitizing effects of flavonoids with hydroxy and/or methoxy groups and structure-activity relationship. *Journal of Pharmacy & Pharmaceutical Sciences: A Publication of the Canadian Society for Pharmaceutical Sciences, Societe Canadienne Des Sciences Pharmaceutiques*, 10(4): 537–46.

Jeong, Y.J., Choi, Y.J., Kwon, H.M., Kang, S.W., Park, H.S. and Lee, M. *et al.* (2005). Differential inhibition of oxidized LDL-induced apoptosis in human endothelial cells treated with different flavonoids. *The British Journal of Nutrition*, 93(5): 581–91.

Kandaswami, C., Lee, L.T., Lee, P.P., Hwang, J.J., Ke, F.C., Huang, Y.T. *et al.* (2005). The antitumor activities of flavonoids. *In vivo,* 19(5): 895–909.

Kawai, Y. (2011). Immunochemical detection of food-derived polyphenols in the aorta: macrophages as a major target underlying the anti-atherosclerotic activity of polyphenols. *Bioscience, Biotechnology and Biochemistry*, 75(4): 609–17. doi:10.1271/ bbb.100785.

Kim, Y.W., Kang, H.E., Lee, M.G., Hwang, S.J., Kim, S.C., Lee, C.H. *et al.* (2009). Liquiritigenin, a flavonoid aglycone from licorice, has a choleretic effect and the ability to induce hepatic transporters and phase-II enzymes. *American Journal of*

Physiology Gastrointestinal and Liver Physiology, 296(2): G372–81. doi:10.1152/ajpgi.90524.2008.

Kris-Etherton, P.M. and Keen, C.L. (2002). Evidence that the antioxidant flavonoids in tea and cocoa are beneficial for cardiovascular health. *Current Opinion in Lipidology*, 13(1): 41–9.

Lahiri-Chatterjee, M., Katiyar, S.K., Mohan, R.R. and Agarwal, R. (1999). A flavonoid antioxidant, silymarin, affords exceptionally high protection against tumor promotion in the SENCAR mouse skin tumorigenesis model. Cancer Research, 59(3): 622–32.

Landi-Librandi, A.P., Caleiro Seixas Azzolini, A.E., de Oliveira, C.A. and Lucisano-Valim, Y.M. (2012). Inhibitory activity of liposomal flavonoids during oxidative metabolism of human neutrophils upon stimulation with immune complexes and phorbol ester. *Drug Delivery*, 19(4): 177–87. doi:10.3109/10717544.2012.679710.

Lau, G.T., Huang, H., Lin, S.M. and Leung, L.K. (2010). Butein downregulates phorbol 12-myristate 13-acetate-induced COX-2 transcriptional activity in cancerous and non-cancerous breast cells. *European Journal of Pharmacology*, 648(1–3): 24–30. doi:10.1016/j.ejphar.2010.08.015.

Lee, J.S., Kang, Y., Kim, J.T., Thapa, D., Lee, E.S. and Kim, J.A. (2012). The anti-angiogenic and anti-tumor activity of synthetic phenylpropenone derivatives is mediated through the inhibition of receptor tyrosine kinases. *European Journal of Pharmacology*, 677(1–3): 22–30. doi:10.1016/j.ejphar.2011.12.012.

Lee, Y.M., Hsieh, K.H., Lu, W.J., Chou, H.C., Chou, D.S., Lien, L.M. *et al.* (2012). Xanthohumol, a prenylated flavonoid from hops (*Humulus lupulus*), prevents platelet activation in human platelets. *Evidence-based Complementary and Alternative Medicine: eCAM*, 2012: 852362. doi:10.1155/2012/852362.

Li, F.Q., Wang, T., Pei, Z., Liu, B. and Hong, J.S. (2005). Inhibition of microglial activation by the herbal flavonoid baicalein attenuates inflammation-mediated degeneration of dopaminergic neurons. *Journal of Neural Transmission*, 112(3): 331–47. doi:10.1007/s00702-004-0213-0.

Li, L., Zeng, J., Gao, Y. and He, D. (2010). Targeting silibinin in the antiproliferative pathway. *Expert Opinion on Investigational Drugs*, 19(2): 243–55. doi:10.1517/13543780903533631.

Li, Y., Ma, C., Qian, M., Wen, Z., Jing, H. and Qian, D. (2014). Butein induces cell apoptosis and inhibition of cyclooxygenase2 expression in A549 lung cancer cells. *Molecular Medicine Reports*, 9(2): 763–7. doi:10.3892/mmr.2013.1850.

Li, Y., Sun, S., Chang, Q., Zhang, L., Wang, G., Chen, W. *et al.* (2013). A strategy for the improvement of the bioavailability and anti-osteoporosis activity of BCS IV flavonoid glycosides through the formulation of their lipophilic aglycone into nanocrystals. *Molecular Pharmaceutics,* 10(7): 2534–42. doi:10.1021/mp300688t.

Lim, E.K., Mitchell, P.J., Brown, N., Drummond, R.A., Brown, G.D., Kaye, P.M. *et al.* (2013). Regiospecific methylation of a dietary flavonoid scaffold selectively enhances IL-1beta production following Toll-like receptor 2 stimulation in THP-1 monocytes. *The Journal of Biological Chemistry*, 288(29): 21126–35. doi:10.1074/jbc.M113.453514.

Lopez-Sanchez, C., Martin-Romero, F.J., Sun, F., Luis, L., Samhan-Arias, A.K., Garcia-Martinez, V. *et al.* (2007). Blood micromolar concentrations of kaempferol afford protection against ischemia/reperfusion-induced damage in rat brain. *Brain Research,* 1182: 123–37. doi:10.1016/j.brainres.2007.08.087.

Lu, P., Mamiya, T., Lu, L.L., Mouri, A., Niwa, M., Hiramatsu, M. *et al.* (2009). Silibinin attenuates amyloid beta (25-35) peptide-induced memory impairments: Implication of inducible nitric-oxide synthase and tumor necrosis factor-alpha in mice. *The Journal of Pharmacology and Experimental Therapeutics*, 331(1): 319–26. doi:10.1124/jpet.109.155069.

Mahapatra, S.K., Chakraborty, S.P., Das, S. and Roy, S. (2009). Methanol extract of *Ocimum gratissimum* protects murine peritoneal macrophages from nicotine toxicity by decreasing free radical generation, lipid and protein damage and enhances antioxidant protection. Oxidative Medicine and Cellular Longevity, 2(4): 222–30. doi:10.4161/oxim.2.4.9000.

Maioli, N.A., Zarpelon, A.C., Mizokami, S.S., Calixto-Campos, C., Guazelli, C.F., Hohmann, M.S. *et al.* (2015). The superoxide anion donor, potassium superoxide, induces pain and inflammation in mice through production of reactive oxygen species and cyclooxygenase-2. *Brazilian Journal of Medical and Biological Research = Revistabrasileira de Pesquisasmedicas e Biologicas*, 48(4): 321–31. doi:10.1590/1414-431X20144187.

Manchope, M.F., Calixto-Campos, C., Coelho-Silva, L., Zarpelon, A.C., Pinho-Ribeiro, F.A., Georgetti, S.R. *et al.* (2016). Naringenin inhibits superoxide anion-induced inflammatory pain: Role of oxidative stress, cytokines, Nrf-2 and the NO-cGMP-PKG-KATP channel signaling pathway. *PloS ONE*, 11(4): e0153015. doi:10.1371/journal.pone.0153015.

Manju, V., Balasubramaniyan, V. and Nalini, N. (2005). Rat colonic lipid peroxidation and antioxidant status: The effects of dietary luteolin on 1,2-dimethylhydrazine challenge. *Cellular & Molecular Biology Letters,* 10(3): 535–51.

Manthey, J.A. (2000). Biological properties of flavonoids pertaining to inflammation. *Microcirculation*, 7(6 Pt 2): S29–34.

McCarty, M.F. (2008). Scavenging of peroxynitrite-derived radicals by flavonoids may support endothelial NO synthase activity, contributing to the vascular protection associated with high fruit and vegetable intakes. *Medical Hypotheses*, 70(1): 170–81. doi:10.1016/j.mehy.2005.09.058.

Meng, X., Munishkina, L.A., Fink, A.L. and Uversky, V.N. (2009). Molecular mechanisms underlying the flavonoid-induced inhibition of alpha-synuclein fibrillation. *Biochemistry,* 48(34): 8206–24. doi:10.1021/bi900506b.

Mercader, A.G. and Pomilio, A.B. (2012). (Iso)flav(an)ones, chalcones, catechins, and theaflavins as anti-carcinogens: Mechanisms, anti-multidrug resistance and QSAR studies. *Current Medicinal Chemistry*, 19(25): 4324–47.

Nisar, A., Malik, A.H. and Zargar, M.A. (2013). *Atropa acuminata* Royle Ex Lindl. blunts production of pro-inflammatory mediators eicosanoids., leukotrienes, cytokines *in vitro* and *in vivo* models of acute inflammatory responses. *Journal of Ethnopharmacology*, 147(3): 584–94. doi:10.1016/j.jep.2013.03.038.

Ozcelik, B., Kartal, M. and Orhan, I. (2011). Cytotoxicity, antiviral and antimicrobial activities of alkaloids, flavonoids, and phenolic acids. *Pharmaceutical Biology*, 49(4): 396–402. doi:10.3109/13880209.2010.519390.

Paquay, J.B., Haenen, G.R., Stender, G., Wiseman, S.A., Tijburg, L.B. and Bast, A. (2000). Protection against nitric oxide toxicity by tea. *Journal of Agricultural and Food Chemistry*, 48(11): 5768–72.

Par, A. and Javor, T. (1984). Alternatives in hepatoprotection: Cytoprotection–influences on mono-oxidase system–free radical scavengers (a review). *Acta Physiologica Hungarica*, 64(3–4): 409–23.

Park, S., Hahm, K.B., Oh, T.Y., Jin, J.H. and Choue, R. (2004). Preventive effect of the flavonoid, wogonin, against ethanol-induced gastric mucosal damage in rats. *Digestive Diseases and Sciences*, 49(3): 384–94.

Patel, S., Akalkotkar, A., Bivona, J.J., Lee, J.Y., Park, Y.K., Yu, M. *et al.* (2016). Vitamin A or E and a catechin synergize as vaccine adjuvant to enhance immune responses in mice by induction of early interleukin-15 but not interleukin-1beta responses. *Immunology*, 148(4): 352–62. doi:10.1111/imm.12614.

Peluso, I., Miglio, C., Morabito, G., Ioannone, F. and Serafini, M. (2015). Flavonoids and immune function in human: A systematic review. *Critical Reviews in Food Science and Nutrition*, 55(3): 383–95. doi:10.1080/10408398.2012.656770.

Rajendran, P., Rengarajan, T., Nandakumar, N., Palaniswami, R., Nishigaki, Y. and Nishigaki, I. (2014). Kaempferol, a potential cytostatic and cure for inflammatory disorders. *European Journal of Medicinal Chemistry*, 86: 103–12. doi:10.1016/j.ejmech.2014.08.011.

Rohdewald, P. (2002). A review of the French maritime pine bark extract (Pycnogenol), a herbal medication with a diverse clinical pharmacology. *International Journal of Clinical Pharmacology and Therapeutics*, 40(4): 158–68.

Romano, B., Pagano, E., Montanaro, V., Fortunato, A.L., Milic, N. and Borrelli, F. (2013). Novel insights into the pharmacology of flavonoids. *Phytotherapy Research: PTR*, 27(11): 1588–96. doi:10.1002/ptr.5023.

Salama, A. and Mueller-Eckhardt, C. (1987). Cianidanol and its metabolites bind tightly to red cells and are responsible for the production of auto-and/or drug-dependent antibodies against these cells. *British Journal of Haematology*, 66(2): 263–6.

Saleem, S., Shaharyar, M.A., Khusroo, M.J., Ahmad, P., Rahman, R.U., Ahmad, K. *et al*. (2013). Anticancer potential of rhamnocitrin 4'-beta-D-galactopyranoside against N-diethylnitrosamine-induced hepatocellular carcinoma in rats. *Molecular and Cellular Biochemistry*, 384(1–2): 147–53. doi:10.1007/s11010-013-1792-6.

Saleh, F., Raghupathy, R., Asfar, S., Oteifa, M. and Al-Saleh, N. (2014). Analysis of the effect of the active compound of green tea (EGCG) on the proliferation of peripheral blood mononuclear cells. BMC Complementary and Alternative Medicine, 14: 322. doi:10.1186/1472-6882-14-322.

Saliou, C., Rihn, B., Cillard, J., Okamoto, T. and Packer, L. (1998). Selective inhibition of NF-kappaB activation by the flavonoid hepatoprotector silymarin in HepG2. Evidence for different activating pathways. *FEBS Letters*, 440(1–2): 8–12.

Sausville, E.A., Zaharevitz, D., Gussio, R., Meijer, L., Louarn-Leost, M., Kunick, C. *et al*. (1999). Cyclin-dependent kinases: Initial approaches to exploit a novel therapeutic target. *Pharmacology & Therapeutics*, 82(2-3): 285–92.

Schmitz, K., Barthelmes, J., Stolz, L., Beyer, S., Diehl, O. and Tegeder, I. (2015). "Disease modifying nutricals" for multiple sclerosis. *Pharmacology & Therapeutics*, 148: 85–113. doi:10.1016/j.pharmthera.2014.11.015.

Shackelford, R.E., Manuszak, R.P., Johnson, C.D., Hellrung, D.J., Link, C.J., Wang, S. (2004). Iron chelators increase the resistance of Ataxia telangiectasia cells to oxidative stress. *DNA Repair*, 3(10): 1263–72. doi:10.1016/j.dnarep.2004.01.015.

Sharma, S., Arif, M., Nirala, R.K., Gupta, R. and Thakur, S.C. (2016). Cumulative therapeutic effects of phytochemicals in *Arnica montana* flower extract alleviated collagen-induced arthritis: inhibition of both pro-inflammatory mediators and oxidative stress. Journal of the Science of Food and Agriculture, 96(5): 1500–10. doi:10.1002/jsfa.7252.

Su, Z.R., Fan, S.Y., Shi, W.G. and Zhong, B.H. (2015). Discovery of xanthine oxidase inhibitors and/or alpha-glucosidase inhibitors by carboxyalkyl derivatization based on the flavonoid of apigenin. *Bioorganic & Medicinal Chemistry Letters*, 25(14): 2778–81. doi:10.1016/j.bmcl.2015.05.016.

Takahashi, T., Baba, M., Nishino, H. and Okuyama, T. (2006). Cyclooxygenase-2 plays a suppressive role for induction of apoptosis in isoliquiritigenin-treated mouse colon cancer cells. *Cancer Letters*, 231(2): 319–25. doi:10.1016/j.canlet.2005.02.025.

Tan, W.F., Lin, L.P., Li, M.H., Zhang, Y.X., Tong, Y.G., Xiao, D. *et al*. (2003). Quercetin, a dietary-derived flavonoid, possesses antiangiogenic potential. *European Journal of Pharmacology*, 459(2-3): 255–62.

Tanaka, T. and Takahashi, R. (2013). Flavonoids and asthma. *Nutrients,* 5(6): 2128–43. doi:10.3390/nu5062128.

Toyoda-Hokaiwado, N., Yasui, Y., Muramatsu, M., Masumura, K., Takamune, M., Yamada, M. *et al*. (2011). Chemopreventive effects of silymarin against 1,2-dimethylhydrazine plus dextran sodium sulfate-induced inflammation-associated carcinogenicity and genotoxicity in the colon of gpt delta rats. *Carcinogenesis,* 32(10): 1512–7. doi:10.1093/carcin/bgr130.

Vezina, A., Chokor, R. and Annabi, B. (2012). EGCG targeting efficacy of NF-kappaB downstream gene products is dictated by the monocytic/macrophagic differentiation status of promyelocytic leukemia cells. *Cancer Immunology, Immunotherapy: CII*, 61(12): 2321–31. doi:10.1007/s00262-012-1301-x.

Vue, B. and Chen, Q.H. (2016). The potential of flavonolignans in prostate cancer management. *Current Medicinal Chemistry*, 23(34): 3925–50.

Wang, H., Zhang, Y., Bai, R., Wang, M. and Du, S. (2016). Baicalin attenuates alcoholic liver injury through modulation of hepatic oxidative stress, inflammation and sonic hedgehog pathway in rats. *Cellular Physiology and Biochemistry: International Journal of Experimental Cellular Physiology, Biochemistry, and Pharmacology*, 39(3): 1129–40. doi:10.1159/000447820.

Wang, J., Qiu, J., Tan, W., Zhang, Y., Wang, H., Zhou, X. *et al.* (2015). Fisetin inhibits *Listeria monocytogenes* virulence by interfering with the oligomerization of listeriolysin O. *The Journal of Infectious Diseases*, 211(9): 1376–87. doi:10.1093/infdis/jiu520.

Zhan, C. and Yang, J. (2006). Protective effects of isoliquiritigenin in transient middle cerebral artery occlusion-induced focal cerebral ischemia in rats. *Pharmacological Research*, 53(3): 303–9. doi:10.1016/j.phrs.2005.12.008.

Zhang, X., Wang, G., Gurley, E.C. and Zhou, H. (2014). Flavonoid apigenin inhibits lipopolysaccharide-induced inflammatory response through multiple mechanisms in macrophages. *PloS ONE*, 9(9): e107072. doi:10.1371/journal.pone.0107072.

6

Molecular Mechanism of Flavonoids Against Ocular Diseases

R. Beema Shafreen[1]* and S. Seema[1]

ABSTRACT

Ocular diseases are emerging recently in all age groups from young to old age. Previously, visual impartment was observed mostly in aged person above 50 years and during certain disease conditions such as cataract, refractive error, glaucoma, macular degeneration, trachoma, childhood blindness and diabetic retinopathy. In this modern world, use of decorative contact lens, eye cosmetics and continuous exposure to electronic devices are reported to be other important factors for ocular infection leading to visual impairment. Hence there is an urgent need to investigate about the multi-targeted compounds that can be used for prevention and treatment of ocular disease. Over the decades, flavonoids are gaining importance in the pharmaceutical arena for their impending health benefits in human. Flavonoids are of key interest for investigation because of their vast availability in human diet for consumption and with different pharmacological actions such as antitumor, anti-inflammatory, antiviral, anti-osteoporotic, antioxidant, anti-aging and antithrombogenic. The multiplicity of pharmacological properties in flavonoids is mainly due to the occurrence of variable phenolic structures. The aetiology of ocular disease is oxidative damage that leads to lower supply of blood to the ocular tissues, hypoxia and other adverse effects leads to increased vascular permeability, leakage of the contents and angiogenesis. Interestingly, flavonoids used for treatment for such diseased conditions were also been investigated against ocular disease. Therefore flavonoids, the multi-factorial compound will be discussed further for their effective role in prevention and treatment of ocular disease.

Key words: Flavanoids, Bacteria, Fungi, Ocular infection, Ocular conditions, Visual impairment, Natural products, World

[1] Molecular Nanomedicine Research Unit, Centre for Nanoscience and Nanotechnology, Sathyabama University, Chennai - 600119, India.

**Corresponding author*: E-mail: beema.shafreen@gmail.com

Health Organization (WHO), Chemokines, Cytokines, Mucin-4 (MUC-4), Quercetin, Epigallocatechin gallate (EGCG), Hesperidin, Endophthalmitis

1. INTRODUCTION

Eyes are the most important organs of our human body that helps us in visualizing the objects. The function of this vital organ is affected due to the major factors such as environmental, microbial, endogenous stress and age which results in diverse spectrum of ocular diseases (Song *et al.*, 2016). A report from the World Health Organization (WHO) in 2015 estimated that approximately 285 million people were suffering from visual impairment worldwide. Among them, 32 million are living blind and 246 million people are at the risk of blindness (Taylor, 2016). According to the estimates 90% of people with visual impairment are recorded from developing countries. However, about 65% of the record shows that people above 50 years of age are visually impaired while this age group encompasses 20% of the world's population (WHO, 2015). Although cataract is an eye condition necessarily associated with ageing, there are other leading causes associated with blindness, including ocular infections due to bacterial, fungal, parasitic and viral agents that leads to granular conjunctivitis (Ridolo *et al.*, 2014), refractive error, macular degeneration (Midena and Pilotto, 2017), pink eye, styes and chalazia, bulging eyes or proptosis, blepharitis and uveitis. According to WHO, about 19 million children are living with visual impairment of which 1.4 million are irreversibly blind and 12 million are visually impaired. Though several treatment methods and precautions are undertaken, still there are people at risk of visual impairment due to chronic eye diseases and ageing processes. Hence bioflavonoids with prominence role in the pharmaceutical arena for their virtue of therapeutic benefits was explored against several ocular disease conditions. Therefore this review will provide the molecular mechanism of disease condition and discuss about the flavonoids that are been used for treatment of ocular diseases.

2. MOLECULAR MECHANISM OF THE DISEASE

Eye being the delicate sensory organ, is exposed with the external world directly and constantly. Many factors such as microbes, environment and stress can trigger the immunological events that can lead to eye infection, disease conditions and visual impairment. Hence the research on understanding the molecular mechanism of the ocular disease can improve the current medication used for treatment of the disease as well as for prevention. In this review the problems in the eye are categorized as Ocular infection, Ocular conditions and visual impairment and discussed in detail.

2.1. Ocular Infection

The widespread of common community-acquired pathogens, usage of contact lens, trauma and immunosuppression are some of the leading cause of ocular infection. The pathogenesis of ocular infection involves a dynamic relationship between host susceptibility and virulence factors. Invading pathogens such as fungi, bacteria, virus and parasite establish the infection either directly by trauma and surgery, or through infected sites and tissue. The infected eye show symptoms of redness of the eye, mucous and watering discharge and remains light sensitive.

2.1.1. *Fungi*

Fungi are recognized as opportunistic pathogens that cause ocular infections such as keratitis, scleritis, canaliculitis, endophthalmitis and orbital cellulitis (Garg, 2012). Ocular fungal infections such as ophthalmic mycoses are important causes of disease condition that leads to blindness and sometimes mortality of the patients. Mycotic keratitis caused by filamentous fungal genera such as *Fusarium, Alternaria*, and *Aspergillus*. *Keratitis* is caused by yeasts like fungi such as *Candida* sp. (Thomas and Kaliamurthy, 2014). These strains are opportunistic that cause infection in patients with dry eye, chronic corneal ulceration and scarring. Once the fungus comes in contact with the corneal stroma of the eye, the immune cells recognize the C-type lectin receptors (CLRs), a pattern recognition receptor of the pathogens and regulate the immune system to clear these pathogens. However, Dectin-1, a natural killer transmembrane signaling receptor on binding of the fungal pathogens induces various cellular functions for killing of the pathogens and produce inflammation by recruiting cytokines and chemokines to the site of infection (Guo and Wu, 2009).

Hyphal production is another important virulence factor that promotes the fungi to invade deep into the tissues and establish the pathogenicity. The signaling cascade activated in response to pH is an essential pathway that leads to the regulation of PacC/Rim101p transcription factor. Thus the activation of the *pacC* genes in fungal species facilitate them to survive in the corneal specific microenvironment and penetrate into the stromal tissues (Hua *et al.*, 2010). Reports have shown that deletion of pacC prevents the invasion of the fungi into the tissues and establish the infection. Thus PacC pathway is identified as potential target to control fungal eye disease.

2.1.2. *Bacteria*

Bacterial pathogens showing resistance to antimicrobial agents play a major role in ocular infection. The key pathogens that are involved in endophthalmitis are coagulase-negative *Staphylococci* and *Streptococcus* species (Mueller and McStay, 2008, Callegan *et al.*, 2013, Deibel and Cowling, 2014). Bacterial keratitis is also frequently caused by *Staphylococcus aureus* and *Pseudomonas aeruginosa* while bacterial conjunctivitis is generally associated with *S. aureus* and *Streptococcus pneumoniae* (Hazlett *et al.*, 2017, Lakhundi *et al.*, 2017). Invading of the bacterial pathogens to ocular region binds to the Toll-like receptors (TLR)-4/5 presented by the corneal macrophages. Thus the binding of the bacterial pathogens reduce the production of cytokines and chemokines (KC/CXCL1) and other Interleukins (IL-α and IL-β) to the site of infection. Expression of inflammasomes (TLR2, TLR4-5 and TLR9, NLRP3 and NLRC4) is necessary for clearance of the bacteria. But during the corneal ulcer there is elevation in inflammasomes that increase the severity and spread of the infection (Zhou *et al.*, 2009). Therefore antimicrobial agents that can inhibit the fast immunological response can indeed control the severity of infection.

2.2. Ocular Conditions

2.2.1. *Allergic conjunctivitis*

An ocular allergic condition has been increased dramatically in the last decades due to numerous factors like cosmetics, pets, air pollution, smoke, dust. (Johnson, 2004, Oh *et al.*, 2016). Ocular allergy is the most common ocular conditions encountered in clinical practice. Molecular mechanism of allergic conjunctivitis involves two stages. The first stage is the sensitization stage, once the environmental antigens are in contact, Th2 immune response is activated and IgE antibodies are produced. In the second stage, the effector phase on encountering with the antigen, histamine is released which leads to the degranulation of mast cells (Stern *et al.*, 2010). The inflammatory response induced by the allergens is the main cause for severity of the conjunctivitis. Oral anti-histamines are commonly used during ocular allergic condition. Due to the adverse effect of the first-generation anti-histamines, the second-generation anti-histamines are recommended for therapy. However, the second-generation anti-histamines can also induce ocular drying which may impair the protective barrier of the ocular tear film and thereby deteriorate the allergic symptoms (Bielory, 2002). Hence there is no evidence for effective treatment of the allergic conjunctivitis. Therefore there is still an augmented search of novel agents that can overcome the inflammatory response caused by the allergens.

2.2.2. *Dry eye disease*

In this modern world, to make life easier and for fun several electronic gadgets are available. The electronic gadget like mobile phones, laptops, tablets and TV directly affect the eye. The content in the electronic screen requires more optical focus which gives more strain for the eyes and are mostly harmful. Dry eye disease is also known as keratoconjunctivitis sicca (KCS) (Galletti *et al.*, 2017). Dry eyes, is a disorder of the tear film which is mainly occurring due to tear deficiency or excessive tear evaporation. Thus dry eye is classified as evaporative dry eye (EDE) and aqueous dry eye (ADE) (Khanal *et al.*, 2009). The limited secretion of oil by the meibomian glands leads to the quick evaporation of tears resulting in EDE. Whereas, in case of ADE the lacrimal gland does not produce the water component leading to concentrated and unstable tear film which cause the damage to the inter-palperbral surface and results in ocular discomfort. During the dry eye syndrome there is increasing level of proinflammatory cytokines. Mucin-4 (MUC-4) is known for clearing function, lubrication and act as barriers to corneal and conjunctival epithelial matrix (Meloni *et al.*, 2011). Increase in the expression of protease such as metallopeptidase which degrades the ocular surface and upregulates the activity of MUC-4 results in deranged corneal epithelial barrier function, corneal desquamation and surface irregularity.

2.2.3. *Cataract*

Cataract is the leading cause of blindness worldwide, associated with age. Cataract is caused with a number of environmental risk factors that includes cigarette smoking, obesity or elevated blood glucose levels, corticosteroid, exposure to UV radiation, oxidation, deamidation, truncations and alcohol consumption (Fig. 1) (Moreau and King, 2013). The aggregates of protein that are accumulated through several pathways on exposure to these risk factors leads to the cumulative damage of lens proteins and cells. Lens proteins are known to undergo a wide variety of alterations with age, due to oxidative, osmotic and other stress factor that leads to cataracts. Lens proteins involve two main crystalline families; βγ-crystallin and α-crystallins. With increase in the age, intermolecular interaction of βγ-crystallin is decreased and they slowly begin to denature and accumulate as precipitate (Basak *et al.*, 2003). The precipitate is bound to α-crystallins, which have chaperone-like activity, to maintain the solubility of βγ-crystallins and reduce the light scattering. Further in the disease condition, α-crystallins binding with the βγ-crystallin remain as insoluble complex that scatters light. Investigations with Mendelian cataract models have shown mutation in crystalline proteins leads to cataract conditions of the eye. The accumulation of denatured crystalline proteins and other short peptides can cause damage to the lens cells (Udupa and Sharma, 2005). The changes in the cellular architecture of the lens lead to the scattering of light which results in cataractous lens.

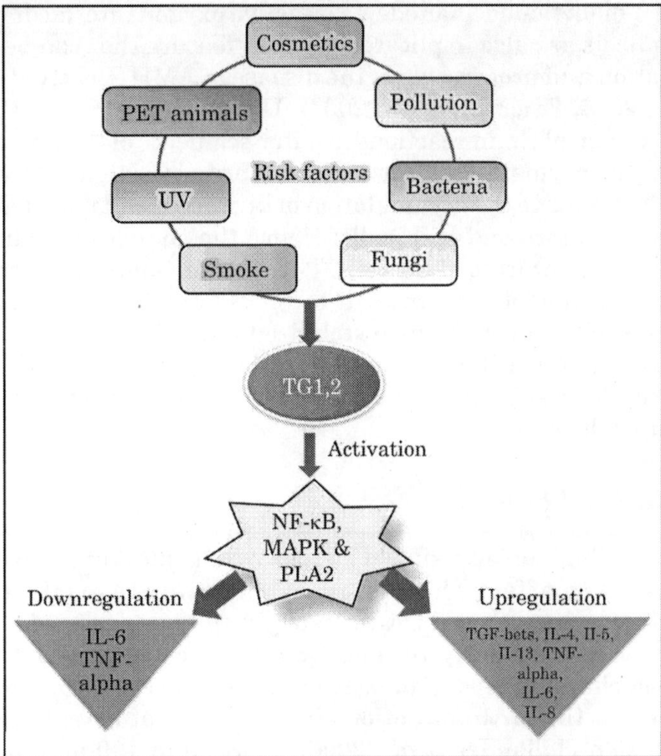

Fig. 1: Risk Factors and molecular mechanism of the immune regulatory factors involved in ocular disease

2.3. Visual Impairment

2.3.1. *Age-related macular degeneration*

Age-related macular degeneration (AMD) is a degenerative disease of the outer retina. AMD is one of the severe leading cause of irreversible visual impairment occurring in people above 50 years of age. There is considerable challenge for treatment of AMD since its etiology is not known and there are only limited treatment options. Old age is identified as the prime risk factor for ADM. Retinal pigmented epithelium (RPE) and photoreceptors are the most affected retinal tissues of AMD disease (Friedman *et al.*, 2004). There are two types of AMD: (i) atrophic form and (ii) disciform macular degeneration. Atrophic form is associated with pigmentary changes in the macula without hemorrhage or scar formation. Disciform macular degeneration is characterized by exudative mound formation and intra-retinal hemorrhage. However, leakage of plasma from small blood vessels in the macula following breakdown of the blood-retinal barrier can lead to macular edema and can endanger vision. Besides age, macular pigmentary change, hypertension, smoking and obesity are other risk factors of AMD.

Importantly, diabetic-macular edema, reactive oxygen intermediates (ROI) and free radicals are also implicated as other feature that can be involved in the initiation and progression of the disease in AMD (Beatty *et al.*, 2000, Ohia *et al.*, 2005, Erickson *et al.*, 2007). Ultraviolet radiation (UV) light initiates free radical chain reactions in outer segments of the photoreceptor and inhibits the normal cellular process that are associated with lysosomal enzymes. This leads to the accumulation of lipofuscin and melanolipofuscin in the photoreceptors and RPE cells. Hence the changes culminate with dysfunction and rupturing of the cells. The mechanism-based therapy such as anti- vascular endothelial growth factor-A (VEGF-A) was used in the earlier stages to treat AMD which stabilized vision in the vast majority of patients. Reports have shown that a mutation in factor XIII (G185T) can deteriorate the response of choroidal neovascularisation during photodynamic therapy.

2.3.2. *Childhood blindness*

Childhood blindness is also known as Leber congenital amaurosis (LCA). LCA rigorously affect the vision of children in early life. The pathogenetic mechanism of LCA was not yet fully understood because of its complexity. Subsequently, the genetic and clinical heterogeneity of LCA was not been characterized (Sahel, 2011). LCA is a rare disorder of retina which occurs at the birth. Mutations in any one of at least 15 genes will cause LCA (den Hollander *et al.*, 2006). More than 400 mutations have been identified related to LCA and approximately 70% of all the LCA cases are related to these mutations. The genes that are frequently mutated are found to be Crumbs homolog 1 (CRB1), centrosomal protein 290 kDa (CEP290; also known as NPHP6), and guanylatecyclase 2D (GUCY2D). The retinal pigment epithelium–(RPE65) gene encodes a retinoid isomerase enzyme necessary for the production of chromophore, which is involved in the formation of the visual pigment of photoreceptors in retina. The proteins that encode LCA-associated genes are also involved in the many retinal function, like photoreceptor morphogenesis, vitamin A cycling, guanine synthesis, phototransduction, and outer segment (OS) phagocytosis (Stone, 2007). Though the LCA-associated genes are preferentially expressed specifically in the retina, two more genes are also identified recently, which is found to be mutated in patients with LCA5, encoding

For Lebercilin (Dharmaraj *et al.,* 2000) and Cep290 (den Hollander *et al.*, 2006). Any mutations that occur in RPE65, can result in 5%–10% of all LCA disorders (Stieger and Lorenz, 2010).

2.3.3. *Uveal melanoma*

Uveal melanoma (UM) is the intraocular malignant tumor seen in adults (Rajpal *et al.*, 1983). Approximately 50% of mortality is observed in patients with metastases occurring in liver. Metastasis involves many processes such as tumor cell adhesion, migration and proteolysis of the extracellular matrix and invasion. The tumor cells undergo intravasation, enter into the vascular and the lymphatic systems, and finally extravasate to invade the secondary sites. Proteolytic enzymes, matrix metalloproteinase (MMP) and plasminogen activators are involved in each step of metastasis. The migration of a malignant cell through extracellular matrix (ECM) and the basement membrane requires proteolytic activities. Thus during uveal melanomas condition the expression of proteins such as MMP-2 and MMP-9, tissue inhibitor of metalloproteases, urokinase plasminogen activator, as well as different integrins are observed. The other conditions are the structural abnormalities on chromosomes 3, 6, and 8q which lead to metastatic death during UM. Previously, there are no reports for predictions of the cytogenetic anomalies associated with the UM. Due to the latest trends in using next generation sequencing non-random mutations in several genes such as GNAQ, GNA11, BAP1 and SF3B1/EIF1AX have been revealed (Dono *et al.*, 2015). Thus the mutations in these genes leads to different levels of expression profiles, which are associated with different classes of tumor formation. There are no postoperative adjuvant therapies obtainable to reduce the threat of metastasis. The only treatment used today is enucleation or radiation therapy. Therefore, new molecular targets are needed to be established that can provide effective treatment modalities in treatment of UM

3. FLAVONOIDS AND DISEASE: POTENTIAL MOLECULAR MECHANISMS INVOLVED

Flavonoids have been documented for multiple actions such as free radical scavenging activity, antibacterial, antifungal, inhibition of nitric oxide production, ROS generating enzymes and chelation of trace elements (Fig. 2). The different classes of flavonoids with such potential role include flavanols, flavones, isoflavones, flavan-3-ols, flavanones and anthocyanidins. There are several reports that apparently discuss about bioflavonoid as potential therapeutic agents with different mechanism of action on ocular disease as well as their effect on the aetiological factors. Hence immense investigations are being carried out to explore new class of flavonoids from medicinal and traditional plant extract for prevention and cure of ocular disease (Table. 1).

Ginkgo leaves are already known for their antioxidant property and used as dietary supplements in different countries. *Ginkgo biloba* extract (GBE) contains two main active ingredients, flavonoids and terpenoids and approximately about 25% of flavone glycosides. Human volunteers with ocular disease were tested with oral dose of 40 mg of GBE, thrice a day and the procedure was repeated for 2 days. The human volunteers consuming GBE showed increased blood flow in the ophthalmic artery. Studies on

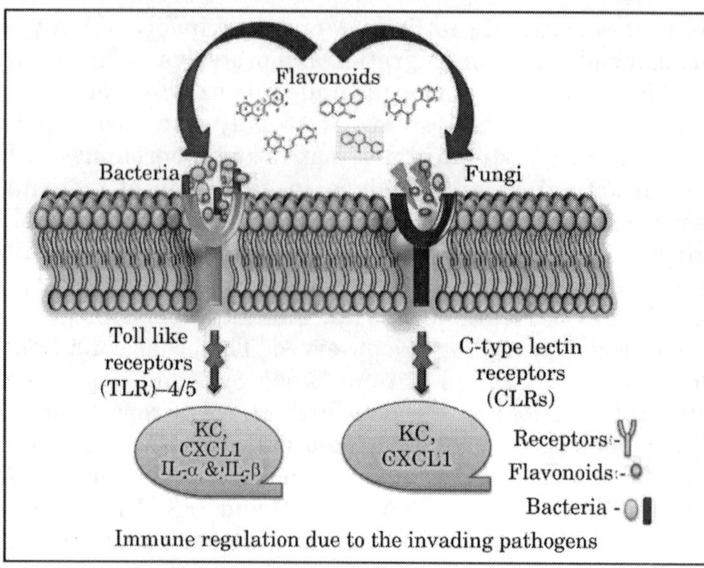

Fig. 2: Schematic representation showing flavonoids as inhibitors against bacterial and fungal pathogens capable of causing ocular infection and the immunomodulatory response.

mammalian cells with GBE indicated protection of cells from nitric oxide reactivity by scavenging the nitric oxide and also prevented their further production. GBE with such potential role is assumed to protect optic nerve degeneration and prevent the loss of retinal ganglion cells in patients suffering from glaucoma, DR, and RP blindness (Chung *et al.*, 1999, Wimpissinger *et al.*, 2007). Therefore, GBE is neuroprotection and would be an interesting component for treatment and prevention of ocular diseases such as glaucoma and other major neurodegenerative retinal pathologies.

Catechins are the major active constituents of green tea, several studies have proposed that green tea extract consumption has beneficiary role in protecting the eyes from oxidative damage and infection. *In vivo* investigation with Sprague – Dawley rats has proved antioxidative effects of catechins in ocular tissues (Chu *et al.*, 2010). Also Sprague – Dawley rat model induced for cataracts with N-methyl-N-nitrosourea (MNU) showed recovery from cataract when treated with catechins (Lee *et al.*, 2011). The apoptosis in cataract lens epithelium was significantly reduced upon treatment with catechins. Epigallocatechin-3 gallate (EGC3g), flavonoid from green tea shows inhibitory effect against bacterial gelatinases. Gelatinases are a class of proteases that are secreted by bacterial pathogens causing ocular infection. EGC3g prevents the invasion of the bacterial pathogens as well as inhibits the gelatinase activity. Gelatinase regulates the production of gelatin which is essential for invasive spreading of the infection. Investigation with *in vivo* model has proved that systemic administration of EGC3g in the invasive keratitis model has significantly

Table 1: Natural products as inhibitors against Ocular disease

Sl. no	*Disease*	*Types*	*Risk factors*	*Symptoms*	*Natural products for treatment*
1.	Dry eye disease	1. Evaporative dry eye 2. Aqueous dry eye	Laser vision surgery, computer and other video displays	Photophobia, blurred vision, Itchy eyes	Human milk
2.	Allergic conjunctivitis	1. Acute allergic conjunctivitis 2. Chronic allergic conjunctivitis	Environment, contact lens	Itching and redness of eye, Light sensitivity	Rose petals, *Calendula officinalis*, *Sassafras albidum*
3.	Cataract	1. Nuclear cataracts 2. Cortical cataracts 3. Posterior cataracts	UV light, Age	Seeing double, blurry vision	Alpha lipoic acid, blue berry fruit, triphala
4.	Glaucoma	1. Open angle glaucoma 2. Angle closure glaucoma	High myopia, diabetes	Headache, nausea and vomiting	*Coleus, Cannabis, Ginkgo leaf.*
5.	Uveal melanoma	1. Iris melanoma 2. Posterior Uveal melanoma	Age, Exposure to UV light	Blurry vision, floaters, Visual field loss	Genistein, *Aloe vera*
6.	Age related macular degeneration	1. Dry macular degeneration 2. Wet macular degeneration	Smoking, obesity	Hallucinations, Blind spots	Dodder seed, lyceum fruit, blue berry fruit.
7.	Childhood blindness		Vitamin deficiency, genetics	Loss of vision	*Asparagus africanuslam*
8.	Herpes keratitis	1. Herpes Simplex type I 2. Herpes Simplex type II	Herpes simplex virus	Tearing, Eye sores, ocular pain	Licorice root, lemon balm, *Hypericum perforatum*
9.	Diabetic retinopathy	1. Non proliferative retinopathy 2. Proliferative retinopathy	Diabetes	Floaters, Impaired color vision.	Pycnogenol, ginkgo leaf, *Cassia tora* seed
10.	Bacterial Keratitis		*Pseudomonas aeroginosa, Staphylococcus aureus*	Eye pain, Light sensitivity, irritation	Barberry root bark, gold thread rhizome, *Coptis chinensis*.
11.	Fungal Keratitis		*Aspergillus* and *candida* sp	Tearing, Redness, photophobia	

reduced the inflammasome migration. Thus EGC3g has been reported as a promising candidate to prevent inflammation and infection of ocular tissues (Blanco *et al.*, 2003). Additionally, Epigallocatechin gallate (EGCG) was tested in AMD induced Sprague-Dawley rat models. *In vivo* models were injected intraperitoneally with sodium iodate to induce degeneration. After 14 days, the histopathological section of the retina showed degeneration of RPE, cone and rod. A series of irregular folding was observed in the outer nuclear layer and the outer regions of the retina leading to the cause for irreversible visual impairment and blindness. The investigation of EGCG along with The ahenon E showed significant reduction of damages in the retinal components. Thus EGCG and Theaphenon E a commercialized product of green tea extract, manufactured under food grade can be used by patients for protection and prevention from oxidative stress related damages (Yang *et al.*, 2016). EGCG has also been revealed as potential agents to protect retinal neuron *in situ* during ischemic reperfusion (Zhang *et al.*, 2007). Therefore it is suggested that catechin would be a better choice of compound that has beneficial role in prevention of AMD and cataract.

Several other neuroprotective flavonoids (3, 6 dihydroxyflavone, 3, 7 dihydroxyflavone, galangin, baicalein, luteolin, fisetin, quercetin, and eriodictyol) were effective on RPE cells in preventing retinal cell death induced by oxidative stress. However the treatment with some of these flavonoids was found to be effective before the RPE cell death. Eriodictyol, investigated with human RPE cells induces the nuclear erythroid 2 - transcription factor and down regulates the heme-oxygenase (*Hox-1*) gene thereby prevents the ROS accumulation and promotes angiogenesis (Johnson *et al.*, 2009).

Quercetin, flavonoid found in a variety of plant, black and green tea, vegetables of *Brassica* sp., and berry fruits is known for their antioxidant property. Quercetin inhibits the sorbitol-aldose reductase, calpain protease production, glycation and epithelial cellular signaling pathways (Chen *et al.*, 2008, Li *et al.*, 2015). In addition, quercetin is also reported with anti-cataract properties that act as inhibitor of sorbitol-aldose reductase pathway. Aldose reductase (AR) are the key enzymes of the sorbitol pathway that contributes to diabetes-associated cataract (Stefek and Karasu, 2011). Hence Quercetin is used as a standard for screening other flavonoids with role in cataract inhibition and aldose-reductase inhibition.

Hesperidin, flavonoid from citrus fruits inhibits the expression of hypoxia-inducible factor-1α (HIF-1α), tumor necrosis factor (TNF-α) and inflammatory cytokine production in the human mast cell line (HMC-1) (Choi *et al.*, 2007). HIF-1α is an important mediator of inflammatory response and one of the major transcriptional activators of vascular endothelial growth factor (VEGF) which plays a critical role in the process of angiogenesis. Thus hesperidin prevents the apoptosis and cell death and can promote the angiogenesis.

Naringenin, flavonoid derived from citrus and grape fruits have reports for their pharmacological properties. Naringenin when used for topical administration (0.5% -1%) in rabbits have shown protection of retinal cells from structural and functional MNU-induced damages (Lin *et al.*, 2014). Narigenin has also potential role in reversing the degeneration of RPE cells induced damage by sodium iodate and choroidal neovascularization induced with laser (Lin *et al.*, 2014). Thus naringenin has been reported as promising flavonoids to treat photoreceptor mediated cell death leading to age-AMD and retinitis pigmentosa (RP).

Genistein, from soybeans was investigated for their pharmacological role in inherited cataract rat (ICR/f) model and for understanding the mechanism of cataractogenesis. The results revealed that dietary supplements for the rats with genistein-containing food has prevented and reversed cataract formation (Floyd *et al.*, 2010). Thus geinstein can be used to prevent or delay lens cataract formation at an early stage of their development.

4. FUTURE PERSPECTIVES

Flavonoids have a wide array of protective actions in the ocular region, including a potential to protect neurons against injury induced by immunological factors and have the ability to suppress inflammation. The effects of flavonoids appear to be underpinned by three common processes. Firstly, flavonoids act as inhibitors of the bacterial and fungal pathogens that can cause ocular infection. Secondly, they interact with critical enzymes of the pathway and activate the signaling cascades in ocular region and further inhibit apoptosis triggered by inflammasomes. Thirdly, they induce beneficial effects on the ocular system leading to changes in ocular blood flow capable of causing angiogenesis and neurogenesis. Hence flavonoids are able to trigger these mechanisms and can act as potential agentd to prevent ocular disease. The consumption of healthy diet such as fruits and vegetables that are rich in flavonoids holds the potential to limit the process of age-dependent degeneration and prevents infection with proper immune regulation. Though flavonoids are being consumed daily through our diet, it is investigated that oral administration of bioflavonoids have limited pharmacological activity on the outer regions of the posterior ocular segment as well as the protection of the retinal ganglionic cells. Therefore it is envisaged that systemic or local administration of bioflavonoids can yield much higher and effective concentrations of the parent bioflavonoids in the ocular tissues and at much lower doses.

Thus flavonoids are of intense interest for developing drug of choice to treat ocular diseases. Furthermore, flavonoids can be used as precursor molecules in the quest to develop new generation drugs that can enhance the protective mechanism for the ocular system.

5. CONCLUSIONS

Flavonoids have been used for the prevention and treatment of various diseases. Previously, flavonoids were not awarded with much scientific consideration. In the recent years, researchers and pharmaceutical companies have raised increasing interest for flavonoids from plants and nutraceuticals. Several major eye diseases in particular, infection due to bacterial and fungal pathogens, conjunctivitis, cataract, AMD, glaucoma, and other retinal pathologies are been investigated with flavonoids for their potential beneficial effects. These diseases can lead to ocular damage, disorder and visual impairment primarily through pathogens, ROS mediated oxidative stress, inflammation, and ocular pressure. Similarly, flavonoids posses several known properties like strong anti-oxidative, anti-inflammatory, and anti-apoptotic properties. Although this review documents with some of the well-known and common flavonoids for treatment of ocular diseases, there are intense interest to screen for new flavonoids classes from other botanical extract that may help with treatment of ocular and other disease as well. Therefore, further investigation of natural plant-derived flavonoids, especially their mechanisms of action, is necessary to harness the full potential of flavonoids to be used as complementary and alternative medicine for major eye diseases.

6. ACKNOWLEDGEMENT

The author's gratefully acknowledge Science and Engineering Research Board (SERB), Department of Science and Technology, Government of India through YSS-SERB [File No.SRYSS/2014/000127].

REFERENCES

Basak, A., Bateman, O., Slingsby, C. *et al.* (2003). High-resolution X-ray crystal structures of human gamma D crystallin (1.25 A) and the R58H mutant (1.15 A) associated with aculeiform cataract. *J. Mol. Biol.,* 328: 1137–1147.

Beatty, S., Koh, H., Phil, M., Henson, D. and Boulton, M. (2000). The role of oxidative stress in the pathogenesis of age-related macular degeneration. *Surv Ophthalmol,* 45: 115–134.

Bielory, L. (2002). Role of antihistamines in ocular allergy. *Am. J. Med.,* 113 (Suppl 9A): 34S–37S.

Blanco, A.R., La Terra Mule, S., Babini, G., Garbisa, S., Enea, V. and Rusciano, D. (2003). (-) Epigallocatechin-3-gallate inhibits gelatinase activity of some bacterial isolates from ocular infection, and limits their invasion through gelatine. *Biochim. Biophys. Acta.,* 1620: 273–281.

Callegan, M., Gregory-Ksander, M., Willcox, M. and Lightman, S. (2013). Ocular inflammation and infection. *Int. J. Inflam.,* 2012: 403520.

Chen, Y., Li, X.X., Xing, N.Z. and Cao, X.G. (2008). Quercetin inhibits choroidal and retinal angiogenesis *in vitro*. *Graefes. Arch. Clin. Exp. Ophthalmol.,* 246: 373–378.

Choi, I.Y., Kim, S.J., Jeong, H.J. *et al.* (2007). Hesperidin inhibits expression of hypoxia inducible factor-1 alpha and inflammatory cytokine production from mast cells. *Mol. Cell. Biochem.,* 305: 153–161.

Chu, K.O., Chan, K.P., Wang, C.C. *et al.* (2010). Green tea catechins and their oxidative protection in the rat eye. *J. Agric. Food Chem.,* 58: 1523–1534.

Chung, H.S., Harris, A., Kristinsson, J.K., Ciulla, T.A., Kagemann, C. and Ritch, R. (1999). *Ginkgo biloba* extract increases ocular blood flow velocity. *J. Ocul. Pharmacol. Ther.,* 15: 233–240.

Deibel, J.P. and Cowling, K. (2014). Ocular inflammation and infection. *Emerg. Med. Clin. North Am.,* 31: 387–397.

den Hollander, A.I., Koenekoop, R.K., Yzer, S. *et al.* (2006). Mutations in the CEP290 (NPHP6) gene are a frequent cause of Leber congenital amaurosis. *Am. J. Hum. Genet.,* 79: 556–561.

Dono, M., Angelini, G., Cecconi, M. *et al.* (2015). Mutation frequencies of GNAQ, GNA11, BAP1, SF3B1, EIF1AX and TERT in uveal melanoma: detection of an activating mutation in the TERT gene promoter in a single case of uveal melanoma. *Br. J. Cancer.,* 110: 1058–1065.

Erickson, K.K., Sundstrom, J.M. and Antonetti, D.A. (2007). Vascular permeability in ocular disease and the role of tight junctions. *Angiogenesis,* 10: 103–117.

Floyd, K.A., Stella, D.R., Wang, C.C., Laurentz, S., McCabe, G.P., Srivastava, O.P. and Barnes, S. (2010). Genistein and genistein-containing dietary supplements accelerate the early stages of cataractogenesis in the male ICR/f rat. *Exp. Eye Res.,* 92: 120–127.

Friedman, D.S., O'Colmain, B.J., Munoz, B. *et al.* (2004). Prevalence of age-related macular degeneration in the United States. *Arch. Ophthalmol.,* 122: 564–572.

Galletti, J.G., Guzman, M. and Giordano, M.N. (2017). Mucosal immune tolerance at the ocular surface in health and disease. *Immunology,*

Garg, P. (2012). Fungal, Mycobacterial, and Nocardia infections and the eye: An update. *Eye (Lond),* 26: 245–251.

Guo, H. and Wu, X. (2009). Innate responses of corneal epithelial cells against *Aspergillus fumigatus* challenge. *FEMS Immunol. Med. Microbiol.,* 56: 88–93.

Hazlett, L., Suvas, S., McClellan, S. and Ekanayaka, S. (2017). Challenges of corneal infections. *Expert. Rev. Ophthalmol.,* 11: 285–297.

Hua, X., Yuan, X. and Wilhelmus, K.R. (2010). A fungal pH-responsive signaling pathway regulating *Aspergillus* adaptation and invasion into the cornea. *Invest Ophthalmol. Vis. Sci.,* 51: 1517–1523.

Johnson, G.J. (2004). The environment and the eye. *Eye (Lond),* 18: 1235–1250.

Johnson, J., Maher, P. and Hanneken, A. (2009). The flavonoid, eriodictyol, induces long-term protection in ARPE-19 cells through its effects on Nrf2 activation and phase 2 gene expression. *Invest. Ophthalmol. Vis. Sci.,* 50: 2398–2406.

Khanal, S., Tomlinson, A. and Diaper, C.J. (2009). Tear physiology of aqueous deficiency and evaporative dry eye. *Optom. Vis. Sci.,* 86: 1235–1240.

Lakhundi, S., Siddiqui, R. and Khan, N.A. (2017). Pathogenesis of microbial keratitis. *Microb. Pathog.,* 104: 97–109.

Lee, S.M., Ko, I.G., Kim, S.E., Kim, D.H. and Kang, B.N. (2011). Protective effect of catechin on apoptosis of the lens epithelium in rats with N-methyl-N-nitrosourea-induced cataracts. *Korean J. Ophthalmol.,* 24: 101–107.

Li, F., Bai, Y., Zhao, M., Huang, L., Li, S., Li, X. and Chen, Y. (2015). Quercetin inhibits vascular endothelial growth factor-induced choroidal and retinal angiogenesis *in vitro. Ophthalmic. Res.,* 53: 109–116.

Lin, J., Sun, J., Wang, Y. *et al.* (2014). Ocular pharmacokinetics of naringenin eye drops following topical administration to rabbits. *J. Ocul. Pharmacol. Ther.,* 31: 51–56.

Lin, J.L., Wang, Y.D., Ma, Y., Zhong, C.M., Zhu, M.R., Chen, W.P. and Lin, B.Q. (2014). Protective effects of naringenin eye drops on N-methyl-N-nitrosourea-induced photoreceptor cell death in rats. *Int. J. Ophthalmol.,* 7: 391–396.

Meloni, M., De Servi, B., Marasco, D. and Del Prete, S. (2011). Molecular mechanism of ocular surface damage: Application to an *in vitro* dry eye model on human corneal epithelium. *Mol. Vis.,* 17: 113–126.

Midena, E. and Pilotto, E. (2017). Microperimetry in age: Related macular degeneration. *Eye (Lond).*

Moreau, K.L. and King, J.A. (2013). Protein misfolding and aggregation in cataract disease and prospects for prevention. *Trends. Mol. Med.,* 18: 273–282.

Mueller, J.B. and McStay, C.M. (2008). Ocular infection and inflammation. *Emerg. Med. Clin. North. Am.,* 26: 57–72, vi.

Oh, J.E., Lee, H.J., Choi, Y.W., Choi, H.Y. and Byun, J.Y. (2016). Metal allergy in eyelid dermatitis and the evaluation of metal contents in eye shadows. *J. Eur. Acad. Dermatol. Venereol.,* 30: 1518–1521.

Ohia, S.E., Opere, C.A. and Leday, A.M. (2005). Pharmacological consequences of oxidative stress in ocular tissues. *Mutat. Res.,* 579: 22–36.

Rajpal, S., Moore, R. and Karakousis, C.P. (1983). Survival in metastatic ocular melanoma. *Cancer,* 52: 334–336.

Ridolo, E., Montagni, M., Caminati, M., Senna, G., Incorvaia, C. and Canonica, G.W. (2014). Emerging drugs for allergic conjunctivitis. *Expert. Opin. Emerg. Drugs,* 19: 291–302.

Sahel, J.A. (2011). Spotlight on childhood blindness. *J. Clin. Invest.,* 121: 2145–2149.

Song, J., Huang, Y.F., Zhang, W.J., Chen, X.F. and Guo, Y.M. (2016). Ocular diseases: Immunological and molecular mechanisms. *Int. J. Ophthalmol.,* 9: 780–788.

Stefek, M. and Karasu, C. (2011). Eye lens in aging and diabetes: Effect of quercetin. *Rejuvenation Res.,* 14: 525–534.

Stern, M.E., Schaumburg, C.S., Dana, R., Calonge, M., Niederkorn, J.Y. and Pflugfelder, S.C. (2010). Autoimmunity at the ocular surface: Pathogenesis and regulation. *Mucosal Immunol.,* 3: 425–442.

Stieger, K. and Lorenz, B. (2010). Gene therapy for vision loss – recent developments. *Discov. Med.,* 10: 425–433.

Stone, E.M. (2007). Leber congenital amaurosis - a model for efficient genetic testing of heterogeneous disorders: LXIV Edward Jackson Memorial Lecture. *Am. J. Ophthalmol,* 144: 791–811.

Taylor, H.R. (2016). The global issue of vision loss and what we can do about it: Jose Rizal Medal 2015. *Asia Pac. J. Ophthalmol. (Phila),* 5: 95–96.

Thomas, P.A. and Kaliamurthy, J. (2014). Mycotic keratitis: epidemiology, diagnosis and management. *Clin. Microbiol. Infect.,* 19: 210–220.

Udupa, E.G. and Sharma, K.K. (2005). Effect of oxidized betaB3-crystallin peptide on lens betaL-crystallin: Interaction with betaB2-crystallin. *Invest Ophthalmol Vis Sci,* 46: 2514–2521.

Wimpissinger, B., Berisha, F., Garhoefer, G., Polak, K. and Schmetterer, L. (2007). Influence of *Ginkgo biloba* on ocular blood flow. *Acta Ophthalmol Scand.,* 85: 445–449.

Yang, Y., Qin, Y.J., Yip, Y.W. *et al.* (2016). Green tea catechins are potent anti-oxidants that ameliorate sodium iodate-induced retinal degeneration in rats. *Sci. Rep.,* 6: 29546.

Zhang, B., Safa, R., Rusciano, D. and Osborne, N.N. (2007). Epigallocatechin gallate, an active ingredient from green tea, attenuates damaging influences to the retina caused by ischemia/reperfusion. *Brain Res.,* 1159: 40–53.

Zhou, Z., Wu, M., Barrett, R.P., McClellan, S.A., Zhang, Y. and Hazlett, L.D. (2009). Role of the Fas pathway in *Pseudomonas aeruginosa* keratitis. *Invest. Ophthalmol. Vis. Sci.,* 51: 2537–2547.

7

Flavonoids in the Treatment of Pulmonary Lung Diseases

SHANMUGARAJ GOWRISHANKAR[1] AND SHUNMUGIAH KARUTHA PANDIAN[1]*

ABSTRACT

Flavonoids are class of polyphenolic compounds that have been classified into flavones, flavonones, catechins and anthocyanins. They are abundant in colored plants and over 4000 flavonoids have been reported from different sources. Recently several reports have documented the beneficial effect of flavonoids such as antiviral, anti-allergic, antitumor, antiplatelet, anti-inflammatory and antioxidant. It include various mechanism of action in biological properties such as scavenging free radicals, chelating metal ions, regulating mitochondrial function, activation of signaling pathways, and modulating inflammatory response. This chapter aims to discuss the effect of different flavonoids in the control of pulmonary lung inflammation and the possible mechanism of action.

Key words: Flavonoids, Pulmonary lung diseases, Lung inflammation, Respiratory diseases, Anti-inflammatory, Anti-oxidant, Rutin, Flavones, Flavonones, Catechins, Anthocyanins, Oxidative stress, Free radicals, ROS, RNS, Anti-allergic, Anti-asthma, Anti-COPD, Anti-ARDS, Vitamin P.

1. INTRODUCTION

For a decade, the rate of pulmonary diseases has been increasing and it has been associated with substantiate morbidity and mortality. Among pulmonary diseases, acute respiratory distress syndrome, asthma and chronic obstructive pulmonary diseases are the most communal and

[1] Department of Biotechnology, Alagappa University, Science Campus, Karaikudi - 630003, Tamil Nadu, India
**Corresponding author*: E-mail: sk_pandian@rediffmail.com

accompanying with increasing rate of death (Bateman *et al.,* 2008). The acute and chronic infections in pulmonary regions have been a major cause for these diseases which could orchestrate a lot of inflammatory mediators (Murphy and O'Byrne, 2010). Inflammation is a cellular process that occurs in the lungs induced by various internal and external agents. Though it has been an important response in the organism, chronic reaction could damage the lungs. Inflammation in lungs involves the activation of inflammatory cells, such as macrophages, neutrophils, eosinophils and lymphocytes. These are the source of different inflammatory mediators like tumor necrosis factor (TNF-α), prostaglandins, histamine, nitric oxide and leukotrienes. The release of these mediators gives signal for the activation of inflammatory process which could act against the symptoms observed in pulmonary diseases. The treatment of the lung diseases often involves the use of anti-inflammatory and anti-oxidant therapies (Kariyawasam *et al.,* 2007).

Since many years, flavonoids have been used in the treatment of inflammatory diseases including pulmonary lung infections for its anti-inflammatory and antioxidant properties (Bravo, 1998). In 1930, a new compound was isolated from orange fruits and believed to be a member of vitamins then it was designated as vitamin P. Research on vitamin-P makes clear that this substance was flavonoids (rutin). Flavonoids are group of natural compound with different phenolic structures and are abundant in fruits, vegetables, grains bark, roots, stems, flowers, wine and tea (Middleton, 1998). They have been a major coloring component of flowers, fruits and leaves (de Groot and Rauen, 1998).

2. CHEMISTRY OF FLAVONOIDS

Chemically, flavonoids have a fifteen-carbon skeleton consisting of two benzene rings linked with the help of heterocyclic pyrene ring. Based on their molecular structure, it has been classified into 4 main groups Table 1.

Table 1: Four major groups of flavonoids with their individual compounds

Group	*Compound*
Flavones	Apigenin, Chrysin, Kaempferol, Luteolin, Myricetin, Rutin, Sibelin, Quercetin
Flavonones	Fisetin, Hesperetin, Narigin, Naringenin, Taxifolin
Catechins	Catechin, Epicatechin, Epigallocatechin gallate
Anthocyanins	Cyanidin, Delphinidin, Malvidin, Pelargonidin, Peonidin, Petunidin

The molecular structure of each group of flavonoids is given in Fig. 1. The different groups of flavonoids differ in the level of oxidation (Middleton,

1998). Flavonoids are also available as glycosides, aglycones, and methylated derivatives. Aglycone is the basic flavonoids structure. It has a six-member ring connected with the benzene ring which is a alpha-pyrone (flavonols and flavanones). The flavonols and flavanones differ by the 3-hydroxyl group and a C2-C3 double bond (Yao *et al.,* 2004). Additionally, flavonoids are hydroxylated in the positions of 3,5,7,2,3′,4′ and 5′ and have methyl ethers and acetyl esters. While the formation of glycosides, the glyosidic linkages are found in the positions 3 or 7 or in the sugar moieties L-rhamnose, D-glucose, glucorhamnose, galactose or arabinose (Yao *et al.,* 2004). A double bond at C2 position creates flavones such as chrysin (Das, 1994), apigenin (Jorgensen, 1993) and rutin (Guardia *et al.,* 2001) as well as isoflavones such as genistin (Pajkrt *et al.,* 1997), genistein (Hesslinger *et al.,* 2009), daidzin (Hantos *et al.,* 2008) and daidzein (Holgate, 1997). The reduction of flavonols produces flavan-3-ols like catechin (Prado *et al.,* 2005), epicatechin (Ricciardolo *et al.,* 2006) and epigallocatechin gallate (Smith *et al.,* 2000) and the colorful anthocyanidins, such as apigenidin and cyaniding (Lin *et al.,* 2002).

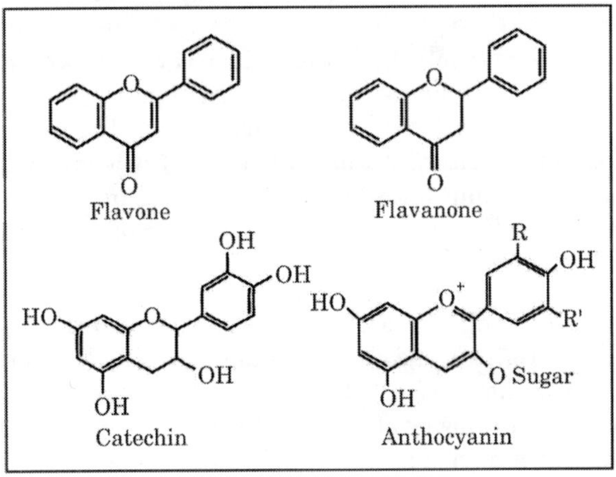

Fig. 1: The molecular structure of different group of flavonoids

3. BIOLOGICAL ACTIVITIES OF FLAVONOIDS IN PROTECTING PULMONARY LUNG INFLAMMATIONS

3.1. Anti-inflammatory Activity of Flavonoids Against Pulmonary Lung inflammation

Inflammation is a dynamic response to cellular damages induced by various physical and chemical factors. An acute inflammatory reaction has a vital role in immune response and protect against injury, chronic inflammation caused by the pathogenesis of autoimmune, neurodegenerative and respiratory diseases. The acute inflammatory response chiefly involves macrophage activation. The activation of macrophages and other immune cells releases pro-inflammatory cytokines such as tumor necrosis factor (TNF-α), interleukins (IL), etc., which elicited the inflammatory cascade by acting on end-organ receptors against injury (Matot and Sprung, 2001, Khazan and Hdayati, 2015).

Cyclooxygenase and lipoxygenase are vital inflammatory mediators. They are involved in the release of arachidonic acid, which is a preparatory for all general inflammatory response. Lipoxygenase found in the neutrophils create chemotactic compound from arachidonic acid, which provoke the release of cytokines. Certain flavonoids like quercetin (Maciel *et al.,* 2013) inhibited both the cyclooxygenase and 5-lipoxygenase pathways to showcase an anti-inflammatory activity (Ferrandiz and Alcaraz, 1991, Laughton *et al.,* 1991). The actual mechanisms by which flavonoids inhibiting these enzymes are still not clear. In addition, inhibiting the eicosanoid biosynthesis is another anti-inflammatory mechanism adopted by flavonoids (Formica and Regelson, 1995). Eicosanoids, like prostaglandins are reported to be involved in several immunological activities (Moroney *et al.,* 1988) and are final product of the cyclooxygenase and lipoxygenase pathways. These phenolic compounds have also inhibited the membrane and cytosolic tyrosine kinase (Formica and Regelson, 1995) and tyrosine 3-monooxygenase kinase which have been involved in the process of enzyme catalysis, transport across the membrane, signal transduction, energy transfer and synthesis. This leads to inhibition of cell growth and proliferation. It also has a potential to degranulate neutrophils and other immune cells which reduced the release of arachidonic acid (Hoult *et al.,* 1994, Tordera *et al.,* 1994).

Flavonoids can suppress the level of COX by interfering the signaling pathways like protein kinase C. NF-κB and tyrosine kinase pathways (Lee *et al.,* 1998, Bastianetto *et al.,* 2000, Lin *et al.,* 2002). Additionally, the anti-inflammatory property of flavonoids are connected with their ability in altering the expression of pro-inflammatory such as NOS, cyclooxygenase, lipoxygenase by modulating the NF-κB, Nrf2/Keapl (Jiang *et al.,* 2012) and mitogen-activated protein kinase (Santangelo *et al.,* 2007, Toledo *et al.,* 2013) pathways. Number of evidences also confirmed that flavonoids modulate the inflammatory cells like T-lyphocytes, TNF-α, interleukin-1 and other controlling enzymes found in the arachidonic acid pathway such as nitric oxide (NO) (Biesalski, 2007, Lopez-Posadas *et al.,* 2008, Cazarolli *et al.,* 2008). The different mechanisms of anti-inflammatory activities of flavonoids were shown in Fig. 2. The flavanols such as quercetin (Soobrattee *et al.,* 2005) and kaempferol (Nijveldt *et al.,* 2001) demonstrated a significant anti-inflammatory activity by suppressing the phospholipase A2, lipoxygenase, cyclooxygenase and thromboxane enzymes through modulating the inducible nitric oxide synthase (iNOS) and resulting in the inhibition of NO (Yoon and Baek, 2005, Santangelo *et al.,* 2007). The same mode of action mechanism was also attributed to apigenin (Jorgensen,

1993), chrysin (Zhang *et al.*, 2014), genistein (Hesslinger *et al.*, 2009) and luteolin (Lien *et al.*, 1999). Furthermore, flavonoids like myricetin (Newman and Cragg, 2007), naringenin (Caltagirone *et al.*, 1997), hesperetin (Croft, 1998) also demonstrated anti-inflammatory activity by inhibiting phospholipase A2 enzyme (Cazarolli *et al.*, 2008). Quercetin inhibits the activity of cyclooxygenase and lipoxygenase metabolites (Robak and Gryglewski, 1996, Kim *et al.*, 1998). Moreover, the flavones chrysin (Das, 1994), luteolin (Lien *et al.*, 1999), and apigenin (Jorgensen, 1993) and the flavonols genistein (Hesslingere *et al.*, 2009), quercetin (Soobrattee *et al.*, 2009), luteolin (Lien *et al.*, 1999), apigenin (Jorgensen, 1993) and rutin (Guardia *et al.*, 2001) have inhibited the pro-inflammatory cytokines such as TNF-α and interlukin-1 (Cazarolli *et al.*, 2001, Nair *et al.*, 2006, Park *et al.*, 2008).

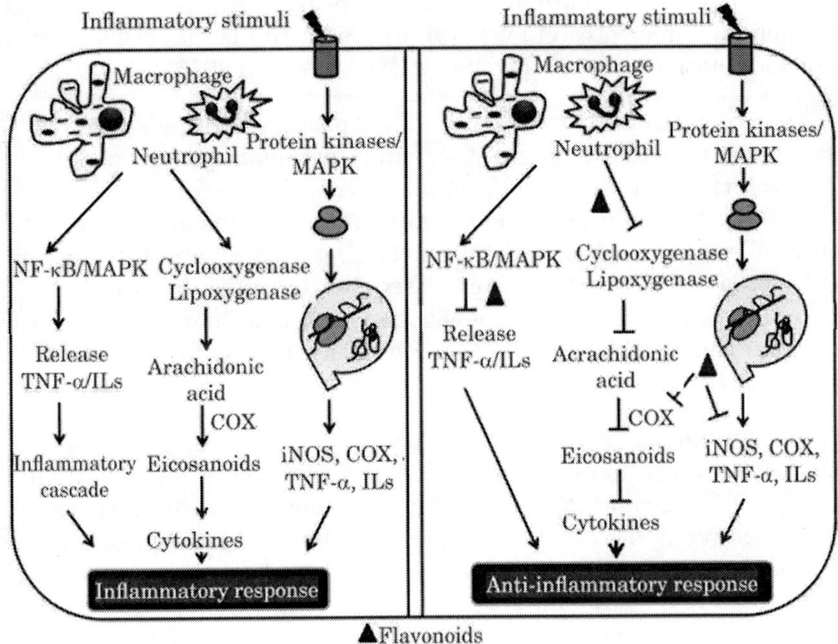

Fig. 2: Graphical representation of different anti-inflammatory mechanisms of flavonoids

3.2. Antioxidant Activity of Flavonoids Against Pulmonary Lung Inflammation

The hallmark property of pulmonary lung diseases is the oxidative stress. Flavonoids have been well documented for its antioxidant activity and it protects free radicals induced cellular injuries (Lago *et al.*, 2014). The activity of any flavonoids is directly associated with the ability of the donation of hydrogen radical from phenolic group and the presence of a lone-pair of electrons in the aromatic ring. The number of hydroxyl groups present in determined the antioxidant activity of non-glycosylated flavonoids (Lago *et al.,* 2014). The less number of hydroxyl group in the chemical structure of Kaempferol determined the low antioxidant activity (Lien *et al.,* 1999, Soobrattee *et al.,* 2005). In addition, the non-glycosylated derivatives like quercetin (Soobrattee *et al.,* 2005), myricetin (Beecher, 2003), luteolin (Lien *et al.,* 1999) and kaempferol (Lago *et al.,* 2014) exhibited a higher antioxidant capacity than the associated flavonoids quercitrin (Bors *et al.,* 1990), astragalin (Noroozi *et al.,* 1998) and rutin (Heim *et al.,* 2002). This suggested that the configuration, number of hydroxyl group and substitution determine the antioxidant activity such as radical scavenging and metal ion chelation potential (Cao *et al.,* 1997, Pandey *et al.,* 2012). The configuration of B ring significantly influenced the scavenging activity of ROS and RNS. The unpaired electron present in the B ring donates hydrogen and an electron to peroxyl, hydroxyl and peroxynitrite radicals promoted relatively stable flavonoids (Mishra *et al.,* 2013).

The action mechanism of antioxidant process include scavenging of ROS, suppression of ROS generation either by chelating elements involved in free radical formation and upregulation of antioxidant defense (Brown *et al.,* 1998). Moreover, some of the antioxidant effects of flavonoids may be the collective result of radical scavenging activity and interfere with the function of enzyme. It suppressed the enzymes involved in ROS production like microsomal monooxygenase, glutathione-S-transferase, mitochondrial succinoxidase, NADH oxidase, and so forth (Kumar and Pandey, 2012).

Lipid peroxidation has been a common significance of oxidative stress. Flavonoids protect lipids from oxidative stress mediated damages (Kumar *et al.,* 2013, Mishra *et al.,* 2013). The reduction of hydroxyl radical and highly reactive hydroxyl radical increases the ROS formation. Owing to the lesser redox potentials (Fl-OH) flavonoids have been thermodynamically reduced the highly oxidizing free radicals like superoxide, peroxyl, alkoxyl and hydroxyl radicals by hydrogen atom donotion (Fig. 3A). The capacity to chelate metal ion determine the ability of flavonoids to inhibit free radical generation (van Acker *et al.,* 1996, Brown *et al.,* 1998). In particular, quercetin is known for its metal chelating and iron-stabilizing potentials. The metal-chelating and stabilization can be achieved by the binding of the trace metal at specific positions of different rings of flavonoids structure (Sekher Pannala *et al.,* 2001) (Fig. 3B). The 3′, 4′-catechol structure in the B ring strongly enhances the inhibition of lipid peroxidation. This special feature of flavonoids makes them effective scavengers of free radicals (Pandey *et al.,* 2012). The oxidation on the B ring of flavonoids in catechol group formed a stable ortho-semiquinone radical which acts as strong scavenger. The lack of oxidation in the flavones leads to the weak scavenging potential (Ratty and Das, 1988).

The heterocycle present in flavonoid contribute to the antioxidant activity by allowing connection between the aromatic rings and the free 3-OH. Removal of 3-OH compromises the scavenging ability of flavonoids (Noroozi *et al.,* 1998). It is hypothesized that B ring OH group form hydrogen bond with the 3-OH, aligning the B ring, heterocycle and A ring. This intramolecular hydrogen bonding and 3′,4′-catechol illustrate the potent antioxidant activity of flavon-3-ols and flavan-3-ols. Mostly the occurrence, position, structure and number of sugar moieties in flavonoids have a vital role in antioxidant activity. Aglycones are reported to be more potent antioxidant than their respective glycoside. Previous study by (Rice-Evans *et al.,* 1996) stated that the antioxidant property of flavonol glycosides decreased with the less number of glycoside moieties in tea. However glycosides are usually weaker antioxidant than aglycones, the bioavailability is increased by glucose moiety. In normal diet, flavonoid glyosidic moieties occur at the 3- or 7- position (Vennat *et al.,* 1994). Increase in the degree of polymerization enhances the activity of procyanidins against a various free radical species. The dimer and trimer of procyanidins have been more effective in scavenging superoxide anion than monomeric flavonoids. Tetramers demonstrated an increased scavenging activity against peroxynitrite and superoxide anion than trimers, while hexamers and heptamers exhibited significantly greater superoxide scavenging properties than trimers and tetramers (Wheeler and Bernard, 1999).

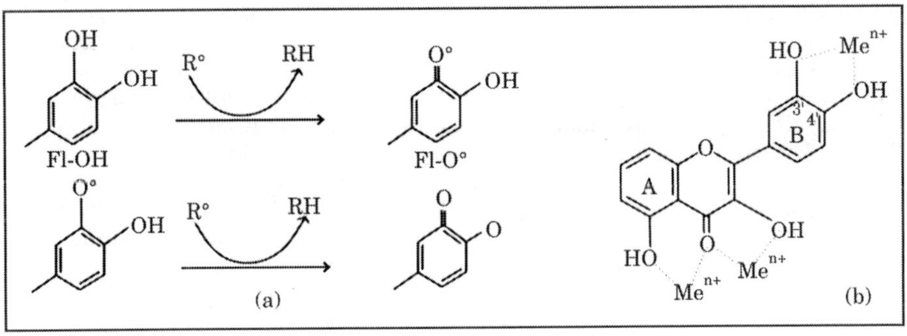

Fig. 3: (A) ROS scavenging effect of flavonoids (Fl-OH) and (B) Binding site for metal ions (Me^{n+} represented the metal ions).

Flavonoids like quercetin (Soobrattee *et al.,* 2005); silibin (Ferrali *et al.,* 1997) and leuteolin (Lien *et al.,* 1999) are the most effective inhibitors of xanthine oxidase (Goya *et al.,* 2016). The ability to chelate metal iron (Goya *et al.,* 2016) and the decreased activation of complement system by flavonoids suppressed the adhesion of inflammatory cells to the endothelium (Prado *et al.,* 2006). Moreover, these compounds interfere with the metabolism of arachidonic acid and inhibit the peroxidase release; this may help to reduce the ROS by neutrophils and α1-antitrypsin activation (Fiander and Schneider, 2000). Notably, some flavonoids have chelate transition metal ions that are responsible for the generation of ROS and inhibit the lipoxygenase reaction. The antioxidant properties of flavonoids have also through the stimulation of antioxidant enzymes. Most of the flavonoids reduce oxidative stress by inducing the glutathione-S-transferase (GST), an enzyme that protect cell from oxidative stress mediated damages (Silva *et al.*, 2002). Table 2 lists the essential flavonoids that have exhibited beneficial activities against lung inflammation and diseases.

Table 2: List represents the essential flavonoids and its beneficial effects on lung diseases

Flavonoids	*Beneficial effect*	*Lung effect*	*References*
Apigenin, Myricetin, Quercetin, Morin, 3,6-Dihydroxy-flavone	Anti-inflammatory/ antioxidant	Anti-allergic	Jorgensen 1993, Soobrattee *et al.*, 2005, Newman and Cragg 2007, Jayaprakasam *et al.*, 2009
Apigenin, Quercetin, Luteolin, Fisetin, Scutellarin, Quercetagetin, Kaempferol-3-O-galactoside, Cirsiliol, Baicalein, Isoliquiritigenin, Liquiritigenin	Anti-inflammatory/ antioxidant	Anti-asthmatic	Shutenko *et al.*, 1999, Fiander and Schneider 2000, Kimata *et al.*, 2000, Silva *et al.*, 2002, Ricciardolo *et al.*, 2006, Rogerio *et al.*, 2007, Wolfe and Liu 2008, Li *et al.*, 2012, Townsend and Emala 2013
Luteolin, Morin, Fisetin, Flavone, Tricetin, Liquritigenin, Isoliquiritigenin, 7,4-Dihydroxyflavone, Liquiritin, Apioside	Anti-inflammatory/ antioxidant	Anti-COPD	Kimata *et al.*, 2000, Johansson *et al.*, 2002, Wolfe and Liu 2008, Weseler *et al.*, 2009, Guan *et al.*, 2011, Li *et al.*, 2012
Quercetin	Anti-inflammatory/ antioxidant	Anti -ARDS	Kalhan *et al.*, 2008

The anti-inflammatory and antioxidant potentials of Sakuranetin, a type of flavonoids have been recently examined in models of lung diseases (Beecher, 2003, Toledo *et al.*, 2013). The results revealed that Sakuranetin has a great deal in treating asthma and other lung diseases by reducing the eosinophilic inflammation. In addition, this reduction in eosinophilic inflammation could be attributed to an inhibition of Th2 cytokines, oxidative stress and NF-κB activity. The different mechanisms of antioxidant activity of flavonoids were shown in Fig. 4.

4. CLINICAL PERSPECTIVES OF FLAVONOIDS APPLICATION IN LUNG DISEASE

Till now, numerous studies have been shown that different types of flavonoids are in controlling lung diseases. Few of the studies have been executed in humans to evaluate their beneficial activity on phytotherapy against lung diseases. Smith *et al.* (2000) demonstrated that the flavonoids improved the functioning of lung in studied 1000 patients. Most studies revealed that the mechanism of action of flavonoids is through the suppression of NF-κB. Therefore, insightful knowledge on molecular mechanism of flavonoids, toxic and adverse effects especially in humans are required.

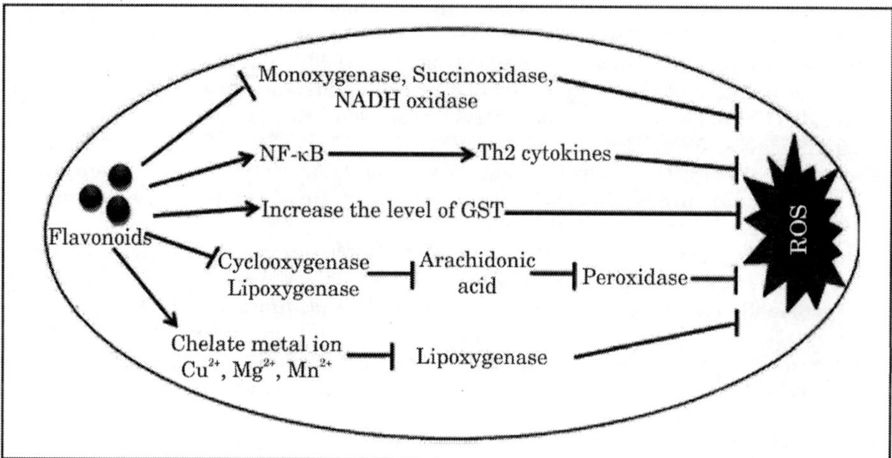

Fig. 4: Graphical representation of different antioxidant mechanisms of flavonoids

5. CONCLUSIONS

This chapter reports that the beneficial activity of flavonoids in lung disease could be attributed to an anti-inflammatory and antioxidant effects. Lung disease is always associated with inflammation and oxidative stress which leads to the loss of its function. To overcome these adverse effects in human, flavonoids have been examined in experimental modes and were found to be favorable by chiefly inhibiting cytokines related with the suppression of several transcription factors. Generally, the key structures features like the unsaturation in the C ring, position and total number of hydroxyl groups, carbonly groups and nonglycosylation of molecules determine the activity of flavonoids. Taking these structural features into consideration, one may infer that the natural products such as flavonoids may perhaps be useful as prototypes in the development of novel therapeutics against several lung diseases. However, insight investigation is required to exhibit the action mechanisms and to determine whether these results can be applicable to human diseases.

REFERENCES

Bastianetto, S., Zheng, W.H. and Quirion, R. (2000). Neuroprotective abilities of resveratrol and other red wine constituents against nitric oxide-related toxicity in cultured hippocampal neurons. *Br. J. Pharmacol.*, 131: 711–720.

Bateman, E.D., Hurd, S.S., Barnes, P.J. *et al.* (2008). Global strategy for asthma management and prevention: GINA executive summary. *Eur. Respir. J.*, 31: 143–178.

Beecher, G.R. (2003). Overview of dietary flavonoids: Nomenclature, occurrence and intake. *J. Nutr.*, 133: 3248S–3254S.

Biesalski, H.K. (2007). Polyphenols and inflammation: Basic interactions. *Curr. Opin. Clin. Nutr. Metab. Care*, 10: 724–728.

Bors, W., Heller, W., Michel, C. and Saran, M. (1990). Flavonoids as antioxidants: Determination of radical-scavenging efficiencies. *Methods Enzymol.*, 186: 343–355.

Bravo, L. (1998). Polyphenols: Chemistry, dietary sources, metabolism, and nutritional significance. *Nutr. Rev.*, 56: 317–333.

Brown, J.E., Khodr, H., Hider, R.C. and Rice-Evans, C.A. (1998). Structural dependence of flavonoid interactions with Cu2+ ions: Implications for their antioxidant properties. *Biochem. J.*, 330(Pt 3): 1173–1178.

Caltagirone, S., Ranelletti, F.O., Rinelli, A. *et al.* (1997). Interaction with type II estrogen binding sites and antiproliferative activity of tamoxifen and quercetin in human non-small-cell lung cancer. *Am. J. Respir. Cell. Mol. Biol.*, 17: 51–59.

Cao, G., Sofic, E. and Prior, R.L. (1997). Antioxidant and prooxidant behavior of flavonoids: Structure-activity relationships. *Free Radic Biol. Med.*, 22: 749–760.

Cazarolli, L.H., Zanatta, L., Alberton, E.H. *et al.* (2008). Flavonoids: Prospective drug candidates. *Mini. Rev. Med. Chem.*, 8: 1429–1440.

Croft, K.D. (1998). The chemistry and biological effects of flavonoids and phenolic acids. *Ann. N.Y. Acad. Sci.*, 854: 435–442.

Das, D.K. (1994). Naturally occurring flavonoids: Structure, chemistry, and high-performance liquid chromatography methods for separation and characterization. *Methods Enzymol.*, 234: 410–420.

De Groot, H. and Rauen, U. (1998). Tissue injury by reactive oxygen species and the protective effects of flavonoids. *Fundam. Clin. Pharmacol.*, 12: 249–255.

Ferrali, M., Signorini, C., Caciotti, B., Sugherini, L., Ciccoli, L., Giachetti, D. and Comporti, M. (1997). Protection against oxidative damage of erythrocyte membrane by the flavonoid quercetin and its relation to iron chelating activity. *FEBS Lett.*, 416: 123–129.

Ferrandiz, M.L. and Alcaraz, M.J. (1991), Anti-inflammatory activity and inhibition of arachidonic acid metabolism by flavonoids. *Agents Actions*, 32: 283–288.

Fiander, H. and Schneider, H. (2000). Dietary ortho phenols that induce glutathione S-transferase and increase the resistance of cells to hydrogen peroxide are potential cancer chemopreventives that act by two mechanisms: The alleviation of oxidative stress and the detoxification of mutagenic xenobiotics. *Cancer Lett.*, 156: 117–124.

Formica, J.V. and Regelson, W. (1995). Review of the biology of Quercetin and related bioflavonoids. *Food Chem. Toxicol.*, 33: 1061–1080.

Goya, L., Martin, M.A., Sarria, B., Ramos, S., Mateos, R. and Bravo, L. Effect of cocoa and its flavonoids on biomarkers of inflammation: Studies of cell culture, animals and humans. *Nutrients*, 8: 212.

Guan, Y., Li, F.F., Hong, L. *et al.* (2011). Protective effects of liquiritin apioside on cigarette smoke-induced lung epithelial cell injury. *Fundam. Clin. Pharmacol.*, 26: 473–483.

Guardia, T., Rotelli, A.E., Juarez, A.O. and Pelzer, L.E. (2001). Anti-inflammatory properties of plant flavonoids. Effects of rutin, quercetin and hesperidin on adjuvant arthritis in rat. *Farmaco.*, 56: 683–687.

Hantos, Z., Adamicza, A., Janosi, T.Z., Szabari, M.V., Tolnai, J. and Suki, B. (2008). Lung volumes and respiratory mechanics in elastase-induced emphysema in mice. *J. Appl. Physiol.*, 105: 1864–1872.

Heim, K.E., Tagliaferro, A.R. and Bobilya, D.J. (2002). Flavonoid antioxidants: Chemistry, metabolism and structure-activity relationships. *J. Nutr. Biochem.*, 13: 572–584.

Hesslinger, C., Strub, A., Boer, R., Ulrich, W.R., Lehner, M.D. and Braun, C. (2009). Inhibition of inducible nitric oxide synthase in respiratory diseases. *Biochem. Soc. Trans.*, 37: 886–891.

Holgate, S.T. (1997). Asthma: A dynamic disease of inflammation and repair. *Ciba. Found. Symp.*, 206: 5–28; *Discussion*, 28–34, 106–110.

Hoult, J.R., Moroney, M.A. and Paya, M. (1994). Actions of flavonoids and coumarins on lipoxygenase and cyclooxygenase. *Methods Enzymol.*, 234: 443–454.

Jayaprakasam, B., Doddaga, S., Wang, R., Holmes, D., Goldfarb, J. and Li, X.M. (2009). Licorice flavonoids inhibit eotaxin-1 secretion by human fetal lung fibroblasts *in vitro*. *J. Agric. Food Chem.*, 57: 820–825.

Jiang, J., Mo, Z.C., Yin, K. *et al.* (2012). Epigallocatechin-3-gallate prevents TNF-alpha-induced NF-kappaB activation thereby upregulating ABCA1 *via* the Nrf2/Keap1 pathway in macrophage foam cells. *Int. J. Mol. Med.*, 29: 946–956.

Johansson, S., Goransson, U., Luijendijk, T., Backlund, A., Claeson, P. and Bohlin, L. (2002). A neutrophil multitarget functional bioassay to detect anti-inflammatory natural products. *J. Nat. Prod.*, 65: 32–41.

Jorgensen, R. (1993). The origin of land plants: A union of alga and fungus advanced by flavonoids? Biosystems, 31: 193–207.

Kalhan, R., Smith, L.J., Nlend, M.C., Nair, A., Hixon, J.L. and Sporn, P.H. (2008). A mechanism of benefit of soy genistein in asthma: Inhibition of eosinophil p38-dependent leukotriene synthesis. *Clin. Exp. Allergy.*, 38: 103–112.

Kariyawasam, H.H., Aizen, M., Barkans, J., Robinson, D.S. and Kay, A.B. (2007). Remodeling and airway hyper responsiveness but not cellular inflammation persist after allergen challenge in asthma. *Am. J. Respir. Crit. Care Med.*, 175: 896–904.

Khazan, M. and Hdayati, M. (2015). The role of nitric oxide in health and diseases. *Scimetr.*, 3: e20987.

Kim, H.P., Mani, I., Iversen, L. and Ziboh, V.A. (1998). Effects of naturally-occurring flavonoids and biflavonoids on epidermal cyclooxygenase and lipoxygenase from guinea-pigs. *Prostaglandins Leukot Essent Fatty Acids*, 58: 17–24.

Kim, H.P., Son, K.H., Chang, H.W. and Kang, S.S. (2004). Anti-inflammatory plant flavonoids and cellular action mechanisms. *J. Pharmacol. Sci.*, 96: 229–245.

Kimata, M., Shichijo, M., Miura, T., Serizawa, I., Inagaki, N. and Nagai, H. (2000). Effects of luteolin, quercetin and baicalein on immunoglobulin E-mediated mediator release from human cultured mast cells. *Clin. Exp. Allergy*, 30: 501–508.

Kumar, S. and Pandey, A.K. (2012). Antioxidant, lipo-protective and antibacterial activities of phyto constituents present in *Solanum xanthocarpum* root. *Int. Rev. Biophys. Chem.*, 3: 42–47.

Kumar, S., Mishra, A. and Pandey, A.K. (2013). Antioxidant mediated protective effect of *Parthenium hysterophorus* against oxidative damage using *in vitro* models. *BMC Complement Altern. Med.*, 13: 120.

Lago, J.H., Toledo-Arruda, A.C., Mernak, M., Barrosa, K.H., Martins, M.A., Tiberio, I.F. and Prado, C.M. (2014). Structure-activity association of flavonoids in lung diseases. *Molecules*, 19: 3570–3595.

Laughton, M.J., Evans, P.J., Moroney, M.A., Hoult, J.R. and Halliwell, B. (1991). Inhibition of mammalian 5-lipoxygenase and cyclo-oxygenase by flavonoids and phenolic dietary additives. Relationship to antioxidant activity and to iron ion-reducing ability. *Biochem Pharmacol.*, 42: 1673–1681.

Lee, S.C., Kuan, C.Y., Yang, C.C. and Yang, S.D. (1998). Bioflavonoids commonly and potently induce tyrosine dephosphorylation/inactivation of oncogenic proline-directed protein kinase FA in human prostate carcinoma cells. *Anticancer Res.*, 18: 1117–1121.

Li, N., Li, Q., Zhou, X.D., Kolosov, V.P. and Perelman, J.M. (2012). The effect of quercetin on human neutrophil elastase-induced mucin 5AC expression in human airway epithelial cells. *Int. Immunopharmacol.*, 14: 195–201.

Lien, E.J., Ren, S., Bui, H.H. and Wang, R. (1999). Quantitative structure-activity relationship analysis of phenolic antioxidants. *Free Radic. Biol. Med.*, 26: 285–294.

Lin, S.Y., Tsai, S.J., Wang, L.H., Wu, M.F. and Lee, H. (2002). Protection by quercetin against cooking oil fumes-induced DNA damage in human lung adenocarcinoma CL-3 cells: Role of COX-2. *Nutr. Cancer.*, 44: 95–101.

Lopez-Posadas, R., Ballester, I., Abadia-Molina, A.C., Suarez, M.D., Zarzuelo, A., Martinez-Augustin, O. and Sanchez de Medina, F. (2008). Effect of flavonoids on rat splenocytes, a structure-activity relationship study. *Biochem. Pharmacol.*, 76: 495–506.

Maciel, R.M., Costa, M.M., Martins, D.B. *et al.* (2013). Antioxidant and anti-inflammatory effects of quercetin in functional and morphological alterations in streptozotocin-induced diabetic rats. *Res. Vet. Sci.*, 95: 389–397.

Matot, I. and Sprung, C.L. (2001). Definition of sepsis. *Intensive. Care. Med.*, 27 (Suppl 1): S3–9.

Middleton, Jr. E. (1998). Effect of plant flavonoids on immune and inflammatory cell function. *Adv. Exp. Med. Biol.*, 439: 175–182.

Mishra, A., Kumar, S. and Pandey, A.K. (2013). Scientific validation of the medicinal efficacy of *Tinospora cordifolia*. *Scientific World J.*, p. 292934.

Mishra, A., Sharma, A.K., Kumar, S., Saxena, A.K. and Pandey, A.K. (2013). *Bauhinia variegata* leaf extracts exhibit considerable antibacterial, antioxidant, and anticancer activities. *Biomed Res. Int.*, p. 915436.

Moroney, M.A., Alcaraz, M.J., Forder, R.A., Carey, F. and Hoult, J.R. (1988). Selectivity of neutrophil 5-lipoxygenase and cyclo-oxygenase inhibition by an anti-inflammatory flavonoid glycoside and related aglycone flavonoids. *J. Pharm. Pharmacol.*, 40: 787–792.

Murphy, D.M. and O'Byrne, P.M. (2010). Recent advances in the pathophysiology of asthma. *Chest,* 137: 1417–1426.

Nair, M.P., Mahajan, S., Reynolds, J.L., Aalinkeel, R., Nair, H., Schwartz, S.A. and Kandaswami, C. (2006). The flavonoid quercetin inhibits proinflammatory cytokine (tumor necrosis factor alpha) gene expression in normal peripheral blood mononuclear cells *via* modulation of the NF-kappa beta system. *Clin. Vaccine. Immunol.*, 13: 319–328.

Newman, D.J. and Cragg, G.M. (2007). Natural products as sources of new drugs over the last 25 years. *J. Nat. Prod.*, 70: 461–477.

Nijveldt, R.J., van Nood, E., van Hoorn, D.E., Boelens, P.G., van Norren, K. and van Leeuwen, P.A. (2001). Flavonoids: A review of probable mechanisms of action and potential applications. Am J Clin Nutr 74: 418–425.

Noroozi, M., Angerson, W.J. and Lean, M.E. (1998). Effects of flavonoids and vitamin C on oxidative DNA damage to human lymphocytes. *Am. J. Clin. Nutr.*, 67: 1210–1218.

Pajkrt, D., van der Poll, T., Levi, M., *et al.* (1997). Interleukin-10 inhibits activation of coagulation and fibrinolysis during human endotoxemia. *Blood*, 89: 2701–2705.

Pandey, A.K., Mishra, A.K. and Mishra, A. (2012). Antifungal and antioxidative potential of oil and extracts derived from leaves of Indian spice plant *Cinnamomum tamala*. *Cell Mol. Biol.* (Noisy-le-grand), 58: 142–147.

Park, H.H., Lee, S., Son, H.Y. *et al.* (2008). Flavonoids inhibit histamine release and expression of proinflammatory cytokines in mast cells. *Arch. Pharm. Res.*, 31: 1303–1311.

Prado, C.M., Leick-Maldonado, E.A., Kasahara, D.I., Capelozzi, V.L., Martins, M.A. and Tiberio, I.F. (2005). Effects of acute and chronic nitric oxide inhibition in an experimental model of chronic pulmonary allergic inflammation in guinea pigs. *Am. J. Physiol. Lung. Cell. Mol. Physiol.*, 289: L677–683.

Prado, C.M., Leick-Maldonado, E.A., Yano, L., Leme, A.S., Capelozzi, V.L., Martins, M.A. and Tiberio, I.F. (2006). Effects of nitric oxide synthases in chronic allergic airway inflammation and remodeling. *Am. J. Respir. Cell. Mol. Biol.*, 35: 457–465.

Ratty, A.K. and Das, N.P. (1988). Effects of flavonoids on nonenzymatic lipid peroxidation: Structure-activity relationship. *Biochem. Med. Metab. Biol.*, 39: 69–79.

Ricciardolo, F.L., Di, Stefano, A., Sabatini, F. and Folkerts, G. (2006). Reactive nitrogen species in the respiratory tract. *Eur. J. Pharmacol.*, 533: 240–252.

Rice-Evans, C.A., Miller, N.J. and Paganga, G. (1996). Structure-antioxidant activity relationships of flavonoids and phenolic acids. *Free. Radic. Biol. Med.*, 20: 933–956.

Robak, J. and Gryglewski, R.J. (1996). Bioactivity of flavonoids. *Pol. J. Pharmacol.*, 48: 555–564.

Rogerio, A.P., Kanashiro, A., Fontanari, C., da Silva, E.V., Lucisano-Valim, Y.M., Soares, E.G. and Faccioli, L.H. (2007). Anti-inflammatory activity of quercetin and isoquercitrin in experimental murine allergic asthma. *Inflamm Res.*, 56: 402–408.

Santangelo, C., Vari, R., Scazzocchio, B., Di Benedetto, R., Filesi, C. and Masella, R. (2007). Polyphenols, intracellular signalling and inflammation. *Ann. Ist Super. Sanita.*, 43: 394–405.

Sekher Pannala, A., Chan, T.S., O'Brien, P.J. and Rice-Evans, C.A. (2001). Flavonoid B-ring chemistry and antioxidant activity: Fast reaction kinetics. *Biochem. Biophys. Res. Commun.,* 282: 1161–1168.

Shutenko, Z., Henry, Y., Pinard, E. *et al.* (1999). Influence of the antioxidant quercetin *in vivo* on the level of nitric oxide determined by electron paramagnetic resonance in rat brain during global ischemia and reperfusion. *Biochem Pharmacol*, 57: 199–208.

Silva, M.M., Santos, M.R., Caroco, G., Rocha, R., Justino, G. and Mira, L. (2002). Structure-antioxidant activity relationships of flavonoids: A re-examination. *Free Radic. Res.,* 36: 1219–1227.

Smith, W.L., DeWitt, D.L. and Garavito, R.M. (2000). Cyclooxygenases: Structural, cellular, and molecular biology. *Annu. Rev. Biochem.*, 69: 145–182.

Soobrattee, M.A., Neergheen, V.S., Luximon-Ramma, A., Aruoma, O.I. and Bahorun, T. (2005). Phenolics as potential antioxidant therapeutic agents: Mechanism and actions. *Mutat Res.*, 579: 200–213.

Toledo, A.C., Sakoda, C.P., Perini, A. *et al.* (2013). Flavonone treatment reverses airway inflammation and remodeling in an asthma murine model. *Br. J. Pharmacol.*, 168: 1736–1749.

Tordera, M., Ferrandiz, M.L. and Alcaraz, M.J. (1994). Influence of anti-inflammatory flavonoids on degranulation and arachidonic acid release in rat neutrophils. *Z Naturforsch C*, 49: 235–240.

Townsend, E.A. and Emala, Sr. C.W. (2013). Quercetin acutely relaxes airway smooth muscle and potentiates beta-agonist-induced relaxation via dual phosphodiesterase inhibition of PLCbeta and PDE4. *Am. J. Physiol. Lung. Cell Mol. Physiol.*, 305: L396–403.

Van Acker, S.A., van den Berg, D.J., Tromp, M.N., Griffioen, D.H., van Bennekom, W.P., van der Vijgh, W.J. and Bast, A. (1996). Structural aspects of antioxidant activity of flavonoids. *Free Radic. Biol. Med.,* 20: 331–342.

Vennat, B., Bos, M.A., Pourrat, A. and Bastide, P. (1994). Procyanidins from tormentil: Fractionation and study of the anti-radical activity towards superoxide anion. *Biol. Pharm. Bull.*, 17: 1613–1615.

Weseler, A.R., Geraets, L., Moonen, H.J. *et al.* (2009). Poly (ADP-ribose) polymerase-1-inhibiting flavonoids attenuate cytokine release in blood from male patients with chronic obstructive pulmonary disease or type 2 diabetes. *J. Nutr.*, 139: 952–957.

Wheeler, A.P. and Bernard, G.R. (1999). Treating patients with severe sepsis. *N. Engl. J. Med.*, 340: 207–214.

Wolfe, K.L. and Liu, R.H. (2008). Structure-activity relationships of flavonoids in the cellular antioxidant activity assay. *J. Agric. Food Chem.*, 56: 8404–8411.

Yao, L.H., Jiang, Y.M., Shi, J., Tomas-Barberan, F.A., Datta, N., Singanusong, R. and Chen, S.S. (2004). Flavonoids in food and their health benefits. *Plant Foods Hum. Nutr.*, 59: 113–122.

Yoon, J.H. and Baek, S.J. (2005). Molecular targets of dietary polyphenols with anti-inflammatory properties. *Yonsei Med. J.*, 46: 585–596.

Zhang, Y., Wang, D., Yang, L., Zhou, D. and Zhang, J. (2014). Purification and characterization of flavonoids from the leaves of *Zanthoxylum bungeanum* and correlation between their structure and antioxidant activity. *PLoS ONE*, 9: e105725.

8

Molecular Mechanisms of the Flavonoids on Cardiac Diseases

D. SARAVANAN[1]*, A. MAHESWARAN[1], J. PADMAVATHY[1] AND P. ANGEL[1]

ABSTRACT

Flavonoids, belonging to the polyphenolic structure are found abundantly in natural products and possess a great mystery in the treatment of various human ailments. The study of bioflavonoids is a complex process as the data available on its molecular structure are very scarce. But it has become an area of research since its contribution to the human well being is on a high edge. Flavonoids are known to possess anti-atherosclerotic activity, anti-inflammatory, antioxidant, antiproliferative, antiplatelet, cholesterol-lowering, antihypertensive effects and provessel function activities. Flavonoids are widely known for its antioxidant activity which is the main criteria for its efficacy in the treatment of various cardiovascular diseases. The biological effects of flavonoids depend on the pharmacokinetic and pharmacodynamic features like chemical structure, administered dose schedule, route of administration, interaction with several key enzymes, signaling cascades involving cytokines and regulatory transcription factors etc. In the present study, we have concentrated our view on the molecular mechanisms of the flavonoids for treating cardiac diseases. Many subclasses of flavonoids, including flavones, flavonols, flavanones, catechins isoflavones, proanthocyanidins, and anthocyanidins contribute much in the treatment of CV diseases. Each subclass of flavonoids seems to possess different molecular mechanism. The probable antioxidant mechanism was by inhibiting the LDL uptake and oxidation, anti-inflammatory action by suppression of cyclooxygenases, prostaglandin E2, and several pro-inflammatory cytokines, including interleukin 1a, 1b, 6, tumor necrosis factor-a. Therefore, in the present work, we have aimed at the collection of all probable molecular

[1]Jaya College of Paramedical Sciences, College of Pharmacy, Thiruninravur, Tamil Nadu, India-602024

**Corresponding author*: E-mail: devasaro@yahoo.co.in

mechanisms by which flavonoids are expected to exhibit its therapeutic activity in various cardiac ailments.

***Keywords*:** Flavonoids, Molecular mechanisms, Cardiovascular ailments.

1. INTRODUCTION

Cardiovascular diseases (CVD) are diseases of the blood vessels or heart, which includes coronary artery diseases like myocardial infarction and angina. Other cardiovascular diseases include congenital heart disease, heart failure, stroke, rheumatic heart disease, hypertensive heart disease, valvular heart disease, peripheral artery disease, aortic aneurysms, venous thrombosis and carditis. An actual mechanism contributing to the cardiovascular diseases differs among the diseases and is doubtful. The most probable reasons for peripheral artery disease, stroke, coronary artery disease and atherosclerosis might be due to lack of exercise, excessive alcohol consumption, obesity, high blood pressure, high blood cholesterol, poor diet, smoking, and diabetes (Nabel, 2003).

CVDs prove to be fatal in most of the cases in several countries. In the year 2008, 30% of all death was caused by cardiovascular diseases. Death attributed to cardiovascular diseases are high in low and middle-income countries as over 80% of all worldwide death from cardiovascular diseases occurred in those countries. Additionally, it is predicted that by the year 2030, every year more than 23 million people will die from cardiovascular diseases. It is prognosticated that 60% of the globe's cardiovascular disease problems arise in South Asian subcontinent despite just accounting for 20% of the globe's population. This can be secondary to a variety of genetic predisposition as well as environmental factors (Morris and Crawford, 1958).

India, one among the mega multifarious center posses over 45,000 plant species. The whole World accounts for about 15,000 to 18,000 plants, 2500 algae, 23,000 fungi, 1800 bryophytes, and 1600 lichens. Around 3000 plants are used in traditional systems of medicines in India. Medicinal plants possess a variety of phytoconstituents necessary for important biological functions and they shield our body against attack from fungi, insects and herbivorous mammals. At least 12,000 such phytoconstituents have been isolated so far (Agarwal *et al.*, 2012). Medicinal plants contain different varieties of phytoconstituents that are used for important biological functions and they defend our body against attack from fungi, insects, and herbivorous mammals. (Lai and Roy, 2004; Fabricant and Farnsworth, 2001). Throughout history, plant materials have served as a reservoir of potential new drugs. 50% of all drugs in clinical use are derived from the natural product. Out of 25 best selling Pharmaceutical drugs, 12 are either natural products or their derivatives. Hence it can be understood that natural products continue to play an important role in drug discovery in pharmaceutical industries and other research organizations.

Phytoconstituents, substances naturally found in fruits, vegetables, and medicinal plants, which are intaken usually as diet exhibits a potential for modulating human metabolism in a favorable way for the prevention of chronic and degenerative diseases (Kamboh *et al.,* 2015). Flavonoids are polyphenols, bioactive, non-nutrient, non-caloric plant constituents found abundantly in natural products which possess a great mystery in the treatment of various human ailments. Flavonoids a big group of plant constituents (which are not synthesized in humans) consists of more than 5,000 hydroxylated polyphenolic compounds which accomplish very important functions in plants, including combating environmental stress such as regulating cell growth and microbial infection; attracting pollinating insects.

The current article describes the potential mechanisms of flavonoids that can be effective for decreasing the chance of cardiovascular disease. Many subclasses of flavonoids could provide the similar familiar health effects.

2. MOLECULAR MECHANISM OF FLAVONOIDS AGAINST CARDIOVASCULAR DISEASES

Chemically, flavonoids have 15 carbon skeletons comprising of three rings such as two phenyl ring (A and B) and one heterocyclic ring (C). The numerous classes of flavonoids are different in the pattern of substitution in the C ring, whereas individual flavonoid within a class differs in the pattern of substitution in the A and B rings. The carbon skeletons can be abbreviated as C_6-C_3-C_6 (Middleton, 1998; Testai, 2015).

Flavonoids (a) occur as glycosides, aglycones and methylated derivatives. The basic structure of flavonoid is aglycone. Flavonoids are divided into various classes based on their molecular structure. The six main groups of flavonoids (Fig. 1) such as flavan3-ols (b), anthocyanidins (c), flavonols (d), flavones (e), flavanones (f) and isoflavones (g) along with best-known members of each group and the food sources (8) are listed in Table 1. The molecular structure of six main groups of flavonoids is also given.

The above major groups of flavonoids differ in their modification of side groups on these rings. The side groups play crucial roles in the function of these compounds since the side group's modification can produce very different activities. Flavonoids can be considered as the king of phytoconstituents available from the plant kingdom. Flavonoids bioavailability and biological activities of human beings seem to be strongly influenced due to their chemical nature (Kumar and Pandey, 2013).

Table 1: Main groups of flavonoids, the individual compounds and their dietary source

Sl. no	*Chemical class*	*Examples*	*Major dietary source*
1	Flavonols	Quercetin, myricetin, rutin, kaempferol	Apple, red wine, tomato, cherry, tea, romaine lettuce, tomatoes, garbanzo beans and onion
2	Flavanols	Catechin, gallocatechin	Apple, bananas, blueberries, peaches, pears and tea
3	Flavones	Apigenin, luteolin, chrysin	Parsley, celery, bell peppers, apples and thyme
4	Isoflavones	Genistein, daidzein, glycitein, formononetin	Legumes and soyabean
5	Flavanones	Naringenin, hesperidin, eriodictyol	Orange, grapefruit
6	Anthocyanidins	delphinidin, cyanidin, pelargonidin, malvidin, petunidin and peonidin	Black beans, oranges, olives, red onion, sweet potato, pomegranates, kidney beans

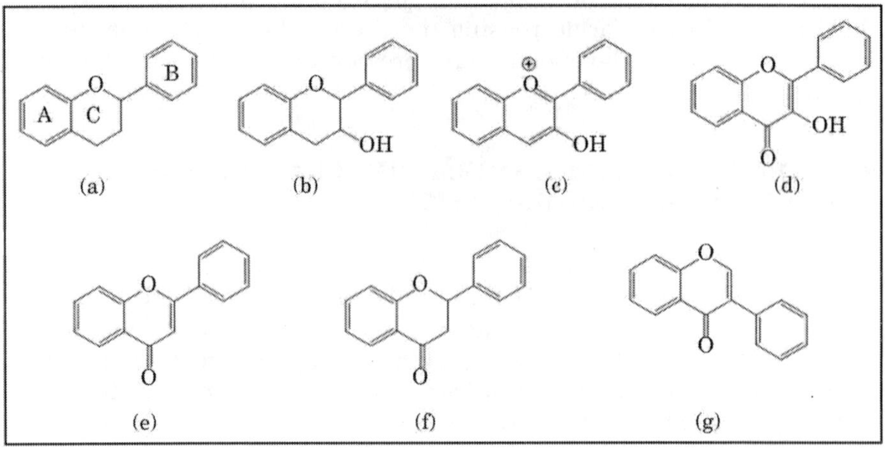

Fig. 1: Structure of flavonoids (a), flavan3-ols (b), anthocyanidins (c), flavonols (d), flavones (e), flavanones (f) and isoflavones (g)

Flavonoids are established bio-molecules possessing powerful pharmacological activities which could be effective in curing the chronic diseases such as CVDs and atherosclerosis (Gross, 2004). CVDs are considered as the major cause of premature death in developed countries and its fundamental pathology is atherosclerosis (Little *et al.,* 2011). Flavonoids are reported to be potentially active in cardiovascular disease prevention usually through improving the nitric oxide bioavailability and decreasing oxidative stress. These polyphenolic compounds have the ability to regulate the expression of a gene associated with metabolism, drug metabolizing enzymes, stress defense, transporter proteins, and detoxification. Their overall effect is protective in overcoming the deleterious effects of cardiovascular risk factors (Dimmeler, 2011; Grassi *et al.,* 2009).

The flavonoids intake serves as a primary prevention as well as benefits the individuals with established cardiovascular diseases by slowing the clinical signs like lowered blood pressure (Hooper *et al.*, 2008; Erlund *et al.*, 2008; Desch *et al.*, 2010), improved endothelial function (Dal-Ros *et al.*, 2011; Schroeter *et al.*, 2006; Heiss *et al.*, 2007), inhibited platelet aggregation (Pearson *et al.*, 2002; Rein *et al.*, 2000; Keevil *et al.*, 2000), decreased low-density lipoprotein oxidation (Mathur *et al.*, 2002; Wan *et al.*, 2001) and reduced inflammatory response (Pan *et al.*, 2010; Mao *et al.*, 2002; Schramm *et al.*, 2003). Flavonoids exhibit several biological effects like anti-hepatotonic, anti-inflammatory and anti-ulcer activity (Bors *et al.*, 1990; Smith *et al.*, 1988). Many of the epidemiological studies showed an inverse association between consumption of polyphenol-rich foods and the risk of cardiovascular diseases (Agarwal, 2011; Manach *et al.*, 2005). Flavonoids contribute in offering cardiovascular health by its anti-inflammatory, antioxidant and free radical scavenging activity, regulation of cellular activities of inflammation related cells and their molecular targets like improvements in endothelial structure and function (Middleton, 1998). Various mechanisms related to use of flavonoids in improving cardiovascular health includes inhibition of low-density lipoprotein oxidation, enhancement of the endothelial function, improving dyslipidemia, reducing the clumping of platelets, inhibiting cardiac hypertrophy, decreasing the blood pressure, free radical scavenging and antioxidant effect (Tangney and Rasmussen, 2013) as shown in Fig. 2.

Consumption of flavonoids from fruits and vegetables is concerned with reduced risk for the development of cardiovascular disease (Nandava *et al.*, 2005). The molecular mechanisms of flavonoids describing these perspectives are still not clear; however existing information shows that flavonoids could exert their effects on cardiovascular risk factors.

2.1. Improves Dyslipidemia

Dyslipidemia, an abnormal level of lipids in the blood is a cause for the most of the cardiovascular diseases and the diet rich in flavonoids can serve as a preventive measure. Atherosclerosis, a disease associated with the hardening and narrowing of the arteries is considered the cause of various cardiovascular diseases like stroke, heart attacks and peripheral vascular disease (Margaret, 2010). Atherosclerosis is the transfer of low density lipoproteins around the endothelium into the artery wall (Grassi *et al.*, 2010). The intimal lipids are entrapped by the modified proteoglycans with hyper-elongated glycosaminoglycan chains (Dadlani *et al.*, 2008; Little *et al.*, 2008), the oxidation of neointimal lipids result in the release of oxidized immunogenic molecular species that initiates a chronic inflammatory process in the vessel wall. Impaired endothelial function followed by inflammation of the blood vessel wall leads to the atherosclerotic lesion which causes myocardial infarction and stroke (Ballinger *et al.*, 2010).

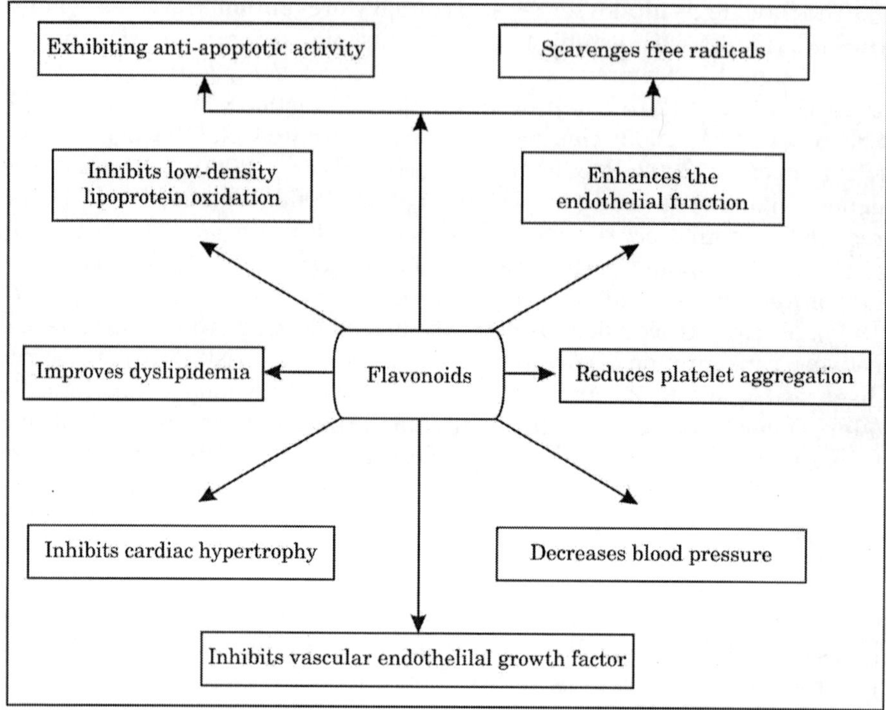

Fig. 2: Molecular mechanism of flavonoids

Flavonoids decrease the progression of atherosclerosis by improving dyslipidemia. The flavonoids responsible for this effect are probably rutin, quercetin, orientin, vitexin and isovitexin (Li *et al.,* 2010).

2.2. Enhances Endothelial Function

The endothelium is the type of epithelium which lines the interior surface of lymphatic vessels and blood vessels. The endothelium plays an important role in maintaining vascular tone, vascular homeostasis, microvascular and cardiovascular health. Dysfunction of endothelium is the important function in the pathogenesis of cardiovascular disease. The endothelial cells synthesize and release the numerous substances such as nitric oxide (NO) and endothelin-1 (ET-1) which causes vascular smooth muscles to dilate or constrict the blood vessel respectively. Nitric oxide is an important regulator of arterial wall tone which can be produced in the endothelial cell by the enzyme endothelial nitric oxide synthase (eNOS). Nitric oxide is a major anti-atherogenic factor in a blood vessel. Decreased availability of NO results in the progression of endothelial dysfunction and atherosclerosis. Endothelial dysfunction can be an important physiopathological mechanism which leads to coronary artery disease as well as atherosclerosis. Flavonoids increase the production of NO by inducing eNOS protein synthase, eNOS gene expression and eNOS activity (Machha and Mustafa, 2005).

2.3. Reduces the Clumping of Platelets

Flavonoids help to reduce the clumping of platelets in our blood and improve the function of our cells that lines the arteries and veins. Platelet clumping is one potential precursor in thrombotic diseases which includes acute myocardial infarction, acute pulmonary embolism and ischemic stroke (Michelson, 2010). Nitric oxide released from the endothelial cells regulates the aggregation of platelets by increasing cyclic guanosine monophosphate (cGMP). But in the CVD s, due to the damage of endothelial cells, the subendothelial matrix and collagen are exposed, which results in the platelet adhesion which is considered to be the crucial step in the formation of platelet rich thrombus. The binding of collagen and von willebrand factor to platelet receptors serves as an initial step for platelet adhesion and activation. Following which, the platelets undergo further activation by releasing their granule contents which include adenosine diphosphate and formation of thromboxane A_2. This process of platelet activation leads to a further conformational change in platelet fibrinogen receptor GPIIbIIIa, which results in platelet aggregation by the formation of bridges between activated platelets (Lüscher and Noll, 1995; Pignatelli *et al.,* 2000; Eisenberg and Ghigliotti, 1999). Polyphenols which shows potent antiplatelet activity are rutin, quercetin, pentamethyl quercetin. The flavonoids and their metabolites show antiplatelet aggregation property by inhibiting protein kinase C activity, formation of thromboxane A_2, exocytosis of dense and alpha granules, intracellular calcium mobilization, platelet spreading and collagen, thrombin-stimulated platelet aggregation signaling pathways (Sheu *et al.,* 2004; Mosawy, 2015).

2.4. Scavenging of Free Radicals

Reactive Oxygen Species (ROS), that is active oxygen species, includes free radicals like superoxide ions (O_2^-) and hydroxyl radicals (OH^-) and non-free radical species (H_2O_2) (Yildrim *et al.,* 2001). The pathological processes of many human ailments like aging, cancers, coronary heart disease, atherosclerosis, Alzheimer's disease, neurodegenerative disorders, cataracts, and inflammation involves ROS (Huang *et al.,* 2005). Body cells and tissues are continually threatened through destruction due to free radicals and reactive oxygen species that are produced through the metabolism of normal oxygen containing compounds in the body. Such free radicals and reactive oxygen species undergo lipid peroxidation. The increased production of reactive oxygen species during the cells and tissue injury leads to consumption and depletion of the endogenous antioxidant compounds such as superoxide catalase, dismutase and glutathione peroxidase, which acts as the key factor for the development of cardiovascular diseases. The best ever property of flavonoids described is its antioxidant property (Nijveldt *et al.,* 2001). The mode of action of flavonoids in preventing the oxidative damage to the cells and tissues is by direct scavenging of the free radicals, decreasing the immobilized leucocytes, oxidation, and stabilization of the reactive oxygen species due to the high reactivity of hydroxyl group of the flavonoids. Flavonoids also act as intracellular antioxidants by inhibiting the enzymes Xanthine oxidase, lipoxygenase, Protein Kinase C, Cyclooxygenase, microsomal monooxygenase and NADPH oxidase (51). Flavonoidal subgroups like flavones, catechins, and flavonols are proved to possess potent antioxidant properties (Nijveldt *et al.,* 2001; Procházková *et al.,* 2011; Rice-Evans *et al.,* 1996; Lobo *et al.,* 2010).

2.5. Inhibits Vascular Endothelial Growth Factor

Vascular Endothelial Growth Factor (VEGF) also known as vascular permeability factor (Santulli, 2013) is a signal protein produced by cells which stimulate vasculogenesis and angiogenesis. It is a system part that restores oxygen supply to the tissues in hypoxia conditions (Birbrair *et al.,* 2015). When it is overexpressed it contributes to a disease state. The family members of VEGF include VEGF-B, Placental growth factors, VEGF-C and VEGF-D, which may be responsible for atherosclerotic plaque formation and in the development of ischemic diseases (Sueishi *et al.,* 1997). Polyphenolic compounds like anthocyanins found in various natural foods inhibit vascular endothelial growth factor, which causes complications with atherosclerotic plaques in the arteries, a factor in cardiovascular disease (Youdim *et al.,* 2002).

2.6. Reduces Blood Pressure

The various subclasses of flavonoids like flavones, flavonols, flavanones, and flavonols modulate blood pressure by restoring endothelial function, either directly, by affecting nitric oxide levels, or indirectly, through other pathways. Flavonoids are also considered to contribute to lowering of blood pressure by inhibiting angiotensin-converting enzymes (ACE) acetylcholine-like and histamine-like mechanisms (Ojeda *et al.,* 2010; Actis-Goretta *et al.,* 2003; Kwon *et al.,* 2010).

2.7. Inhibition of LDL Oxidation

Low density lipoprotein (LDL), is considered as an important factor for atherosclerosis (Ross, 1993; Steinberg *et al.,* 1989). The accumulation of LDL in arterial intima is the primary step in atherosclerosis. Oxidized LDL increases the susceptibility for developing atherosclerosis. Oxidized LDL deposits in the human coronary arteries followed by plaque formation and plaque growth. Oxidized LDL may also be responsible for the development of coronary arterial diseases. Nitric oxide (NO) is generated by macrophages and endothelial cells in our body by the use of enzyme nitric oxide synthase. The minimum concentration of nitric oxide is necessary for the dilation of blood vessels, but higher concentrations can lead to oxidative damage. On this condition, the activated macrophages enhance the generation of both nitric oxide and superoxide anions simultaneously. The generated nitric oxide reacts with superoxide anions to give the peroxynitrite that can directly oxidize LDL's, causing irreversible damage to the cell membrane. LDL is very important for the structural integrity of cells, when LDL is oxidized they can promote inflammation that can lead to coronary artery disease. Flavonoid scavenges free radicals and so that they are no longer available to react with nitric oxide, leading to slight damage of cell membrane (Vaya, 2003). Further, the oxidation of LDL can also occur by lipoxygenase. Flavonoids, on the other hand, inhibit lipoxygenase (Terao *et al.,* 1994; Yoshimoto *et al.,* 1983; Laughton *et al.,* 1991) thereby preventing the oxidation of LDL, leading to the decrease in the development of atherosclerosis. Flavonoids that are proved to inhibit the LDL oxidation are flavonol quercetin, flavan-3-ols epicatechin, flavones, morin, pelargonidin, genistein, naringin, apigenin etc (Da Silva *et al.,* 2000; Safari and Shiek, 2003).

2.8. Inhibits Cardiac Hypertrophy

Cardiac hypertrophy is the thickening of the myocardium (heart muscle) which leads to a reduction in the size of the chambers of the heart such as right and left ventricles (Bendall *et al.,* 2002). Oxidative stress forms a major reason for Cardiac hypertrophy and cardiac fibrosis (Sano *et al.,* 2001; Zhang *et al.,* 2012; Li *et al.,* 2002; Takimoto and Kass, 2007; Liang and Gardner, 1999). A common reason for cardiac hypertrophy is increased blood pressure either in the body or lungs. The additional work of pumping blood against the increased pressure leads to the ventricle to thicken over time (Sun *et al.,* 2016). Many studies have proved that the flavonoids like luteolin, catechins of plant origin can serve to inhibit cardiac hypertrophy.

2.9. Exhibiting Anti-apoptotic Activity

The significant cardioprotective activity of flavonoids may be partly attributed due to its anti-apoptotic activity. Apoptosis is programmed cell death. The evidence shows that oxidative stress, calcium overload and energy depletion following ischemia acts as stimulators for apoptosis in myocardium leading to myocardial infarction. Flavonoids inhibit apoptosis in myocardial tissues and thereby rescue normal cells. The mechanism by which the flavonoids are considered to exhibit the antiapoptotic properties are by inhibition of pro-apoptotic factors JNK and C-JUN, decrease in oxidative stress, free radical scavenging activity, inhibition of activation of caspase pathway and restoration of mitochondrial functions (Aoki *et al.*, 2001; Hockenbery *et al.*, 1993).

3. MOLECULAR MECHANISM OF SUBCLASS OF FLAVONOIDS

3.1. Promethoxylated Flavones

Promethoxylated flavones (Fig. 3) such as tangeritin (h) and nobiletin (i) found in tangerine, sour orange, sweet orange, and grapefruit prevent metabolic syndrome. Metabolic syndrome is a group of risk factors which increases the risk of diabetes and heart disease. The major risk factors for metabolic syndrome are hypertension, cholesterol abnormalities, insulin resistance and central obesity. Obesity leads to insulin resistance that has been suggested as a most important fundamental reason for dyslipidemia, atherosclerosis, and hypertension (Kopelman, 2000).

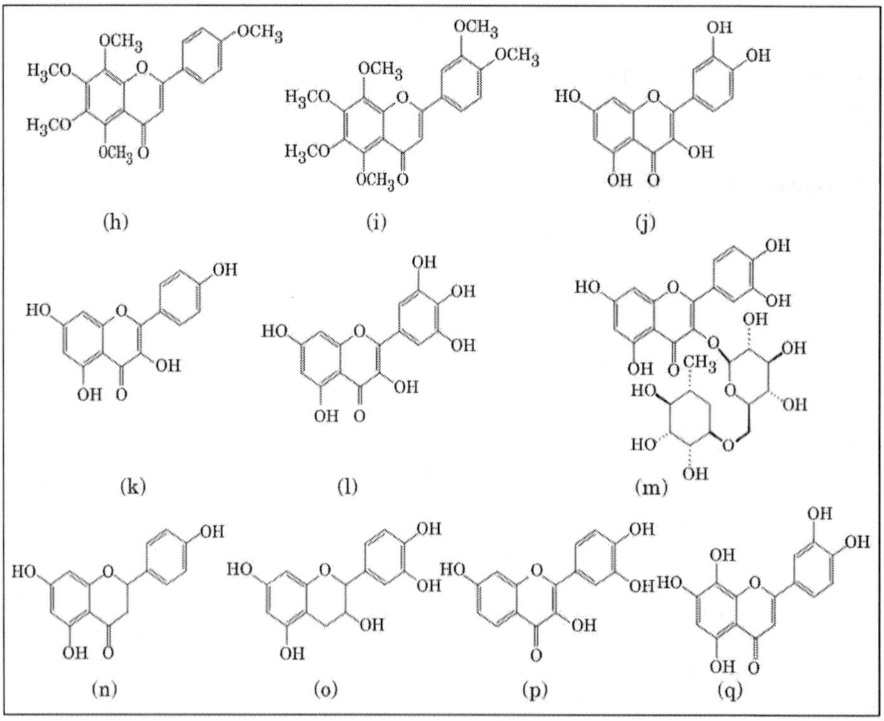

OCH_3 OCH_3 H_3CO H_3CO OCH_3 O O

(h)

OCH_3 OCH_3 OCH_3 H_3CO H_3CO OCH_3 O O

(i)

OH OH HO O OH OH O

(j)

OH HO O OH OH O

(k)

OH OH OH HO O OH OH O

(l)

OH OH HO O OH O OH CH_3 OH HO O O OH HO O OH

(m)

OH HO O OH O

(n)

OH HO O OH OH OH

(o)

OH HO O OH OH O

(p)

OH OH OH HO O OH O

(q)

Fig. 3: Structure of tangeritin (h), nobiletin (i), quercetin (j), kaempferol (k), myricetin (l), rutin (m), naringenin (n), catechin (o), fisetin (p) and gossypetin (q)

The citrus flavonoids, nobiletin, and tangeritin are proved to possess a significant antithrombotic property by the inhibition of human platelet activation, inhibition of platelet granule secretion, modulation of intracellular calcium mobilization, reduction of platelet adhesion and thrombus formation, elevation of platelet cGMP (Vaiyapuri *et al.,* 2015). They also seem to possess the antihypertensive activity and antioxidant activity by increasing the bioavailable nitric oxide and scavenging of reactive oxygen species (Ikemura1 *et al.,* 2012).

3.2. Quercetin

Quercetin, (3', 4', 3, 5, 7-pentahydroxy flavone), a unique flavonoid belonging to subclass flavonols has positive health benefits in the treatment of cardiovascular diseases. It is found in many of the common foods like apples, tea, onion, nuts, berries, cauliflower, cabbage etc (Lakhanpal and Rai, 2007). Quercetin (**j**) improves the endothelium-dependent vasorelaxation in the aorta, decreases systolic blood pressure, reduces cardiac hypertrophy in animal models (Duarte *et al.,* 2001; García-Saura *et al.,* 2005). Quercetin (Fig. 3) can also be considered as an alternative drug for atherosclerosis, CVD like hypertension and obesity. A few plant species with a high content of quercetin are *Allium fistulosam, Camellia sinensis, Calamus scipionum, Centella asiatica, Moringa oleifera, Hypericum perforatum* and *Hypericum hircinum* (Salvamani *et al.,* 2014). It also seems to possess antioxidant activity, direct free radical scavenging action, inducible nitric oxide synthase inhibitory action, Xanthine oxidase inhibitory action and decreases leukocyte immobilization.

3.3. Kaempferol

Kaempferol (**k**), a secondary metabolite and a natural flavonol derived from plants are found widely in the families of Pteridophyta, Pinophyta, and Angiospermae. It is found in the common foods like apples, grapes, tomatoes, green tea, potatoes, onion, broccoli, cucumber, lettuce, green beans peaches, blackberries, spinach etc (Calderon-Montaño *et al.,* 2011; Liu, 2013; Kim and Choi, 2013). The consumption of kaempferol (Fig. 3) rich foods reduces the risk of cardiovascular diseases. It increases endothelium-dependent vasorelaxation in a coronary artery, prevents endothelial injuries and oxidative damage in cells. It lessens the severity of vascular inflammation to prevent atherosclerosis.

3.4. Myricetin

Myricetin (l), a natural flavonol present in medicinal plants, vegetables, tea, berries, and fruits is reported to possess cardioprotective action through antioxidant, antiplatelet, antihypertensive, antithrombotic and anti-atherosclerotic activity (Santhakumar *et al.,* 2013; Rice, 2014; Kratz *et al.,* 2013; Salvamani *et al.,* 2014). The plant species of *Calamus scipionum, Aloe vera, Myrica cerifera, Moringa oleifera* and *Chrysobalanus icaco* is reported to possess high content of myricetin (Fig. 3).

3.5. Rutin

Rutin (m), a bioflavonoid found in buckwheat bran, black tea, citrus fruits is proved to possess various cardioprotective activities. Rutin possesses the antioxidant activity, free radical scavenging activity, and anti-atherosclerotic activity. Thereby, it serves as an effective cardioprotectant for the treatment of hypertension, atherosclerosis. The plant source of rutin (Fig. 3) includes *Ruta graveolens, Flos hippocastani, Phyllanthus amarus* and *Rhus cotinus* (Salvamani *et al.,* 2014).

3.6. Naringenin

Naringenin (n), a substituted flavanone, is reported to possess poor antioxidant property compared to other flavonoids. Naringenin inhibits oxidation of LDL by inhibiting Lipooxygenase, COX, and MPO. It possesses antithrombotic, anti-inflammatory and vasodilatory effect in atherosclerosis (Salvamani *et al.,* 2014; Luiz da Silva *et al.,* 1998; de Whalley *et al.,* 1990; Fremont *et al.,* 1998; Hayek *et al.,* 1997; Santos *et al.,* 1999). The plant sources rich in naringenin (Fig. 3) are *Solanum lycopersicum, Citrus fruits, Mentha citrata* and flowers of *Acacia podalyriifolia*.

3.7. Catechin

Catechin (o), a flavonol, is known to possess a preventive effect in cardiovascular disease atherosclerosis, by its antioxidant property. It effectively scavenges free radical, inhibits lipid peroxidation and modulates the cell signaling pathway that causes the reduction of inflammation, increase the platelet aggregation and increase the vascular reactivity (Stangl *et al.,* 2007). Catechins are present in many plant sources (Fig. 3) which includes *Betula pendula, Betula pubescens, Argania spinosa, Cassia fistula* and *Cocos nucifera* (Salvamani *et al.,* 2014).

3.8. Fisetin

Fisetin (p), a flavan- 3-ol, is found to be widely distributed in vegetables and fruits like apple, strawberry, cucumber, grapes, and onion. It possesses strong antioxidant, anti-inflammatory, antiproliferative activity. Fisetin (Fig. 3) prevents the LDL oxidation through macrophages and also acts as a scavenger for free radical in LDL oxidation that additionally prevents the oxidative enzymes on macrophages. It's protective role in atherosclerosis is under research. Rich plant Sources of fisetin are *Gleditsia triacanthos,*

Butea frondosa, Quebracho colorado, Rhus verniciflua, Curcuma longa, Acacia berlandieri and *Acacia greggii* (Arai *et al.*, 2000; Salvamani *et al.*, 2014).

3.9. Gossypetin

Gossypetin (q), a hexahydroxyflavone has its source from *Hibiscus* species. It suppresses oxidation of LDL, reduces oxidative stress and prevents atherosclerosis, decreases systolic blood pressure and pulse pressure. Gossypetin (Fig. 3) is also found in the plant species like *Hibiscus rosa-sinensis, Hibiscus esculentus, Hibiscus vitifolius, Acacia constricta, Empetrum nigrum, Fremontia californica, Fagonia cretica* and *Thespesia populnea* (Harborne, 1969; Salvamani *et al.*, 2014).

4. FUTURE IMPLICATIONS

The study of flavonoids is complicated due to the heterogeneousness of different molecular structures as well as the lack of data on the bioavailability of flavonoids. Moreover, inadequate methods are available for determination of oxidative damage *in-vivo* and the measurement of objective endpoints continues to be a difficult task. Many epidemiological studies have shown that the regular intake of flavonoids in our diet is associated with improved cardiovascular prognosis. The flavonoids contribution to the prevention of the cardiovascular diseases is mainly due to the antioxidant properties, antihypertensive property, and antiatherosclerotic property. Further research has to be focused on the use of the natural flavonoids for the prevention of cardiovascular diseases which can at a high rate decrease the cardiovascular disease mortality. Due to the side effects of the available drugs, research can be pinpointed towards the development of natural flavonoids based drugs for the treatment of cardiovascular ailments, which will be a boon to the human society.

5. CONCLUSIONS

A variety of flavonoids compounds are widely available in the plants demonstrate various effects which can avoid the development of cardiovascular diseases such as coronary artery diseases like myocardial infarction and angina and other cardiovascular diseases like congenital heart disease, heart failure, stroke, rheumatic heart disease, hypertensive heart disease, valvular heart disease, peripheral artery disease, aortic aneurysms, venous thrombosis and carditis. Future research is concentrated on the function of flavonoids on signaling pathway and human metabolism included over the treatment of CVD's. This can serve as an assistance to find out the various methods for enhancing other therapeutic approaches for CVD's.

Because there's an urge for this alternative natural therapy due to the side effects of existing CVS drugs, flavonoid based drugs can serve as an asset for the prevention of CVDs.

6. ACKNOWLEDGEMENT

The authors are thankful to the authorities of Jaya College of Paramedical Sciences, College of Pharmacy for providing support to the study and other facilities.

REFERENCES

Actis-Goretta, L., Ottaviani, J.I., Keen, C.L. and Fraga, C.G. (2003). Inhibition of angiotensin converting enzyme (ACE) activity by flavan-3-ols and procyanidins. *FEBS Lett.*, 555(3): 597–600.

Agarwal, A.D. (2011). Pharmacological activities of flavonoids: A review. *Int. J. Pharm. Sci. Nanotech.*, 4(2): 1394–1398.

Agarwal, P., Fatima, A. and Singh, P.P. (2012). Herbal medicine scenario in India and European countries. *J. Pharmacog. Phytochem.*, 1(4): 88.

Aoki, M., Nata, T., Morishita, R., Matsushita, H., Nakagami, H., Yamamoto, K., Yamazaki, K., Nakabayashi, M., Ogihara, T. and Kaneda, Y. (2001). Endothelial apoptosis induced by oxidative stress through activation of NF-κB: Antiapoptotic effect of antioxidant agents on endothelial cells. *Hypertension*, 38(1): 48–55.

Arai, Y., Watanabe, S., Kimira, M., Shimoi, L., Mochizuki, R. and Kinae, N. (2000). Dietary intakes of flavonols, flavones and isoflavones by Japanese women and the inverse correlation between quercetin intake and plasma LDL cholesterol concentration. *J. Nutr.*, 130(9): 2243–2250.

Ballinger, M.L., Osman, N., Hashimura, K., De Haan, J.B., Jandeleit-Dahm, K., Allen, T., Tannock, L.R., Rutledge, J.C. and Little, P.J. (2010). Imatinib inhibits vascular smooth muscle proteoglycan synthesis and reduces LDL binding *in vitro* and aortic lipid deposition *in vivo*. *J. Cell Mol. Med.*, 14(6B): 1408–1418.

Bendall, J.K., Cave, A.C., Heymes, C., Gall, N., Shah, A.M. (2002). Pivotal role of a gp91 (phox)-containing NADPH oxidase in angiotensin II-induced cardiac hypertrophy in mice. *Circulation*, 105(3): 293–296.

Birbrair, A., Zhang, T., Wang, Z.M., Messi, M.L., Mintz, A. and Delbono, O (2015). Pericytes at the intersection between tissue regeneration and pathology. *Clin. Sci. (Lond)*, 128(2): 81–93.

Bors, W., Heller, W., Michel, C. and Saran, M. (1990). Flavonoids as antioxidants: Determination of free radical scavenging efficiencies. *Methods Enzymol.*, 186: 343–355.

Calderon-Montaño, J.M., Burgos-Moron, E., Perez-Guerrero, C. and Lopez-Lazaro, M. (2011). A review on the dietary flavonoid kaempferol. *Mini. Rev. Med. Chem.*, 11(4): 298–344.

Da Silva, E.L., Abdalla, D.S.P. and Terao, J. (2000). Inhibitory effect of flavonoids on low-density lipoprotein peroxidation catalyzed by mammalian 15-lipoxygenase, *IUBMB Life*, 49(4): 289–295.

Dadlani, H., Ballinger, M.L., Osman, N., Getachew, R. and Little, P.J. (2008). Smad and p38 MAP kinase-mediated signaling of proteoglycan synthesis in vascular smooth muscle. *J. Biol. Chem.*, 283(12): 7844–7852.

Dal-Ros, S., Zoll, J., Lang, A.L., Auger, C., Keller, N., Bronner, C., Geny, B. and Schini-Kerth, V.B. (2011). Chronic intake of red wine polyphenols by young rats prevents aging-induced endothelial dysfunction and decline in physical performance: Role of NADPH oxidase. *Biochem. Biophys. Res. Commun.*, 404(2): 743–749.

De Whalley, C.V., Rankin, S.M., Hoult, J.R.S., Jessup, W., Leake, D.S. (1990). Flavonoids inhibit the oxidative modification of low density lipoproteins by macrophages. *Biochem Pharmacol.*, 39(11): 1743–1750.

Desch, S., Schmidt, J., Kobler, D., Sonnabend, M., Eitel, I., Sareban, M., Rahimi, K., Schuler, G. and Thiele, H. (2010). Effect of cocoa products on blood pressure: Systematic review and meta-analysis. *Am. J. Hypertens.*, 23(1): 97–103.

Dimmeler, S. (2011). Cardiovascular disease review series. *EMBO Mol. Med.,* 3(12): 697.

Duarte, J., Perez-Palencia, R., Vargas, F., Ocete, M.A., Pérez-Vizcaino, F., Zarzuelo, A. and Tamargo, J. (2001). Antihypertensive effects of the flavonoid quercetin in spontaneously hypertensive rats. *Br. J. Pharmacol.*, 133(1): 17–124.

Eisenberg, P.R. and Ghigliotti, G. (1999). Platelet-dependent and procoagulant mechanisms in arterial thrombosis. *Int. J. Cardiol.*, 68 (Suppl 1): S3–S10.

Erlund, I., Koli, R., Alfthan, G., Marniemi, J., Puukka, P., Mustonen, P., Mattila, P. and Jula, A. (2008). Favorable effects of berry consumption on platelet function, blood pressure, and HDL cholesterol. *Am. J. Clin. Nutr.*, 87(2): 323–331.

Fabricant, D.S. and Farnsworth, N.R. (2001). The value of plants used in traditional medicine for drug discovery. *Environ. Health Perspect.,* 109(1): 69–75.

Fremont, L., Gozzelino, M.T., Franchi, M.P. and Linard, A. (1998). Dietary flavonoids reduce lipid peroxidation in rats fed polyunsaturated or monounsaturated fat diets. *J. Nutr.*, 128(9): 1495–1502.

García-Saura, M.F., Galisteo, M., Villar, I.C., Bermejo, A., Zarzuelo, A., Vargas, F., Duarte, J. (2005). Effects of chronic quercetin treatment in experimental renovascular hypertension. *Mol. Cell Biochem.*, 270(1–2): 147–155.

Grassi, D., Desideri, G. and Ferri, C. (2010). Flavonoids: Antioxidants against atherosclerosis. *Nutrients*, 2(8): 889–902.

Grassi, D., Desideri, G., Ferri, L., Aggio, A. and Tiberti, S. (2009). Oxidative stress, endothelial dysfunction and prevention of cardiovascular diseases. *Agro. Food Ind. Hi-Tech*, 20: 8–11.

Gross, M. (2004). Flavonoids and cardiovascular disease. *Pharm Bio.*, 42(Suppl 1): 21–35.

Harborne, J.B. (1969). Gossypetin and herbacetin as taxonomic markers in higher plants. *Phytochemistry,* 8(1): 177–183.

Hayek, T., Fuhrman, B., Vaya, J., Rosenblat, M., Belinky, P., Coleman, R., Elis, A. and Aviram, M. (1997). Reduced progression of atherosclerosis in apolipoprotein E-deficient mice following consumption of red wine, or its polyphenols quercetin or catechin, is associated with reduced susceptibility of LDL to oxidation and aggregation. *Arterioscler Thromb. Vasc. Biol.*, 17(11): 2744–2752.

Heiss, C., Finis, D., Kleinbongard, P., Hoffmann, A., Rassaf, T., Kelm, M., Sies, H. (2007). Sustained increase in flow-mediated dilation after daily intake of high-flavanol cocoa drink over 1 week. *J. Cardiovasc. Pharmacol.*, 49(2): 74–80.

Hockenbery, D.M., Olivai, Z.N., Yin, X.M., Milliman, C.I. and Korsmeyer, S.J. (1993). *Bcl-2* functions in an antioxidant pathway to prevent apoptosis. *Cell.*, 75(2): 241–251.

Hooper, L., Kroon, P.A., Rimm, E.B., Cohn, J.S., Harvey, I., Le Cornu, K.A., Ryder, J.J., Hall, W.L. and Cassidy, A. (2008). Flavonoids, flavonoid-rich foods and cardiovascular risk: A meta-analysis of randomized controlled trials. *Am. J. Clin. Nutr.*, 88(1): 38–50.

Huang, D.H., Chen, C., Lin, C. and Lin, Y. (2005). Antioxidant and antiproliferative activities of water spinach (*Ipomoea aquatica* Forsk) constituents. *Bot. Bull. Acad. Sci.*, 46: 99–106.

Ikemural, M., Sasaki, Y., Giddings, J.C. and Yamamoto, J. (2012). Protective effects of nobiletin on hypertension and cerebral thrombosis in stroke-prone spontaneously hypertensive rats (SHRSP). *Food Nutr. Sci.*, 3(11): 1539–1546.

Kamboh, A.A., Arain, M.A., Mughal, M.J., Zaman, A., Arain, Z.M., Soomro, A.H. (2015). Flavonoids: Health promoting photochemical for animal productions-a review. *J. Anim. Health Prod.*, 3(1): 6.

Keevil, J.G., Osman, H.E., Reed, J.D. and Folts, J.D. (2000). Grape juice, but not orange juice or grapefruit juice, inhibits human platelet aggregation. *J. Nutr.*, 130(1): 53–56.

Kim, S.H. and Choi, K.C. (2013). Anti-cancer effect and underlying mechanism(s) of kaempferol, a phytoestrogen, on the regulation of apoptosis in diverse cancer cell models. *Toxicol. Res.*, 29(4): 229–234.

Kopelman, P.G. (2000). Obesity as a medical problem. *Nature,* 404(6778): 635–643.

Kratz, M., Baars, T. and Guyenet, S. (2013). The relationship between high-fat dairy consumption and obesity, cardiovascular, and metabolic disease. *Eur. J. Nutr.*, 52(1): 1–24.

Kumar, S. and Pandey, A.K. (2013). Chemistry and biological activities of flavonoids: An overview. *Scientific World J.*, 2013: 16.

Kwon, E.K., Lee, D.Y., Lee, H., Kim, D.O., Baek, N.I., Kim, Y.E. and Kim, H.Y. (2010). Flavonoids from the buds of *Rosa damascena* inhibit the activity of 3-hydroxy-3-methylglutaryl-coenzyme a reductase and angiotensin I-converting enzyme. *J. Agric. Food Chem.*, 58(2): 882–6.

Lai, P.K. and Roy, J. (2004). Antimicrobial and chemopreventive properties of herbs and spices. *Curr. Med. Chem.*, 11(11): 1451–60.

Lakhanpal, P. and Rai, D.K. (2007). Quercetin: A versatile flavonoid. *Internet Journal of Medical Update*, 2(2): 22–37.

Laughton, M.J., Evans, P.A., Moroney, M.A., Hoult, J.R.S., Halliwell, B. (1991). Inhibition of mammalian 5-lipoxygenas e and cyclo-oxygenase by flavonoids and phenolic dieatary additivies: Relationship to antioxidant activity and to iron ion-reducing ability. *Biochem Pharmacol*, 42(9): 1673–1681.

Li, D., Li, X.L. and Ding, X.L. (2010). Composition and antioxidative properties of the flavonoid-rich fractions from tartary buckwheat grains. *Food Sci. Biotechnol.*, 19(3): 711–716.

Li, J.M., Gall, N.P., Grieve, D.J., Chen, M., Shah, A.M. (2002). Activation of NADPH oxidase during progression of cardiac hypertrophy to failure. *Hypertension*, 40(4): 477–484.

Liang, F. and Gardner, D.G. (1999). Mechanical strain activates BNG gene transcription through a p38/NF-kappaB-dependent mechanism. *J. Clin. Invest.*, 104(11): 1603–12.

Little, P.J., Chait, A., Bobik, A. (2011). Cellular and cytokine-based inflammatory processes as novel therapeutic targets for the prevention and treatment of atherosclerosis. *Pharmacol. Ther.*, 131(3): 255–268.

Little, P.J., Osman, N. and O'Brien, K.D. (2008). Hyperelongated biglycan: The surreptitious initiator of atherosclerosis. *Curr. Opin. Lipidol.*, 19(5): 448–454.

Liu, R.H. (2013). Health-promoting components of fruits and vegetables in the diet. Adv. Nutr., 4(3): 384S–92S.

Lobo, V., Patil, A., Phatak, A. and Chandra, N. (2010). Free radicals, antioxidants and functional foods: Impact on human health. *Pharmacogn Rev.*, 4(8): 118–126.

Luiz da Silva, E.L., Tsushida, T. and Terao, J. (1998). Inhibition of mammalian 15-lipoxygenase-dependent lipid peroxidation in low-density lipoprotein by quercetin and quercetin monoglucosides. *Arch Biochem. Biophys.*, 349(2): 313–320.

Lüscher, T.F. and Noll, G. (1995). The pathogenesis of cardiovascular disease: Role of the endothelium as a target and mediator. *Atherosclerosis*, 118(Suppl 1): S81–S90.

Machha, A. and Mustafa, M.R. (2005). Chronic treatment with flavonoids prevents endothelial dysfunction spontaneouly hypertensive rat aorta. *J. Cardiovasc. Pharmacol.*, 46(1): 36–40.

Manach, C., Masur, A. and Scalbert, A. (2005). Polyphenols and prevention of cardio vascular diseases. *Curr. Opin. Lipidol.*, 16(1): 77–84.

Mao, T.K., Van De Water, J., Keen, C.L., Schmitz, H.H. and Gershwin, M.E. (2002). Modulation of TNF-alpha secretion in peripheral blood mononuclear cells by cocoa flavanols and procyanidins. *Dev. Immunol.*, 9(3): 135–141.

Margaret, C. (2010). Burden: Mortality, morbidity and risk factors. *Global Status Report on Non Communicable Diseases*, pp. 9–31.

Mathur, S., Devaraj, S., Grundy, S.M. and Jialal, I. (2002). Cocoa products decrease low density lipoprotein oxidative susceptibility but do not affect biomarkers of inflammation in humans. *J. Nutr.*, 132(12): 3663–3667.

Michelson, A.D. (2010). Antiplatelet therapies for the treatment of cardiovascular disease. *Nat. Rev. Drug Discov.*, 9(2): 154–169.

Middleton, E.J. (1998). Effect of plant flavonoids on immune and inflammatory cell function. *Adv. Exp. Med. Bio.*, 439: 175–182.

Morris, J.N. and Crawford, M.D. (1958). Coronary heart disease and physical activity of work. *Br. Med. J.*, 2(5111): 1485–1496.

Mosawy, S. (2015). Effect of the flavonol quercetin on human platelet function: A review. *Food Public Health*, 5(1): 1–9.

Nabel, E.G. (2003). Cardiovascular disease. *N. Engl. J. Med.*, 349: 60–72.

Nandava, M., Ojha, S.K. and Arya, D.S. (2005). Protective role of flavonoids in cardio vascular diseases. *Natural Product Radiance*, 4(3): 166–176.

Nijveldt, R.J., van Nood, E., van Hoorn, D.E., Boelens, P.G., van Norren, K. and van Leeuwen, P.A. (2001). Flavonoids: A review of probable mechanisms of action and potential applications. *Am. J. Clin. Nutr.*, 74(4): 418–25.

Ojeda, D., Jiménez-Ferrer, E., Zamilpa, A., Herrera-Arellano, A., Tortoriello, J. and Alvarez, L. (2010). Inhibition of angiotensin converting enzyme (ACE) activity by the anthocyanins delphinidin-and cyanidin-3-O-sambubiosides from *Hibiscus sabdariffa*. *J. Ethnopharmacol.*, 127(1): 7–10.

Pan, M.H., Laia, A.C.S., Ho, C.T. (2010). Anti-inflammatory activity of natural dietary flavonoids. *Food Funct.*, 1(1): 15–31.

Pearson, D.A., Paglieroni, T.G., Rein, D., Wun, T., Schramm, D.D., Wang, J.F., Holt, R.R., Gosselin, R., Schmitz, H.H. and Keen, C.L. (2002). The effects of flavanol-rich cocoa and aspirin on *ex vivo* platelet function. *Thromb. Res.*, 106(4–5): 191–197.

Pignatelli, P., Pulcinelli, F.M., Celestini, A., Lenti, L., Ghiselli, A., Gazzaniga, P.P. and Violi, F. (2000). The flavonoids quercetin and catechin synergistically inhibit platelet function by antagonizing the intracellular production of hydrogen peroxide. *Am. J. Clin. Nutr.*, 72(5): 1150–5.

Procházková, D., Bousová, I. and Wilhelmová, N. (2011). Antioxidant and prooxidant properties of flavonoids. *Fitoterapia*, 82(4): 513–23.

Rein, D., Paglieroni, T.G., Wun, T., Pearson, D.A., Schmitz, H.H., Gosselin, R., Keen, C.L. (2000). Cocoa inhibits platelet activation and function. *Am. J. Clin. Nutr.*, 72(1): 30–35.

Rice, B.H. (2014). Dairy and cardiovascular disease: A review of recent observational research. *Curr. Nutr. Rep.*, 3(2): 130–138.

Rice-Evans, C.A., Miller, N.J. and Paganga, G. (1996). Structure-antioxidant activity relationships of flavonoids and phenolic acids. *Free Radic Biol. Med.*, 20(7): 933–956.

Ross, R. (1993). The pathogenesis of atherosclerosis: A perspective for the 1990s. *Nature*, 362(6423): 801–809.

Safari, M.R. and Shiek, N. (2003). Effect of some flavonoids on the susceptibility of low density lipoprotein to oxidative modification. *Prostaglandins Leukot Essent Fatty Acids*, 69(1): 73–7.

Salvamani, S., Gunasekaran, B., Shaharuddin, N.A., Ahmad, S.A. and Shukor, M.Y. (2014). Antiartherosclerotic effects of plant flavonoids. *BioMed Res. Int.*, 2014: 480258.

Sano, M., Fukuda, K., Sato, T., Kawaguchi, H., Suematsu, M., Matsuda, S., Koyasu, S., Matsui, H., Yamauchi-Takihara, K., Harada, M., Saito, Y. and Ogawa, S. (2001). ERK and p38 MAPK, but not NF-kappaB, are critically involved in reactive oxygen species-mediated induction of IL-6 by angiotensin II in cardiac fibroblasts. *Circ. Res.*, 89(8): 661–669.

Santhakumar, A.B., Bulmer, A.C. and Singh, I. (2013). A review of the mechanisms and effectiveness of dietary polyphenols in reducing oxidative stress and thrombotic risk. *J. Hum. Nutr. Diet.*, 27(1): 1–21.

Santos, K.F.R., Oliveira, T.T., Nagem, T.J., Pinto, A.S. and Oliveira, M.G.A. (1999). Hypolipidaemic effects of naringenin, rutin, nicotinic acid and their associations. *Pharmacol Res.*, 40(6): 493–496.

Santulli, G. (2013). Angiogenesis insights from a systematic overview. New York: Nova Science.

Schramm, D.D., Karim, M., Schrader, H.R., Holt, R.R., Kirkpatrick, N.J., Polagruto, J.A., Ensunsa, J.L., Schmitz, H.H. and Keen, C.L. (2003). Food effects on the absorption and pharmacokinetics of cocoa flavanols. *Life Sci.*, 73(7): 857–869.

Schroeter, H., Heiss, C., Balzer, J., Kleinbongard, P., Keen, C.L., Hollenberg, N.K., Sies, H., Kwik-Uribe, C., Schmitz, H.H. and Kelm, M. (2006). (-)-Epicatechin mediates beneficial effects of flavanol-rich cocoa on vascular function in humans. *Proc. Natl. Acad. Sci. USA*, 103(4): 1024–1029.

Sheu, J.R., Hsiao, G., Chou, P.H., Shen, M.Y. and Cho, D.S. (2004). Mechanism involved in the antiplatelet activity of rutin, a glycoside of the flavonol quercetin in human platelets. *J. Agric. Food Chem.*, 52(14): 4414–4418.

Smith, P.D.S., Thomas, P., Scurr, J.H. and Dormandy, J.A. (1980). Causes of various ulceration, a new hypothesis. *Br. Med. J.*, (*Clin. Res. Ed.*), 96(6638): 1726–1727.

Stangl, V., Dreger, H., Stangl, K. and Lorenz, M. (2007). Molecular targets of tea polyphenols in the cardiovascular system. *Cardiovasc Res* 2007; 73(2): 348–358.

Steinberg, D., Parthasarathy, S., Carew, T.E., Khoo, J.C. and Witztum, J.L. (1989). Beyond cholesterol: Modifications of low-density lipoprotein that increase its atherogenicity. *N. Engl. J. Med.*, 320(14): 915–924.

Sueishi, K., Yonemitsu, Y., Nakagawa, K., Kaneda, Y., Kumamoto, M. and Nakashima, Y. (1997). Atherosclerosis and angiogenesis. Its pathophysiological significance in humans as well as in an animal model induced by the gene transfer of vascular endothelial growth factor. *Ann. N. Y. Acad. Sci.*, 811: 311–22; 322–4.

Sun, G.W., Qiu, Z.D., Wang, W.N., Sui, X. and Sui, D.J. (2016). Flavonoids extraction from propolis attenuates pathological cardiac hypertrophy through PI3K/AKT signaling pathway. *Evid. Based Complement. Alternat. Med.*, 2016: 6281376.

Takimoto, E. and Kass, D.A. (2007). Role of oxidative stress in cardiac hypertrophy and remodeling. *Hypertension*, 49(2): 241–248.

Tangney, C.C. and Rasmussen, H.E. (2013). Polyphenols, inflammation and cardio vascular diseases. *Curr. Atheroscler. Rep.*, 15(5): 324.

Terao, J., Piskula, M. and Yao, Q. (1994). Protective effect of epicatechin, epicatechin gallate, and quercetin on lipid peroxidation in phospholipid bilayers. *Arch. Biochem. Biophys.*, 308(1): 278–284.

Testai, L. (2015). Flavonoids and mitochondrial pharmacology: A mew paradign for cardio protection. *Life. Sci.*, 135: 68–76.

Vaiyapuri, S., Roweth, H., Ali, M.S., Unsworth, A.J., Stainer, A.R., Flora, G.D., Crescente, M., Jones, C.I., Moraes, L.A. and Gibbins, J.M. (2015). Pharmacological actions of nobiletin in the modulation of platelet function. *Br. J. Pharmacol.*, 172(16): 4133–4145.

Vaya, J., Mahmood, S., Goldblum, A., Aviram, M., Volkova, N., Shaalan, A., Musa, R. and Tamir, S. (2003). Inhibition of LDL oxidation by flavonoids in relation to their structure and calculated enthalpy. *Phytochemistry*, 62(1): 89–99.

Wan, Y., Vinson, J.A., Etherton, T.D., Proch, J., Lazarus, S.A. and Kris-Etherton, P.M. (2001). Effects of cocoa powder and dark chocolate on LDL oxidative susceptibility and prostaglandin concentrations in humans. *Am. J. Clin. Nutr.*, 74(5): 596–602.

Yildrim, A., Oktay, M. and Bilaloçlu, V. (2001). The antioxidant activity of leaves of *Cydonia vulgaris*. *Turk. J. Med. Sci.*, 31: 23–27.

Yoshimoto, T., Furukawa, M., Yamamoto, S., Horie, T. and Watanabe-Kohno, S. (1983). Flavonoids: Potent inhibitors of arachidonate 5-lipoxygenase. *Biochem. Biophys. Res. Commun.*, 116(2): 612–618.

Youdim, K.A., McDonald, J., Kalt, W. and Joseph, J.A. (2002). Potential role of dietary flavonoids in reducing microvascular endothelium vulnerability to oxidative and inflammatory insults (small star, filled). *J. Nutr. Biochem.*, 13: 282–8.

Zhang, W., Chen, X.F., Huang, Y.J., Chen, Q.Q., Bao, Y.J. and Zhu, W. (2012). 2,3,4',5-Tetrahydroxystilbene-2-O-beta-D-glucoside Inhibits angiotensin II-induced cardiac fibroblast proliferation through suppression of reactive oxygen species-ERK1/2 pathway. *Clin. Exp. Pharmacol. Physiol.*, 39(5): 429–437.

9

Molecular Mechanisms Underlining Anti-infective Potential of Flavonoids

VIJAY KOTHARI[1]*, SAKSHI SHARMA[1], DEEPA SHAHI[1] AND DIVYA GAJERA[1]

ABSTRACT

Infectious microorganisms have been one of the forefront challenges before the mankind since antiquity. The rapid emergence of the multidrug resistant phenotypes among pathogens has only raised the magnitude and severity of this challenge. This persuades the researchers to keep searching for novel and more effective antimicrobial / anti-infective agents. Many phytocompounds have been reported for their anti-pathogenic potential, of which flavonoids are an important category. This chapter provides an overview of the flavonoids reported for their anti-infective properties, and also peeps into the molecular mechanisms underlining the antimicrobial potential of some of them, giving an insight on their mode of action. Antimicrobial flavonoids may have multiple cellular targets, rather than only one specific site of action.

Key words: Anti-infective, Antimicrobial, Flavonoids, Quorum Sensing, Quercetin

1. INTRODUCTION

Flavonoids are widely distributed plant compounds, with a wide spectrum of biological effects. This review focuses on their anti-infective potential, which is of importance in context of the serious challenge of antimicrobial resistance staring in the face of human race. After taking an overview of the problem of antibiotic-resistance among infectious microbes, and antimicrobial potential of different types of plant metabolites, this review moves onto anti-infective potential of flavonoids specifically, followed by

[1] Institute of Science, Nirma University, Ahmedabad, India
**Corresponding author*: E-mail: vijay.kothari@nirmauni.ac.in; vijay23112004@yahoo.co.in

description of the molecular mechanisms involved in antimicrobial action of flavonoids.

2. OVERVIEW OF THE PROBLEM OF ANTIMICROBIAL RESISTANCE (AMR)

Misuse and overuse of antimicrobial chemotherapeutics started soon after they entered into widespread use for infection control. Promiscuous antibiotic usage practices boosted the quick emergence of resistance among the pathogens. Prevalence of AMR among major microbial pathogens of humans and animals has allowed the complications of morbidity, mortality, extended hospitalization and healthcare expenses to exacerbate. Among the most threatening bacterial pathogens are methicillin/vancomycin-resistant *Staphylococcus aureus* (MRSA/VRSA), multidrug-resistant (MDR) *Mycobacterium tuberculosis*, vancomycin resistant enterococci (VRE), and extended spectrum beta-lactamase (ESBLs) producing bacteria. We obviously cannot manage without effective antibiotics, and owing to this 'selection pressure' in form of continuous antibiotic use, the emergence of novel MDR phenotypes of pathogens will also remain aregular phenomenon (Medina and Pieper, 2016). Multidrug resistance can be described as the insensitivity or resistance of a microbe to the administered antimicrobial agents (which are structurally not related and do not have an overlap of their molecular targets) despite earlier sensitivity to it (Tanwar *et al.*, 2014).

Among the examples of most notorious drug-resistant pathogens *Pseudomonas aeruginosa* sits at the forefront. It is inherently resistant to a considerable number of antimicrobials such as ampicillin, amoxicillin, amoxicillin/clavulanate, first-generation cephalosporins, second-generation antimicrobials like cefotaxime and ceftriaxone, nalidixic acid, and trimethoprim. Moreover, it effortlessly acquires resistance to new antibacterial agents by mutation or acquisition of non-self genetic material. MDR phenotypes of *P. aeruginosa* resistant to at least four classes of antibiotics *i.e.,* third-generation cephalosporins, fluoroquinolones, aminoglycosides, and carbapenems have been reported. Selection pressure imposed by the antimicrobial therapy itself can be said to be the driving force for the rapid emergence of MDR strains (Porras-Gómez *et al.,* 2012). Another instance where MDR phenotypes are looming as a big threat is that of tuberculosis. The causative agent *M. tuberculosis* is referred to as MDR if it can not be controlled by rifampicin and isoniazid. When compared to drug-susceptible tuberculosis, treatment for MDR tuberculosis extends for 18-24 months, is less efficacious, and noticeably more toxic (Millard *et al.,* 2015).

3. ANTIMICROBIAL *VS.* ANTI-INFECTIVE STRATEGY

One of the major limitations of the traditional antimicrobial therapy is that by putting the target pathogen in a 'either die or develop resistance to survive' condition, it imposes a strong selection pressure on them to mutate into a resistant phenotype. An alternative approach seems to be that of targeting the pathogenicity rather than the pathogen. This can be achieved by attenuating the virulence of the pathogenic population without necessarily killing them. This anti-infective approach is likely to exert lesser selection pressure on the target pathogenic microbial populations. Among the potential targets of such anti-infective agents are the microbial quorum sensing (QS) circuit, siderophore production, efflux pumps, antibiotic-degrading enzymes, genes coding for toxin production, hemolysis, biofilm formation, etc. These anti-infective agents may be used either alone or in combination with conventional microbicidal antibiotics. Some polyherbal formulations capable of modulating bacterial QS have been demonstrated to possess significant anti-infective potential *in vitro* as well as *in vivo* (Palep *et al.,* 2016). Such bioactive polyherbal formulations can also have certain flavonoids as their active ingredients.

4. PHYTOCOMPOUNDS AS ANTIMICROBIALS AND/OR ANTI-INFECTIVES

"Eat leeks in March and wild garlic in May, and all the year after the physicians may play."

– Traditional Welsh rhyme (Tyler, 1987)

Plants in nature are continuously exposed to pathogenic and non-pathogenic microbes, and it is not illogical to expect them to synthesize different protective compounds with antimicrobial potential. Most of the currently used antibiotics have come from the microbial kingdom. Antimicrobial phytocompounds can be expected to differ significantly from their microbial counterparts with respect to structure as well as mode of action. It may take some time and effort for the pathogenic microbes to develop resistance against any novel antimicrobial structure of plant origin. Investigation on antimicrobial phytocompounds with lesser side-effects to the host can help in effective management of the AMR challenge (Parekh and Chanda, 2007). There are many plant species mentioned in traditional medicine literature of different ancient cultures, which are very much likely to be safe and cost-effective (Ghosh *et al.,* 2008; Kumar and Pandey, 2013). The antimicrobial phytocompounds can mainly be divided into two classes: Phytoalexins and Phytoanticipins (Table 1).

With a current estimated count of 250,000 to 500,000 (Borris, 1996) the plant kingdom has had been a source of bioactive formulations since ancient times. As back as sixty thousand years ago, Neanderthals used hollyhock (*Alcea* spp.), as famous ornamental plants (Thomson, 1978). Even without precisely knowing the biosynthetic pathways of the plants, and ones inside human body influenced by plant formulations, herbal remedies have been

Table 1: Two major classes of antimicrobial phytocompounds

Phytoalexins	***Phytoanticipins***
• Low molecular weight compounds that are produced in response to microbial, herbivorous or other external stimuli (VanEtten *et al.*, 1994)	• Produced in plants prior to infection or from pre-existing compounds after infection (Van Etten *et al.*, 1994)
• Synthesized *de novo*; as opposed to being released by, for example, hydrolytic activity (Dixon *et al.*, 2001)	• Define as "pre-formed infectional inhibitors" (Dixon *et al.*, 2001)
• Include simple prenylpropanoid derivatives, flavonoids, isoflavonoids, terpenes, polyketides, pterocarpans, sulfur-containing indole derivatives and coumarins (Grayer and Harborne, 1995; Ibraheem *et al.*, 2010).	• Include glycosides, glucosinolates and saponins that are usually stored in the vacuoles of plant cells (Morrissey and Osbourn, 1999)

used for alleviating a large number of ailments. They have been claimed to possess a variety of biological activities including anti-inflammatory, anti-pyretic, nutritional, wound-healing, anti-spasmodic, anti-diabetes, cardioprotective, etc (Michael, 1998). For example, *Alcea rosea* is used as medicine for prophylaxis and treatment of respiratory disease, gastrointestinal tract (GI) complications, urinary tract infection (UTI), for countering against excess stomach acid, and peptic ulceration. Its root contains starch, mucilage, pectin, flavonoids (chiefly kaempferol, quercetin, and diosmetin glycosides), phenolic acid like syringic, caffeic, salicyclic, vanillic, and p-coumaric acids, sucrose, and tannins (Khare, 2008).

Plant products can broadly be categorized as primary and secondary metabolites on the basis of their indispensability for the survival of the plants (Molyneux *et al.,* 2007). Use of chemicals of plant origin is gaining popularity owing to numerous studies reporting their biological effects. The role of phytocompounds as therapeutics, functional foods, and nutraceuticals become more relevant in context of the efficacy of microbial source of antibiotics getting bit fadedaway due to AMR (Klink, 1997). A brief overview of antimicrobials properties of different classes of plant metabolites, including flavonoids, is presented below. Anti-infective potential of flavonoids has been dealt in more detail in later part of this review.

***Alkaloids*:** Alkaloids obtained from *Strychnos potatorum L.f.* (Loganiaceae) seeds, were reported for their antimicrobial activity against gram-positive, gram-negative, acid-fast bacteria and fungi at 100 and 200 µg/ml. Their inhibitory activity against *Proteus vulgaris*, *S. aureus, Salmonella typhimurium, V. cholerae, M. tuberculosis, A. niger* and *C. albicans* has also been reported (Patra, 2012). Berberine is an important example of antimicrobial alkaloids. Its efficacy against *Trypanosomes* and *Plasmodia* is believed to owe to its ability of intercalating with DNA (Cowan, 1999).

***Coumarins*:** They are the benzopyrones in which pyrone rings are fused with benzenes (Rao, 2015). Antimicrobial compounds like novobiocin and chlorobiocin have coumarin skeleton and are the growth inhibitors of *A. niger* and *Candida albicans* mycelia. Some coumarin derivatives possess antiviral activity including that against HIV (Al-Majedy *et al.,* 2017).

***Flavonoids*:** Many of the flavonoids are synthesized by plants as secondary metabolites in response to infection by a phytopathogenic microbe, and accordingly many flavonoids have been reported for their antimicrobial potential (Özçelik *et al.,* 2008). Flavonoids are a category of phenolic compounds, are synthesized by phenylpropanoid pathway (Du *et al.,* 2011). They have been shown to exert effect on different gram-negative and gram-positive bacteria, and also to possess anti-allergic, anti-cancer, and anti-inflammatory effect (Okoye *et al.*, 2015). Owing to their wide distribution in different plant parts, flavonoids are the largest group of naturally occurring phenolic phytochemicals, (Pretorius, 2003; Cushnie and Lamb, 2005). Flavonoids make a large part of dietary intake and the array of their antimicrobial activities spans from antibacterial and antiviral, to antifungal (Özçelik *et al.,* 2008), and hence it is recommended to have a diet rich in vegetables and fruits making enough flavonoids available (Huang *et al.,* 2016), as flavonoids are present in most of the photosynthetic organisms (Havsteen, 1983). The structural skeleton of flavonoids is derived from benzo-g-pyrone (Havsteen, 2002). Flavonoids and their corresponding aglycones like eriodictyol aglycone and naringenin were shown to be effective against MRSA infection when used in conjunction with neomycin and amikacin (Barreto *et al.,* 2014). Combination of flavonoids like rutin, morin, quercetin, with different antibiotics (ampicillin, amoxicillin, cefixime, ceftriaxone, vancomycin, methicillin) also proved effective against MRSA (Amin, 2015). Flavonoids also have an inhibitory influence against intestinal pathogens *Vibrio cholerae*, *Shigella* spp. and some viruses (Godstime, 2014).

***Phenolic compounds*:** The single substituted phenolic compounds like cinnamic acid and caffeic acids are very commonly found in herbs like tarragon, thyme, propolis etc. They have been reported for their antiviral (Silva-Carvalho *et al.*, 2015), antibacterial (Guzman, 2014) or antifungal (Sardi, 2016) properties. Phenolic compounds exert their effect by inhibiting critical pathway enzymes, by oxidizing products, either by non-specific interactions of sulfhydryl groups present in them or by other structural-activity relationship. Cinnamic acid was shown as an inhibitor of the activity of the benzoate 4-hydroxylase enzyme, which is involved in detoxification of benzoates in fungi (Korošec, 2014). Antimicrobial potency of essential oils can also stem from their phenolic constituents. For example, eugenol in clove oils is effective against dermatophytosis causing fungus *Trichophyton rubrum* (Hamini-Kadar *et al.*, 2014). The 4-hydroxylated stilbenes have been shown to exert antibacterial activity against *B. brevis* (Albert *et al.,* 2011). Resveratrol is believed to possess weak antimicrobial activity, but it is the precursor for synthesizing more active derivatives like pterostilbene and viniferins, which are having stronger antimicrobial activity compared to resveratrol (Chalal *et al.,* 2014). Wood-associated polyphenols, particularly pinosylvin, are effective against food pathogens and spoilage organisms. Their mechanism of action seems to be destabilization of the outer membrane of gram-negative bacteria, and interaction with the cell membrane (Plumed-Ferrer, 2013).

***Quinones*:** They are aromatic compounds with ketone functional groups. Quinones have an antihemorrhagic role in form of vitamin K. They are a source of free radicals which can form stable complex with amino acids of microbial origins thereby blocking essential pathways, DNA intercalation, alkylation, induction of DNA strand breaks or inhibition of special proteins or enzymes such as topoisomerases, and hence are potent antibacterial and anti-fungal compounds (Rahmoun, 2013). Nitrogen substituted derivatives of quinones exerted antibacterial activity against *S. aureus* and *Mycobacterium luteum*, and antifungal activity against *Candida tenuis* and *Aspergillus niger* (Mickevièienë, 2015).

***Tannins*:** A tannin or tannoid is any polyphenolic compound which can precipitate proteins, amino acids or alkaloids by binding to them. They are omnipresent in plants and are astringent in nature with a molecular weight in the range 500-3000 Da (Haslam, 1996). Polymeric tannins present in green tea are potent antioxidants and possess bactericidal activity (Kaur *et al.*, 2015). Antimicrobial activity of tannins can be attributed to their ability to prevent cell adhesions, inhibition of enzymes, inactivation of cellular transport proteins and biofilm formation by blocking QS in microbial colonies (Trentin *et al.*, 2013). Tannins have been noted for their efficacy against *Clostridium perfringens* induced necrotic enteritis (Carrasco *et al.*, 2016). Tannic acid proved better than gallic acid with respect to bactericidal activity against food borne bacteria *Shewanella putrefaciens* (Widsten, 2014). Tannin derivatives which are constituents of mango leaves and fruits could exert inhibitory effect against bacterial species like *Shigella flexneri*, *Pseudomonas fluorescens*, *Escherichia coli*, *Staphylococcus aureus* and *Bacillus* spp. (Mustapha *et al.,* 2014).

***Terpenoids*:** Terpenes are the chemicals made of isoprene backbone and form terpenoids when combined with oxygen. Artemisinin is a sesquiterpene lactone, which is a highly effective antimalarial compound, and was recently implicated as anti-cancer compound too (Das, 2015). Monoterpenes were reported to inhibit the growth of dermatophytes and yeasts, owing to their affinity for ergosterol, relating their mode of action to cell membrane destabilization (Miron, 2014). Essential oil terpenes have both antibacterial and antioxidant activities, as confirmed by electron microscopic studies (Zengin and Baysal, 2014). Monoterpenes like beta-pinene and limonene which are part of many essential oils have antiviral activities especially against Herpes Simplex Virus type-1 (HSV-1) (Astani and Schnitzler, 2014).

5. FLAVONOIDS AS ANTIMICROBIAL PLANT COMPOUNDS

Flavonoids are present in almost every part of plants including fruits, vegetables, flowers, and stems (Harborne, 1999), and even in wines and honey (Grange, 1990). They protect plants from ultraviolet radiation and from fungal infections when present in leaves (Harborne, 1999). The flavonoids may get classified according to their origin in the biosynthetic cycle or as end products of any physiological pathway *e.g.,* chalcones, flavanones, 3-flavanols, flavan-3,4-diols, anthocyanidins, flavonols, flavones, proanthocyanidins, isoflavones *etc.* High degree of structural variety among a particular class of metabolites can make it difficult for the pathogens to become completely resistant to that whole class. There are approximately 4000 types of flavonoid compounds known, of which quercetin, kaempferol and quercitrin are the most common flavonoids present in about 70% of vascular plants. A wide range of medicinal properties have been attributed to different flavonoids, including antitumor (Harborne, 2000), antioxidant, enzyme inhibitors, antimicrobial, anti-inflammatory, and antiallergic (Harborne, 1999). Flavonoids as plant pigments of red, blue and purple colour. Since long, without knowing their precise mode of action, flavonoids rich crude plant preparations have been used by practitioners of traditional medicine for treatment of many human diseases. For illustration, the plant *Tagetes minuta* (containing quercetagetin-7-arabinosyl-galactoside) are used majorly in Argentine folk medicines to treat infectious diseases (Cushnie and Lamb, 2005). Propolis (Bee glue) balm was introduced by Hippocrates for treatment of sores and ulcers (Fearnley, 2001). The bioactive ingredients in propolis which possesses antimicrobial activity are flavonoids including galangin and pinocembrin (Huang *et al.,* 2014). Similarly, the flavone baicalin contained in *Scutellaria baicalensis* Georgi is the main chemical component of traditional Chinese medicine Huang-chin possessing activity against oral bacteria (Tsao *et al.*, 1982). Baicalein has also been noted for anti-viral and anti-inflammatory activities (Liu *et al.,* 2015). Flavonoids and their corresponding aglycones like eriodictyol aglycone and naringenin are effective against gram-negative bacteria (Mandalari *et al.*, 2007). The mode of action of the flavonoid aglycones including eriodictyol, hesperetin and naringenin as explored through fractional inhibitory concentration (FIC) isobolograms studies seems to be involving synergistic and antagonistic interactions of flavonoids (Olasupo *et al.,* 2004). *In vivo* studies have proved anti-cancer activity of the flavonoid quercetin, against the group I carcinogen *Helicobacter pylori* (Gonzalez-Segovia *et al.,* 2008). Flavonoids are reportedly having anti-inflammatory activities owing to their ability to block enzymes involved in free radical generation, like cyclooxygenases, lipoxygenases, and nitric oxide synthase (Izzi *et al.*, 2012). Extracts from *Flos Rosae Chinensis* were reported to be active against fluconazole-resistant *Candida albicans*, and flavonoids (kaempferol, kaempferol-3-O-a-L-arabinoside, kaempferol-3-O-a-L-rhamnoside, quercetin, and quercetin-3-O-a-L-arabinoside) were indicated among the major bioactive compounds of this extract (Zhang *et al.*, 2017).

Flavonoids like rutin, morin, and quercetin have been shown to be effective against MRSA, when administered along with antibiotics like ampicillin, amoxicillin, cefixime, ceftriaxone, vancomycin, or methicillin (Amin, 2015).

Sugarcane bagasse is a rich source of flavonoids, that showed bacteriostatic activities against foodborne pathogens like *S. aureus, Listeria monocytogenes, E. coli,* and *S. typhimurium* which are susceptible to polyphenolic compounds (Zhao, 2015). The glycosides of flavonoids obtained from *Polygonum capitatum*, a Chinese herb usually used for urological disorders, confer protection against inflammation caused by *H. pylori* infections (Zhang, 2015). Flavonoids like isoquercitrin-6-*O*-4-hydroxybenzoate and quercetin-3-*O*-β-rhamnoside obtained from *Ficus exasperata*, a deciduous African tree, inhibited growth of gram-positive bacteria (Taiwo and Igbeneghu, 2014). Hesperidin and its aglycone, hesperetin are important flavonoids obtained from citrus fruits and they are suggested to be effective antimicrobials with a proposed role in bacterial membrane disruption (Iranshahi, 2015). A flavonoid, entadanin showed strong antimicrobial activity against *S. typhimurium* with minimum inhibitory concentration (MIC) of 1.56 µg/mL (Dzoyem *et al.*, 2017). *Phyllanthus emblica* (L.) is a plant known to possess antifungal, antiviral and antibacterial activities. Its transcriptomic analysis has also been done, with particular focus on genes involved in flavonoid biosynthesis (Kumar *et al.,* 2016).

Hitherto a wide variety of flavonoids have been reported for their antimicrobial potential against multiple pathogens. Few examples of their antibacterial, antifungal, and antiviral activity are presented through Tables 2 to 4 (Sandhar *et al.*, 2011; Kumar and Pandey, 2013; Hosein *et al.,* 2014; Ahmad, *et al.*, 2015).

Table 2: Flavonoids with antibacterial property

Sl. no.	*Flavonoid compound*	*Effective against*
1	Apigenin	*Streptococcus pyogenes, S. jaccalis, S. viridans, Enterobacter cloacae, Vibrio cholerae, E. faecalis, E. coli, S. aureus, P. aeruginosa, B. cereus, B. subtilis, Klebsiella pneumoniae, Salmonella typhimurium*
2	Baicalin	*S. aureus, P. aeruginosa*
3	Bartramia flavone	*E. cloacae, E. aerogenes, P. aeruginosa*
4	Catechins	*Vibrio cholerae, Streptococcus mutans, Shigella*
5	Chrysin	*S. jaccalis, S. pneumoniae, E. coli, S. baris*
6	Datisetin	*Proteus vulgaris*
7	Hydroxyethylrutoside	*Clostridium perfringens*
8	Iso-liquiritigenin	*S. aureus*
9	Licochalcones A and C	*S. aureus* and *Micrococcus luteus.*
10	Lucenin	*E. cloacae, E. aerogenes, P. aeruginosa*
11	Naringenin and Sophoraflavanone G	MRSA and Streptococcus

Table 2: (*Contd...*)

Table 2: (*Contd...*)

Sl. no.	*Flavonoid compound*	*Effective against*
12	Quercetin	*Staphylococcus aureus, Bacillus subtilis, B. cereus, Escherichia coli, Helicobacter pylori, Pseudomonas aeruginosa, P. fluorescens, Enterobacter aerogens*
13	Rutin	*Bacillus anthracis, P. aeruginosa, K. pneumoniae, E. coli, S. typhimurium, B. cereus*
14	Robinetin, Myricetin, and (–)-Epigallocatechin	*Proteus vulgaris*
15	Saponarine	*P. aeruginosa, E. cloacae, E. aerogenes,*
16	5,7-dimethoxyflavan one-42-O-B-D-glucopyranoside	*K. pneumoniae*
17	5-Hydroxyflavanones and 5-Hydroxyiso-flavanones	*S. mutans, S. sobrinus*

Table 3: Flavonoids with antiviral property

Sl. no.	*Flavonoid compound*	*Effective against*
1	Acacetin	Influenza viruses
2	Apigenin	Influenza virus, Enteovirus-71, Hepatitis C virus (HCV), Immunodeficiency virus infection, Herpes Simplex Virus (HSV) type, Auzesky virus
3	Galangin	HSV type
4	Ladanein	HCV
5	Liquiritigenin	HCV
6	Luteolin	Auzesky virus
7	Naringenin	HCV
8	Naringin	Respiratory syncytial virus
9	Orientin	Parainfluenza type 3 virus
10	Quercetin	HCV, HSV, Polio virus, Rabies virus, Parainfluenza virus, Mengo virus, Pseudorabies virus
11	Rutin	Parainfluenza virus, Influenza virus
12	Vitexin	Para influenza type 3 virus

Table 4: Flavonoids with antifungal property

Sl. no.	*Flavonoid compound*	*Effective against*
1	Galangin	*Candida albicans, Aspergillus tamarii, A. flavus, Cladosporium sphaerospermum, Penicillium digitatum, Penicillium italicum*
2	5,7,4-trihydroxy-8-methyl-6-(3-methyl-[2-butenyl])-(2*S*)-flavanon	*C. albicans*
3	6,7,42 -trihydroxy-32,52 dimethoxy-flavone,5,52-dihydroxy-8,22,42 trimethoxyflavone,5,7,42-trihydroxy-32,52 dimethoxyflavone	*A. flavus*
4	7-hydroxy-3,4-(methylenedioxy) flavan	*C. albicans*

6. MOLECULAR MECHANISMS UNDERLINING ANTIMICROBIAL POTENTIAL OF SOME OF THE FLAVONOIDS

Though an exceedingly large number of plant extracts (including those rich in flavonoid content) and purified phytocompounds have been reported for their *in vitro* antimicrobial activity against a multitude of pathogenic microorganisms, relatively small number of them have been validated for their *in vivo* efficacy, and the molecular mechanism explaining their mode of action has been elucidated for still a smaller number of these bioactive plant products. Different flavonoids can be targeting different sites in susceptible pathogens such as cell membrane or cell wall by interacting through hydrogen bonds, resulting in altered morphology/physiology-leading to cellular damage (Shehadi *et al.*, 2014). Fig. 1 presents an overview of the anti-infective spectrum of flavonoids.

Flavonol, flavan-3-ol and flavone classes of compounds are believed to act as inhibitors of energy metabolism; whereas flavolan and flavonols cause damage to the cytoplasmic membrane. Isoflavones interrupt nucleic acid synthesis (Ahmad *et al.*, 2015). These phenolic compounds can exert their toxic effect against susceptible pathogens by targeting certain enzyme's active site or by reacting with sulfhydryl groups of enzymes leading to enzyme denaturation. Flavonoids like glabridinare potent inhibitors of DNA gyrase, and dihydrofolate reductase, which forms the basis for their activity against *H. pylori* (Wang, 2014).

As flavonoids are part of routine diet, it is not illogical to think that they can affect the human health and immunity by influencing composition of the gut microbiome. Human microbiome has now been accepted as a major factor in determining susceptibility of the host to various disease conditions and microbial infections. Imbalance of the gut microbiota composition can bring the host immunity in a compromised state, and put the host at risk. Flavonoids being a substantial part of human diet, they do confer some protection against microbial infections (Hollman, 2004). A recent *in vitro* study (Huang *et al.*, 2016) showed that different flavonoids can shape unique gut microbiota profile. Quercetin and catechin could significantly stimulate Actinobacteria, while inhibiting Bacteroidetes. Catechin had a suppressive effect on Firmicutes and Fusobacteria. To understand the interaction of flavonoids with the gut microbial community, it is necessary to know how flavonoids are absorbed and metabolized inside human system. Structural feature of the flavonoids is a decisive factor in determining whether they will be absorbed from the small intestine or required to go to the colon before absorption can happen (Hollman, 2004). It is considered that 90-95% polyphenols of total intake can enter colonic region without absorption (Huang *et al.*, 2016).

Despite the widely known antimicrobial potential of flavonoids, not many efforts are reported to decode their mode of action at the molecular level.

One of the reasons is that elucidation of molecular mechanisms demands use of high-end equipment and technology for investigation at genomic, transcriptomic, proteomic, and/or metabolomics level, and all investigators may not have access to such sophisticated labs. Further these experiments are quite cost-intensive. Table 5 lists mode of action of few antimicrobial flavonoids.

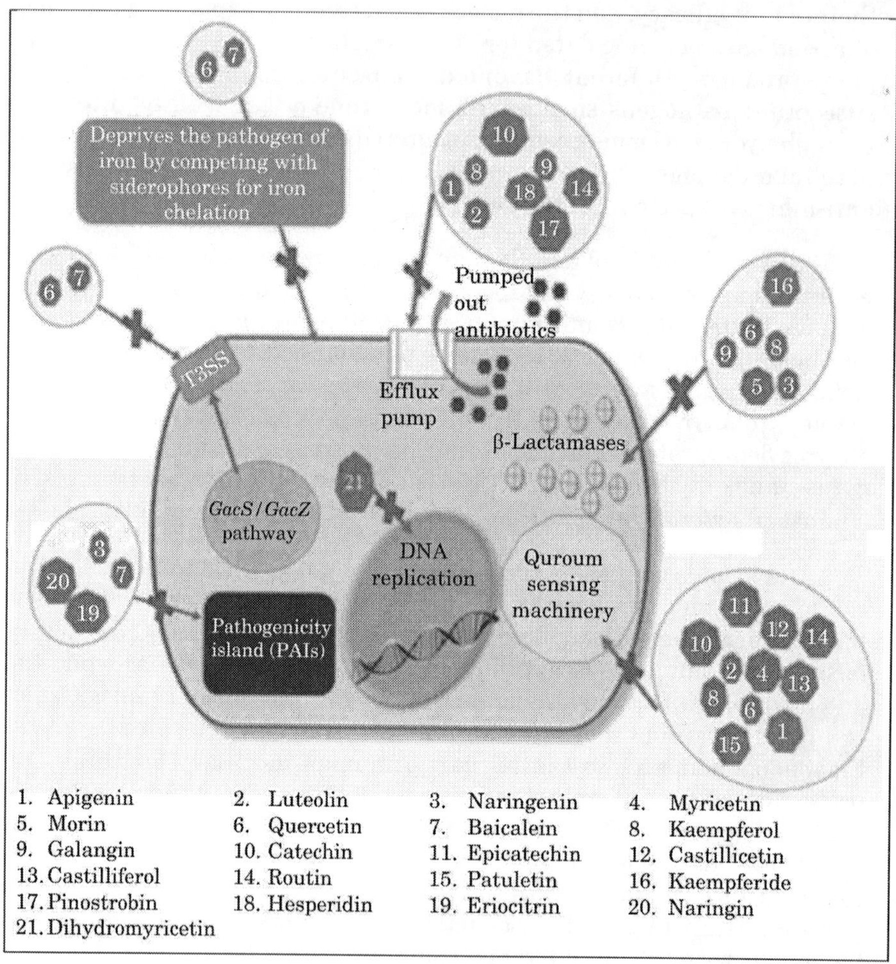

Fig. 1: Anti-infective spectrum of flavonoids. This figure depicts a summary of various targest of anti-infective flavonoids, inside a bacterial cell. Antimicrobial flavonoids can have multiple cellular targets, and not necessarily one particular site of action. (Denny *et al.*, 2002; Vandepuputte *et al*, 2010; Vikram *et al.*, 2011; Eumkeb *et al.*, 2012; Vasavi *et al.*, 2014; Filocamo *et al.*, 2015; Abreu *et al.*, 2015; Christena *et al.*, 2015; Randhwa *et al.*, 2016; Siriwong *et al.*, 2016; Tsou *et al.*, 2016; Vasavi *et al.*, 2016; Orhan, 2017)

Table 5: Suggested mode of action of certain antimicrobial flavonoids

Sl. no	*Flavonoid compound*	*Type of antimicrobial activity*	*Mechanism*	*Effective against*	*References*
1	Baicalin	Antiviral	Interaction between HIV-1 envelope protein sit; blocks entry of virus in human peripheral blood mononuclear cells	HIV virus	Park *et al.,* 2009
2	Thearubigin	Antibacterial	Neutralizes bacterial toxin by covalently binding with it	*Clostridium tetani*	Ahmad, A. *et al.*, 2015
3	Epigallocatechin gallate (EGCG)		Increases endogenous oxidative stress	*E. coli*	Xiong *et al.,* 2017
4	Naringenin		Inhibits biofilm formation	*V. harveyi, E. coli*	Vikram *et al.,* 2010
5	Apigenin				
6	Kaempferol				
7	Curcumin		Diminishes pyocyanin production, and biofilm formation; Reduces protease and elastase activities; Was shown to reduce infectivity of the test pathogen towards *Arabidopsis thaliana* and *C. elegans*	*P. aeruginosa* PA01	Truchado *et al.,* 2015

6.1. Flavonoids as Antibacterial Compounds

There are many examples of flavonoid rich plant extracts being used in folk medicine for treatment of bacterial infections (Ahmad *et al.,* 2015), but their mode of action has not been understood completely. For example, flavonoid containing roots of *Inula racemosa*, exhibits hypolipidemic, antifungal and antimicrobial properties, and are used in traditional Indian and Chinese medicine (Mohan and Gupta, 2017). Flavonoid profile of many medicinal plants can overlap, and hence it will be useful to understand mode of action of individual flavonoid molecules. These molecules when simultaneously present in some plant extract, may interact among themselves, producing a different type and/or level of biological effect. Xiao *et al.* (2014) identified five enzymes: DNA gyrase, fumarate reductase flavoprotein, dihydroorotate dehydrogenase, dihydrofolate reductase, and NADH-dependent enoyl-ACP reductase of *E. coli* as potential targets of nineteen antimicrobial flavonoids, through comparative genomics and molecular modeling. This finding was validated by molecular docking. By using comparative genomic studies, authors found homologous targets between *E. coli* and human gut microbiota. The "3-O-galloyl or 3-O-glycosides" side chain of flavonoids was shown to be responsible for the activity against these enzymes.

S. aureus, a major infectious agent, is estimated to cause 241,000 illnesses per year in the United States (Kadariya *et al.,* 2014). *S. aureus* strains resistant to methicillin and/or vancomycin has become a nightmare for clinicians. Recently, a flavonoid namely 2R, 3R-Dihydromyricetin (DMY) was shown to be effective against *S. aureus*. It registered a MIC value of 0.125 mg/mL (0.39 mM), and MBC (minimum bactericidal concentration) value of 0.25 mg/mL (0.78 mM). DMY was shown to rupture the cell wall of *S. aureus*, decrease the membrane fluidity, and interfere with membrane lipids and proteins. Cellular function was inhibited by DMY's binding on DNA groove of *S. aureus* (Wu *et al.,* 2016).

Many bacteria acquire resistance against beta-lactam antibiotics by producing the β – lactamases (Boussoualim *et al.,* 2011; Ahmad *et al.,* 2015). Six flavonoid compounds: 5,7-dimethoxyflavanone-4'-*O*- β -D-glucopyranosid, 5,7-dimethoxyflavanone-4'-*O*-[2"-*O*-(5'"-*O*-trans-cinnamoyl)-β-D-apiofuranosyl]-β-D-glucopyranoside, naringenin-7-*O*-β-D-glucopyranoside, 5,7,3'-trihydroxy-flavanone-4'-*O*-β -D-glucopyranoside, rutin, and nicotiflorin were shown to be effective at 32 and 64 µg/mL against ESBL producing MDR *Klebsiella pneumoniae* (Özçelik *et al.,* 2008). Kinetics study with different flavonoids showed that quercitrin, morin, naringenin, myricetin, kaempferol and rutin inhibit β-lactamase of *E. coli* K18 strain in a non-competitive manner. Few other flavonoids namely fisetine, flavone, quercetin, catechin and gossypin inhibit β-lactamases in uncompetitive manner. One reason for such kind of inhibition can be the position of the hydroxyl (-OH) group in flavonoids (Boussoualim *et al.,* 2011). Recently it was observed that quercetin inhibits growth of amoxicillin-resistant *Staphylococcus epidermidis* (ARSE) when prescribed with amoxicillin, by synergistically blocking peptidoglycan synthesis and β-lactamases activity (Siriwong *et al.,* 2016). *Stenotrophomonas maltophilia,* a gram-negative, nosocomial pathogen is resistant to numerous antibiotics, due to its ability to produce both metallo- L-lactamases (MBLs) and a non-metallo (serine)-L-lactamase. Galangin (3,5,7-trihydroxy-flavone) was found to block the activity of partially purified MBL from *S. maltophilia* (Denny *et al.,* 2002).

Peptic ulcer and duodenal ulcer causing *Helicobacter pylori* infect more than 50% of the world population. Urease production, flagellar motility, and most importantly *vac*A and *cag*A are the major virulence factors contributing to its survival in harsh stomach conditions, and its pathogenicity. Many plant products including flavonoids possess anti *H. pylori* activity. Quercetin 3-methyl ether can inhibit *H. pylori* at 3.9–62.5 µg/mL; cabreuvin can do it at 7.8 µg/mL; whereas kaempferol registered MBC of 6 µg/mL (Wang *et al.*, 2014)

Quite a few flavonoids have been reported for their anti-diarrheal potential. Their antimicrobial potency against the diarrhea casing microbes seems to stem from their ability to inactivate microbial adhesins, and thereby complexing with the microbial cell wall, besides inactivating enzymes. Mechanism underlining the anti-diarrhoeal potential of flavonoids is believed to involve inhibition of release of autocoids and prostaglandins, inhibition of contractions caused by spasmogens, stimulating normalization of the deranged water transport across the mucosal cells, and inhibition of GI release of acetylcholine (Pandey and Kumar, 2013). Some flavonoids exert their anti-infective potential by neutralizing bacterial toxins. Change in protein (toxin) structure upon flavonoid binding, leaves it incapable of interacting with the target cell membrane receptor. Catechins neutralize *S. aureus* toxin both *in vitro* and *in vivo* (Ahmad *et al.,* 2015), and can inactivate cholera toxin too (Kumar and Pandey, 2013). Anthrax lethal factor produced by *B. anthracis* is obstructed by epigallocatechin- 3-gallate (ECGC). Probably the Zn atom of this toxin binds to the phenyl ring of epicatechin-3-gallate, resulting in inactivation of the toxin (Ahmad *et al.,* 2015).

One of the general mechanisms how pathogens resist antibiotics is through the efflux pumps, which can pump the antibiotic and other toxic substances, out of the bacterial cell. Since the substrate specificity of efflux pumps is somewhat loose, a single efflux pump can make bacteria resistant to a broad range of chemically and structurally diverse compounds (Stavri *et al.,* 2006). Some flavonoids have been reported of being capable of inhibiting bacterial efflux pumps. Flavonoids apigenin and luteolin seem to be capable of acting as Efflux Pump Inhibitors (EPI) against MRSA (Brown *et al.,* 2015). Pinostrobin, besides being capable of synergizing with ciprofloxacin against a wide range of gram-positive as well as gram-negative organisms, also can act as an EPI. This nutraceutical compound was shown to inhibit efflux pump in *S. aureus,* biofilm formation by *E. coli* and *P. aeruginosa,* and to decrease their membrane permeability (Christena *et al.,* 2015). While some flavonoids can act as EPI, microbes do possess efflux pumps capable of pumping flavonoids out. One of the four major efflux pump families, is the RND family, which confer resistance against flavonoids, on various pathogens. The major flavonoid resisting efflux pumps are MexAB-OprM from *Pseudomonas syringae*, *Acr*AB from *Erwinia amylovora*, *Acr*D from *Erwinia chrysanthemi*, *Ife*AB from *Agrobacterium tumefaciens*, XagID2689 from *Xanthomonas axonopodis*, SmeDEF from *S. maltophilia*, EmrAB from *Sinorhizobium meliloti* and BjG30 from *Bradyrhizobium japonicum.*

Secretion systems of the pathogenic microbes form a very important part of their arsenal. Through these secretion systems, particularly type III and type IV secretions systems (*i.e.* T3SS and T4SS), pathogens inject their virulence factors into the host cells. Some flavonoids are able to inhibit the *Gac*S/*Gac*A pathways which regulate T3SS (Alcalde-Rico *et al.*, 2016). Quercetin and its structurally similar flavonoids and baicalein have recently been reported to induce their antibacterial response by inactivating *S. typhimurium* pathogenicity island-1 (SPI-1) encoded T3SS effectors, and also by inactivating translocases, thereby inhibiting the bacterial entry into epithelial cells (Tsou *et al.*, 2016).

For successful survival in the host, pathogens have to ensure enough iron availability, and they achieve this goal through the iron-chelators called siderophores. Flavonoids like quercetin, baicalein and its glycoside, obtained from *Coriander sativa* extracts were shown to exhibit antibacterial activity against *Pseudomonas syringae* by depriving this pathogen of iron (Jayasinghe *et al.*, 2015).

Flavonoids have also been tested for synergistic effect with conventional antibiotics against some clinically important strains. Synergistic action can enhance the susceptibility of pathogens against the conventional antibiotics. Quercetin, morin, and rutin with other antibiotics *i.e.* ampicillin, amoxicillin, cephradine, imipenem, ceftriaxone, and methicillin showed synergism effect against *S. aureus* (Amin *et al.*, 2015).

6.1.1. *Flavonoids as QS modulators*

Cell density based intercellular communication among bacteria is called quorum sensing. QS regulates expression of a notable part of bacterial genome, including that coding for virulence. Hence QS is being viewed as a useful target for novel anti-infective agents. For an overview of the basic elements of bacterial QS machinery, reader may refer to Joshi *et al.* (2010) and Koh *et al.* (2013). *Rosa rugosa* tea polyphenol extract consisting about 61.03% flavonoids, is able to inhibit QS-regulated violacein production in *Chromobacterium violaceum* by 87.56%, and biofilm formation in *P. aeruginosa* by 72.90%, in concentration dependent manner (Zhang *et al.*, 2014). Naringenin displayed nonspecific QS inhibitory action against *E. coli* O157:H7. It could hinder biofilm formation by *E. coli* O157:H7 and *Vibrio harveyi* by interfering with AI-2-mediated signalling (Vikram *et al.*, 2010). Quercetin was shown to be an effective QS inhibitor against *P. aeruginosa*. At 16 µg/mL, it could down-regulate expression of *las*I, *las*R, *rhl*I and *rhl*R genes by 34, 68, 57 and 50 percent, respectively (Ouyang *et al.*, 2016). Another flavonoid, catechin from *Combretum albiflorum* bark extract was also shown to down-regulate expression of QS-regulated virulence traits in *P. aeruginosa* (Vandeputte *et al.*, 2010). Catechin and salicylic acid can modulate bacterial QS to varying extent against different organisms. Catechin can inhibit violacein production in *C. violaceum* CVO26 by acting as a QS disruptor. It can also inhibit biofilm formation and elastase production in *P. aeruginosa* PAO1 by interfering with AI reception (Martín-Rodríguez *et al.*, 2015). Flavanones, naringenin and morin down-regulate the QS regulated traits like protease and elastase activity, and hemolysin, besides disrupting biofilm formation in *P. aeruginosa* PAO1 (Martín-Rodríguez *et al.,* 2016). Naringenin can interfere both with AI production and formation of C4-HSL-RIhR complex, when tested against *C. violaceum* CVO26 and *P. aeruginosa* PAO1 (Martín-Rodríguez *et al.,* 2015).

Flavanones (naringenin, eriodictyol and taxifolin) can reduce the production of pyocyanin and elastase in *P. aeruginosa* without inhibiting growth. Naringenin and taxifolin reduced the expression of different QS-controlled genes (lasI, lasR, rhlI, rhlR, lasA, lasB, phzA1, rhlA) in *P. aeruginosa* PAO1. Naringenin dramatically reduced the production of AHLs driven by the *lasI* and *rhlI* gene products. Using biosensors based on mutant strains deficient for autoinduction, it was shown that Q S inhibition by naringenin besides being a consequence of reduced production of autoinduction compounds also stems from a defect in the functioning of the RlhR–C4-HSL complex (Vandeputte *et al.*, 2011).

Among nine different flavonoids isolated from *Piper delineatum*, (-)-2S-7,5'-dihydroxy-5,3'-dimethoxyflavonone, and 2',4',4-trihydroxy-3,6'-dimethoxychalcone could inhibit QS in *V. harveyi* without affecting growth up to 500 µg/mL. Furthermore, employing the mutant strain of *V. harveyi*, molecular target was indicated downstream *Lux*O for these flavonoids. (Martín-Rodríguez *et al.,* 2015). QS-regulated traits such as hemolysis, biofilm formation, and virulence, were found to be down regulated in *S. aureus,* when challenged with trans-stilbene and resveratrol at10 µg/mL. Trans-stilbene and resveratrol inhibited *S. aureus* virulence *in vivo* assay too, performed with the nematode *Caenorhabditis elegans* as host. This worm is usually killed by *S. aureus.* Transcriptome analysis determined that trans-stilbene suppressed α-hemolysin (*hla*) gene and intercellular adhesion locus (*ica*A and *ica*D) in *S. aureus.* Vitisin B, a stilbenoid at concentration of 1 µg/mL is reported to reduce the hemolytic potential of *S. aureus* (Lee *et al.,* 2014).

6.2. Flavonoids as Antiviral Compounds

Viral agents of infection like HIV, hepatitis, avian and swine influenza strains remain among the difficult problems in the field of healthcare (Rider *et al.,* 2011). Enterovirus 71 (EV71), an RNA virus is responsible for neurological diseases like brainstem encephalitis, or acute flaccid paralysis. Till now no effective treatment or vaccine is being developed against EV71. 7-Hydroxyisoflavone was shown to display antiviral activity against this virus. It hinders RNA and protein synthesis in a dose-dependent manner. 7-hydroxyisoflavone obstructs at an early step of EV71 replication (Wang *et al.,* 2013).

Extract of *Melastoma malabathricum*, containing flavonoids namely rutin, quercetin and quercitrin, was shown to exert antiviral activity against

Measles, and HSV-1 (Nazlina *et al.,* 2007). Quercetin probably inhibits reverse transcriptase of Measles virus, and target an early stage of replication of HSV-1. Quercetin can also inhibits Zika virus by targeting the protein 'NS2B-NS3', essential for its replication, through allosteric inhibition. This was validated by molecular docking of quercetin with NS2B-NS3 protien (Lim *et al.,* 2016). It may be noted that at present no vaccine is available against Zika virus.

7. FUTURE PERSPECTIVES

Flavonoids are bioactive molecules widely distributed among the members of plant kingdom, and also form a notable part of human diet in the form of fruits and vegetables. Different flavonoids have been reported for a variety of biological effects of therapeutic relevance, including the antimicrobial/ anti-infective effects. Flavonoids are attractive molecules from a phytopharmaceutical and nutraceutical perspective. In-depth investigations on their interaction with pathogenic microorganisms at the molecular level are required to realize their anti-infective potential for the human benefit. Studies on their bioavailability and metabolism inside human systems are also needed. Many of them are pharmacologically active against infections caused in oral cavity (Gau *et al.*, 2016). Flavonoids are chiefly found as glycosides in medicinal drugs. The importance of oral hydrolysis of flavonoid glycosides by β-glycosidases has been revealed through various studies. The secretion of bioactive aglycones, which act as anti-bacterial and anti-oxidant is vital during decomposition of flavonoids (Gau *et al.*, 2016). Flavonoids are being viewed as useful chemotherapeutics, since they possess attractive features likewide distribution in nature, amenable to easy detection owing to their stability *in vivo* as well as after isolation, ease of chromatographic detection, etc (Pretorius, 2003). Bioavailability of some of them *e.g.* isoflavones, is also sufficiently high (Hollman, 2004). Some of the bioactive flavonoids may be present at low concentrations in their producing plants, and hence researchers are trying to construct genetically modified bacterial strains for fermentative production of flavonoids by incorporating artificial gene cluster containing enzymes for flavonoid biosynthesis into the recombinant bacteria. *E. coli, Streptomyces venezuelae, Phellinus igniarius* and *S. cerevisiae* have been shown to be satisfactory bacterial systems for incorporation of phenylpropanoid pathways of the plants (Du *et al.*, 2011).

Flavonoids have generated enough interest in the research community, and there are numerous reports on biological activities of these phytocompounds, either in pure form or as part of some extract. However, validation of their biological effects *in vitro* and *in vivo*, and deciphering their mode of action at molecular level is required for their wider acceptance for therapeutic use. Flavonoids may not confer all their benefit through their activity against pathogens; part of the beneficial effect may arise from their immune-modulatory influence on human system, and/or their interaction with gut microbial community. Future investigations to unfold interesting findings on these issues will certainly boost our confidence in flavonoids as useful bioactive molecules of high therapeutic relevance.

8. CONTRIBUTION NOTE

All authors contributed to this manuscript equally.

REFERENCES

Ahmad, A., Kaleem, M., Ahmed, Z. and Shafiq, H. (2015). Therapeutic potential of flavonoids and their mechanism of action against microbial and viral infections–A review. *Food Research International,* 77: 221–35. doi: 10.1016/j.foodres.2015.06.021.

Albert, S., Horbach, R., Deising, H.B., Siewert, B. and Csuk, R. (2011). Synthesis and antimicrobial activity of stilbene derivatives. *Bioorganic and Medicinal Chemistry,* 19(17): 5155–66. doi.org/10.1016/j.bmc.2011.07.015.

Alcalde-Rico, M., Hernando-Amado, S., Blanco, P. and Martínez, J.L. (2016). Multidrug efflux pumps at the crossroad between antibiotic resistance and bacterial virulence. *Frontiers in Microbiology*, 7(1483). doi: 10.3389/fmicb.2016.01483

Al-Majedy, Y.K., Kadhum, A.A., Al-Amiery, A.A. and Mohamad, A.B. (2017). Coumarins: The antimicrobial agents. *Systematic Reviews in Pharmacy,* 8(1): 62–70. doi: 10.1186/s12906-015-0580-0.

Amin, M.U., Khurram, M., Khattak, B. and Khan, J. (2015). Antibiotic additive and synergistic action of rutin, morin and quercetin against methicillin resistant *Staphylococcus aureus. BMC Complementary and Alternative Medicine,* 15(1): 59. doi: 10.1186/s12906-015-0580-0.

Astani, A. and Schnitzler, P. (2014). Antiviral activity of monoterpenes beta-pinene and limonene against herpes simplex virus *in vitro. Iranian Journal of Microbiology,* 6(3): 149–155.

Borris, R.P. (1996). Natural products research: Perspectives from a major pharmaceutical company. *Journal of Ethnopharmacology. Ethnopharmacol. Elsevier BV.*, 51: 29–38. doi: 10.1016/0378-8741(95)01347-4.

Boussoualim, N., Meziane-Cherif, D. and Baghiani, A. (2011). Kinetic study of different flavonoids as inhibitors of beta-lactamase enzyme. *African Journal of Biochemistry Research,* 5(10): 321–27.

Brown, A.R., Ettefagh, K.A., Todd, D., Cole, P.S., Egan, J.M., Foil, D.H., Graf, T.N., Schindler, B.D., Kaatz, G.W. and Cech, N.B. (2015). A mass spectrometry-based assay for improved quantitative measurements of efflux pump inhibition. *Plos One*, 10(5): e0124814. doi: 10.1371/journal.pone.0124814.

-Carvalho, R., Baltazar, F. and Almeida-Aguiar, C. (2015). Propolis: A complex natural product with a plethora of biological activities that can be explored for drug development. *Evidence-Based Complementary and Alternative Medicine,* 2015. doi: 10.1155/2015/206439.

Chalal, M., Klinguer, A., Echairi, A., Meunier, P., Vervandier-Fasseur, D. and Adrian, M. (2014). Antimicrobial activity of resveratrol analogues. *Molecules,* 19(6): 7679–88. doi: 10.3390/molecules19067679

Christena, L.R., Subramaniam, S., Vidhyalakshmi, M., Mahadevan, V., Sivasubramanian, A. and Nagarajan, S. (2015). Dual role of pinostrobin-a flavonoid nutraceutical as an efflux pump inhibitor and antibiofilm agent to mitigate food borne pathogens. *Royal Society of Chemistry,* 5(76): 61881–7. doi: 10.1039/C5RA07165H.

Christena, L.R., Subramaniam, S., Vidhyalakshmi, M., Mahadevan, V., Sivasubramanian, A. and Nagarajan, S. (2015). Flavonoid nutraceutical as an efflux pump inhibitor and antibiofilm agent to mitigate food borne pathogens. *Royal Society of Chemistry*, 5(76): 61881–7.

Cowan, M.M. (1999). Plant products as antimicrobial agents. *Clinical Microbiology Reviews*, 12(4): 564–82.

Cushnie, T.T. and Lamb, A.J. (2005). Antimicrobial activity of flavonoids. *International Journal of Antimicrobial Agents*, 26(5): 343–56. doi: 10.1016/j.ijantimicag.2005.09.002.

Das, A.K. (2015). Anticancer effect of antimalarial artemisinin compounds. *Annals of Medical and Health Sciences Research*, 5(2): 93–102. doi: 10.4103/2141-9248.153609.

Denny, B.J., Lambert, P.A. and West, P.W. (2002). The flavonoid galangin inhibits the L1 metallo-β-lactamase from *Stenotrophomonas maltophilia*. *Federation of Europen Microbiological Societies*, 208(1): 21–4. doi: 10.1016/S0378-1097(01)00580-8.

Diaz Carrasco, J.M., Redondo, L.M., Redondo, E.A., Dominguez, J.E., Chacana, A.P. and Fernandez Miyakawa, M.E. (2016). Use of plant extracts as an effective manner to control *Clostridium perfringens* induced necrotic enteritis in poultry. *BioMed. Research International*, 2016. doi: 10.1155/2016/3278359.

Dixon, R.A. (2001). Natural products and plant disease resistance. *Nature*, 411(6839): 843–7. doi:10.1038/35081178.

Du, F., Zhang, F., Chen, F., Wang, A.,Wang, Q., Yin, X. and Wang, S. (2011). Advances in microbial heterologous production of flavonoids. *African Journal of Microbiology Research*, 5(18): 2566–74. doi: 10.5897/AJMR11.394.

Dzoyem, J.P., Melong, R., Tsamo, A.T., Tchinda, A.T., Kapche, D.G., Ngadjui, B.T., McGaw, L.J. and Eloff, J.N. (2017). Cytotoxicity, antimicrobial and antioxidant activity of eight compounds isolated from *Entada abyssinica* (Fabaceae). *BioMed. Central Research Notes*, 10(1): 118. doi: 10.1186/s13104-017-2441.

Eumkeb, G., Siriwong, S., Phitaktim, S., Rojtinnakorn, N. and Sakdarat, S. (2012). Synergistic activity and mode of action of flavonoids isolated from smaller galangal and amoxicillin combinations against amoxicillin resistant *Escherichia coli*. *Journal of Applied Microbiology*, 112(1): 55–64. doi: 10.1111/j.1365-2672.2011.05190.

Fearnley, J. (2001). Bee propolis: Natural healing from the hive. Souvenir.

Filocamo, A., Bisignano, C., Ferlazzo, N., Cirmi, S., Mandalari, G. and Navarra, M. (2015). *In vitro* effect of bergamot (*Citrus bergamia*) juice against *cag* A-positive and-negative clinical isolates of *Helicobacter pylori*. *BMC Complementary and Alternative Medicine*, 15(1): 256. doi: 10.1186/s12906-015-0769-2.

Gau, J., Furtmüller, P.G., Obinger, C., Prévost, M., Van Antwerpen, P., Arnhold, J. and Flemmig, J. (2016). Flavonoids as promoters of the (pseudo-) halogenating activity of lactoperoxidase and myeloperoxidase. *Free Radical Biology and Medicine*, 97: 307–19. doi: 10.1016/j.freeradbiomed.2016.06.026.

Ghosh, A., Das, B.K., Roy, A., Mandal, B. and Chandra, G. (2008). Antibacterial activity of some medicinal plant extracts. *Journal of Natural Medicines*, 62(2): 259–62. doi:10.1007/s11418-007-0216.

Gonzαlez-Segovia, R., Quintanar, J.L., Salinas, E., Ceballos-Salazar, R., Aviles-Jiménez, F. and Torres-López, J. (2008). Effect of the flavonoid quercetin on inflammation and lipid peroxidation induced by *Helicobacter pylori* in gastric mucosa of *guinea pig*. *Journal of Gastroenterology*, 43(6): 441. doi: 10.1007/s00535-008-2184-7.

Grange, J.M. and Davey, R.W. (1990). Antibacterial properties of propolis (bee glue). *Journal of the Royal Society of Medicine*, 83(3): 159–60.

Grayer, R.J. and Harborne, J.B. (1994). A survey of antifungal compounds from higher plants. *Phytochemistry*, 37(1): 19–42. doi: 10.1016/0031-9422(94)85005-4.

Guzman, J.D. (2014). Natural cinnamic acids, synthetic derivatives and hybrids with antimicrobial activity. *Molecules*, 19(12): 19292–349. doi: 10.3390/molecules191219292.

Hamini-Kadar, N., Hamdane, F., Boutoutaou, R., Kihal, M. and Henni, J.E. (2014). Antifungal activity of clove (*Syzygium aromaticum* L.) essential oil against phytopathogenic fungi of tomato (*Solanum lycopersicum* L.) in Algeria. *Journal of Experimental Biology and Agricultural Sciences*, 2(5): 447–54.

Harborne, J.B. and Baxter, H. (1999). The handbook of natural flavonoids. Volume 1 and Volume 2. John Wiley and Sons.

Harborne, J.B. and Williams, C.A. (2000). Advances in flavonoid research since 1992. *Phytochemistry,* 55(6): 481–504. doi: 10.1016/S0031-9422(00)00235-1.

Haslam, E. (1996). Natural polyphenols (vegetable tannins) as drugs: Possible modes of action. *Journal of Natural Products,* 59(2): 205–15. doi: 10.1021/np960040.

Havsteen, B. (1983). Flavonoids, a class of natural products of high pharmacological potency. *Biochem. Pharmacol.*, 32(7): 1141–8. doi: 10.1016/0006-2952(83)90262-9.

Havsteen, B.H. (2002). The biochemistry and medical significance of the flavonoids. *Pharmacology & Therapeutics,* 96(2): 67–202. doi: 10.1016/S0163-7258(02)00298.

Hollman, P.C. (2004). Absorption, bioavailability, and metabolism of flavonoids. *Pharmaceutical Biology,* 42(sup1): 74–83. doi: 10.1080/13880200490893492.

Hosein, F.M., Abbasabadi, Z., Reza, S.A., Abdollahi, M. and Rahimi, R. (2014). A comprehensive review of plants and their active constituents with wound healing activity in traditional Iranian medicine. *Wounds: A Compendium of Clinical Research and Practice*, 26(7): 197–206.

Huang, J., Chen, L., Xue, B., Liu, Q., Ou, S., Wang, Y. and Peng, X. (2016). Different flavonoids can shape unique gut microbiota profile *in vitro*. *Journal of Food Science,* 81(9): H2273–9. doi: 10.1111/1750-3841.13411.

Huang, S., Zhang, C.P., Wang, K., Li, G.Q. and Hu, F.L. (2014). Recent advances in the chemical composition of propolis. *Molecules*, 19(12): 19610–32. doi: 10.3390/molecules191219610.

Ibraheem, F., Gaffoor, I. and Chopra, S. (2010). Flavonoid phytoalexin-dependent resistance to anthracnose leaf blight requires a functional yellow seed1 in *Sorghum bicolor*. *Genetics*, 184(4): 915–26. doi: 10.1534/genetics.109.111831.

Iranshahi, M., Rezaee, R., Parhiz, H., Roohbakhsh, A., Soltani, F. (2015). Protective effects of flavonoids against microbes and toxins: The cases of hesperidin and hesperetin. *Life Sciences,* 137: 125–32. doi: 10.1016/j.lfs.2015.07.014.

Izzi, V., Masuelli, L., Tresoldi, I., Sacchetti, P., Modesti, A., Galvano, F. and Bei, R. (2012). The effects of dietary flavonoids on the regulation of redox inflammatory networks. *Frontiers in Bioscience*, 17: 2396–418.

Jayasinghe, S.U., Siriwardhana, A.S. and Karunaratne, V.E. (2015). Natural iron sequestering agents: Their roles in nature and therapeutic potential. *International Journal of Pharmacy and Pharmaceutical Sciences*, 7(9): 8–12.

Joshi, P., Wadhwani, T., Bahaley, P. and Kothari, V. (2010). Microbial Chit-Chat: Quorum Sensing. *The IUP Journal of Life Sciences,* 4(1): 59–72.

Kadariya, J., Smith, T.C. and Thapaliya, D. (2014). *Staphylococcus aureus* and staphylococcal food-borne disease: An ongoing challenge in public health. *BioMed Research International,* 2014. doi: 10.1155/2014/827965.

Kaur, H.P., Kaur, S. and Rana, S. (2015). Antibacterial activity and phytochemical profile of Green Tea, Black Tea and Divya Peya Herbal Tea. *Int. J. International Journal of Pure & Applied Bioscience.*, 3(3): 117–23. doi: 10.4103/0974-8490.89748.

Khare, C.P. (2008). Indian medicinal plants: An illustrated dictionary. Springer Science & Business Media.

Klink, B. (1997). Alternative medicines: Is natural really better. *Drug Top.*, 141(2): 99–100.

Koh, C.L., Sam, C.K., Yin, W.F., Tan, L.Y., Krishnan, T., Chong, Y.M. and Chan, K.G. (2013). Plant-derived natural products as sources of anti-quorum sensing compounds. *Sensors,* 13(5): 6217–28. doi: 10.3390/s130506217

Korošec, B., Sova, M., Turk, S., Kraševec, N., Novak, M., Lah, L., Stojan, J., Podobnik, B., Berne, S., Zupanec, N., Bunc, M. (2014). Antifungal activity of cinnamic acid derivatives involves inhibition of benzoate 4 hydroxylase (CYP53). *Journal of Applied Microbiology*, 116(4): 955–66. doi: 10.1111/jam.12417.

Kumar, A., Kumar, S., Bains, S., Vaidya, V., Singh, B., Kaur, R., Kaur, J. and Singh, K. (2016). *De novo* transcriptome analysis revealed genes involved in flavonoid and vitamin C biosynthesis in *Phyllanthus emblica* (L.). *Frontiers in Plant Science*, 7: 1610. doi. 10.3389/fpls.2016.01610.

Kumar, S. and Pandey, A.K. (2013). Chemistry and biological activities of flavonoids: An overview. *The Scientific World Journal,* 2013: 162750. doi: 10.1155/2013/162750.

Lee, K., Lee, J.H., Ryu, S.Y., Cho, M.H. and Lee, J. (2014). Stilbenes reduce *Staphylococcus aureus* hemolysis, biofilm formation, and virulence. *Foodborne Pathogens and Disease*, 11(9): 710–7. doi: 10.1089/fpd.2014.1758.

Lim, L., Roy, A. and Song, J. (2016). Identification of a Zika NS2B-NS3pro pocket susceptible to allosteric inhibition by small molecules including qucertin rich in edible plants. *BioRxiv,* pp. 078543. doi: 10.1101/078543.

Liu, T.Y., Gong, W., Tan, Z.J., Lu, W., Wu, X.S., Weng, H., Ding, Q., Shu, Y.J., Bao, R.F., Cao, Y. and Wang, X.A. (2015). Baicalein inhibits progression of gallbladder cancer cells by down regulating ZFX. *Plos One*, 10(1): e0114851. doi: 10.1371/journal.pone.0114851.

Mandalari, G., Bennett, R.N., Bisignano, G., Trombetta, D., Saija, A., Faulds, C.B., Gasson, M.J. and Narbad, A. (2007). Antimicrobial activity of flavonoids extracted from bergamot (*Citrus bergamia* Risso) peel, a byproduct of the essential oil industry. *Journal of Applied Microbiology,* 103(6): 2056–64. doi:10.1111/j.1365-2672.2007.03456.x.

Martín-Rodríguez, A.J., Quezada, H., Becerril, G., Maeda, V.P., Wood, T.K. and García-Contreras, R. (2016). Recent advances in novel antibacterial development. 3(1): 3–10. doi: 10.2174/9781681081533116020003.

Martín-Rodríguez, A.J., Ticona, J.C., Jiménez, I.A., Flores, N., Fernández, J.J. and Bazzocchi, I.L. (2015). Flavonoids from *Piper delineatum* modulate quorum-sensing-regulated phenotypes in *Vibrio harveyi*. *Phytochemistry*, 117: 98–106. DOI: 10.1016/j.phytochem.2015.06.006.

Medeiros Barreto, H., Cerqueira Fontinele, F., Pereira de Oliveira, A., Arcanjo, D.D., Cavalcanti dos Santos, B.H., de Abreu, A.P., Douglas Melo Coutinho, H., Alves Carvalho da Silva, R., Oliveira de Sousa, T., Freire de Medeiros, M.D. and Lopes Citó, A.M. (2014). Phytochemical prospection and modulation of antibiotic activity *in vitro* by *Lippia origanoides* HBK in methicillin resistant *Staphylococcus aureus*. *BioMed Research International,* 2014: 305610. doi: 10.1155/2014/305610.

Medina, E. and Pieper, D.H. (2016). Tackling Threats and Future Problems of Multidrug-Resistant Bacteria. How to Overcome the Antibiotic Crisis: Facts, Challenges, Technologies and Future Perspectives. pp. 3–33. doi: 10.1007/82_2016_492.

Michael (1999). Alkaloids: Biochemistry, ecology, and medicinal applications. *Journal of Natural Products*, 62(4): 664–664. doi: 10.1021/np980259j.

Mickevièienë, K., Baranauskaitë, R., Kantminienë, K., Stasevych, M., Komarovska-Porokhnyavets, O. and Novikov, V. (2015). Synthesis and antimicrobial activity of N-substituted-β-amino acid derivatives containing 2-hydroxyphenyl, benzo phenoxazine and quinoxaline moieties. *Molecules,* 20(2): 3170–89. doi: 10.3390/molecules20023170.

Millard, J., Ugarte-Gil, C. and Moore, D.A. (2015). Multidrug resistant tuberculosis. *British Medical Journal*, 350: h882. doi: 10.1136/bmj.h882.

Miron, D., Battisti, F., Silva, F.K., Lana, A.D., Pippi, B., Casanova, B., Gnoatto, S., Fuentefria, A., Mayorga, P. and Schapoval, E.E. (2014). Antifungal activity and mechanism of action of monoterpenes against dermatophytes and yeasts. *Revista Brasileira de Farmacognosia,* 24(6): 660–7. Doi: 10.1016/j.bjp.2014.10.014.

Mohan, S. and Gupta, D. (2017). Phytochemical analysis and differential *in vitro* cytotoxicity assessment of root extracts of *Inula racemosa*. *Biomedicine & Pharmacotherapy,* 89: 781–95. doi: 10.1016/j.biopha.2017.02.053.

Molyneux, R.J., Lee, S.T., Gardner, D.R., Panter, K.E. and James, L.F. (2007). Phytochemicals: The good, the bad and the ugly? *Phytochemistry,* 68(22): 2973–85. doi: 10.1016/j.phytochem.2007.09.004.

Mustapha, A.A., Enemali, M.O., Olose, M., Owuna, G., Ogaji, J.O., Idris, M.M. and Aboh, V.O. (2014). Phytoconstituents and antibacterial efficacy of Mango (*Mangifera indica*) leave extracts. *Journal of Medicinal Plants Studies,* 2(5): 19–23.

Nazlina, I., Norha, S., Noor Zarina, A.W. and Ahmad, I.B. (2008). Cytotoxicity and antiviral activity of *Melastoma malabathricum* extracts. *Malays J. Appl. Biol.*, 37: 53–5.

Okoye, F.B., Sawadogo, W.R., Sendker, J., Aly, A.H., Quandt, B., Wray, V., Hensel, A., Esimone, C.O., Debbab, A., Diederich, M. and Proksch, P. (2015). Flavonoid glycosides from *Olax mannii*: Structure elucidation and effect on the nuclear factor kappa B pathway. *Journal of Ethnopharmacology,* 176: 27–34. doi: 10.1016/j.jep.2015.10.019.

Olasupo, N.A., Fitzgerald, D.J., Narbad, A. and Gasson, M.J. (2004). Inhibition of *Bacillus subtilis* and *Listeria innocua* by nisin in combination with some naturally occurring organic compounds. *Journal of Food Protection*, 67(3): 596–600. doi:10.4315/0362-028X-67.3.596

Omojate Godstime, C., Enwa Felix, O., Jewo Augustina, O. and Eze Christopher, O. (2014). Mechanisms of antimicrobial actions of phytochemicals against enteric pathogens–a review. *Journal of Pharmaceutical, Chemical and Biological Sciences*, 2(2): 77–85.

Orhan, I.E. (2012). *Centella asiatica* (L.) Urban: From traditional medicine to modern medicine with neuroprotective potential. *Evidence-based Complementary and Alternative Medicine,* 2012. doi: 10.1155/2012/946259.

Osbourn, A.E. (1996). Preformed antimicrobial compounds and plant defense against fungal attack. *The Plant Cell*, 8(10): 1821–183. doi: 10.1105/tpc.8.10.1821.

Ouyang, J., Sun, F., Feng, W., Sun, Y., Qiu, X., Xiong, L., Liu, Y. and Chen, Y. (2016). Quercetin is an effective inhibitor of quorum sensing, biofilm formation and virulence factors in *Pseudomonas aeruginosa*. *Journal of Applied Microbiology,* 120: 966–974. doi: 10.1111/jam.13073.

Özçelik, B., Orhan, D.D., Özgen, S. and Ergun, F. (2008). Antimicrobial activity of flavonoids against extended-spectrum β-lactamase (ESβL)-producing *Klebsiella pneumoniae*. *Tropical Journal of Pharmaceutical Research*, 7(4): 1151–7. doi.org/10.4314/tjpr.v7i4.14701.

Palep, H., Kothari, V. and Patil, S. (2016). Quorum Sensing inhibition: A new antimicrobial mechanism of *Panchavalkal*, an Ayurvedic formulation. *Bombay Hospital Journal*, 58(2): 198–204.

Pandey, A.K. and Kumar, S. (2013). Perspective on plant products as antimicrobial agents: A review. *Pharmacologia,* 4: 469–80. doi: 10.5567/pharmacologia 2013.469.480.

Parekh, J. and Chanda, S. (2007). *In vitro* antimicrobial activity and phytochemical analysis of some Indian medicinal plants. *Turkish Journal of Biology,* 31(1): 53–8. doi: 10.1016/j.ejar.2013.01.005.

Park, I.W., Han, C., Song, X., Green, L.A., Wang, T., Liu, Y., Cen, C., Song, X., Yang, B., Chen, G. and He, J.J. (2009). Inhibition of HIV-1 entry by extracts derived from traditional Chinese medicinal herbal plants. *BMC Complementary and Alternative Medicine,* 9(1): 29. doi: 10.1186/1472-6882-9-29.

Patra, A.K. (2012). An overview of antimicrobial properties of different classes of phytochemicals. *Dietary Phytochemicals and Microbes*, doi: 10.1007/978-94-007-3926-01.

Plumed-Ferrer, C., Väkeväinen, K., Komulainen, H., Rautiainen, M., Smeds, A., Raitanen, J.E., Eklund, P., Willför, S., Alakomi, H.L., Saarela, M. and von Wright, A. (). The antimicrobial effects of wood-associated polyphenols on food pathogens and spoilage organisms. *International Journal of Food Microbiology,* 164(1): 99–107. doi: 10.1016/j.ijfoodmicro.2013.04.001.

Porras-Gómez, M. and Vega-Baudrit, J. (2012). Overview of multidrug-resistant *Pseudomonas aeruginosa* and novel therapeutic approaches. *Journal of Biomaterials and Nanobiotechnology,* 3(04): 519. doi: 10.4236/jbnb.2012.324053.

Pretorius, J.C. (2003). Flavonoids: A review of its commercial application potential as anti-infective agents. *Current Medicinal Chemistry-Anti-Infective Agents,* 2(4): 335–53. doi: 10.2174/1568012033482971.

Rahmoun, N.M., Boucherit-Atmani, Z., Benabdallah, M., Boucherit, K., Villemin, D. and Choukchou-Braham, N. (2013). Antimicrobial activities of the henna extract and some synthetic naphthoquinones derivatives. *American Journal of Medical and Biological Research,* 1(1): 16–22. doi: 10.12691/ajmbr-1-1-3.

Randhawa, H.K., Hundal, K.K., Ahirrao, P.N., Jachak, S.M. and Nandanwar, H.S. (2016). Efflux pump inhibitory activity of flavonoids isolated from *Alpinia calcarata* against methicillin-resistant *Staphylococcus aureus*. *Biologia,* 71(5): 484–93. doi: 10.1515/biolog-2016-0073.

Rider, T.H., Zook, C.E., Boettcher, T.L., Wick, S.T., Pancoast, J.S. and Zusman, B.D. (2011). Broad-spectrum antiviral therapeutics. *Plos ONE*, 6(7): e22572. doi: 10.1371/journal.pone.0022572.

Sandhar, H.K., Kumar, B., Prasher, S., Tiwari, P., Salhan, M. and Sharma, P. (2011). A review of phytochemistry and pharmacology of flavonoids. *Internationale Pharmaceutica Sciencia,* 1(1): 25–41.

Sardi, J.D., Gullo, F.P., Freires, I.A., de Souza Pitangui, N., Segalla, M.P., Fusco-Almeida, A.M., Rosalen, P.L., Regasini, L.O. and Mendes-Giannini, M.J. (2016). Synthesis, antifungal activity of caffeic acid derivative esters, and their synergism with fluconazole and nystatin against *Candida spp. Diagnostic Microbiology and Infectious Disease*, 86(4): 387–91. doi: 10.1016/j.diagmicrobio.2016.08.002.

Shehadi, M., Awada, F., Oleik, R., Chokr, A., Hamze, K., Hamdan, H.A., Harb, A. and Kobaissi, A. (2014). Comparative analysis of the anti-bacterial activity of four plant extracts. *International Journal of Current Research and Academic Review,* 2(6): 83–94.

Siriwong, S., Teethaisong, Y., Thumanu, K., Dunkhunthod, B. and Eumkeb, G. (2016). The synergy and mode of action of quercetin plus amoxicillin against amoxicillin-resistant *Staphylococcus epidermidis*. *BMC Pharmacology and Toxicology*, 17(1): 39. doi: 10.1186/s40360-016-0083-8.

Stavri, M., Piddock, L.J. and Gibbons, S. (2007). Bacterial efflux pump inhibitors from natural sources. *Journal of Antimicrobial Chemotherapy*, 59(6): 1247–60. doi: 10.1093/jac/dkl460.

Taiwo, B.J. and Igbeneghu, O.A. (2014). Antioxidant and antibacterial activities of flavonoid glycosides from *Ficus exasperata* Vahl-Holl (moraceae) leaves. *African Journal of Traditional, Complementary and Alternative Medicines,* 11(3): 97–101. doi: 10.4314/ajtcam.v11i3.14

Tanwar, J., Das, S., Fatima, Z. and Hameed, S. (2014). Multidrug resistance: An emerging crisis. *Interdisciplinary Perspectives on Infectious Diseases,* 2014(541340). doi: 10.1155/2014/541340.

Thomson (1978). Medicines from the Earth. McGraw-Hill Book Co., Maidenhead, United Kingdom.

Thomson, W.A. and Schultes, R.E. (1978). Medicines from the Earth. McGraw-Hill.

Trentin, D.S., Silva, D.B., Amaral, M.W., Zimmer, K.R., Silva, M.V., Lopes, N.P., Giordani, R.B. and Macedo, A.J. (2013). Tannins possessing bacteriostatic effect impair *Pseudomonas aeruginosa* adhesion and biofilm formation. *Plos ONE*, 8(6): e66257. doi: 10.1371/journal.pone.0066257.

Truchado, P., Larrosa, M., Castro-Ibáñez, I. and Allende, A. (2015). Plant food extracts and phytochemicals: Their role as quorum sensing inhibitors. *Trends in Food Science & Technology*, 43(2): 189–204. doi: 10.1016/j.tifs.2015.02.009

Tsao, T.F., Newman, M.G., Kwok, Y.Y. and Horikoshi, A.K. (1982). Effect of Chinese and western antimicrobial agents on selected oral bacteria. *Journal of Dental Research*, 61(9): 1103–6. doi: 10.1177/00220345820610091501.

Tsou, L.K., Lara-Tejero, M., RoseFigura, J., Zhang, Z.J., Wang, Y.C., Yount, J.S., Lefebre, M., Dossa, P.D., Kato, J., Guan, F. and Lam, W. (2016). Antibacterial flavonoids from medicinal plants covalently inactivate type III protein secretion substrates. *Journal of the American Chemical Society,* 138(7): 2209–18. doi: 10.1021/jacs.5b11575.

Vandeputte, O.M., Kiendrebeogo, M., Rajaonson, S., Diallo, B., Mol, A., El Jaziri, M. and Baucher, M. (2010). Identification of catechin as one of the flavonoids from *Combretum albiflorum* bark extract that reduces the production of quorum-sensing-controlled virulence factors in *Pseudomonas aeruginosa* PAO1. *Applied and Environmental Microbiology,* 76(1): 243–53. doi: 10.1128/AEM.01059-09.

Vandeputte, O.M., Kiendrebeogo, M., Rasamiravaka, T., Stevigny, C., Duez, P., Rajaonson, S., Diallo, B., Mol, A., Baucher, M., El Jaziri, M. (2011). The flavanone naringenin reduces the production of quorum sensing-controlled virulence factors in *Pseudomonas aeruginosa* PAO1. *Microbiology*, 157(7): 2120–32. doi: 10.1099/mic.0.049338-0.

VanEtten, H.D., Mansfield, J.W., Bailey, J.A. and Farmer, E.E. (1994). Two Classes of Plant Antibiotics: Phytoalexins versus" Phytoanticipins". *The Plant Cell,* 6(9): 1191. doi: 10.1105/tpc.6.9.1191.

Vasavi, H.S., Arun, A.B. and Rekha, P.D. (2014). Anti quorum sensing activity of *Psidium guajava* L. flavonoids against *Chromobacterium violaceum* and *Pseudomonas aeruginosa* PAO1. *Microbiology and Immunology*, 58(5): 286–93. doi: 10.1111/1348-0421.12150.

Vasavi, H.S., Arun, A.B. and Rekha, P.D. (2016). Anti-quorum sensing activity of flavonoid-rich fraction from *Centella asiatica* L. against *Pseudomonas aeruginosa* PAO1. *Journal of Microbiology, Immunology and Infection*, 49(1): 8–15. doi: 10.1016/j.jmii.2014.03.012.

Vikram, A., Jayaprakasha, G.K., Jesudhasan, P.R., Pillai, S.D. and Patil, B.S. (2010). Suppression of bacterial cell–cell signalling, biofilm formation and type III secretion system by citrus flavonoids. *Journal of Applied Microbiology,* 109(2): 515–27. doi: 10.1111/j.1365-2672.2010.04677.

Vikram, A., Jesudhasan, P.R., Jayaprakasha, G.K., Pillai, S.D., Jayaraman, A. and Patil, B.S. (2011). Citrus flavonoid represses *Salmonella* pathogenicity Island 1 and motility in *S. Typhimurium* LT2. *International Journal of Food Microbiology*, 145(1): 28–36. doi: 10.1016/j.ijfoodmicro.2010.11.013.

Wang, H.Q., Meng, S., Li, Z.R., Peng, Z.G., Han, Y.X., Guo, S.S., Cui, X.L., Li, Y.H. and Jiang, J.D. (2013). The antiviral effect of 7-hydroxyisoflavone against *Enterovirus* 71 *in vitro*. *Journal of Asian Natural Products Research*, 15(4): 382–9. doi: 10.1080/10286020.2013.770737.

Wang, Y.C. (2014). Medicinal plant activity on *Helicobacter pylori* related diseases. *World Journal of Gastroenterol*, 20(30): 10368–82. doi: 10.3748/wjg.v20.i30.10368.

Widsten, P., Cruz, C.D., Fletcher, G.C., Pajak, M.A. and McGhie, T.K. (2014). Tannins and extracts of fruit byproducts: Antibacterial activity against food-borne bacteria and antioxidant capacity. *Journal of Agricultural and Food Chemistry*, 62(46): 11146–56. doi: 10.1021/jf503819t.

Wu, Y., Bai, J., Zhong, K., Huang, Y. and Gao, H. (2016). A dual antibacterial mechanism involved in membrane disruption and DNA binding of 2R, 3R-dihydromyricetin from pine needles of *Cedrus deodara* against *Staphylococcus aureus*. *Food Chemistry,* 218: 463–70. doi: 10.1016/j.foodchem.2016.07.090.

Xiao, Z.T., Zhu, Q. and Zhang, H.Y. (2014). Identifying antibacterial targets of flavonoids by comparative genomics and molecular modeling. *Open Journal of Genomics,* 3(1). doi: 10.13055/ojgen311.140317.

Xiong, L.G., Chen, Y.J., Tong, J.W., Huang, J.A., Li, J., Gong, Y.S. and Liu, Z.H. (2017). Tea polyphenol epigallocatechin gallate inhibits *Escherichia coli* by increasing endogenous oxidative stress. *Food Chemistry*, 217: 196–204. doi: 10.1016/j.foodchem.2016.08.098.

Zengin, H. and Baysal, A.H. (2014). Antibacterial and antioxidant activity of essential oil terpenes against pathogenic and spoilage-forming bacteria and cell structure-activity relationships evaluated by SEM microscopy. *Molecules*, 19(11): 17773–98. doi: 10.3390/molecules191117773.

Zhang, J., Rui, X., Wang, L., Guan, Y., Sun, X. and Dong, M. (2014). Polyphenolic extract from *Rosa rugosa* tea inhibits bacterial quorum sensing and biofilm formation. *Food Control,* 42: 125–31. doi: 10.1016/j.foodcont.2014.02.001.

Zhang, L., Lin, H., Liu, W., Dai, B., Yan, L., Cao, Y. and Jiang, Y.Y. (2017). Antifungal activity of the ethanol extract from *Flos Rosae Chinensis* with activity against Fluconazole-resistant Clinical *Candida. Evidence-Based Complementary and Alternative Medicine,* 2017(4780746). doi: 10.1155/2017/4780746.

Zhang, S., Mo, F., Luo, Z., Huang, J., Sun, C. and Zhang, R. (2015). Flavonoid glycosides of *Polygonum capitatum* protect against inflammation associated with *Helicobacter pylori* infection. *Plos ONE*, 10(5): e0126584. doi: 10.1371/journal.pone.0126584.

Zhao, Y., Chen, M., Zhao, Z. and Yu, S. (2015). The antibiotic activity and mechanisms of sugarcane (*Saccharum officinarum L.*) bagasse extract against food-borne pathogens. *Food Chemistry,* 185: 112–8. doi: 10.1016/j.foodchem.2015.03.120.

10

Molecular Mechanism of the Flavonoids Against Kidney Disorders

Athira K.V.[1*], Pavan Kumar Samudrala[1] and Mangala Lahkar[1,2]

ABSTRACT

Kidney disease burden is growing at an alarming rate nowadays. Nephropathy usually arises as a complication of Type 1 or 2 diabetes, high blood pressure, certain infections as well as cancer and toxicity induced by agents like antibiotics, cytotoxic drugs, heavy metals and toxic metabolites. The putative mechanisms of induction of nephrotoxicity are still not validated, however; oxidative stress, inflammation and apoptosis seem to play a crucial role. With the past quanta of research focusing on the identification of nephroprotective components of medicinal plants, flavonoids have emerged as promising candidates. The protective effects of flavonoids in biological systems are ascribed to their antioxidant and anti-inflammatory capacity. Accordingly, they were able to interfere with the activation of pathways associated with renal damage such as oxidative-nitrosative-endoplasmic reticulum stress, mitochondrial dysfunction, inflammation, immune activation and apoptosis. Adoption of sound clinical translation strategies are needed to bring flavonoids into clinical application.

Key words: Flavonoids, Kidney, Nephrotoxicity, Oxidative stress, Inflammation, Apoptosis

[1] Department of Pharmacology & Toxicology, National Institute of Pharmaceutical Education and Research (NIPER)-Guwahati, Assam – 781032, India.

[2] Department of Pharmacology, Gauhati Medical College, Guwahati, Assam – 781032, India.

**Corresponding author*: E-mail: athiravenu88@gmail.com

1. INTRODUCTION

Renal disease burden is growing at an alarming rate nowadays. Kidney disorders usually arises as a complication of Type 1 or 2 diabetes, high blood pressure, certain infections, cancer and toxicity induced by certain drugs and toxicants. The renal impairments range from acute renal failure, rhabdomyolysis, obstructive nephropathy, hyperlipoproteinemia, lipoprotein nephropathy and glomerular damage to chronic renal failure and hemodialysis (Singh *et al.,* 2006). In the United States, acute kidney injury (AKI) has a prevalence ranging from 1% (in total population) to 7.1% (in total hospitalized patients) along with a mortality rate of 10-80% (Ratliff *et al.,* 2016). Further, >10% of adults have chronic kidney disease (CKD), with 30% of individuals with age >65 years experiencing some form of kidney failure. However, the treatment for kidney diseases has not progressed much in the past, since the introduction of dialysis (Ratliff *et al.,* 2016). This is, in part, due to poor understanding of the molecular mechanisms behind development and progression of kidney disorders. The experimental evidence supports the view that oxidative stress, inflammation and apoptosis play a key role in the pathophysiologic processes of renal diseases. With the past quanta of research focusing on the identification of nephroprotective components of medicinal plants, flavonoids have emerged as promising candidates.

2. MOLECULAR MECHANISM OF THE FLAVONOIDS AGAINST KIDNEY DISORDERS

2.1. Molecular Mechanisms Involved in the Therapeutic Effect of Flavonoids Against Diseases Affecting Kidney

Research in the past has revealed beneficial role of flavonoids against diseases affecting kidney (Fig.1), principally diabetic nephropathy, ischemia-reperfusion-induced renal injury, rhabdomyolysis-induced myoglobinuric acute renal failure and lupus nephritis.

2.1.1. *Diabetic nephropathy*

Diabetes mellitus (DM) is the major concern among the diseases affecting kidney. DM is a complex endocrine metabolic disorder associated with the body's inability to control blood glucose level and is characterized by insulin resistance, impaired insulin signaling, β-cell dysfunction and altered lipid metabolism. The complications of DM include macrovascular diseases like cardiovascular disease, stroke and peripheral vascular disease, as well as microvascular complications like retinopathy, neuropathy and nephropathy that lead to decreased quality of life and increased rate of mortality (Santaguida *et al.,*2005; Evans *et al.,* 2002; Spranger *et al.,* 2003; Testa *et al.,* 2016).

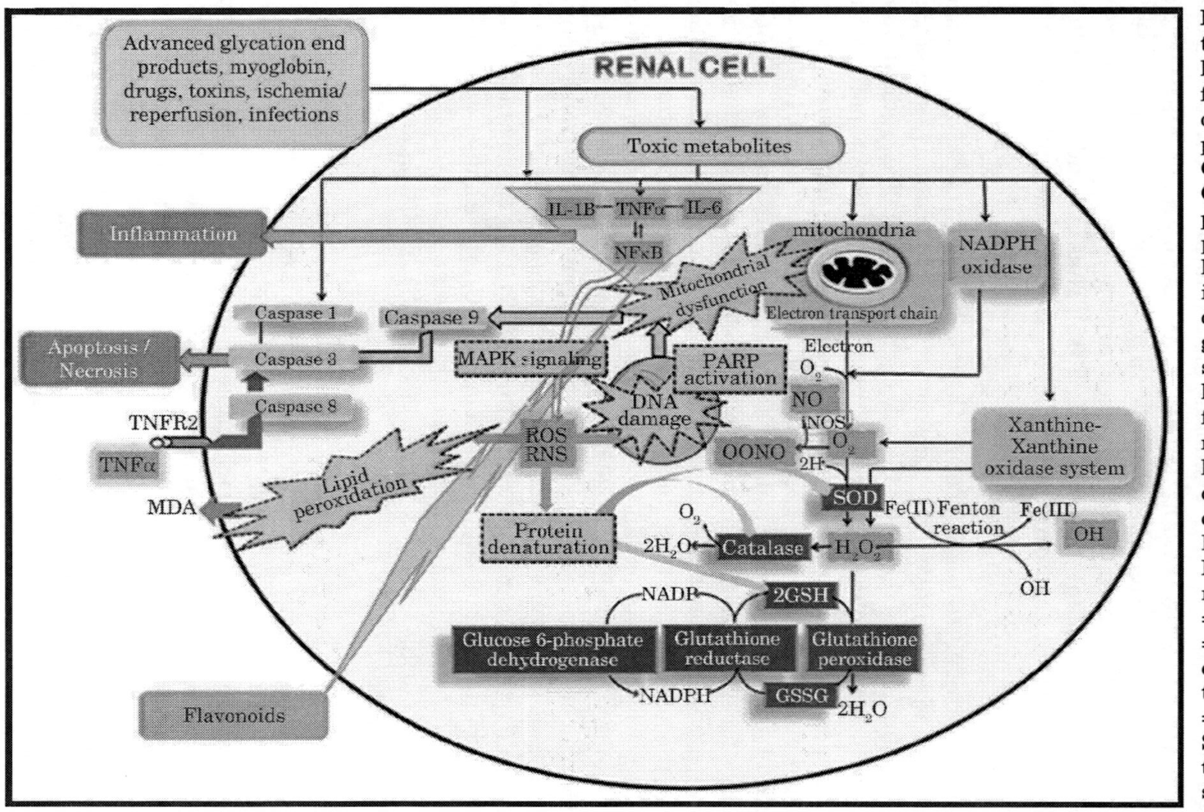

Fig. 1: Pictorial representation of the possible mechanism of intervention of flavonoids against kidney disorders; Where ER=endoplasmic reticulum stress, GSH=reduced glutathione, GSSG=glutathione disulphide, H_2O_2= hydrogen peroxide, IL-1b=interleukin-1b, IL-6=interleukin-6, iNOS= inducible nitric oxide synthase, MAPK=mitogenactivated protein kinases, MDA=malondialdehyde, NADPH=reduced form of nicotinamide adenine dinucleotide phosphate (NADP), NF-kB=nuclear factor kappa-light-chain-enhancer of activated B cells, NO=nitric oxide, Nrf2= nuclear factor erythroid 2 related factor 2, OH• =hydroxyl radical, ONOO- =per-oxynitrite, O_2•-=super-oxide anion, RNS=reactive nitrogen species, ROS =reactive oxygen species, SOD= super-oxide dismutase, TNF-a=tumor necrosis factor-a, TNFR2=tumor necro-sis factor receptor2

Diabetic nephropathy (DN) is a progressive and irreversible kidney disease that is characterized by initial hyperfiltration, albuminuria, expansion of mesangial matrix, interstitial fibrosis, thickening of basement membranes and renal cell damage (Al-Waili *et al.,* 2017). The symptoms include weight loss, polyuria, polydipsia and polyphagia (Balasubashini *et al.,* 2004). It affects 40% of the diabetic patients and is the leading cause of CKD and end stage renal disease (Rizvi *et al.,* 2014; Aruoma *et al.,* 2007). Reduction of blood pressure, normalizing blood sugar and controlling dyslipidemia are the main strategies in clinical practice to ameliorate albuminuria and to treat diabetic patients with DN (Al-Waili *et al.,* 2017; Vasavada and Agarwal, 2005; Go and Jones, 2008). However, these interventions do not prevent progression to end stage renal disease, which requires medical attentions like dialysis or even kidney transplant (Agarwal *et al.,* 2015). Thus DN and renal failure continues to present an enormous burden on the economics of health care management.

The downstream consequences of chronic hyperglycemia such as the formation of advanced glycation end products (AGEs), oxidative stress and inflammation underlie the intricate pathogenesis of DN. Free radicals and AGEs are involved in the structural changes in diabetic nephropathy such as glomerulosclerosis, interstitial fibrosis and tubular atrophy, consequently affecting kidney function (Al-Waili *et al.,* 2017; Agarwal *et al.,* 2015). In the presence of AGEs, glomerular podocytes upregulate the expression of RAGE (receptors for AGEs) triggering multiple intracellular signal transduction cascades, particularly oxidative stress *via* NADPH oxidase and inflammation through the activation of the proinflammatory transcription factor nuclear factor kappa-light-chain-enhancer of activated B cells (NF-κB), contributing to renal injury (Agarwal *et al.,* 2015; Bierhaus and Nawroth, 2009). The translocation of mature NF-κBp65 subunit to nucleus initiates transcription of several genes that play a pivotal role in the pathogenesis of DN, such as those encoding transforming growth factor-beta (TGF-β), chemokine ligand2 (CCL2) and intercellular adhesion molecule (ICAM) (Ahad *et al.,* 2014). Activation of Protein kinase C (PKC), extracellular signal–related kinase (ERK), and inducible nitric oxide synthase (iNOS) are also associated with DN (Al-Waili *et al.,* 2017).

Inhibitors of these mechanisms have been found to offer significant nephroprotection in various experimental models of diabetes. Flavonoids are the most promising in this category with their capability to modulate multiple pathways involved in DN (Table 1), even having the potential to control diabetes as a whole (Vinayagam and Xu, 2015). A particularly innovative approach was used by J Singh *et al.,* who used a mixture of flavonoids chrysin and baicalin to improve antioxidant and anti-inflammatory potential. Baicalin and chrysin combined treatment showed strong protective effects against diabetic tubular injury by suppressing reactive oxygen species (ROS) generation, mitochondrial depolarization, AGEs and apoptosis (Singh *et al.,* 2017).

Recent studies have accentuated the role of TGF-5β 1/smads signaling in DN. TGF-5β1 is a major mediator of renal fibrosis because of its ability to stimulate the accumulation of glomerular extracellular matrix (ECM) protein and increase the thickness of glomerular basement membrane, leading to glomerulosclerosis and proteinuria. TGF-5β 1/smads signaling is highly activated in DN. TGF-5β1 can also up-regulate type IV collagen in all glomerular cell types (Yan *et al.,* 2016). Excessive deposition of type IV collagen is an established feature associated with diabetic glomerulopathy (Huang *et al.,* 2009). Hydroxyproline, an amino acid integrated in ECM as a sign of the tissue fibrosis, is also increased in DN (Qi *et al.,* 2011). In the TGF-5β1/smad signaling pathway, the binding of TGF-5β1 to TGFBR1 activates phosphorylation of smad2 and smad3. The phosphorylated smad2 and smad3 binds to the common smad4 to form the smad complex which regulate the downstream gene transcription. let-7a, belonging to microRNA let-7 family that is reported to participate in many diseases including kidney diseases, is also proposed to negatively regulate TGF-5β 1/smads signaling by targeting TGFBR1. This pathway could provide novel therapeutic targets for DN as revealed by the capability of naringenin to ameliorate kidney injury and inhibit mesangial cells proliferation and accumulation of ECM in DN by regulating let-7a/TGFBR1 (Yan *et al.,* 2016).

Another prominent target include a group of enzymes called matrix metalloproteinases (MMPs) that controls the remodeling of ECM in both normal and pathological conditions. MMPs are a family of structurally and functionally related zinc endopeptidases that are capable of *in-vitro* and *in-vivo* degradation of all kinds of ECM protein components, such as interstitial basement membrane collagen, proteoglycans, fibronectin and laminin, and hence implicated in connective tissue remodelling processes associated with various pathological conditions (Bissell, 1998; Kamalakkannan and Prince, 2006). The activity of MMPs is tightly regulated by tissue inhibitors of MMPs (TIMPs), and the MMP/TIMP ratio is critical for coordinating matrix production and degradation (Vincenti, 2001). Flavonoids are capable of modulating MMPs as evident from the rutin's ability to decrease the content of collagen and hydroxyproline and maintain the balance between MMPs/ TIMPs by increasing the activity of MMPs and decreasing the levels of TIMPs in the kidney of STZ-induced diabetic rats (Kamalakkannan and Prince, 2006).

Apart from this, some other risk factors like genetic alterations and increased blood pressure also play a causal role in DN (Bowden, 2002). Hence management of DN centers on aggressive antihypertensive treatment (target blood pressure 130/80 mm Hg) and inhibition of the rennin-angiotensin aldosterone system (RAAS) (Aruoma *et al.,* 2007). As activation of RAAS has a major role in the pathogenesis of DN, inhibition of this system by angiotensin-converting enzyme (ACE) inhibitors or angiotensin receptor blockers (ARBs) is used currently for the management of DN.

However, it fails to contain the progression to end stage renal disease in a large proportion of patients. In such a context, addition of silymarin to RAAS inhibitors was found beneficial (Fallahzadeh *et al.,* 2012). Thus the supplementation of flavonoids has shown remarkable benefits in mitigating DN through their potential to interfere in the multiple pathways involved in pathogenesis (Table 1).

Table 1: Schematic representation of the nephroprotective mechanisms of flavonoids against experimental models of diabetic nephropathy

Flavonoid	*Dose, duration and route of administration*	*Animal model*	*Diabetes induction; dose and route*	*Key findings*	*References*
Catechin (31.7% of epigallocatechin gallate, 15.7% of epigallocatechin, 10.0% of epicatechin gallate, and 8.5% of epicatechin)	5 mg daily in drinking water for 12 weeks	Sprague-Dawley rats	Streptozotocin (STZ) 80 mg/kg, i.p.	↓ in 24 h urinary albumin excretion rate, ↓ in interstitial fibrosis in the kidney	(Hase *et al.,* 2006)
Chrysin	40 mg/kg/day for 16 weeks post-induction of diabetes, i.g.	Wistar rats	Animals were fed with high fat diet (HFD, 60% calories from fat and 70% animal fat) initially for five weeks followed by a low dose of STZ 35 mg/kg, i.p.	↓ in renal dysfunction and oxidative stress, ↓ in renal tumor necrosis factor (TNF)-α expression and nuclear factor kappa-light-chain-enhancer of activated B cells (NF-κB) activation, improved renal pathology, ↓ in transforming growth factor-beta (TGF-β) fibronectin and collagen-IV protein expressions in renal tissues, ↓ in the serum levels of pro-inflammatory cytokines, interleukin (IL)-1β and IL-6	(Ahad *et al.,* 2014)
A mixture of flavonoids chrysin and baicalin	75 mg and 10 mg/kg of baicalin and chrysin respectively for 60 days,	Wistar rats; Normal rat kidney tubular epithelial cell line (NRK	STZ 65 mg/kg, i.p. 15 min after the administration of nicotin-	↓ in protein levels of inducible nitric oxide synthase (iNOS), protein kinase C (PKC) and ↑ in inhibitor of kappa B (IκB), ↓ in AGEs and their receptor proteins (RAGE),	(Singh *et al.,* 2017)

Table 1: (*Contd...*)

Table 1: (*Contd...*)

Flavonoid	*Dose, duration and route of administration*	*Animal model*	*Diabetes induction; dose and route*	*Key findings*	*References*
	oral	52E)	amide 110 mg/kg, i.p.; methylglyoxal induced cytotoxicity	↓ in renal tubular injuries, ↓ in kidney dysfunction	
Fisetin	0.05% ad *libitum* beginning at 6 weeks of age till 24 weeks of age (diabetic mice received ~40 mg /kg/day)	C57BL/6-Ins2^{Akita} (Akita) mice (Model of Type 1 diabetes)	-	↓ in kidney hypertrophy and albuminuria, ↓ in proteins glycated by methylglyoxal in the blood, kidney and brain, ↑ in glyoxalase 1 enzyme activity, ↑ in the expression of the rate-limiting enzyme for the synthesis of glutathione (GSH), a co-factor for glyoxalase 1, ↓ in the expression of RAGE, serum amyloid A and serum C-reactive protein, markers of protein oxidation, glycation and inflammation	(Maher *et al.*, 2011)
Hesperidin	50, 100 and 200 mg/kg for 4 weeks (after 4 weeks of diabetes induction), oral	Sprague-Dawley rats	Animals were fed with a combination of high fat emulsion (HFE) and HFD for 2 weeks, followed by administration of STZ 35 mg/kg, i.p.	↓ in creatinine and urea nitrogen, ↓ in renal hypertrophy, hyperfiltration and microalbuminuria, ↓ in oxidative stress, ↓ in basement membrane thickening and mesangial expansion	(Jain and Somani, 2014)
Icariin	80 mg/kg, administered for 8 weeks from 5th to 12th week, i.g.	Sprague-Dawley rats	STZ 40 mg/kg, i.v.	↓ in serum creatinine and blood urea nitrogen (BUN), ↑ in superoxide dismutase (SOD), ↓ in malondialdehyde (MDA) and hydroxyproline (Hyp) in the kidney tissue, ↓ in glomerular pathology, ↓ in proteins levels of TGF-β1 and type IV collagen	(Qi *et al.*, 2011)
Luteolin	200 mg/kg, i.g.	Sprague-Dawley rats	STZ 70 mg /kg, i.p.	↓ in serum BUN, creatinine and 24 h urinary protein, ↑ in SOD activity, ↓ in MDA	(Wang *et al.*, 2011)

Table 1: (*Contd...*)

Table 1: (*Contd...*)

Flavonoid	*Dose, duration and route of administration*	*Animal model*	*Diabetes induction; dose and route*	*Key findings*	*References*
				content, ↑ in expression of Heme Oxygenase-1 (HO-1) protein	
Myricetin	6 mg/kg every 12 h for 10 days (beginning 16 weeks after diabetes induction), i.p.	Wistar rats	STZ 50 mg /kg, i.p.	↓ in glomerulosclerosis, ↓ in BUN, urinary volume and protein, ↑ in creatinine clearance, ↑ in glutathione peroxidase (GPX) and ↓ in xanthine oxidase activities	(Ozcan *et al.*, 2012)
	0.5,1.0 and 1.5 mg/kg for 4 weeks, i.p.	Wistar rats	STZ 40 mg /kg, i.p. followed by cadmium in the dose of 100 ppm as cadmium chloride given in drinking water	1 mg/kg exhibited prominent renoprotective effect including ↓ in urea, creatinine, uric acid and BUN in plasma, ↑ in the levels of urinary urea, creatinine and uric acid, ↓ in urinary albumin and urine volume	(Kandasamy and Ashok Kumar, 2012)
Naringenin	50 mg/kg for 7 days (beginning two days after the alloxan injection), i.p.	Swiss mice	alloxan 75 mg/kg, i.v.	↓ in renal lipid peroxidation, ↓ in histopathological changes in kidney	(Sirovina *et al.*, 2016)
	50 mg/kg for 6 weeks, oral; 100–1000 μmol /L	Sprague-Dawley rats; Mouse glomerular mesangial cell (MMC) line	Animals were fed with a high -sugar-high-fat diet for 5 weeks, followed by administration of STZ 30 mg /kg, i.p.; 25 mmol/L glucose	↓ in 24 h urinary protein, ↑ in creatinine clearance ratio, ↓ in mesangial cell proliferation, ↓ in the deposition of extracellular matrix, inhibited TGF-β 1/smads signaling activation by upregulating let-7a	(Yan *et al.*, 2016)
Quercetin	10 mg/kg for 4 weeks	Sprague-Dawley	STZ 45 mg/kg, i.v.	↓ in serum creatinine and BUN, ↓ in urine output and	(Anjaneyulu and Chopra,

Table 1: (*Contd...*)

Table 1: (*Contd...*)

Flavonoid	*Dose, duration and route of administration*	*Animal model*	*Diabetes induction; dose and route*	*Key findings*	*References*
	(after 4 weeks of diabetes induction), oral	rats		urinary albumin excretion, ↓ in MDA, ↑ in GSH, SOD and catalase	2004)
	10 mg/kg per day for 4 weeks (after 6 weeks of STZ injections), oral	C57BL/6J mice	STZ 100 mg/kg for 3 days, i.p.	↓ in polyuria, proteinuria and plasma levels of uric acid, urea and creatinine, ↓ in glomerulosclerosis, ↓ in oxidative stress and apoptosis	(Gomes *et al.*, 2014)
	10 mg/kg per day for 4 weeks (after 6 weeks of STZ injections), oral	apoE–/– mice	STZ 100 mg/kg for 3 days, i.p.	↓ in polyuria, creatininemia and proteinuria, normalization of the index of glomerulosclerosis and kidney weight /bodyweight	(Gomes *et al.*, 2015)
Rutin	100 mg/kg for 45 days, i.g.	Wistar rats	STZ 50 mg/kg, i.p.	↓ in Hyp and collagen, ↓ in activity of matrix metalloproteinases (MMPs), ↓ in levels of tissue inhibitors of MMPs (TIMPs) in the kidney matrix	(Kamalakkannan and Prince, 2006)
Silymarin	100 mg/kg for 4 weeks (after 4 weeks of diabetes induction), oral	Sprague-Dawley rats	STZ 60 mg/kg, i.p.	↓ in renal tissue thiobarbituric acid reactive species (TBARS) and ↓ in catalase and GPX	(Vessal *et al.*, 2010)
	200 mg/kg for 9 weeks (20 days after alloxan administration), oral	Wistar rats	Alloxan 150 mg/kg, s.c.	↓ in renal tissue damage, ↑ in the activity and expression of SOD, catalase and GPX	(Soto *et al.*, 2010)
	60 and 120 mg/kg for 60 days	Wistar rats	STZ 60 mg/kg and nicotinamide 120 mg/kg, i.m.	↓ in urine volume, serum creatinine, serum uric acid, and urine albumin, ↓ in histopathological alterations	(Sheela *et al.*, 2013)

2.1.2. *Ischemia-reperfusion (I/R)-induced renal injury*

Ischemia/reperfusion (I/R) of an organ or tissue is cellular injury triggering a complex cascade of biochemical events that affect the structure and function of almost every organelle and subcellular system of affected cells (Eldaif *et al.,* 2010). Renal ischemia is a common cause of acute renal failure and occurs frequently in hospitalized patients. Ischemic renal cell injury occurs during shock, cardiovascular surgery, renal transplantation, delayed graft function or graft rejection (Singh and Chopra, 2004). It is characterized by decreased renal blood flow and glomerular filtration rate, extensive tubular damage, tubular cell necrosis, glomerular injury, and signs of tubular obstruction with cell debris (Tanner and Steinhausen, 1976; Finn, 1981; Barnes *et al.,* 1981). Current therapy is limited to supportive measures and preventive strategies, none of which have been definitively shown to alter the overall mortality rate.

The pathophysiology of renal injury involves numerous potential mediators and hence is very complex. When oxygen is supplied to the kidney by reperfusion following ischemia, the formation of oxygen radical might exceed the cellular detoxification capacity of the kidneys (Singh *et al.,* 2005). This can result in development of oxidative stress which may further injure tubular cells by activating inflammatory pathways. The major mediators of I/R induced renal damage include ROS, reactive nitogen species (RNS), purine metabolites, neutrophil accumulation, up-regulation of major histocompatibility complex (MHC) antigens, inflammatory cytokines, chemokines and adhesion molecules, vasoactive substance (endothelin, angiotensin II) and release of lytic enzymes (Waz *et al.,* 1998; Nonoliguric, 1993; Bonventre, 1988; Shoskes, 1998). ROS interacts with proteins, lipids, and nucleic acids leading to lipid peroxidation of biological membranes, which in turn, impacts enzymatic processes such as ion pump activity and damage DNA, thereby inhibiting transcription and repair (Chatterjee *et al.,* 1999; Chatterjee *et al.,* 2000; Singh and Chopra, 2004). The progression of these mechanisms in the presence of compromised cellular antioxidant defense components leads to cell death. Various flavonoids such as catechin, naringin, quercetin and silymarin have been found promising against rodent model of I/R induced renal injury (Table 2). They were found to exert protective effect *via* attenuation of oxidative stress as well as inflammatory pathway mediated renal damage.

2.1.3. *Rhabdomyolysis-induced myoglobinuric acute renal failure*

Rhabdomyolysis is a clinical syndrome in which injury to the skeletal muscle results in leakage of intracellular contents from myocytes into the circulation. As muscles account for approximately 40% of total body mass, it is affected by a wide variety of toxic, infectious, inflammatory and metabolic insults (Beetham, 2000). Rhabdomyolysis is associated with intrinsic muscle dysfunction (including trauma, burns, intrinsic muscle disease, excessive physical exertion), metabolic disorders, hypoxia, drugs, toxins, infections, temperature extremes, and idiopathic disorders. The accompanying complications include disseminated intravascular coagulation, hyperkalemia and other metabolic imbalances, acute renal failure (ARF), and acute cardiomyopathy (Chander *et al.,* 2003).

In general, about 10–40% of patients with rhabdomyolysis develop some degree of acute renal failure. This accounts for 2–15% of all cases of ARF (Beetham, 2000). While half of the cases are mild in degree and are responsive to volume repletion, the remaining are more severe with a clinical course typical of acute tubular necrosis (Chander *et al.,* 2002). Stress and the catalytic effect of redox-active iron are considered key mediators of renal injury. Following rhabdomyolysis, myoglobin is released into the systemic circulation and is further discharged into the renal tubules, initiating the renal injury process. Myoglobin is considered to mediate renal injury through oxidant as well as non-oxidant mechanism. Besides causing tubular obstruction, it causes heme-iron-mediated lipid peroxidation which in turn affects the tubular fluid flow dynamics and renal clearance of heme proteins. Even in the absence of heme protein precipitation, tubular injury may result from the lipid peroxidation caused by tubular cell heme-loading and the release of catalytically active iron through the continuous bathing of the tubular cells in myoglobin filtrate. The renal injury results from renal vasoconstriction, direct cytotoxicity, and cast formation. Hypovolemia and metabolic acidosis aggravates the damage through facilitation of tubular precipitation of myoglobin, therefore, form the basis for fluid-alkaline-diuresis therapy (Chander *et al.,* 2003; Singh *et al.,* 2004b).

The intramuscular administration of hypertonic glycerol induces myolysis, hemolysis and intravascular volume depletion, and is the most widely used animal model of myoglobinuric ARF (Chander *et al.,* 2003; Singh *et al.,* 2004b). Preclinical experiments in this model has revealed the potential of flavonoids such as catechin, naringin and proanthocyanidins for use in myoglobinuric acute renal failure (Table 2). Their ability to attenuate ARF was based on their virtue to scavenge free radical and improve renal antioxidant status.

2.1.4. *Lupus nephritis (LN)*

Lupus nephritis (LN) is an inflammation of the kidneys caused by systemic lupus erythematosus (SLE), a prototypic autoimmune disease characterized by the development of autoantibodies directed against nuclear and cellular components and the activation of inflammatory cascades, resulting in multisystem organ damage (Chung *et al.,* 2014). Development of SLE is thought to be secondary to genetic and epigenetic predisposition which promotes autoreactive T and B cell survival following exposure to appropriate environmental stimuli. Autoantibodies and autoreactive cells can be present in a quiescent state of low disease activity. However, SLE patients will experience episodes of disease flare during which inflammation of various organs results in permanent damage (Clark *et al.,* 2015).

LN account for significant morbidity and mortality and results from glomerular immune complex deposition and inflammation involving autoantibodies, autoreactive T and B cells, macrophages, dendritic cells, cytokines and chemokines (Clark *et al.,* 2015). The deposition of the immune complex triggers a cascade of events in the inflammatory response that are accompanied by the generation of ROS, which play a pivotal role in both acute and chronic glomerular injuries in lupus nephritis patients. ROS mediates lipid oxidation, oxidative DNA damage and protein oxidation in lupus patients. Accordingly the redox sensitive transcription factors, nuclear factor erythroid 2 related factor 2 (Nrf2) and NF-κB are thought to be involved in the pathophysiology of lupus (Jiang *et al.,* 2014; Kovacic and Jacintho 2003; Morgan *et al.,* 2007; Tsai *et al.,* 2011; Kang *et al.,* 2009).

Murine lupus models have been widely used to dissect disease pathogenesis as well as for the evaluation of protective agents against the complications of lupus. Lupus prone SFN1 mice and (NZB/W) F1 mice have helped to reveal the mechanisms of flavonoids such as apigenin and epigallocatechin-3-gallate that can be used for protection against the development of LN (Table 2).

Table 2: Schematic representation of the nephroprotective mechanisms of flavonoids against experimental models of ischemia-reperfusion-induced renal injury, rhabdomyolysis-induced myoglobinuric acute renal failure and lupus nephritis

Flavonoid	*Dose, duration and route of administration*	*Animal model*	*Diabetes induction; dose and route*	*Key findings*	*References*
Ischemia-reperfusion-induced renal injury					
Catechin	40 mg/kg twice daily for 4 days and 2 h prior to ischemia/reperfusion on 5th day	Sprague-Dawley rats	Renal ischemia was instituted by using 2 different sets of protocols. 1) both the renal pedicles were occluded 2) only left renal pedi-	↓ in renal dysfunction (↓ in BUN and creatinine), ↓ in morphological alterations, ↓ in oxidative stress (↓ in TBARS, ↑ in GSH, glutathione reductase (GR), catalase and SOD activities)	(Singh *et al.,* 2005)

Table 2: (*Contd...*)

Table 2: (*Contd...*)

Flavonoid	*Dose, duration and route of administration*	*Animal model*	*Diabetes induction; dose and route*	*Key findings*	*References*
			cle was occluded after right nephrectomy. Ischemia lasted 45 min and was followed by reperfusion for 24 h.		
Naringin	400 mg/kg 60 min prior to ischemia, oral	Sprague-Dawley rats	Renal ischemia was instituted by using 2 different sets of protocols. 1) both the renal pedicles were occluded 2) only left renal pedicle was occluded after right nephrectomy. Ischemia lasted 45 min and was followed by reperfusion for 24 h.	↓ in renal dysfunction (↓ in BUN and creatinine), ↓ in morphological alterations, ↓ in oxidative stress (↓ in TBARS, ↑ in GSH, GR catalase and SOD activities)	(Singh and Chopra, 2004)
Quercetin	1-30 mg/kg 2 h before surgery, i.p.	F344 rats	Unilateral ischemia-reperfusion in the left kidney (left renal pedicle occluded for 30 min, reperfusion confirmed visually and	↓ in serum creatinine, improved renal histology, ↓ in gene expression of the chemokines (Regulated on Activation, Normal T Cell Expressed and Secreted (RANTES), monocyte chemoattractant protein-1 (MCP-1)) and macrophage-associated cytokine allograft inflammatory factor (AIF)	(Shoskes, 1998)

Table 2: (*Contd...*)

Table 2: (*Contd...*)

Flavonoid	*Dose, duration and route of administration*	*Animal model*	*Diabetes induction; dose and route*	*Key findings*	*References*
			right kidney removed)		
Rutin	1 g/kg 1 h before ischemia, i.p.	Wistar rats	Left renal pedicle was occluded for 45 min to induce ischemia followed by 3h of reperfusion	↓ in plasma nitrite/nitrate and cyclic guanosine monophosphate (cGMP) levels in the kidneys, ↓ in positive staining for iNOS and 3-nitrotyrosine (3-NT) in the kidneys	(Korkmaz and Kolankaya, 2013)
Silymarin (dried extract of *Silybum marianum*)	100 mg/kg for 7 days before ischemia, oral	Wistar rats	45 min of bilateral ischemia followed by 24 h of reperfusion	↑ in kidney function (↓ in serum urea, creatinine and cystatin C levels), ↑ in serum and tissue antioxidant enzymes levels (SOD, GPX), ↓ in tissue oxidant product levels (↓ in serum and tissue MDA), nitric oxide and protein carbonyl)	(Turgut *et al.*, 2008)
Rhabdomyolysis-induced myoglobinuric acute renal failure					
Catechin	40 mg/kg twice a day for 4 days, oral	Wistar rats	8 ml/kg hypertonic glycerol as a divided dose into the hind limbs on 5th day, i.m.	↓ in renal function (↓ in serum creatinine and BUN, ↑ in creatinine and urea clearance), ↓ in renal oxidative stress (↓ in MDA, ↑ in GSH, activity of catalase, GR and SOD)	(Chander *et al.*, 2003)
Naringin	100, 200 and 400 mg/kg, oral	Wistar rats	8 ml/kg hypertonic glycerol as a divided dose into the hind limbs on 5th day, i.m.	↓ in renal dysfunction (↓ in plasma creatinine and BUN, ↑ in creatinine and urea clearance), ↓ in renal oxidative stress (↓ in renal MDA levels, ↑ in GSH, enzymatic activity of catalase, GR and SOD)	(Singh *et al.*, 2004a)
Proanthocyanidins (catechin 35.7%, epicatechin 24.2%, procyanidins B1-	20 mg/kg immediately following glycerol and daily in the next 3 days, i.p.	Wistar rats	50% (v/v) glycerol 8 ml/kg, i.m.	↓ in blood urea and serum creatinine, ↑ in kidney cortex dipeptidylpeptidase IV activity, ↓ in kidney cortex MDA, improved renal histology	(Stefanovic *et al.*, 2000)

Table 2: (*Contd...*)

Table 2: (*Contd...*)

Flavonoid	*Dose, duration and route of administration*	*Animal model*	*Diabetes induction; dose and route*	*Key findings*	*Referencesz*
B4 27.4%, procyanidin C1 12.7%)					
Proanthocyanidin-BP1	20 mg/kg 24 hours before glycerol and daily in the next 4 day, i.p.	Wistar rats	50% (v/v) glycerol 8 ml/kg, i.m.	↓ in volume density of tubular lumen and cast formations, ↓ in renal dysfunction	(Avramovic *et al.*, 1999)
Lupus associated severe nephritis					
Apigenin	3, 6 or 20 mg/kg for 40 weeks, i.p.	Lupus-prone SNF 1 mice	-	↓ in proteinuria, ↓ in renal histopathology features, inhibited autoantigen presentation for expansion of autoreactive Th1 and Th17 cells, inhibited NF-κB and cyclo-oxygenase (COX)-2	(Kang *et al.*, 2009)
Epigallocatechin-3-gallate	120 mg/kg daily for 22 weeks, oral	Lupus prone New Zealand black/white (NZB/W) F1 mice	-	↓ in proteinuria, renal function impairment and renal lesions, ↑ in renal nuclear factor erythroid 2 related factor 2 (Nrf2) and GPX activity, ↓ in renal oxidative stress, NF-κB activation, and Nucleotide-binding domain, Leucine-Rich Repeat, Pyrin domain containing proteins (NLRP)3 mRNA/protein expression and protein levels of mature caspase-1, inter-leukin (IL)-1β, and IL-18, ↑ in splenic regulatory T (Treg) cell activity	(Tsai *et al.*, 2011)

2.2. Molecular Mechanisms Involved in the Therapeutic Effect of Flavonoids Against Drug Induced Toxicity in Kidney

A number of therapeutic agents can adversely affect the kidney resulting in acute renal failure, chronic interstitial nephritis and nephritic syndrome. These generally include potent drugs belonging to the category of analgesics, antibiotics, immunosuppressants and cytotoxic agents. Iodinated contrast media (ICM), used in radiographic diagnostic and interventional procedures is also reported to induce nephrotoxicity. Flavonoids are emerging as prominent nephroprotective compounds whose supplementation can help in mitigation of nephrotoxicity associated with agents such as cisplatin, acetaminophen, adriamycin, cyclosporine, daunorubicin, gentamicin, imipenem, methotrexate and ICM. In fact, a vast quanta of research has been undertaken to elucidate the mechanisms of flavonoids against nephrotoxicity induced by cisplatin.

2.2.1. *Cisplatin induced nephrotoxicity*

Cisplatin (cis-diamminedichloroplatinum(II)), a cytotoxic platinum derivative acting as an alkylating agent, is one of the most effective and widely used drug for treatment of solid tumors, including head and neck, ovarian, testicular, lung, and breast cancers (Delord *et al.,* 2009; Go and Adjei, 1999). Unfortunately, the clinical utility of cisplatin in cancer therapy is limited by its dose dependent side effects on normal tissues. Acute renal injury and varying degrees of renal dysfunction are experienced by about 28 to 36% of patients after an initial dose of cisplatin (Basnakian *et al.,* 2005). High dose of cisplatin is needed for effective treatment, predominantly in ovarian and colorectal cancer (Ozols and Young, 1985). Even the low dose repeated chemotherapeutic cycles can affect renal functions by their cumulativity, thereby compromising the patients' quality of life (Ozols and Young, 1985; Dkhil *et al.,* 2013). Despite the development of preventive strategies and numerous trials for protective agents, cisplatin induced nephrotoxicity are inadequately controlled.

Kidney is predominantly affected by cisplatin because of three factors: membrane transporter mediated uptake of cisplatin in kidney, metabolism of cisplatin to potent nephrotoxin in renal cells, and kidney being the major route of cisplatin excretion. Cisplatin reacts with nucleophilic sites in DNA forming monoadducts as well as intra- and interstrand cross links. The damage in DNA signals mitochondrial mechanisms activating caspase-dependent pathways to cause cell death. High concentrations of cisplatin induce necrosis in proximal tubule cells, whereas lower concentrations induce apoptosis through a caspase-9-dependent pathway. Engagement of a cell surface receptor with extracellular tumor necrosis factor (TNF)-α also activates caspase 8. Cisplatin increases NFκB binding activity which in turn can lead to heightened expression of TNF-α. TNF-α mediates the upregulation of IL-1β, IL-6, RANTES, MCP-1 and macrophage inflammatory protein 2 (MIP-2), which promotes migration of inflammatory cells into the renal parenchyma. A rise in TNF-α level not only activate apoptotic pathways causing resultant renal cell damage, but also produce oxidative sress through sensitization of infiltrating leukocytes which respond by increased oxidant formation. There exists a remarkable cross talk between the processes of oxidative stress and inflammation; thereby which oxidative stress beyond the physiological threshold mediates TNF-α production by activation of NF-κB. Thus it is hypothesized that the accumulation of cisplatin in renal tissues leads to massive oxidative stress, which in turn causes inflammatory damage to the tubular epithelium, which spreads to the renal microvasculature, impeding the blood flow by evoking ischemic injury, and decreasing the glomerular filtration rate with resultant acute renal failure (Yao *et al.*, 2007; Chirino and Pedraza-Chaverri, 2009). However, regardless of its toxicity, cisplatin remains to be one of the most commonly used chemotherapeutic drug due to its therapeutic efficacy and hence, novel management strategies are being explored that can offer protection from its toxicity.

In recent years, flavonoids have received considerable attention as a dietary supplement to abate nephrotoxic side effects of cisplatin. For instance, drinking of green tea polyphenol (Ahn *et al.*, 2014), and feeding of honey, the remarkably flavonoid-rich sources; offered protection to kidney against cisplatin nephrotoxicity (Hamad *et al.*, 2015). In a similar pattern, numerous flavonoids exhibited significant nephroprotective mechanisms against toxicity induced by cisplatin, essentially involving attenuation of renal damage mediated by oxidative stress, inflammation and/or apoptosis (Table 3).

2.2.2. *Acetaminophen*

Acetaminophen or paracetamol is a widely used analgesic and antipyretic drug. Its analgesic activity is due to either inhibition of prostaglandin synthesis or *via* an active metabolite, p-aminophenol, influencing cannabinoid receptors (Anderson, 2008). The major problem with this medication is misuse through intentional or unintentional ingestion of supratherapeutic dosages (Bond *et al.*, 2003). For example, cancer patients on chemotherapy receive higher doses of acetaminophen to relieve pain (Nassar *et al.*, 2009). Overdose of acetaminophen is encountered commonly and is often associated with hepatic and renal damage (Ghosh and Sil, 2007; Nelson, 1995). Although nephrotoxicity is less common than hepatotoxicity, acute renal failure can occur even in the absence of liver injury and can even lead to death (Ahmad *et al.*, 2012).

At therapeutic doses, acetaminophen is primarily metabolized *via* glucuronidation and sulfuration reactions occurring primarily in the liver, and results in water-soluble metabolites that are excreted *via* kidney. A minor pathway through CYP450 had been also reported to yield a highly reactive metabolite, N-acetyl-p-benzoquinonimine (NAPQI). This metabolite is generally stabilized through conjugation with glutathione (GSH) and eliminated *via* the kidney. However, at overdosage, the essential routes become saturated and the production of NAPQI exceeds the capacity to detoxify it. The excess NAPQI then bind to cellular proteins and initiate lipid peroxidation, leading to renal and hepatic damage associated with oxidative stress (Ahmad *et al.*, 2012; Ojo *et al.*, 2006; Hart *et al.*, 1994; Yousef *et al.*, 2010).

Table 3: Schematic representation of the nephroprotective mechanisms of flavonoids against experimental models of cisplatin-induced nephrotoxicity

Flavonoid	*Dose, duration and route of administration*	*Animal model*	*Cisplatin dose and route of administration*	*Key findings*	*References*
Apigenin	5, 10, 20 µM	Human renal proximal tubular epithelial (HK-2) cell line	40 µM	↓ in apoptosis, ↓ in caspase-3 activity, Poly (ADP-ribose) polymerase (PARP) cleavage, phosphorylation and expression of p53, ↑ in Protein kinase B (Akt) phosphorylation	(Ju *et al.*, 2015)
	5, 10 and 20 mg/kg for 3 days, i.p.	BALB/c mice	20 mg/kg, i.p.	↓ in BUN, GPX and SOD, ↓ in TNF-α, IL-1β and TGF-β in the kidneys, ↓ in the activations of Cytochrome P450 - 2E1 (CYP2E1), phospho (NF-κB) p65 and phospho-P38 mitogen-activated protein kinases (P38MAPK), improved renal histology	(He *et al.*, 2016)
	3 mg/kg for 3 days, i.p.	Wistar albino mice	7.5 mg/kg for 3 days, i.p.	↓ in BUN, serum creatinine, caspase-3, TNF-α, IL-6, COXI and COXII and MDA levels, ↑ in GSH level and catalase activity, improvement in renal histopathology	(Hassan *et al.*, 2017)
Baicalein	50 mg/kg for 15 days, oral	BALB/C mice	20 mg/kg, i.p.	↓ in renal oxidative stress, improved kidney injury and function, ↓ in expression of iNOS, TNF-α, IL-6 and mononuclear cell infiltration and concealed redox-sensitive transcription factor NF-κB activation *via* reduced DNA-binding activity, inhibitor of IκBα phosphorylation and p65 nuclear translocation in kidneys, ↓ in p38 MAPK, extracellular signal-regulated kinase (ERK)1/2 and c- Jun N-terminal kinase (JNK) phosphorylation in kidneys, ↓ in the amount of total and nuclear accumulation of Nrf2 and downstream target protein, heme oxygenase (HO)-1 in kidneys, preserved mitochondrial respiratory enzyme activities, ↓ in	(Sahu *et al.*, 2015)

Table 3: (*Contd...*)

Table 3: (*Contd...*)

Flavonoid	*Dose, duration and route of administration*	*Animal model*	*Cisplatin dose and route of administration*	*Key findings*	*References*
				apoptosis by suppressing p53 expression, Bax/Bcl-2 imbalance, cytochrome c release and activation of caspase-9, caspase-3 and PARP	
Ellagic acid	10 mg/kg for 10 days, oral	Sprague-Dawley rats	7 mg/kg, i.p.	↓ in plasma creatinine, urea and calcium levels, ↓ in oxidative stress markers and pathological changes	(Atessahín *et al.*, 2007)
	10 and 30 mg/kg for 9 days, oral	Sprague-Dawley rats	6 mg/kg, i.p.	dose of 30 mg/kg : ↓ in body weight, water intake, urine output, renal total antioxidant and GSH concentration, ↓ in relative kidney weight, plasma creatinine and BUN, ↓ in necrotic lesions in the renal cortical area, ↑ in expression of clusterin and kidney injury molecule-1	(Al-Kharusi *et al.*, 2013)
Epigallo-catechin-3-gallate	100 mg/kg for 2 days, oral	Wistar rats	7 mg/kg, i.p.	↑ in levels of Nrf2, HO-1, ↓ in levels of NF-κB and hydroxynonenal (an oxidative stress marker), ↑ in renal activities of antioxidant enzymes (catalase, SOD, GPX) and GSH	(Sahin *et al.*, 2010)
	100 mg/kg at 30 min before and 48 h after cisplatin injection, i.p.	C57/BL6 mice	20 mg/kg, i.p.	ameliorated histopathological changes, ↓ in serum creatinine and BUN, ↓ in TUNEL-positive cells, inhibited the expression of the ligand of death receptor Fas, apoptosis regulator Bax and tumor-suppressor protein p53, ↑ in the expression of Bcl-2	(Zou *et al.*, 2014)
	100 mg/kg for 2 days, i.p.; 10 μM	C57BL/6 mice; HK-2 cell line	20 mg/kg, i.p.; 60 μM	↓ in renal dysfunction (↓ in serum creatinine and BUN), improved cisplatin induced kidney structural damages (↓ in tubular dilatation, cast formation, granulovaculoar degeneration and tubular cell necrosis), ↓ in mitochondrial oxidative stress, ↓ in impaired activities of mitochondrial electron transport	(Pan *et al.*, 2015)

Table 3: (*Contd...*)

Table 3: (*Contd...*)

Flavonoid	*Dose, duration and route of administration*	*Animal model*	*Cisplatin dose and route of administration*	*Key findings*	*References*
				chain enzyme complexes, ↑ in GPX manganese superoxide dismutase (Mn-SOD) in mitochondria, ↓ in inflammation (TNF-α and IL-1β), ↓ in accumulation of NF-κB in nuclear fraction, p53 induction, and apoptotic cell death (caspase 3 activity and DNA fragmentation); ↓ in apoptotic cell death and mitochondrial reactive oxygen species (ROS) in HK-2 cell line	
	100 mg/kg at 30 min before and 48 h after cisplatin injection, i.p.	C57/BL6 mice	20 mg/kg, i.p.	↓ in renal dysfunction (↓ in renal index, serum creatinine and BUN), ↓ in renal tubular damage, ↓ in endoplasmic reticulum (ER) stress-induced apoptosis (↓ in expression of phosphorylated ERK, glucose-regulated protein 78 (GRP78), caspase-12)	(Chen *et al.*, 2015)
Eriodictyol	10, 20, 40 mg/kg for 3 days, i.p.	BALB/c mice	20 mg/kg, i.p.	↓ in BUN, creatinine, MDA and ROS, ↓ in production of TNF-α, and IL-1β in kidney tissues, ↑ in the activities of SOD, catalase and GPX, ↑ in expression of Nrf2/HO-1 and ↓ in NF-κB activation	(Li *et al.*, 2016)
Fisetin	0.625 and 1.25 mg/kg for 7 days, i.p.	Sprague-Dawley rats	5 mg/kg, i.p.	↓ in serum biomarkers of renal damage (BUN and creatinine), ↓ in degree of histopathological alterations and oxidative stress, ↓ in IκBα degradation and phosphorylation, ↓ in NF-κB p65 nuclear translocation, ↓ in TNF-α, iNOS and myeloperoxidase (MPO) activities, ↓ in cytochrome c translocation, ↓ in the expression of pro-apoptotic proteins (Bax, cleaved caspase-3, cleaved caspase-9 and p53), ↑ in Bcl-2, ↓ in renal and phagocyte NADPH oxidase activity and expression, ↓ in res-	(Sahu, Kalvala, *et al.*, 2014)

Table 3: (*Contd...*)

Table 3: (*Contd...*)

Flavonoid	*Dose, duration and route of administration*	*Animal model*	*Cisplatin dose and route of administration*	*Key findings*	*References*
				piratory enzyme activities and ↑ in mitochondrial antioxidants	
Genistein	10 mg/kg for 3 days, oral; 25 µg /ml	C57BL/6 mice; HK-2 cell line	20 mg/kg, i.p.; 1 µg/ml	↓ in ROS production, ↓ in the expression of intercellular adhesion molecule-1 and monocyte chemoattractant protein-1 proteins, ↓ in the translocation of the NF-κB p65 into the nucleus, ↓ in infiltration of macrophages, ↓ in apoptosis by regulating p53 induction in kidney; ↓ in ROS production, ↑ in GSH, ↓ in NF-κBp65 levels, ↓ in NF-κB-DNA binding	(Sung *et al.*, 2008)
Hesperidin	100 and 200 mg/kg for 10 days, oral	Wistar rats	7.5 mg/kg, i.p.	↓ in oxidative stress/lipid peroxidation, ↓ in inflammation (infiltration of leukocytes and pro-inflammatory cytokine), ↓ in apoptosis/necrosis (caspase-3 activity with DNA damage), ↓ in nitric oxide expression, improved renal function	(Sahu *et al.*, 2013)
	200 mg/kg for 14 days, oral	Sprague-Dawley rats	5 mg/kg, i.p.	restoration of kidney function (↓ in serum sodium, BUN, serum creatinine, total sodium and potassium excreted in urine) and oxidative stress biomarkers (↓ in MDA, ↑ in GSH and SOD), ↓ in histopathological changes	(Kamel *et al.*, 2014)
	200 mg/kg for 10 days, oral	Wistar rats	7 mg/kg, i.p.	↓ in oxidative stress and nitric oxide level, ↑ in catalase activity, and ↓ in MPO activity	(Kaltalioglu and Coskun-Cevher, 2016)
Hidrosmin	0.3, 1, 3 g/kg for 6 days, oral	Wistar rats	6 mg/kg, i.v.	↓ in cisplatin-induced loss in body weight, ↓ in cisplatin-induced increase in kidney wet weight, ↓ in plasma levels of urea nitrogen and creatinine	(Corcostegui *et al.*, 1998)
Isoliquiritigenin	1 mg/kg for 15	CT-26 mouse colon	5 mg/kg for 15 days,	↓ in the size of the solid tumors without any detectable	(Lee *et al.*, 2008)

Table 3: (*Contd...*)

Table 3: (*Contd...*)

Flavonoid	*Dose, duration and route of administration*	*Animal model*	*Cisplatin dose and route of administration*	*Key findings*	*References*
	days, oral	cancer cell-inoculated BALB/c mice	*i.p*	induction of nephrotoxicity (↓ in serum creatinine, BUN, nitric oxide, renal lipid peroxidation)	
Licochalcone A	1 mg/kg for 15 days, oral	CT-26 mouse colon cancer cell-inoculated BALB/c mice	5 mg/kg for 15 days, i.p.	↓ in the size of the solid tumors without any detectable induction of nephrotoxicity (↓ in serum creatinine, BUN, nitric oxide and renal lipid peroxidation, ↓ in GSH)	(Lee *et al.*, 2008)
Luteolin	50 mg/kg for 3 days, oral	C57BL/6 mice	20 mg/kg, i.p.	↓ in renal dysunction, ↓ in tubular cell damage, ↓ in oxidative stress, ↓ in apoptosis *via* ↓ in the levels of p53 and its phosphorylation, p53-responsive pro-apoptotic factor, (PUMA-α), Bax and caspase-3	(Kang *et al.*, 2011)
	10 mg/kg for 3 days, i.p.	BALB/cN mice	10 or 20 mg/kg, i.p.	↓ in histological and biochemical changes, ↓ in platinum levels, ↓ in oxidative/nitrosative stress, ↓ in inflammation (↓ in NF-κB, TNF-α and COX-2) and apoptosis in the kidneys	(Domitrovis *et al.*, 2013)
Morin	50 and 100 mg/kg for 6 days, oral	Swiss albino mice	20 mg/kg, i.p.	↓ in body weight loss, mortality, functional and structural alterations of kidney, ↑ in cellular antioxidant defense components (GSH, MDA, nitrite), ↓ in TNF-α, IL-1β and IL-6	(KV *et al.*, 2016)
	50 mg/kg for 10 days, oral	Wistar rats	7 mg/kg, i.p.	↓ in oxidative stress, ↑ in nitric oxide level, catalase activity, ↓ in MPO activity	(Kaltalioglu and Coskun-Cevher 2016)
Myricetin	3 mg/kg for 3 days, i.p.	Wistar Albino mice	7.5 mg/kg for 3 days, i.p.	↓ in BUN, serum creatinine, caspase-3, TNF-α, IL-6, CO-XI, COXII and MDA levels, ↑ in GSH level and catalase activity, improvement in renal histopathology	(Hassan *et al.*, 2017)
Naringin	20, 50 or 100 mg/kg body weight for	Wistar rats	5 mg/kg/week for 5 consecutive weeks;	↓ in renal markers, lipid peroxidation, protein and DNA oxidation, ROS formation, TNF-α and nitrite levels, ↓ in	(Chtourou *et al.*, 2016)

Table 3: (*Contd...*)

Table 3: (*Contd...*)

Flavonoid	*Dose, duration and route of administration*	*Animal model*	*Cisplatin dose and route of administration*	*Key findings*	*References*
	5 consecutive weeks; oral		i.p.	renal expressions of NF-κB, iNOS, caspase-3 and p53, improvement in histological changes	
Naringenin	20 mg/kg for 10 days, oral	Wistar rats	7 mg/kg, i.v.	↓ in serum urea and creatinine concentrations, ↓ in polyuria, ↓ in body weight loss, ↓ in reduction in urinary fractional sodium excretion and glutathione S-transferase (GST) activity, ↑ in creatinine clearance, improvement in renal anti-oxidant defense system (SOD, GPX, and catalase)	(Badary *et al.*, 2005)
Nobiletin	1.25, 2.5 and 5 mg/kg for 10 days, i.p.	Wistar rats	8 mg/kg, i.p.	↓ in renal dysfunction (↓ in serum creatinine and BUN levels), ↑ in renal anti-oxidant status (↓ in MDA level, ↑ in GSH, SOD and catalase), ↓ in activation of apoptotic pathways (↓ in Bax, caspase-3 and DNA damage, ↑ in Bcl-2), ↓ in tubular injury	(Malik *et al.*, 2015)
Quercetin	100, 200, 500 μM	cultured tubular epithelial cells (LLC-PK1)	400 μM	↓ in the extent of cell damage	(Kuhlmann *et al.*, 1998)
	50 mg/kg 48, 24, and 1 h before cisplatin injection	Wistar rats	5 mg/kg, i.p.	↓ in plasma creatinine, tubular cell necrosis and immunostaining for vimentin, α-smooth muscle actin, fibronectin, ED1, NF-κB and JNK in the renal cortex and outer medulla	(Francescato *et al.*, 2004)
	50 mg/kg 24 and 1 h before cisplatin injections and repeated daily for 2, 5 or 20 subsequent da-	Wistar rats	5 mg/kg, i.p.	By day 5, cisplatin caused structural alterations in the renal cortex and outer medulla, characteristic of acute tubular necrosis, and by day 20, histological features of chronic nephropathy such as interstitial fibrosis, tubular atrophy and dilatation were observed, quercetin treatment	(Behling *et al.*, 2006)

Table 3: (*Contd...*)

Table 3: (*Contd...*)

Flavonoid	*Dose, duration and route of administration*	*Animal model*	*Cisplatin dose and route of administration*	*Key findings*	*References*
	ys, oral			attenuated the above alterarations along with ↓ in lipid peroxidation, urine volume and plasma creatinine levels and ↑ in urine osmolality	
	50 mg/kg for 9 days, i.p.	Breast adenocarcinoma (13762 Mat B-III) cells inoculated Fischer F344 rats	4 mg/kg, i.p.	↑ in renal blood flow and glomerular filtration rate, ↓ in tubular necrosis/apoptosis and lipid peroxidation, ↑ in endogenous antioxidant systems, ↓ in expression of inflammation markers and caspase-3 activity	(Sanchez-Gonzalez *et al.*, 2011)
	100 mg/kg for consecutive 30 days, oral	Albino rats	2 mg/kg for 5 mutual days, i.p.	↓ in free radical production, ↑ in the activity of catalase, SOD, GPX and GR as well their genes expression, ↑ in vitamin E, vitamin C and GSH levels	(Almaghrabi, 2015)
Rutin	75 and 150 mg/kg for 21 days, oral	Wistar rats	7 mg/kg b for 3 days, i.p.	↓ in oxidative stress, ↓ in caspase-3, TNF-α and NF-κB protein expression levels, restoration of histopathological changes	(Arjumand *et al.*, 2011)
	30 mg/kg for 14 days, oral	Sprague-Dawley rats	5 mg/kg, i.p.	restoration of kidney function (↓ in serum sodium, BUN, serum creatinine, total sodium and potassium excreted in urine) and oxidative stress biomarkers (↓ in MDA, ↓ in GSH and SOD), ↓ in histopathological changes	(Kamel *et al.*, 2014)
Silbinin	0.2 g/kg, i.v.; 0.05 mg ml^{-1} or 0.005 mg ml^{-1}	Wistar rats; human testicular cancer cell lines H12. 1, 577LM, 1777NR CI-A	5 mg/kg, i.v.; 3 to 30000 nmol	↓ in glomerular (↓ in serum creatinine and urea level) and tubular kidney toxicity (excretion of brush-border enzymes and magnesium); no interference with the anti-tumour activity of cisplatin *in vitro*	(Bokemeyer *et al.*, 1996)
	0.2 g/kg, i.v., 1 h before cisplatin	Wistar rats	5 mg/kg, i.v.	↑ in creatinine clearance, ↓ in proteinuria, ↓ in impairment of proximal tubular function (enzymuria and magnesium wasting), ↓ in	(Gaedeke *et al.*, 1996)

Table 3: (*Contd...*)

Table 3: (*Contd...*)

Flavonoid	*Dose, duration and route of administration*	*Animal model*	*Cisplatin dose and route of administration*	*Key findings*	*References*
				morphological alterations observed in the S3-segment of the proximal tubule	
Silymarin	50 mg/kg, i.p.	Sprague-Dawley rats	5 mg/kg, i.p.	Pretreatment with silymarin caused ↓ in cisplatin induced histological and ultrastructural changes	(Abdelmeguid *et al.*, 2010)
	25-200 µM	HK-2, lung carcinoma H460 and melanoma G361 cells	25 and 100 µM	Offered protection against cisplatin-induced cell death in a dose-dependent manner in HK-2, no significant change on cisplatin-induced cell death in H460 cells but potentiated cisplatin-induced apoptosis in G361 cells	(Ninsontia *et al.*, 2011)
Tangeretin	100 mg/kg for 7 days, oral; 200 µM	Wistar rats; Hep3B, MCF-7 & HCT-116 human cancer cell lines	7.5 mg/kg, i.p.; 2 µM	↓ in the levels of serum creatinine and BUN, reversed histopathologic alterations, ↓ in renal oxidative stress (↓ in lipid peroxides, nitric oxide and Nrf2 levels with concomitant ↓ in GSH and GPX), ↓ in inflammatory response (↓ in activated NF-κB p65 protein expression, iNOS and TNF-α, ↓ in IL-10), ↓ in the expression of caspase-3; ↓ in cytotoxic actions of cisplatin in Hep3B and HCT-116 human cancer cell lines	(Arab *et al.*, 2016)

With concerted scientific efforts directed into developing therapeutic or prophylactic agents to protect against acetaminophen toxicity, flavonoids have shown promising results primarily by virtue of their antioxidant potential (Table 4).

2.2.3. *Adriamycin*

Adriamycin or doxorubicin is an anthracycline anticancer agent (Blum and Carter, 1974). The clinical use of adriamycin is delimited by severe cytotoxic side effects including cardiotoxicity and nephrotoxicity. The mechanism of adriamycin-induced cardiotoxicity and nephrotoxicity is most likely mediated by the formation of an iron–anthracycline complex that generates free radicals, which in turn, causes diverse oxidative damage on critical cellular components and membrane lipids in the plasma membranes and mitochondria (Fadillioglu *et al.*, 2004; Malarkodi *et al.*, 2003; El-Shitany *et al.*, 2008). Accordingly amelioration of oxidative stress acted to offer protection from adriamycin nephrotoxicity when rats were treated with silymarin (Table 4).

2.2.4. *Cyclosporine*

Cyclosporine is a potent immunosuppressant agent, commonly used to prevent rejection of transplanted organs (Borel *et al.*, 1996). Even though cyclosporine is widely used in organ transplantation and autoimmune diseases, the side effects on cardiovascular and renal tissues limits its application. The acute form of cyclosporine nephrotoxicity is characterized by reduced glomerular filtration rate and renal blood flow. It is dose dependent, mostly reversible and appears to be related to afferent arteriolar vasoconstriction, possibly mediated by imbalance between renal vasoconstrictors (catecholamines, angiotensin II, endothelin, thromboxane, platelet activating factor), and vasodilators (prostaglandins, nitric oxide). The chronic form is characterized by structural changes in the kidney and appears as tubulointerstitial fibrosis of a striped pattern in arteriolopathy of the afferent arterioles, tubular atrophy, and glomerulosclerosis (Campistol and Sacks, 2000; Tariq *et al.*, 2000; Bennett 1996; Andoh *et al.*, 1996).

The intricate pathophysiology is not fully illustrated, however considers oxidative stress as a major causative factor (Anjaneyulu *et al.*, 2003). ROS can be derived directly from cyclosporine or during its metabolism by the CYP450 system (Ahmed *et al.*, 1995). Cyclosporine can also induce renal nerve activity resulting in vasoconstriction in the kidney *via* blocking the mitochondrial calcium release leading to an increase in intracellular free calcium (Diederich *et al.*, 1994; Moss *et al.*, 1985). Flavonoids are capable of exerting nephroprotective potential against the toxicity induced by cyclosporine by combating oxidative stress insults. (Table 4)

2.2.5. *Daunorubicin*

Daunorubicin is another anthracycline anticancer agent. Its clinical use is limited by the incidence of undesirable systemic toxicity, particularly nephrotoxicity and cardiotoxicity, leading to renal dysfunction and congestive heart failure. The pathogenetic mechanisms behind daunorubicin-induced nephrotoxicity is not fully known and approaches are being tried to minimize the associated risks. Oxidative stress coupled with inflammatory pathways, ER stress, MAPK/ ERK1/2 signaling, activation of NF-κB, peroxisome proliferator activated receptors (PPAR) and RAAS may underlie the intricate pathogenesis of daunorubicin-induced nephrotoxicity. Oxidative or inflammatory stress activate angiotensin II to mediate induction of nephrotoxicity *via* angiotensin II type I receptor (AT1R). Renal failure is manifested as hypertrophy of renal cells, increased renal microvascular pressure, induction of apoptosis, presence of ROS, podocyte autophagy and inflammation. Endothelin (ET)1 may also play an important role in the pathophysiology of renal dysfunction. Activation of the ET receptor type A (ETAR) and ET receptor type B (ETBR) promotes oxidative stress and a compromised free radical scavenging ability (Arozal *et al.,* 2011; Esteban *et al.,* 2004; Karuppagounder *et al.,* 2015). The beneficial role of flavonoids against daunorubicin-induced nephrotoxicity was proved by naringenin which demonstrated an ability to improve renal function *via* attenuation of AT1R, ERK1/2-NFκB p65 signaling pathways (Table 4).

2.2.6. *Gentamicin*

Gentamicin is an aminoglycoside antibiotic effective against infections caused by Gram-negative aerobes (Negrette-Guzmán *et al.,* 2013). Despite possessing numerous benefits such as rapid bactericidal action, low incidence of bacterial resistance and low cost, complications arise from dose-dependent side effects such as ototoxicity and nephrotoxicity (Sahu, Tatireddy, *et al.,* 2014; Fouad *et al.,* 2014). Even after strict monitoring of serum drug concentrations and maintenance of fluid volume, about 30% of gentamicin-treated patients develop nephrotoxicity (Shifow *et al.,* 2000). Indeed, gentamicin nephrotoxicity accounts for 10–15% of all cases of ARF (Mathew, 1992). Gentamicin-induced nephrotoxicity is characterized by renal cellular destruction, necrosis and apoptosis mainly in the proximal tubule, eventually leading to AKI and dysfunction. The specificity of gentamicin for renal toxicity could be related to its preferential accumulation in the renal proximal convoluted tubules (Humes and Weinberg, 1986). The underlying mechanisms may include increased generation of ROS, increased lipid peroxidation and depletion of antioxidant defenses in the renal cells. Oxidative stress may be coupled with renal inflammation mediated by monocytes/macrophage infiltration, NF-κB activation along with the release of pro-inflammatory cytokines and chemokines. Further, apoptosis/necrosis of renal tubular epithelial cells, mitochondrial dysfunction and activation of renal MMPs are proposed to be involved in gentamicin-induced nephrotoxicity (Lee *et al.,* 2012; Bae *et al.,* 2014; Sahu, Tatireddy, *et al.,* 2014; Fouad *et al.,* 2014). Studies have revealed the ability of flavonoids in mitigating gentamicin-induced nephrotoxicity *via* amelioration of oxidative/nitrosative stress, inflammation and apoptosis mediated damage (Table 4).

2.2.7. *Imipenem*

Imipenem is a β-lactam antibiotic. When imipenem is administered alone, it is metabolized by a brush-border enzyme called dehydropeptidase I in proximal tubule. The metabolites of imipenem are very toxic and cause proximal tubular necrosis. The mechanisms of injury include (a) transport into the tubular cell mediated by organic anion transporter (OAT) expressed at the basolateral membrane of renal proximal tubules, (b) acylation of target proteins, causing respiratory toxicity by inactivation of mitochondrial anionic substrate carriers and (c) lipid peroxidation (Tune, 1997). Cilastatin, an inhibitor of dehydropeptidase I, is usually administered along imipenem allowing the drug to be excreted unchanged in the urine. Morin was found to exert beneficial role in reducing the nephrotoxicity of imipenem, at least in part, *via* the inhibition of OAT3-mediated renal excretion of imipenem (Table 4).

2.2.8. *Methotrexate*

Methotrexate is a cytotoxic chemotherapeutic agent and immune system suppressant. It is required in high doses for the treatment of a variety of childhood and adult cancers (Widemann and Adamson, 2006; Widemann *et al.,* 2014). Since more than 90% of methotrexate is excreted unchanged *via* the kidneys, at high doses it may induce renal failure (Henderson *et al.,* 1965). Methotrexate-induced nephrotoxicity can be life threatening because, it further leads to delayed elimination of methotrexate, and the resulting sustained, elevated circulating drug level may aggravate other related toxicities. The methotrexate-induced nephrotoxicity is believed to be mediated by two primary mechanisms (a) induction of crystal nephropathy, which occurs when methotrexate and its metabolites precipitate within the renal tubules, (b) direct tubular toxicity, mediated by oxidative stress. Thus methotrexate-induced toxicity in kidney is characterized by increase in free radicals, increased MPO activity, depletion in endogenous antioxidant defense components as well as activation of inflammatory mediators and neutrophil infiltration. Despite the use of preventive measures such as administration of pharmacokinetically guided leucovorin, urinary alkalinization and intravenous hydration, methotrexate-induced nephrotoxicity continues to occur (Perazella and Moeckel, 2010; Perazella 1999; Devrim *et al.,* 2005; Kolli *et al.,* 2009; Dabak and Kocaman, 2015). Among several experimental studies conducted for the prevention of methotrexate-induced nephrotoxicity, silymarin was found promising with its ability to decrease renal tubular apoptosis (Table 4).

2.2.9. *Iodinated contrast media*

Iodinated contrast media (ICM) is used in radiographic diagnostic and interventional procedures. It can be nephrotoxic when combined with potentially nephrotoxic agents, or in patients with comorbid illness, such as diabetic nephropathy. It is characterized by the presence of tubular necrosis, tubular epithelial damage, hyaline casts and hemorrhagic casts. The AKI mediated by ICM leads to a condition known as contrast-induced nephropathy (CIN). While the incidence of CIN is approximately 2% in patients without risk factors, it may range between 9 and >50% in people with mild-to-moderate renal impairment and DM. With 1% of patients experiencing CIN requiring dialysis, it has led to increased medical care costs and increased mortality. CIN is currently reported as the third most common cause of hospital-acquired renal failure (Palabiyik *et al.,* 2017; Jorgensen 2013; Seeliger *et al.,* 2012; Sadat 2013).

The pathogenesis of CIN is not fully elucidated, but recent studies point towards a combination of toxic and ischemic injury to the renal tubular cells. Reduced renal blood flow, direct cytotoxic effects, auto- and paracrine factors perturbing renal hemodynamics, altered rheological properties affecting renal hemodynamics and tubulodynamics and increased hypoxia mediated damage are the probable underlying mechanisms of CIN. Oxidative stress, the perturbation of the balance between pro-oxidants and antioxidants may underline the pathology of CIN (Jorgensen 2013; Seeliger *et al.,* 2012; Palabiyik *et al.,* 2017).

Protection of the renal tubules from prolonged contact with CM is the goal of prevention, as permanent damage can occur at the time of contact. Sodium bicarbonate and N-acetyl cysteine (NAC) are used to prevent an acidic environment and formation of free radicals in the renal tubules. Major preventive strategies include adequate hydration of the patient, discontinuation of nephrotoxic drugs before CM administration and NAC and vitamins C and E treatment. Even though some compounds such as infliximab and simvastatin have been shown to ameliorate CIN; there is no available standard prophylactic or therapeutic agent for this condition. Antioxidant protection is expected to preserve at the level of the glomerulus and reduce systemic inflammatory effects (Jorgensen, 2013; Palabiyik *et al.,* 2017). Hence flavonoids are a promising category of agents that could offer protection. Evidently, epigallocatechin-3-gallate treatment was found to markedly attenuate CIN-induced oxidative stress and inflammatory damage (Table 4).

2.3. Molecular Mechanisms Involved in the Therapeutic Effect of Flavonoids Against Occupational/Environmental Nephrotoxins Induced Damage in Kidney

In recent years, human exposure to a vast array of industrial and environmental chemicals has risen dramatically owing to the exponential increase of their use in several industrial, pharmaceutical, agricultural, domestic and technological applications. Amongst this some chemicals enter into the body by dermal contact, inhalation or ingestion of contaminated drinking water and redistribute itself to the entire organ systems of the body. Those agents affecting the kidney are called nephrotoxins and their manifestations include acute renal injury, chronic renal changes that may

Table 4: Schematic representation of the nephroprotective mechanisms of flavonoids against experimental models of drug induced nephrotoxicity

Flavonoid	*Dose, duration and route of administration*	*Animal model*	*Drug dose and route of administration*	*Key findings*	*References*
Acetaminophen					
Hesperidin	100 and 200 mg/kg for 14 days, oral	Wistar rats	750 mg/kg for 14 days, oral	↓ in serum BUN and creatinine, ↑ in the activity of GSH, GST, GR, GPX and catalase, ↓ in apoptotic death and inflammation in renal tubular cells, manifested by a ↓ in the expression of caspase-3, caspase-9, NF-κB, iNOS, kidney injury molecule 1 (Kim-1) and ↑ in Bcl-2 expression	(Ahmad *et al.*, 2012)
Quercetin	20 mg/kg for 15 days, oral	Wistar rats	650 mg/kg for 15 days, oral	↓ in TBARS, ↑ in GPX, GST, SOD and catalase activities, ↑ in GSH content, ↑ in plasma total protein, albumin and globulin, ↓ in urea and creatinine	(Yousef *et al.*, 2010)
Adriamycin					
Silymarin	50 mg/kg silymarin 7 days before adriamycin and daily thereafter throughout the study (30 days), i.p.	Albino rats	10 mg/kg, i.p.	↓ in plasma creatinine and urea, ↓ in MDA and ↑ in GSH in kidney, ↓ in renal tubular damage	(El-Shitany *et al.*, 2008)
Cyclosporine					
Catechin	50 and 100 mg/kg for 21 days, oral	Wistar rats	20 mg/kg for 20 days, s.c.	Dose dependent effects, 50 mg/kg: ↓ in serum creatinine, ↑ in GSH 100 mg/kg: ↓ in serum creatinine, BUN and ↑ in creatinine and urea clearance, ↓ in lipid peroxidation, ↑ in SOD, GSH and catalase in kidney	(Anjaneyulu *et al.*, 2003)
Quercetin	0.5 and 2 mg/kg 24 h before and con-	Albino rats	20 mg/kg for 21 days, s.c.	↓ in TBARS, ↑ in renal function (↓ in plasma creatinine and BUN, ↑ in creatinine and urea clearance), atten-	(Satyanarayana *et al.*, 2001)

Table 4: (*Contd...*)

Table 4: (*Contd...*)

Flavonoid	*Dose, duration and route of administration*	*Animal model*	*Drug dose and route of administration*	*Key findings*	*References*
	currently with cyclosporine for 21 days, i.p.			uated renal morphological alterations (striped interstitial fibrosis, arteriopathy, glomerular basement thickening, tubular vacuolization and hyaline casts)	
Quercetin formulated into a novel self-emulsifying drug delivery system	50 mg/kg, oral Prophylactic group: from day 1 to 3 Therapeutic group: day 1 to 6	Swiss mice	5 mg/kg, i.p. Prophylactic group: from day 4 to 6 Therapeutic group: on day 1	↓ in serum BUN and creatinine	(Jain *et al.*, 2013)
Daunorubicin					
Naringenin	20 mg/kg daily after daunorubicin administration (1 week from the start of the the experiment) and continued for 6 weeks, oral	Sprague-Dawley rats	3 mg/kg thrice with 48 h interval between each injection for one week to get a cumulative dose of 9 mg/kg, i.v.	↓ in renal dysfunction (↓ in BUN, serum creatinine), ↓ in histopathogical abnormalities, ↑ in peroxisome proliferator activated receptor (PPAR)γ and ↓ in angiotensin II type I receptor (AT1R), endothelin (ET)1, ET receptor type A (ETAR), phosphorylated ERK 1/2, phophosphorylated NF-κB p65, ER stress and apoptosis (↓ in renal GRP78, C/Eb p-homologous protein (CHO P), cleaved caspase-7 and caspase -12 levels) as well as inflammatory (interferon (IFN)γ, IL-6, TNFR1 and COX2) markers	(Karuppagounder *et al.*, 2015)
Gentamicin					
Morin	50, 100 and 200 mg/kg, oral (Prophylactic group: day 1 to 18, treatment groups: day 4 to 18)	Sprague-Dawley rats	100 mg/kg for 5 days (4th day to 8th day), s.c.	Dose dependent effects, Treatment groups:↓ in weight loss and kidney/body weight ratio, ↓ in serum creatinine and BUN levels, ↓ in ROS and ↑ in levels of GSH, SOD, catalase and total protein levels Prophylactic group: same as above except lack of signifi-	(Jonnalagadda *et al.*, 2013)

Table 4: (*Contd...*)

Table 4: (*Contd...*)

Flavonoid	*Dose, duration and route of administration*	*Animal model*	*Drug dose and route of administration*	*Key findings*	*References*
				cant reduction of ROS and tissue nitrite levels	
Naringin	50 and 100 mg/kg for 7 days, oral	Sprague-Dawley rats	120 mg/kg for 7 consecutive days, i.p.	Reinstated mitochondrial function, ↓ in renal antioxidant levels, ↓ in TNF-α, IL-6 and NF-κB p65, ↓ in NF-κB-DNA binding and MPO activity, ↓ in cleaved caspase 3, Bax and p53 protein expression, ↑ in Bcl-2 protein expression, ↓ in renal histolopathological alterations	(Sahu, Tatireddy, *et al.*, 2014)
Naringenin	50 mg/kg for 8 days, oral	Sprague-Dawley rats	80 mg/ kg for 8 days, i.p.	↓ in serum creatinine, ↓ in renal MDA, nitric oxide and IL-8, ↓ in renal histopathological alterations, ↓ in kim-1, vascular endothelial growth factor, iNOS and caspase-9, ↑ in survivin expression	(Fouad *et al.*, 2014)
Quercetin	50 mg/kg for 7 days, oral	Wistar rats	80 mg/ kg for 7 days, i.p.	↓ in renal dysfunction (↓ in BUN and creatinine), ↓ in oxidative stress (↓ in TBA-RS, ↑ in GSH, SOD and catalase activities, ↓ in histopathological alterations	(Abdel-Raheem *et al.*, 2009)
Imipenem					
Morin	12, 25 and 50 mg/kg, oral; 100 μM	Albino Rabbits; Madin-Darby canine kidney (MDCK) cells over-expressing human organic anion transporter 1 and 3 (MDCK/ hOAT1 or MDCK/ hOAT3)	200 mg/kg, i.v.; 1-10 mM	↓ in renal histopathological damage, Imipenem induced cytotoxicity only in MDCK/ hOAT3 cells which was ↓ in presence of morin (*i.e.* inhibition of OAT3-mediated cellular uptake)	(Lim *et al.*, 2008)

Table 4: (*Contd...*)

Table 4: (*Contd...*)

Flavonoid	*Dose, duration and route of administration*	*Animal model*	*Drug dose and route of administration*	*Key findings*	*References*
Methotrexate					
Silymarin	300 mg/kg for 5 days, i.p.	Sprague-Dawley rats	20 mg/kg, i.p.	↓ in histopathologic alterations (dilated Bowman's space, inflammatory cell infiltration, glomerular and peritubular vascular congestion and swelling of renal tubular epithelium cells), ↓ in apoptotic cell death in renal tubules	(Dabak and Kocaman 2015)
Iodinated contrast media					
Epigallocatechin-3-gallate	50 and 100 mg/kg for 4 days, oral	Wistar rats	25% glycerol at a single dose of 10 ml/kg, i.m., after 24 h iohexol CM was administered into the tail vein of the animals at a single dose of 10 ml/kg over a period of 2 min, i.v.	Both doses : ↓ in renal dysfunction (↓ in serum creatinine and BUN), ↓ in oxidative stress, ↓ in TNF-α and NF-κB mRNA expression, attenuated kidney damage	(Palabiyik *et al.*, 2017)

lead to end-stage renal failure and renal malignancy. Exposure may be over a long period of time or limited to a single event and can vary from minute quantities to cumulative and very high doses. Exposure to environmental toxicants is prominent in point source areas such as mining, foundries and smelters, and other metal-based industrial operations. Prominent among environmental/occupational nephrotoxins are heavy metals such as cadmium (Cd), lead (Pb) and mercury (Hg), metalloid such as arsenic (As), Ferric nitrilotriacetate (Fe-NTA) and carbon tetrachloride (CCl_4) (Bradl 2005; He *et al.,* 2005; Tchounwou *et al.,* 2012). Heavy metals are capable of inducing toxicity even at a low level of exposure. The kidney plays a principal role in the toxicokinetics of these agents, since it serves as a major excretory and osmoregulatory organ with a larger perfusion and hence becomes the site of increased exposure owing to accumulation during urinary elimination. As these toxicants are capable of generating ROS during metabolic activation processes, oxidative stress may be one of the key mechanisms behind their nephrotoxicity (Ratnaike, 2003; Lin *et al.*, 2008; Prabu and Muthumani, 2012; Renugadevi and Prabu, 2009; Vijayaprakash *et al.*, 2013). Accordingly, among the approaches practiced to ameliorate the toxicity induced by environmental/occupational nephrotoxins include the use of agents with powerful antioxidant properties. Preclinical experimental models have thrown light into the profound potential of flavonoids in offering nephroprotection from these agents (Table 5).

2.3.1. *Arsenic*

Arsenic (As) toxicity in kidney is manifested as tubular necrosis, inflammatory cell infiltration, tubular degeneration, hemorrhage, swelling of tubules and vacuolization (Prabu and Muthumani, 2012). As exerts its toxic effects through several mechanisms, the most significant of which is the reversible reaction with sulfhydryl groups especially vicinal dithiols. The binding of As to thiol containing amino acid residues in proteins leads to the inhibition of activities of several enzymes by As (Kokilavani *et al.*, 2005). As *via* induction of NADPH oxidase, iNOS and downregulation of Nrf2 mediates oxidative damage at the molecular and cellular level causing lipid peroxidation, enhanced oxidation of proteins, enzymes as well as DNA, disruption of mitochondrial respiratory chain and apoptosis, leading to proximal tubular damage (Lin *et al.*, 2008; Li *et al.*, 2010; Sinha *et al.*, 2008; Chou *et al.*, 2004). As also decreases the activities of membrane bound total ATPases in the kidney leading to a decrease in sodium efflux, thereby altering membrane permeability, which in turn leads to the leakage of Ca^{2+} ions into cells thereby potentiating irreversible cell destruction (Finotti and Palatini, 1986). Further, As can mediate the activation of NF-κB signaling pathway to mediate inflammatory insults in renal cells (Prabu and Muthumani, 2012). Flavonoids such as naringin/naringenin, quercetin and silibinin have demonstrated remarkable nephroprotective mechanisms to attenuate As nephrotoxicity (Table 5).

2.3.2. *Cadmium*

Cadmium (Cd) has a long biological half life of 15 years, making it a cumulative toxin in liver and kidney (Norberg and Nishiyama, 1972). Cadmium nephrotoxicity principally involves the proximal tubules and is believed to be irreversible at advanced stages (Ahn *et al.*, 1999). Even kidney stones and glomerular damage are reported in those with occupational exposure (Hu 2000). The nephrotoxic action of Cd is attributed to the Cd–metallothionein complex released from the damaged liver cells, which gets filtered through the glomerulus into the urinary space where it gets endocytosed by the proximal tubular cells and on degradation by the lysosomes release Cd (Morales *et al.*, 2006). The released Cd in turn stimulates the production of metallothionein in proximal tubular cells, directly damaging the integrity of microvilli and intracellular vesicles and indirectly inhibiting the transporter activity *via* changes in the membrane fluidity due to oxidative stress and increased lipid peroxidation by binding with membrane phospholipids and targeting various intracellular proteins and membrane transporters at the cytoplasmic side by binding to their reactive SH-groups (Renugadevi and Prabu, 2009, 2010).

Although several chelating agents and antagonists are utilized to reduce the Cd toxicity, their application is limited by undesirable side effects and ineffectiveness in chronic cases (Nordberg, 1984). As antioxidant therapy has been reported promising, flavonoids such as naringenin and quercetin have shown capacity to mitigate Cd nephrotoxicity *via* amelioration of damages inflicted by oxidative stress (Table 5).

2.3.3. *Lead*

Lead (Pb) nephrotoxicity appears to be primarily localized in the kidney tubule and is manifested as progressive glomerular and tubular alterations, such as renal tubular epithelial cell necrosis, leukocyte infiltration and tubular epithelial cell pyknosis, excessive urinary excretion of amino acids, glucose and phosphate, natriuresis, kaliuresis and intranuclear body inclusion (Moneim *et al.,* 2011; O'Flaherty *et al.,* 1986). These are associated with increased serum levels of Pb or decreased Pb re-absorption caused by disrupted enzymes and energy production systems and in part by the failure in the ion pump transport of kidney tubules cells (Moneim *et al.,* 2011; Jadhav *et al.,* 2007). Pb induced excessive ROS production and activation of intracellular signaling pathways (such as MAPK, TGF-β1, NF-κB) leading to increased cytokine production are assumed to be the key pathophysiologic mechanisms of Pb nephrotoxicity (Gloire *et al.,* 2006; Zuscik *et al.,* 2002; Liu *et al.,* 2010; Liu *et al.,* 2012). Pb can also induce DNA injury in the kidney resulting in caspase-3 dependent apoptosis. Accordingly, the nephroprotective activity of quercetin against Pb nephrotoxicity was related to the attenuation of renal oxidative stress, inflammation as well as apoptosis (Table 5).

2.3.4. *Mercury*

Mercury (Hg) nephrotoxicity is reflected as reabsorptive and secretary defects principally in the proximal tubules (Al-Madani *et al.,* 2009). Hg has a high affinity for cellular cysteine thiols and hence affects oxidative function (Clarkson, 1997). Exposure to mercuric compounds induces oxidative stress characterized by accumulation of lipid peroxidation products, increase in production of ROS/RNS, decrease in antioxidant enzymes and reduction in ATP content (Nava *et al.,* 2000; Vijayaprakash *et al.,* 2013). Flavonoids like ellagic acid, hesperidin, kaempferol, lespeflan and morin have shown ability to reverse these mechanisms thereby offering protection against Hg nephrotoxicity (Table 5).

2.3.5. *Ferric nitrilotriacetate (Fe-NTA)*

Nitrilotriacetic acid (NTA) is an aminotricarboxylic acid chelating agent, which forms water-soluble chelate complexes with several metal cations including iron at neutral pH (Singh, Chander, and Chopra, 2004a). Because of its ability to chelate calcium and magnesium ions, the trisodium salt is used in laundry detergents as a "builder" to replace phosphates, the use of which has been restricted by legislation in some countries owing to their contribution to the eutrophication of lakes and ponds (Anderson *et al.*, 1985). However, Fe-NTA is reported to induce acute nephrotoxicity and renal cellular carcinoma. Renal damage is assumed to be caused by the elevation of free serum iron concentration, following its reduction at the luminal side of the proximal tubule, generating ROS, leading to lipid peroxidation and subsequent oxidative damage (Hamazaki *et al.*, 1985; Liu *et al.*, 1991). Naringin and rutin was found to have beneficial effect against Fe-NTA induced nephrotoxicity by suppressing renal oxidative stress mediated damage (Table 5).

2.3.6. *Carbon tetrachloride*

Carbon tetrachloride (CCl_4) is an industrial solvent, cleaner, and degreaser. Its capability to induce hepatic injury has been widely investigated. However, it was demonstrated that liver is not the only target organ of CCl_4 toxicity, the toxic trichloromethyl radicals (CCl_3^- and/or CCl_3OO^-) was also generated in other tissues, including brain, lungs, kidney, testis and blood affecting their structure and function (Hermenean *et al.*, 2013). Kidney is particularly susceptible owing to the presence of common xenobiotic metabolizing enzymes, mainly localized in proximal tubular cells (Lock and Reed, 1998). The initial step in biotransformation of CCl_4 is reductive dehalogenation, which results in formation of reactive radicals (Slater, 1982). Excessive formation of radicals initiates lipid peroxidation which on progression ends in overwhelming the antioxidant defense system. This along with mitochondrial dysfunction and reduction in lysosomal integrity leads to mesangial cell fibrogenesis and tubulointerstitial fibrosis, affecting renal function (Hermenean *et al.*, 2013). Supplementation of hesperidin and naringenin were found to decrease CCl_4 induced nephrotoxicity by suppressing oxidative stress mediated renal damage (Table 5).

Table 5: Schematic representation of the nephroprotective mechanisms of flavonoids against experimental models of occupational/environmental nephrotoxins-induced renal damage

Flavonoid	*Dose, duration and route of administration*	*Animal model*	*Nephrotoxin dose and route of administration*	*Key findings*	*References*
Arsenic					
Naringin	20, 40, and 80 mg/kg for 28 days, oral	Sprague-Dawley rats	Sodium arsenite dissolved in normal saline at a dose of 5 mg/kg for 28 days, oral	↓ in kidney dysfunction (↓ in serum creatinine, ↑ in urine creatinine, BUN, uric acid and creatinine clearance), ↓ in renal oxido-nitrosative stress, dose-dependent ↓ in renal KIM-1, caspase-3, TGF-β, and TNF-α mRNA expression, improved histopathological alterations	(Adil *et al.*, 2015)
Naringenin	20 and 50 mg/kg for 28 days, oral	Wistar rat	Arsenic trioxide in normal saline at a dose of 2 mg/kg for 28 days, oral	Dose-dependent activity, ↓ in renal dysfunction (↓ in levels of serum urea, uric acid and creatinine), ↓ in oxidative stress (↓ in lipid peroxidation, ↑ in GSH, GPX, GST, SOD and catalase), ↓ in renal histopathological changes	(Mershiba *et al.*, 2013)
Quercetin	0.2 mmol/kg for 5 days, oral	Swiss mice	25-ppm sodium arsenite in drinking water for 12 months	↓ in renal TBARS level, protection of inhibited blood δ-aminolevulinic acid dehydratase activity and depletion of arsenic level from target organs	(Mishra and Flora, 2008)
Silibinin	75 mg/kg for 4 weeeks, oral	Wistar rat	Sodium arsenite 5 mg/kg for 4 weeks, oral	↓ in renal dysfunction (↓ in serum urea, uric acid and creatinine, ↑ in creatinine clearance, ↑ in levels of urea, uric acid and creatinine in urine), ↓ in levels of lipid peroxidation markers (TBARS and lipid hydroperoxides) and protein carbonyl, ↑ in non-enzymatic antioxidants (↑ in total sulfhydryl groups, GSH, vitamin C and vitamin E) and enzymatic antioxidants (↑ in SOD, GPX, GST and catalase), ↑ in GSH metbolizing enzymes (GR and glutathione-6-phosphate	(Prabu and Muthumani, 2012)

Table 5: (*Contd...*)

Table 5: (*Contd...*)

Flavonoid	*Dose, duration and route of administration*	*Animal model*	*Nephrotoxin dose and route of administration*	*Key findings*	*References*
				dehydrogenase (G6PD)), ↑ in membrane bound ATPases, preserved the normal histological architecture of the renal tissue, ↓ in caspase-3 mediated tubular cell apoptosis and NADPH oxidase, iNOS and NF-κB over expression, ↑ in renal Nrf2 expression	
Cadmium					
Naringenin	25 and 50 mg/kg for 4 weeks, oral	Wistar rat	Cadmium chloride in sterile physiological saline at the dose of 5 mg/kg for 4 weeks, oral	25 and 50 mg/kg: ↓ in renal dysfunction (↓ in levels of serum urea, uric acid and creatinine, ↑ in creatinine clearance), ↓ in oxidative stress (↓ in TBARS, lipid hydroperoxides and protein carbonyl content, ↑ in total sulphydryl group, GSH, vitamin C, vitamin E, SOD, catalase, GSH, GPX, GST, GR and G6PD), attenuated histopathological changes 50 mg/kg: ↓ in Toxicity, preserved the normal histological architecture of the renal tissue	(Renugadevi and Prabu, 2009)
Quercetin	50 mg/kg/day, 5 times/week beginning from the fourth week, i.p.	Wistar rats	Aqueous solution of cadmium chloride at a dose of 1.2 mg Cd/kg/day, 5 times/week during nine weeks, s.c.	↓ in renal dysfunction, ↓ in tubular lesions, ↓ in plasma TBARS, ↑ in total plasma antioxidants and renal SOD and GR activities	(Morales *et al.*, 2006)
	50 mg/kg for 4 weeks, oral	Wistar rats	Cadmium chloride in sterile physiological saline at the dose of 5 mg/kg for	↓ in renal dysfunction (↓ in levels of serum urea, uric acid and creatinine, ↓ in creatinine clearance), ↓ in oxidative stress (↓ in TBARS, lipid hydroperoxides and protein carbonyl content, ↓ in	(Renugadevi and Prabu, 2010)

Table 5: (*Contd...*)

Table 5: (*Contd...*)

Flavonoid	*Dose, duration and route of administration*	*Animal model*	*Nephrotoxin dose and route of administration*	*Key findings*	*References*
			4 weeks, oral	total sulphydryl group, GSH, vitamin C, vitamin E, SOD, catalase, GSH, GPX, GST, GR and G6PD), attenuated histopathological changes	
Lead					
Quercetin	10 mg/kg for 10 weeks, oral	Wistar rats	Aqueous solution of lead acetate at a concentration of 500 mg Pb/l as the only drinking fluid for 10 weeks	↓ in renal dysfunction, ↓ in ROS level, GSH/GSSG ratio and 8-hydroxydeoxyguanosine levels, ↑ in Cu/Zn-SOD, catalase and GPX activities, ↓ in apoptosis, attenuated histotopathologic changes	(Liu *et al.*, 2010)
	25 and 50 mg/kg for 75 days, oral	Wistar rats	Aqueous solution of lead acetate at a concentration of 500 mg Pb/l of drinking water for 75 days	Exhibited dose dependent activity, ↓ in renal dysfunction (↓ in serum uric acid, urea, creatinine), ↓ in renal ROS production, attenuated histopathological changes, ↓ in renal lead content, ↓ in renal inflammation (↓ in TNF-α, IL-1β, IL-6, COX-2, NF-κB), ↓ in MAPK signaling (↓ in ERK1/2, JNK1/2, p38 MAPK)	(Liu *et al.*, 2012)
Mercury					
Ellagic acid	5 mg/kg for 7 days, oral	Albino rats	Mercuric chloride 1.23 mg/kg in 0.9% NaCl for 7 days, i.p.	↓ in lipid peroxidation, ↑ in GSH, GPX, catalase and SOD activities in the kidney	(Bharathi and Jagadeesan, 2014)
Hesperidin	5 mg/kg for 7 days, oral	Albino rats	Mercuric chloride 1.23 mg/kg in 0.9% NaCl for 7 days, i.p.	↓ in lipid peroxidation, ↑ in GSH, GPX, catalase and SOD activities in the kidney	(Bharathi and Jagadeesan, 2014)
Kaempferol	100 mg/kg for a period of 28 successive days, oral	Wistar rats	Mercuric chloride 1 mg/kg weekly thrice for 1 mon-	↓ in renal dysfunction (blood urea, serum creatinine, uric acid), ↓ in renal oxidative stress (↓ in lipid peroxidation, ↑ in the levels of serum pro-	(Vijayaprakash *et al.*, 2013)

Table 5: (*Contd...*)

Table 5: (*Contd...*)

Flavonoid	*Dose, duration and route of administration*	*Animal model*	*Nephrotoxin dose and route of administration*	*Key findings*	*References*
			th, i.p.	tein, nucleic acids, enzymic and non-enzymic antioxidants)	
Lespeflan	1 ml/kg	Spraque Dawley rats	Mercuric chloride in a dose of 3 mg/kg, i.p.	↓ in acute uremic syndrome (↓ in urea and creatinine levels in blood plasma), ↑ in kidney transamidinase activity	(Nikolic and Sokolovic, 2004)
Morin	200 mg/kg from 6th to 15th day, i.p.	Wistar rats	Mercuric chloride dissolved in 0.9% saline at a dose of 5 mg/kg for 5 days, i.p.	↓ in serum urea, uric acid and creatinine, improvement in renal histopathology	(Venkatesan *et al.*, 2010)
Ferric nitrilotriacetate (Fe-NTA)					
Naringin	100, 200, and 400 mg/kg, oral	Wistar rats	Ferric nitrate (0.16 mmol/kg body weight) soution mixed with a 4 fold molar excess of disodium salt of Nitrilotriacetic acid (NTA) (0.64 mmol/kg body weight), pH adjusted to 7.4, administered at the dose of 8 mg Fe/kg, i.p.	Improvement in renal architecture and renal function, ↓ in renal oxidative stress (↓ in TBARS, ↑ in catalase, SOD and GR)	(Singh *et al.*, 2004a)
Rutin	50 µmol/kg at different times before or after Fe-NTA in experiment	ICR mice	300 mM Ferric nitrate enneahydrate and 600 mM NTA were mixed	↓ in renal lipid peroxidation, ↓ in formation of hydroxyl radical spin adduct of 5,5-dimethyl-1-pyrroline-N-oxide suggesting capability to scavenge ROS, exhibited ability to chelate ferric ions to ↓ oxida-	(Shimoi *et al.*, 1997)

Table 5: (*Contd...*)

Table 5: (*Contd...*)

Flavonoid	*Dose, duration and route of administration*	*Animal model*	*Nephrotoxin dose and route of administration*	*Key findings*	*References*
	1 and 50 μmol/kg 30 min after each Fe-NTA treatment in experiment 2		at the volume ratio of 1:2 (molar ratio 1:4) and pH adjusted to 7.4 with sodium hydrogen carbonate and administered at the dose of 7 mg Fe/kg in experiment 1 and 2 mg Fe/kg for the first 3 days and 3 mg Fe/kg for 12 days (5 days a week) in experiment 2, i.p.	tive renal damage	
Carbon tetrachloride					
Hesperidin	100 and 200 mg/kg for 10 days, oral	Wistar rats	2 ml/kg (40% v/v in olive oil) on 8th day, s.c.	↓ in TBARS levels, ↑ in GSH, SOD and catalase levels	(Tirkey *et al.*, 2005)
Naringenin	50 mg/kg for 7 days, oral	Swiss mice	10 mmol/kg in 50% olive oil (1:1) on the 8th day, i.p.	↓ in oxidative stress (↓ in MDA, ↑ in SOD, catalase, GSH, GPX), improvement in renal histopathology (↓ in glomerular and tubular degenerations, vascular congestion, necrosis and fatty changes), ↓ in collagen deposition and TGF-β1 expression in the mesangial cells of the glomeruli and tubulointerstitial areas, ↓ in ultrastructural alterations in proximal and distal tubular epithelial cells	(Hermenean *et al.*, 2013)

3. FUTURE PERSPECTIVES

The preclinical leads for the application of flavonoids in kidney disorders are enormous. In comparison, there are only few clinical trials directed towards the clinical translation of these promising compounds. It is noteworthy that direct extrapolation of preclinical data to humans is not possible and similar outcomes cannot be expected because of the differences in age, sex, genetic makeup, dosing levels, duration, regimen with respect to disease inducing agents, route of administration, pharmacokinetic parameters, safety profile, formulation aspects, clinically relevant stage of disease, diversity among human participants in clinical trials, co-morbidities and concurrent medication profiles (Athira *et al.,* 2016). Particularly, the solubility and bioavailability of flavonoids are a major concern in product development. Moreover the criteria and design of clinical trials can significantly alter the outcomes. For example, numerous preclinical studies have demonstrated remarkable nephroprotective property of silymarin against cisplatin-induced nephrotoxicity (Shahbazi *et al.,* 2012). In agreement, administration of silymarin tablets 140 mg/bid seven days before cisplatin administration reduced cisplatin nephrotoxicity in 60 adult patients with malignancy (Momeni *et al.,* 2015). However, a clinical trial in 58 cancer patients randomized to silymarin (420 mg) or placebo plus chemotherapy (cisplatin 50-60 mg/m^2, 5-fluorouracil mg/m^2, docetaxel 60-80 mg/m^2 every 21 days) for 63 day after inclusion reported that silymarin could not prevent cisplatin-induced decline in renal function (Shahbazi *et al.,* 2015). This calls for a much needed scientific refinement of the experiments. With collective integration in the research, flavonoids could be brought into the forefront as clinically effective, safe and better tolerated nephroprotective agents from their promising preclinical results.

4. CONCLUSIONS

In conclusion, the current evidences project flavonoids as the emerging class of compounds for use in disorders of kidney. Their nephroprotective potential could be attributed to their antioxidant as well as anti-inflammatory properties. Accordingly they were able to interfere with the activation of pathways associated with renal damage such as oxidative-nitrosative-endoplasmic reticulum stress, mitochondrial dysfunction, inflammation, immune activation and apoptosis. The primary advantage with the flavonoids is their safety profile which permits the use of high doses. Refined scientific strategies need to be undertaken for successful clinical translation.

REFERENCES

Abdel Moneim Ahmed, E., Dkhil Mohamed, A. and Saleh Al-Quraishy (2011). 'The protective effect of flaxseed oil on lead acetate-induced renal toxicity in rats'. *Journal of Hazardous Materials*, 194: 250–55.

Abdelmeguid Nabila, E., Chmaisse Hania, N. and Zeinab Abuo, N.S. (2010). 'Protective effect of silymarin on cisplatin-induced nephrotoxicity in rats'. *Pak. J. Nutr.*, 9: 624–36.

Abdel-Raheem, Ihab Talat, Ahmed Ali Abdel-Ghany and Gamal Abdallah Mohamed (2009). 'Protective effect of quercetin against gentamicin-induced nephrotoxicity in rats (Pharmacology)'. *Biological & Pharmaceutical Bulletin*, 32: 61–67.

Adil, Mohammad, Kandhare Amit, D., Asjad Visnagri, and Bodhankar Subhash, L. (2015). 'Naringin ameliorates sodium arsenite-induced renal and hepatic toxicity in rats: Decisive role of KIM-1, Caspase-3, TGF-β, and TNF-α'. *Renal Failure*, 37: 1396–407.

Agarwal Namrata, Pritam Sadhukhan, Sukanya Saha and Sil Parames, C. (2015). 'Therapeutic Insights against oxidative stress induced diabetic nephropathy: A review'. *Journal of Autoimmune Disorders*.

Ahad Amjid, Ajaz Ahmad Ganai, Mohd Mujeeb and Waseem Ahmad Siddiqui (2014). 'Chrysin, an anti-inflammatory molecule, abrogates renal dysfunction in type 2 diabetic rats'. *Toxicology and Applied Pharmacology*, 279: 1–7.

Ahmad Shiekh Tanveer, Wani Arjumand, Sana Nafees, Amlesh Seth, Nemat Ali, Summya Rashid and Sarwat Sultana (2012). 'Hesperidin alleviates acetaminophen induced toxicity in Wistar rats by abrogation of oxidative stress, apoptosis and inflammation'. *Toxicology Letters*, 208: 149–61.

Ahmed Sohail, S., Napoli Kimberly, L. and Strobel Henry, W. (1995). 'Oxygen radical formation during cytochrome P450-catalyzed cyclosporine metabolism in rat and human liver microsomes at varying hydrogen ion concentrations', *Molecular and Cellular Biochemistry*, 151: 131–40.

Ahn Do Whan, Young Mook Kim, Kyoung Ryong Kim and Yang Saeng Park (1999). 'Cadmium binding and sodium-dependent solute transport in renal brush-border membrane vesicles'. *Toxicology and Applied Pharmacology*, 154: 212–18.

Ahn Tae-Gyu, Han-Kyoung Kim, So-Won Park, Soo-Ah Kim, Byoung-Rai Lee and Sei Jun Han (2014). 'Protective effects of green tea polyphenol against cisplatin-induced nephrotoxicity in rats'. *Obstetrics & Gynecology Science*, 57: 464–70.

Al-Kharusi, N., Babiker, H.A., Al-Salam, S., Waly, M.I., Nemmar, A., Al-Lawati, I., Yasin, J., Beegam, S. and Ali, B.H. (2013). 'Ellagic acid protects against cisplatin-induced nephrotoxicity in rats: a dose-dependent study'. *Eur. Rev. Med. Pharmacol Sci.*, 17: 299–310.

Al-Madani, W.A., Siddiqi, N.J. and Alhomida, A.S. (2009). 'Renal toxicity of mercuric chloride at different time intervals in rats'. *Biochemistry Insights*, 2: 37.

Almaghrabi Omar Abdulhakeem (2015). 'Molecular and biochemical investigations on the effect of quercetin on oxidative stress induced by cisplatin in rat kidney'. *Saudi Journal of Biological Sciences*, 22: 227–31.

Al-Waili Noori, Hamza Al-Waili, Thia Al-Waili and Khelod Salom (2017). 'Natural antioxidants in the treatment and prevention of diabetic nephropathy; A potential approach that warrants clinical trials'. *Redox Report*, 1–20.

Anderson Brian, J. (2008). 'Paracetamol (Acetaminophen): Mechanisms of action'. *Pediatric Anesthesia*, 18: 915–21.

Anderson Robert, L., Bishop William, E., Campbell Robert, L. and Becking George, C. (1985). 'A review of the environmental and mammalian toxicology of nitrilotriacetic acid'. *CRC Critical Reviews in Toxicology*, 15: 1–102.

Andoh Takeshi, F., Burdmann Emmanuel, A., Nora Fransechini, Houghton Donald, C. and Bennett William, M. (1996). 'Comparison of acute rapamycin nephrotoxicity with cyclosporine and FK506'. *Kidney International*, 50: 1110–17.

Anjaneyulu Muragundla and Kanwaljit Chopra (2004). 'Quercetin, an anti oxidant bioflavonoid, attenuates diabetic nephropathy in rats'. *Clinical and Experimental Pharmacology and Physiology*, 31: 244–48.

Anjaneyulu Muragundla, Naveen Tirkey and Kanwaljit Chopra (2003). 'Attenuation of cyclosporine-induced renal dysfunction by catechin: Possible antioxidant mechanism', *Renal Failure*, 25: 691–707.

Arab Hany, H., Mohamed Wafaa, R., Barakat Bassant, M. and Arafa, El-Shaimaa A. (2016). 'Tangeretin attenuates cisplatin-induced renal injury in rats: Impact on the inflammatory cascade and oxidative perturbations'. *Chemico-Biological Interactions*, 258: 205–13.

Arjumand Wani, Amlesh Seth and Sarwat Sultana (2011). 'Rutin attenuates cisplatin induced renal inflammation and apoptosis by reducing NFκB, TNF-α and caspase-3 expression in wistar rats'. *Food and Chemical Toxicology*, 49: 2013–21.

Arozal Wawaimuli, Kenichi Watanabe, Veeraveedu, Punniyakoti T., Meilei Ma, Thandavarayan Rajarajan, A., Vijayakumar Sukumaran, Kenji Suzuki, Makoto Kodama and Yoshifusa Aizawa. (2011). 'Telmisartan prevents the progression of renal injury in daunorubicin rats with the alteration of angiotensin II and endothelin-1 receptor expression associated with its PPAR-γ agonist actions'. *Toxicology*, 279: 91–99.

Aruoma Okezie, I., Neergheen Vidushi, S., Theeshan Bahorun and Jen, L-S. (2007). 'Free radicals, antioxidants and diabetes: embryopathy, retinopathy, neuropathy, nephropathy and cardiovascular complications'. *Neuroembryology and Aging*, 4: 117–37.

Ate°°ahín Ahmet, Ali Osman Çeríba°i, Abdurrauf Yuce, Özgür Bulmus and Gürkan Çikim (2007). 'Role of ellagic acid against cisplatin induced nephrotoxicity and oxidative stress in rats'. *Basic & Clinical Pharmacology & Toxicology*, 100: 121–26.

Athira, K.V., Rajaram Mohanrao Madhana and Mangala Lahkar (2016). 'Flavonoids, the emerging dietary supplement against cisplatin-induced nephrotoxicity'. *Chemico-Biological Interactions*, 248: 18–20.

Athira, K.V., Rajaram Mohanrao Madhana, Eshvendar Reddy Kasala, Pavan Kumar Samudrala, Mangala Lahkar and Ranadeep Gogoi (2016). 'Morin hydrate mitigates cisplatin induced renal and hepatic injury by impeding oxidative/nitrosative stress and inflammation in mice'. *Journal of Biochemical and Molecular Toxicology*, 30: 571–79.

Avramovic Verica, Predrag Vlahovic, Dragan Mihailovic and Vlaclisav Stefanovic (1999). 'Protective effect of a bioflavonoid proanthocyanidin-BP1 in glycerol-induced acute renal failure in the rat: Renal stereological study'. *Renal Failure*, 21: 627–34.

Badary Osama, A., Sahar Abdel-Maksoud, Ahmed Wafaa, A. and Owieda Gehan, H. (2005). 'Naringenin attenuates cisplatin nephrotoxicity in rats'. *Life Sciences*, 76: 2125–35.

Bae Eun Hui, In Jin Kim, Soo Yeon Joo, Eun Young Kim, Joon Seok Choi, Chang Seong Kim, Seong Kwon Ma, JongUn Lee and Soo Wan Kim (2014). 'Renoprotective effects of the direct renin inhibitor aliskiren on gentamicin-induced nephrotoxicity in rats'. *Journal of the Renin-Angiotensin-Aldosterone System*, 15: 348–61.

Balasubashini, M., Rukkumani, R., Viswanathan, P. and Menon Venugopal, P. (2004). 'Ferulic acid alleviates lipid peroxidation in diabetic rats'. *Phytotherapy Research*, 18: 310–14.

Barnes, J.L., Osgood, R.W., Reineck, H.J. and Stein, J.H. (1981). 'Glomerular alterations in an ischemic model of acute renal failure'. *Laboratory Investigation; A Journal of Technical Methods and Pathology*, 45: 378–86.

Basnakian Alexei, G., Apostolov Eugene, O., Xiaoyan Yin, Markus Napirei, Hans Georg Mannherz and Shah Sudhir, V. (2005). 'Cisplatin nephrotoxicity is mediated by deoxyribonuclease I'. *Journal of the American Society of Nephrology*, 16: 697–702.

Beetham, R. (2000). 'Biochemical investigation of suspected rhabdomyolysis'. *Annals of Clinical Biochemistry*, 37: 581–87.

Behling Estela, B., Sendão Milena, C., Francescato Heloísa, D.C., Antunes Lusβnia, M.G., Costa Roberto, S. and Bianchi Maria de Lourdes, P. (2006). 'Comparative study of multiple dosage of quercetin against cisplatin-induced nephrotoxicity and oxidative stress in rat kidneys'. *Pharmacological Reports,* 526–32.

Bennett William, M. (1996). 'Mechanisms of acute and chronic nephrotoxicity from immunosuppressive drugs'. *Renal Failure*, 18: 453–60.

Bharathi Erusan and Ganesan Jagadeesan (2014). 'Antioxidant potential of hesperidin and ellagic acid on renal toxicity induced by mercuric chloride in rats'. *Biomedicine & Preventive Nutrition*, 4: 131–36.

Bierhaus, A. and Nawroth, P.P. (2009). 'Multiple levels of regulation determine the role of the receptor for AGE (RAGE) as common soil in inflammation, immune responses and diabetes mellitus and its complications'. *Diabetologia*, 52: 2251–63.

Blum Ronald, H. and Carter Stephen, K. (1974). 'Adriamycin: A new anticancer drug with significant clinical activity'. *Annals of Internal Medicine*, 80: 249–59.

Bokemeyer, C., Fels, L.M., Dunn, T., Voigt, W., Gaedeke, J., Schmoll, H.J., Stolte, H. and Lentzen, H. (1996). 'Silibinin protects against cisplatin-induced nephrotoxicity without compromising cisplatin or ifosfamide anti-tumour activity'. *British Journal of Cancer*, 74: 2036.

Bonventre Joseph, V. (1988). 'Mediators of ischemic renal injury'. *Annual Review of Medicine*, 39: 531–44.

Borel Jean, F., Götz Baumann, Ian Chapman, Peter Donatsch, Alfred Fahr, Mueller Edgar, A. and Jean-Marie Vigouret (1996). '*In vivo* pharmacological effects of ciclosporin and some analogues'. *Advances in Pharmacology*, 35: 115–246.

Bowden Donald, W. (2002). 'Genetics of diabetes complications'. *Current Diabetes Reports*, 2: 191–200.

Bradl Heike (2005). *Heavy metals in the environment: Origin, interaction and remediation* (Academic Press).

Campistol Josep, M. and Sacks Steven, H. (2000). 'Mechanisms of nephrotoxicity', *Transplantation*, 69: SS5–SS10.

Chander Vikas, Devinder Singh and Kanwaljit Chopra (2002). 'Attenuation of glycerol-induced acute renal failure in rats by trimetazidine and deferoxamine'. *Pharmacology*, 67: 41–48.

Chatterjee Prabal, K., Kai Zacharowski, Salvatore Cuzzocrea, Mike Otto and Christoph Thiemermann (2000). 'Inhibitors of poly (ADP-ribose) synthetase reduce renal ischemia-reperfusion injury in the anesthetized rat *in vivo*', *The FASEB Journal*, 14: 641–51.

Chatterjee Prabal, K., Salvatore Cuzzocrea and Christoph Thiemermann (1999). 'Inhibitors of poly (ADP-ribose) synthetase protect rat proximal tubular cells against oxidant stress'. *Kidney International*, 56: 973–84.

Chen Binbin, Guangyi Liu, Peimei Zou, Xing Li, Qiufa Hao, Bei Jiang, Xiangdong Yang and Zhao Hu (2015). 'Epigallocatechin-3-gallate protects against cisplatin-induced nephrotoxicity by inhibiting endoplasmic reticulum stress-induced apoptosis'. *Experimental Biology and Medicine*, 240: 1513–19.

Chirino Yolanda, I. and José Pedraza-Chaverri (2009). 'Role of oxidative and nitrosative stress in cisplatin-induced nephrotoxicity'. *Experimental and Toxicologic Pathology*, 61: 223–42.

Chou Wen-Chien, Chunfa Jie, Kenedy Andrew, A., Jones Richard, J. Trush Michael, A. and Dang Chi, V. (2004). 'Role of NADPH oxidase in arsenic-induced reactive oxygen species formation and cytotoxicity in myeloid leukemia cells'. *Proceedings of the National Academy of Sciences of the United States of America*, 101: 4578–83.

Chtourou Yassine, Baktha Aouey, Sonia Aroui, Mohammed Kebieche and Hamadi Fetoui. (2016). 'Anti-apoptotic and anti-inflammatory effects of naringin on cisplatin-induced renal injury in the rat'. *Chemico-Biological Interactions*, 243: 1–9.

Chung Sharon, A., Brown Elizabeth, E., Williams Adrienne, H., Ramos Paula, S., Berthier Celine, C., Tushar Bhangale, Alarcon-Riquelme Marta, E., Behrens Timothy, W., Criswell Lindsey, A. and Deborah Cunninghame Graham. (2014). 'Lupus nephritis susceptibility loci in women with systemic lupus erythematosus'. *Journal of the American Society of Nephrology*: ASN, 2013050446.

Clark Kaitlyn, L., Reed Tamra, J., Wolf Sonya, J., Lori Lowe, Hodgin Jeffrey, B. and Michelle Kahlenberg, J. (2015). 'Epidermal injury promotes nephritis flare in lupus-prone mice'. *Journal of Autoimmunity*, 65: 38–48.

Clarkson, T. (1997). 'The toxicology of mercury'. *Crit. Rev. Clin. Lab. Sci.*, 34(4): 369–403. *Find this article online.*

Corcostegui, R., Labeaga, L., Arteche, J.K. and Orjales, A. (1998). 'Protective effect of hidrosmin against cisplatin induced acute nephrotoxicity in rats'. *Pharmacy and Pharmacology Communications*, 4: 465–67.

Dabak Durrin Ozlem, and Nevin Kocaman. (2015). 'Effects of silymarin on methotrexate-induced nephrotoxicity in rats'. *Renal Failure*, 37: 734–39.

Delord Jean-Pierre, Christian Puozzo, Florence Lefresne, and Roland Bugat (2009). 'Combination chemotherapy of vinorelbine and cisplatin: A phase I pharmacokinetic study in patients with metastatic solid tumors'. *Anticancer Research*, 29: 553–60.

Devrim Erdinç, Recep Çetin, Bülent Kýlýçoðlu, Imge Ergüder, B., Aslýhan Avcý and Ýlker Durak (2005). 'Methotrexate causes oxidative stress in rat kidney tissues', *Renal Failure*, 27: 771–73.

Diederich Dennis, Joseph Skopec, Alice Diederich and Fu-Xiang Dai (1994). 'Cyclosporine produces endothelial dysfunction by increased production of superoxide' *Hypertension*, 23: 957–61.

Dkhil Mohamed, A., Saleh Al-Quraishy, Aref Ahmed, M., Othman Mohamed, S., El-Deib Kamal, M. and Abdel Moneim Ahmed, E. (2013). 'The potential role of *Azadirachta indica* treatment on cisplatin-induced hepatotoxicity and oxidative stress in female rats'. *Oxidative Medicine and Cellular Longevity*, 2013.

Domitroviæ Robert, Olga Cvijanoviæ, Ester Pernjak Pugel, Gordana Blagojeviæ Zagorac, Hana Mahmutefendiæ and Marko Škoda (2013). 'Luteolin ameliorates cisplatin-induced nephrotoxicity in mice through inhibition of platinum accumulation, inflammation and apoptosis in the kidney'. *Toxicology*, 310: 115–23.

Eldaif Shady, M., Deneve Jeremiah, A., Ning Ping Wang, Rong Jiang, Mario Mosunjac, Mutrie Christopher, J., Guyton Robert, A., Zhi Qing Zhao and Jakob Vinten Johansen (2010). 'Attenuation of renal ischemia–reperfusion injury by postconditioning involves adenosine receptor and protein kinase C activation'. *Transplant International*, 23: 217–26.

El-Shitany Nagla, A., Sahar El-Haggar and Karema El-Desoky (2008). 'Silymarin prevents adriamycin-induced cardiotoxicity and nephrotoxicity in rats'. *Food and Chemical Toxicology*, 46: 2422–28.

Emeigh Hart, S.G., Beierschmitt William, P., Stuart Wyand, D., Khairallah Edward, A. and Cohen Steven, D. (1994). 'Acetaminophen nephrotoxicity in CD-1 mice: I. Evidence of a role for *in situ* activation in selective covalent binding and toxicity'. *Toxicology and Applied Pharmacology*, 126: 267–75.

Esteban Vanesa, Oscar Lorenzo, Mónica Rupérez, Yusuke Suzuki, Sergio Mezzano, Julia Blanco, Mathias Kretzler, Takeshi Sugaya, Jesús Egido and Marta Ruiz-Ortega (2004). 'Angiotensin II, *via* AT1 and AT2 receptors and NF-κB pathway, regulates the inflammatory response in unilateral ureteral obstruction'. *Journal of the American Society of Nephrology*, 15: 1514–29.

Evans Joseph, L., Goldfine Ira, D. Maddux Betty, A. and Grodsky Gerold, M. (2002). 'Oxidative stress and stress-activated signaling pathways: A unifying hypothesis of type 2 diabetes'. *Endocrine Reviews*, 23: 599–622.

Fadillioglu Ersin, Emin Oztas, Hasan Erdogan, Murat Yagmurca, Sadik Sogut, Muharrem Ucar and Kemal Irmak, M. (2004). 'Protective effects of caffeic acid phenethyl ester on doxorubicin induced cardiotoxicity in rats'. *Journal of Applied Toxicology*, 24: 47–52.

Fallahzadeh Mohammad Kazem, Banafshe Dormanesh, Mohammad Mahdi Sagheb, Jamshid Roozbeh, Ghazal Vessal, Maryam Pakfetrat, Yahya Daneshbod, Eskandar Kamali-Sarvestani and Lankarani Kamran, B. (2012). 'Effect of addition of silymarin to renin-angiotensin system inhibitors on proteinuria in type 2 diabetic patients with overt nephropathy: A randomized, double-blind, placebo-controlled trial'. *American Journal of Kidney Diseases*, 60: 896–903.

Finn William, F. (1981). 'Nephron heterogeneity in polyuric acute renal failure'. *Journal of Laboratory and Clinical Medicine,*

Finotti, P. and Palatini, P. (1986). 'Reduction of erythrocyte (Na+-K+) ATPase activity in type 1 (insulin-dependent) diabetic subjects and its activation by homologous plasma', *Diabetologia*, 29: 623–28.

Fouad Amr, A., Albuali Waleed, H., Ahmed Zahran and Wafaey Gomaa (2014). 'Protective effect of naringenin against gentamicin-induced nephrotoxicity in rats'. *Environmental Toxicology and Pharmacology*, 38: 420–29.

Francescato Helo, Iacute sa D Coletta, Coimbra Terezila, M., Costa Roberto, S. and Bianchi Maria de, L.P. (2004). 'Protective effect of quercetin on the evolution of cisplatin-induced acute tubular necrosis'. *Kidney and Blood Pressure Research*, 27: 148–58.

Gaedeke, J., Fels, L.M., Bokemeyer, C., Mengs, U., Stolte, H. and Lentzen, H. (1996). 'Cisplatin nephrotoxicity and protection by silibinin'. *Nephrology Dialysis Transplantation*, 11: 55–62.

Ghosh Ayantika and Sil Parames, C. (2007). 'Anti-oxidative effect of a protein from *Cajanus indicus* L. against acetaminophen-induced hepato-nephro toxicity'. *Journal of Biochemistry and Molecular Biology*, 40: 1039.

Gloire Geoffrey, Sylvie Legrand-Poels and Jacques Piette (2006). 'NF-κB activation by reactive oxygen species: Fifteen years later'. *Biochemical Pharmacology*, 72: 1493–505.

Go Ronald, S. and Adjei Alex, A. (1999). 'Review of the comparative pharmacology and clinical activity of cisplatin and carboplatin'. *Journal of Clinical Oncology*, 17: 409–22.

Go Young-Mi, and Jones Dean, P. (2008). 'Redox compartmentalization in eukaryotic cells'. *Biochimica et Biophysica Acta (BBA)-General Subjects*, 1780: 1273–90.

Gomes Isabele Beserra Santos, Marcella Leite Porto, Maria Carmen Lopes Ferreira Silva Santos, Bianca Prandi Campagnaro, Agata Lages Gava, Silvana Santos Meyrelles, Thiago Melo Costa Pereira and Vasquez Elisardo, C. (2015). 'The protective effects of oral low-dose quercetin on diabetic nephropathy in hypercholesterolemic mice'. *Frontiers in Physiology*, 6: 247.

Gomes Isabele, B.S., Porto Marcella, L., Santos Maria Carmen, L.F.S., Campagnaro Bianca, P. Pereira Thiago, M.C., Meyrelles Silvana, S. and Vasquez Elisardo, C. (2014). 'Renoprotective, anti-oxidative and anti-apoptotic effects of oral low-dose quercetin in the C57BL/6J model of diabetic nephropathy'. *Lipids in Health and Disease*, 13: 184.

Hamad Rania, Calpurnia Jayakumar, Punithavathi Ranganathan, Riyaz Mohamed, El Hamamy Mahmoud, M.I., Dessouki Amina, A., Abdelazim Ibrahim and Ganesan Ramesh (2015). 'Honey feeding protects kidney against cisplatin nephrotoxicity through suppression of inflammation'. *Clinical and Experimental Pharmacology and Physiology*, 42: 843–48.

Hamazaki Shuji, Shigeru Okada, Yoshihito Ebina and Osamu Midorikawa (1985). 'Acute renal failure and glucosuria induced by ferric nitrilotriacetate in rats'. *Toxicology and Applied Pharmacology*, 77: 267–74.

Hase Michiyo, Tetsuya Babazono, Sachiko Karibe, Naohide Kinae and Yasuhiko Iwamoto. (2006). 'Renoprotective effects of tea catechin in streptozotocin-induced diabetic rats', *International Urology and Nephrology*, 38: 693.

Hassan Samar, M., Khalaf Marwa, M., Sadek Sawsan, A. and Abo-Youssef Amira, M. (2017). 'Protective effects of apigenin and myricetin against cisplatin-induced nephrotoxicity in mice'. *Pharmaceutical Biology*, 55: 766–74.

He Xuexiu, Chunmei Li, Zhengkai Wei, Jingjing Wang, Jinhua Kou, Weijian Liu, Mingyu Shi, Zhengtao Yang and Yunhe Fu. (2016). 'Protective role of apigenin in cisplatin-induced renal injury'. *European Journal of Pharmacology*, 789: 215–21.

He Zhenli, L., Yang Xiaoe, E. and Stoffella Peter, J. (2005). 'Trace elements in agroecosystems and impacts on the environment', *Journal of Trace Elements in Medicine and Biology*, 19: 125–40.

Henderson Edward, S., Adamson Richard, H., Charlene Denham and Oliverio Vincent, T. (1965). 'The metabolic fate of tritiated methotrexate'. *Cancer Research*, 25: 1008–17.

Hermenean Anca, Aurel Ardelean, Miruna Stan, Hildegard Herman, Ciprian-Valentin Mihali, Marieta Costache and Anca Dinischiotu (2013). 'Protective effects of naringenin on carbon tetrachloride-induced acute nephrotoxicity in mouse kidney'. *Chemico-Biological Interactions*, 205: 138–47.

Hu Howard (2000). 'Exposure to metals', *Primary care: Clinics in Office Practice*, 27: 983–96.

Huang Wen-Yan, Zu-Guo Li, Horea Rus, Xiaoyan Wang, Jose Pedro, A. and Shi-You Chen (2009). 'RGC-32 mediates transforming growth factor-β-induced epithelial-mesenchymal transition in human renal proximal tubular cells'. *Journal of Biological Chemistry*, 284: 9426–32.

Humes, H.D. and Weinberg, J.M. (1986). 'Toxic nephropathies', *The Kidney*, 2: 1491–532.

Jadhav, S.H., Sarkar, S.N., Patil, R.D. and Tripathi, H.C. (2007). 'Effects of subchronic exposure *via* drinking water to a mixture of eight water-contaminating metals: A biochemical and histopathological study in male rats'. *Archives of Environmental Contamination and Toxicology*, 53: 667–77.

Jain Dilpesh, P. and Somani, Rahul S. (2014). 'Hesperidin ameliorates streptozotocin and high fat diet induced diabetic nephropathy in rats'. *Journal of Experimental and Integrative Medicine*, 4: 261–67.

Jain Sanyog, Jain Amit, K., Milind Pohekar and Kaushik Thanki (2013). 'Novel self-emulsifying formulation of quercetin for improved *in vivo* antioxidant potential: Implications for drug-induced cardiotoxicity and nephrotoxicity'. *Free Radical Biology and Medicine*, 65: 117–30.

Jiang Tao, Fei Tian, Hongting Zheng, Whitman Samantha, A., Yifeng Lin, Zhigang Zhang, Nong Zhang and Zhang Donna, D. (2014). 'Nrf2 suppresses lupus nephritis through inhibition of oxidative injury and the NF-κB-mediated inflammatory response'. *Kidney International*, 85: 333–43.

Jonnalagadda, V.P., Srinivas Pittala, Mangala Lahkar and Vattikundala Pradeep (2013). 'Ameliorative effect of morin hydrate, a flavonoid against gentamicin induced oxidative stress and nephrotoxicity in sprague-dawley rats'. *Int. J. Pharm. Pharm. Sci.*, 6: 851–56.

Jorgensen, Ann L. (2013). 'Contrast-induced nephropathy: Pathophysiology and preventive strategies'. *Critical Care Nurse*, 33: 37–46.

Ju Sung Min, Jun Gue Kang, Jun Sang Bae, Hyun Ock Pae, Yeoung Su Lyu, and Byung Hun Jeon (2015). 'The flavonoid apigenin ameliorates cisplatin-induced nephrotoxicity through reduction of p53 activation and promotion of PI3K/Akt pathway in human renal proximal tubular epithelial cells'. *Evidence-Based Complementary and Alternative Medicine*, 2015.

Kaltalioglu Kaan and Sule Coskun-Cevher (2016). 'Potential of morin and hesperidin in the prevention of cisplatin-induced nephrotoxicity'. *Renal Failure*, 38: 1291–99.

Kamalakkannan, N. and Prince, P. (2006). 'The influence of rutin on the extracellular matrix in streptozotocin induced diabetic rat kidney' *Journal of Pharmacy and Pharmacology*, 58: 1091–98.

Kamel Kamel, M., Abd El Raouf, Ola, M., Metwally Salwa, A., Abd El Latif, Hekma, A. and El sayed Mostafa, E. (2014). 'Hesperidin and rutin, antioxidant citrus flavonoids, attenuate cisplatin induced nephrotoxicity in rats'. *Journal of Biochemical and Molecular Toxicology*, 28: 312–19.

Kandasamy Neelamegam and Natarajan Ashokkumar (2012). 'Myricetin, a natural flavonoid, normalizes hyperglycemia in streptozotocin-cadmium-induced experimental diabetic nephrotoxic rats'. *Biomedicine & Preventive Nutrition*, 2: 246–51.

Kang Hee-Kap, Diane Ecklund, Michael Liu and Datta Syamal, K. (2009). 'Apigenin, a non-mutagenic dietary flavonoid, suppresses lupus by inhibiting autoantigen presentation for expansion of autoreactive Th1 and Th17 cells'. *Arthritis Research & Therapy*, 11: R59.

Kang Kyung Pyo, Sung Kwang Park, Duk Hoon Kim, Mi Jeong Sung, Yu Jin Jung, Ae Sin Lee, Jung Eun Lee, Kunka Mohanram Ramkumar, Sik Lee and Moon Hyang Park. (2011). 'Luteolin ameliorates cisplatin-induced acute kidney injury in mice by regulation of p53-dependent renal tubular apoptosis'. *Nephrology Dialysis Transplantation*, 26: 814–22.

Karuppagounder Vengadeshprabhu, Somasundaram Arumugam, Rajarajan Amirthalingam Thandavarayan, Vigneshwaran Pitchaimani, Remya Sreedhar, Rejina Afrin, Meilei Harima, Hiroshi Suzuki, Kenji Suzuki and Masahiko Nakamura (2015). 'Naringenin ameliorates daunorubicin induced nephrotoxicity by mitigating AT1R, ERK1/2-NFκB p65 mediated inflammation'. *International Immunopharmacology*, 28: 154–59.

Kokilavani Vedagiri, Muthuswamy Anusuya Devi, Kumarasamy Sivarajan and Chinnakkannu Panneerselvam (2005). 'Combined efficacies of dl-α-lipoic acid and meso 2, 3 dimercaptosuccinic acid against arsenic induced toxicity in antioxidant systems of rats'. *Toxicology Letters*, 160: 1–7.

Kolli, W.K., Premila Abraham, Bina Isaac and Dhayakani Selvakumar (2009). 'Neutrophil infiltration and oxidative stress may play a critical role in methotrexate-induced renal damage'. *Chemotherapy*, 55: 83–90.

Korkmaz, Aslý and Dürdane Kolankaya (2013). 'Inhibiting inducible nitric oxide synthase with rutin reduces renal ischemia/reperfusion injury'. *Can. J. Surg*, 56: 7.

Kovacic Peter and Jacintho Jason, D. (2003). 'Systemic lupus erythematosus and other autoimmune diseases from endogenous and exogenous agents: Unifying theme of oxidative stress'. *Mini Reviews in Medicinal Chemistry*, 3: 568–75.

Kuhlmann Martin, K., Ernst Horsch, Gunther Burkhardt, Martina Wagner and Hans Köhler (1998). 'Reduction of cisplatin toxicity in cultured renal tubular cells by the bioflavonoid quercetin' *Archives of Toxicology*, 72: 536–40.

Lee Chang Ki, Seung Hwa Son, Kwang Kyun Park, Jung Han Yoon Park, Soon Sung Lim and Won Yoon Chung (2008). 'Isoliquiritigenin inhibits tumor growth and protects the kidney and liver against chemotherapy-induced toxicity in a mouse xenograft model of colon carcinoma'. *Journal of Pharmacological Sciences*, 106: 444–51.

Lee Chang Ki, Seung Hwa Son, Kwang Kyun Park, Jung Han Yoon Park, Soon Sung Lim, Sook Hyang Kim and Won Yoon Chung (2008). 'Licochalcone a inhibits the growth of colon carcinoma and attenuates cisplatin induced toxicity without a loss of chemotherapeutic efficacy in mice'. *Basic & Clinical Pharmacology & Toxicology*, 103: 48–54.

Lee In-Chul, Sung-Hwan Kim, Sang-Min Lee, Hyung-Seon Baek, Changjong Moon, Sung-Ho Kim, Seung-Chun Park, Hyoung-Chin Kim and Jong-Choon Kim (2012). 'Melatonin attenuates gentamicin-induced nephrotoxicity and oxidative stress in rats'. *Archives of Toxicology*, 86: 1527–36.

Li Cheng-zhen, Hai-hong Jin, Hong-xin Sun, Zhong-zhe Zhang, Jia-xin Zheng, Shu-hua Li, and Seong-ho Han (2016). 'Eriodictyol attenuates cisplatin-induced kidney injury by inhibiting oxidative stress and inflammation'. *European Journal of Pharmacology*, 772: 124–30.

Li Yuan, Min Ling, Yuan Xu, Shoulin Wang, Zhong Li, Jianwei Zhou, Xinru Wang and Qizhan Liu (2010). 'The repressive effect of NF-κB on p53 by Mot-2 is involved in human keratinocyte transformation induced by low levels of arsenite'. *Toxicological Sciences*, kfq109.

Lim Sung-Chul, Young-Bin Im, Chun-Sik Bae, Song Iy Han, Se-Eun Kim and Hyo-Kyung Han (2008). 'Protective effect of morin on the imipenem-induced nephrotoxicity in rabbits'. *Archives of Pharmacal Research*, 31: 1060–65.

Lin Aijun, Xuhong Zhang, Yong Guan Zhu and Fang Jie Zhao (2008). 'Arsenate induced toxicity: Effects on antioxidative enzymes and DNA damage in *Vicia faba*'. *Environmental Toxicology and Chemistry*, 27: 413–19.

Lina Santaguida, P., Cynthia Balion, Dereck Hunt, Katherine Morrison, Hertzel Gerstein, Parminder Raina, Lynda Booker and Hossein Yazdi (2005). 'Diagnosis, prognosis, and treatment of impaired glucose tolerance and impaired fasting glucose'. *Evid. Rep. Technol. Assess. (Summ)*, 128.

Liu Chan-Min, Jie-Qiong Ma and Yun-Zhi Sun (2010). 'Quercetin protects the rat kidney against oxidative stress-mediated DNA damage and apoptosis induced by lead'. *Environmental Toxicology and Pharmacology*, 30: 264–71.

Liu Chan-Min, Yun-Zhi Sun, Jian-Mei Sun, Jie-Qiong Ma and Chao Cheng (2012). 'Protective role of quercetin against lead-induced inflammatory response in rat kidney through the ROS-mediated MAPKs and NF-κB pathway'. *Biochimica et Biophysica Acta (BBA)-General Subjects*, 1820: 1693–703.

Liu Miao, Shigeru Okada and Teruyuki Kawabata (1991). 'Radical-promoting" free" iron level in the serum of rats treated with ferric nitrilotriacetate: Comparison with other iron chelate complexes'. *Acta Medica Okayama*, 45: 401–08.

Lock Edward, A. and Reed Celia, J. (1998). 'Xenobiotic metabolizing enzymes of the kidney'. *Toxicologic Pathology*, 26: 18–25.

Maher Pamela, Richard Dargusch, Ehren Jennifer, L., Shinichi Okada, Kumar Sharma and David Schubert (2011). 'Fisetin lowers methylglyoxal dependent protein glycation and limits the complications of diabetes'. *PLoS ONE*, 6: e21226.

Malarkodi Kumaravel Palanichamy, Andithangal Venkatesan Balachandar and Palaninathan Varalakshmi (2003). 'The influence of lipoic acid on adriamycin-induced hyperlipidemic nephrotoxicity in rats' *Molecular and Cellular Biochemistry*, 247: 139–45.

Malik Salma, Jagriti Bhatia, Kapil Suchal, Nanda Gamad, Amit Kumar Dinda, Yogender Kumar Gupta and Dharamvir Singh Arya (2015). 'Nobiletin ameliorates cisplatin-induced acute kidney injury due to its anti-oxidant, anti-inflammatory and anti-apoptotic effects'. *Experimental and Toxicologic Pathology*, 67: 427–33.

Mathew, T.H. (1992). 'Drug-induced renal disease'. *The Medical Journal of Australia*, 156: 724–28.

Mershiba Sam Daniel, Velayutham Dassprakash, M. and Sundara Dhakshinamurthy Saraswathy (2013). 'Protective effect of naringenin on hepatic and renal dysfunction and oxidative stress in arsenic intoxicated rats' *Molecular Biology Reports*, 40: 3681–91.

Milton Prabu, S. and Muthumani, M. (2012). 'Silibinin ameliorates arsenic induced nephrotoxicity by abrogation of oxidative stress, inflammation and apoptosis in rats'. *Molecular Biology Reports*, 39: 11201–16.

Mishra Deepshikha and Flora, S.J.S. (2008). 'Quercetin administration during chelation therapy protects arsenic-induced oxidative stress in mice'. *Biological Trace Element Research*, 122: 137–47.

Momeni Ali, Ali Hajigholami, Shohreh Geshnizjani and Soleiman Kheiri (2015). 'Effect of silymarin in the prevention of cisplatin nephrotoxicity'. *A Clinical Trial Study*.

Montgomery Bissell, D. (1998). 'Hepatic fibrosis as wound repair: A progress report'. *Journal of Gastroenterology*, 33: 295–302.

Morales, A.I., Vicente-Sanchez, C., Santiago Sandoval, J.M., Egido, J., Mayoral, P., Arévalo, M.A., Fernández-Tagarro, M., López-Novoa, J.M. and Pérez-Barriocanal, F. (2006). 'Protective effect of quercetin on experimental chronic cadmium nephrotoxicity in rats is based on its antioxidant properties'. *Food and Chemical Toxicology*, 44: 2092–100.

Morgan Philip, E., Sturgess Allan, D., Annemarie Hennessy and Davies Michael, J. (2007). 'Serum protein oxidation and apolipoprotein CIII levels in people with systemic lupus erythematosus with and without nephritis'. *Free Radical Research*, 41: 1301–12.

Moss Nicholas, G., Powell Susan, L. and Falk Ronald, J. (1985). 'Intravenous cyclosporine activates afferent and efferent renal nerves and causes sodium retention in innervated kidneys in rats'. *Proceedings of the National Academy of Sciences*, 82: 8222–26.

Nassar Inthisham, Thanikachalam Pasupati, John Paul Judson and Ignacio Segarra (2009). 'Reduced exposure of imatinib after coadministration with acetaminophen in mice'. *Indian Journal of Pharmacology*, 41: 167.

Nava Mayerly, Freddy Romero, Yasmir Quiroz, Gustavo Parra, Lizette Bonet and Bernardo Rodríguez-Iturbe (2000). 'Melatonin attenuates acute renal failure and oxidative stress induced by mercuric chloride in rats' *American Journal of Physiology-Renal Physiology*, 279: F910–F18.

Negrette-Guzmán Mario, Sara Huerta-Yepez, Omar Noel Medina-Campos, Zyanya Lucía Zatarain-Barrón, Rogelio Hernández-Pando, Ismael Torres, Edilia Tapia and José Pedraza-Chaverri (2013). 'Sulforaphane attenuates gentamicin-induced nephrotoxicity: Role of mitochondrial protection'. *Evidence-Based Complementary and Alternative Medicine*, 2013.

Nelson Sidney, D. (1995). 'Mechanisms of the formation and disposition of reactive metabolites that can cause acute liver injury'. *Drug Metabolism Reviews*, 27: 147–77.

Nikolic Jelenka and Dusan Sokolovic (2004). 'Lespeflan, a bioflavonoid, and amidinotransferase interaction in mercury chloride intoxication'. *Renal Failure*, 26: 607–11.

Ninsontia Chuanpit, Kanittha Pongjit, Chatchai Chaotham and Pithi Chanvorachote (2011). 'Silymarin selectively protects human renal cells from cisplatin-induced cell death'. *Pharmaceutical Biology*, 49: 1082–90.

Nonoliguric, A.R.F. (1993). 'Pathophysiology of experimental nonoliguric acute renal failure'. *Kidney International*, 43: 513–21.

Norberg Gunnar, F. and Keitaro Nishiyama (1972). 'Whole-body and hair retention of cadmium in mice: Including an autoradiographic study on organ distribution'. *Archives of Environmental Health: An International Journal*, 24: 209–14.

Nordberg Gunnar, F. (1984). 'Chelating agents and cadmium toxicity: Problems and prospects', *Environmental Health Perspectives*, 54: 213.

O'Flaherty Ellen, J., Adams Wayne, D., Hammond Paul, B. and Elizabeth Taylor. (1986). 'Resistance of the rat to development of lead induced renal functional deficits'. *Journal of Toxicology and Environmental Health, Part A Current Issues*, 18: 61–75.

Ojo, O.O., Kabutu, F.R., Bello, M. and Babayo, U. (2006). 'Inhibition of paracetamol-induced oxidative stress in rats by extracts of lemongrass (*Cymbopogon citratus*) and green tea (*Camellia sinensis*) in rats'. *African Journal of Biotechnology*, 5.

Ozcan Filiz, Aslý Ozmen, Bahar Akkaya, Yakup Aliciguzel and Mutay Aslan (2012). 'Beneficial effect of myricetin on renal functions in streptozotocin-induced diabetes', *Clinical and Experimental Medicine*, 12: 265–72.

Ozols Robert, F. and Young Robert, C. (1985). 'High-dose cisplatin therapy in ovarian cancer', *Semin Oncol*, 12: 21–30.

Palabiyik Saziye Sezin, Busra Dincer, Elif Cadirci, Irfan Cinar, Cemal Gundogdu, Beyzagul Polat, Muhammed Yayla and Zekai Halici (2017). 'A new update for radiocontrast-induced nephropathy aggravated with glycerol in rats: The protective potential of epigallocatechin-3-gallate'. *Renal Failure*, 39: 314–22.

Pan Hao, Jun Chen, Kezhen Shen, Xueping Wang, Ping Wang, Guanghou Fu, Hongzhou Meng, Yimin Wang and Baiye Jin (2015). 'Mitochondrial modulation by Epigallocatechin 3-Gallate ameliorates cisplatin induced renal injury through decreasing oxidative/ nitrative stress, inflammation and NF-kB in mice'. *PloS ONE*, 10: e0124775.

Perazella Mark, A. (1999). 'Crystal-induced acute renal failure'. *The American Journal of Medicine*, 106: 459–65.

Perazella Mark, A. and Moeckel, Gilbert W. (2010). "Nephrotoxicity from chemotherapeutic agents: Clinical manifestations, pathobiology, and prevention/therapy." In *Seminars in nephrology*, Elsevier. pp. 570–81.

Qi Min-You, Hao-Ran Liu, Yan-hui Su and Su-Qing Yu. (2011). 'Protective effect of Icariin on the early stage of experimental diabetic nephropathy induced by streptozotocin *via* modulating transforming growth factor β 1 and type IV collagen expression in rats'. *Journal of Ethnopharmacology*, 138: 731–36.

Randall Bond, G., Wiegand Christopher, B. and Hite Ladonna, K. (2003). 'The difficulty of risk assessment for hepatic injury associated with supra-therapeutic acetaminophen use'. *Veterinary and Human Toxicology*, 45: 150–53.

Ratliff Brian, B., Wasan Abdulmahdi, Rahul Pawar and Wolin Michael, S. (2016). 'Oxidant mechanisms in renal injury and disease', *Antioxidants & Redox Signaling*, 25: 119–46.

Ratnaike Ranjit Nihal. (2003). 'Acute and chronic arsenic toxicity'. *Postgraduate Medical Journal*, 79: 391–96.

Renugadevi, J. and Milton Prabu, S. (2009). 'Naringenin protects against cadmium-induced oxidative renal dysfunction in rats'. *Toxicology*, 256: 128–34.

Renugadevi, J. and Milton Prabu, S. (2010). 'Quercetin protects against oxidative stress-related renal dysfunction by cadmium in rats'. *Experimental and Toxicologic Pathology*, 62: 471–81.

Rizvi Saliha, Syed Tasleem Raza, and Farzana Mahdi (2014). 'Association of genetic variants with diabetic nephropathy'. *World J. Diabetes*, 5: 809–16.

Sadat Umar (2013). 'Radiographic contrast-media-induced acute kidney injury: Pathophysiology and prophylactic strategies'. *ISRN Radiology*, 2013.

Sahin Kazim, Mehmet Tuzcu, Hasan Gencoglu, Ayhan Dogukan, Mustafa Timurkan, Nurhan Sahin, Abdullah Aslan, and Omer Kucuk (2010). 'Epigallocatechin-3-gallate activates Nrf2/HO-1 signaling pathway in cisplatin-induced nephrotoxicity in rats'. *Life Sciences*, 87: 240–45.

Sahu Bidya Dhar, Anil Kumar Kalvala, Meghana Koneru, Jerald Mahesh Kumar, Madhusudana Kuncha, Shyam Sunder Rachamalla and Ramakrishna Sistla (2014). 'Ameliorative effect of fisetin on cisplatin-induced nephrotoxicity in rats *via* modulation of NF-κB activation and antioxidant defence'. *PLoS ONE*, 9: e105070.

Sahu Bidya Dhar, Jerald Mahesh Kumar and Ramakrishna Sistla (2015). 'Baicalein, a bioflavonoid, prevents cisplatin-induced acute kidney injury by up-regulating antioxidant defenses and down-regulating the MAPKs and NF-κB pathways'. *PloS ONE*, 10: e0134139.

Sahu Bidya Dhar, Madhusudana Kuncha, Jeevana Sindhura, G. and Ramakrishna Sistla (2013). 'Hesperidin attenuates cisplatin-induced acute renal injury by decreasing oxidative stress, inflammation and DNA damage'. *Phytomedicine*, 20: 453–60.

Sahu Bidya Dhar, Srujana Tatireddy, Meghana Koneru, Borkar Roshan, M., Jerald Mahesh Kumar, Madhusudana Kuncha, Srinivas, R. and Ramakrishna Sistla (2014). 'Naringin ameliorates gentamicin-induced nephrotoxicity and associated mitochondrial dysfunction, apoptosis and inflammation in rats: Possible mechanism of nephroprotection'. *Toxicology and Applied Pharmacology*, 277: 8–20.

Sanchez-Gonzalez, Penelope, D., Francisco, J., Lopez-Hernandez, Fernando Perez-Barriocanal, Morales Ana, I. and Lopez-Novoa Jose, M. (2011). 'Quercetin reduces cisplatin nephrotoxicity in rats without compromising its anti-tumour activity'. *Nephrology Dialysis Transplantation,* gfr195.

Satyanarayana, P.S., Singh, D. and Chopra, K. (2001). 'Quercetin, a bioflavonoid, protects against oxidative stress-related renal dysfunction by cyclosporine in rats'. *Methods Find Exp. Clin. Pharmacol.*, 23: 175–81.

Seeliger Erdmann, Mauricio Sendeski, Rihal Charanjit, S. and Persson, Pontus B. (2012). 'Contrast-induced kidney injury: Mechanisms, risk factors, and prevention'. *European Heart Journal*, 33: 2007–15.

Shahbazi Foroud, Sanambar Sadighi, Simin Dashti Khavidaki, Farhad Shahi, Mehrzad Mirzania, Alireza Abdollahi and Mohammad Hossein Ghahremani (2015). 'Effect of silymarin administration on cisplatin nephrotoxicity: Report from A Pilot, Randomized, Double Blinded, Placebo Controlled Clinical Trial', *Phytotherapy Research*.

Shahbazi Foroud, Simin Dashti-Khavidaki, Hossein Khalili and Mahboob Lessan-Pezeshki (2012). 'Potential renoprotective effects of silymarin against nephrotoxic drugs: A review of literature', *Journal of Pharmacy & Pharmaceutical Sciences*, 15: 112–23.

Sheela Nagarajan, Manonmani Alvin Jose, Duraiswami Sathyamurthy and Balasubramanian Nandha Kumar (2013). 'Effect of silymarin on streptozotocin-nicotinamide-induced type 2 diabetic nephropathy in rats'. *Iranian Journal of Kidney Diseases*, 7: 117.

Shifow, A.A., Kumar, K.V., Naidu, M.U.R. and Ratnakar, K.S. (2000). 'Melatonin, a pineal hormone with antioxidant property, protects against gentamicin-induced nephrotoxicity in rats'. *Nephron*, 85: 167–74.

Shimoi Kayoko, Bingrong Shen, Shinya Toyokuni, Rika Mochizuki, Michiyo Furugori and Naohide Kinae (1997). 'Protection by α G Rutin, a water soluble antioxidant flavonoid, against renal damage in mice treated with ferric nitrilotriacetate'. *Cancer Science*, 88: 453–60.

Shoskes Daniel, A. (1998). 'Effect of bioflavonoids quercetin and curcumin on ischemic renal injury: A new class of renoprotective agents1'. *Transplantation*, 66: 147–52.

Singh Devinder and Kanwaljit Chopra. (2004). 'The effect of naringin, a bioflavonoid on ischemia-reperfusion induced renal injury in rats'. *Pharmacological Research*, 50: 187–93.

Singh Devinder, Rajnendrapal Kaur, Vikas Chander and Kanwaljit Chopra. (2006). 'Antioxidants in the prevention of renal disease'. *Journal of Medicinal Food*, 9: 443–50.

Singh Devinder, Vikas Chander and Kanwaljit Chopra (2004a). 'Protective effect of naringin, a bioflavonoid on ferric nitrilotriacetate-induced oxidative renal damage in rat kidney', *Toxicology*, 201: 1–8.

Singh Devinder, Vikas Chander and Kanwaljit Chopra (2004b). 'Protective effect of naringin, a bioflavonoid on glycerol-induced acute renal failure in rat kidney'. *Toxicology*, 201: 143–51.

Singh Devinder, Vikas Chander and Kanwaljit Chopra (2005). 'Protective effect of catechin on ischemia-reperfusion-induced renal injury in rats'. *Pharmacol. Rep.*, 57: 70–76.

Singh Jyotsna, Chaudhari, Bhushan P. and Poonam Kakkar. (2017). 'Baicalin and chrysin mixture imparts cyto-protection against methylglyoxal induced cytotoxicity and diabetic tubular injury by modulating RAGE, oxidative stress and inflammation'. *Environmental Toxicology and Pharmacology*, 50: 67–75.

Singh Vikas Chander and Kanwaljit Chopra (2003). 'Catechin, a natural antioxidant protects against rhabdomyolysis-induced myoglobinuric acute renal failure'. *Pharmacological Research*, 48: 503–09.

Sinha Mahua, Prasenjit Manna and Sil Parames, C. (2008). 'Arjunolic acid attenuates arsenic-induced nephrotoxicity'. *Pathophysiology*, 15: 147–56.

Sirovina Damir, Nada Oršoliæ, Gordana Gregoroviæ and Marijana Zovko Konèiæ (2016). 'Naringenin ameliorates pathological changes in liver and kidney of diabetic mice: A preliminary study/Naringenin reducira histopatološke promjene u jetri i bubregu miševa s dijabetesom'. *Archives of Industrial Hygiene and Toxicology*, 67: 19–24.

Slater, T.F. (1982). "Lipid peroxidation." *In*: Portland Press Limited.

Soto, C., Pérez, J., García, V., Uría, E., Vadillo, M. and Raya, L. (2010). 'Effect of silymarin on kidneys of rats suffering from alloxan-induced diabetes mellitus'. *Phytomedicine*, 17: 1090–94.

Spranger Joachim, Anja Kroke, Matthias Möhlig, Kurt Hoffmann, Bergmann, Michael Ristow, Heiner Boeing and Pfeiffer Andreas, F.H. (2003). 'Inflammatory cytokines and the risk to develop type 2 diabetes'. *Diabetes*, 52: 812–17.

Stefanovic Vladisav, Vojin Savic, Predrag Vlahovic, Tatjana Cvetkovic, Stevo Najman and Marina Mitic-Zlatkovic (2000). 'Reversal of experimental myoglobinuric acute renal failure with bioflavonoids from seeds of grape'. *Renal Failure*, 22: 255–66.

Sung Mi Jeong, Duk Hoon Kim, Yu Jin Jung, Kyung Pyo Kang, Ae Sin Lee, Sik Lee, Won Kim, Munkhtugs Davaatseren, Jin-Taek Hwang and Hyun-Jin Kim (2008). 'Genistein protects the kidney from cisplatin-induced injury', *Kidney international*, 74: 1538-47.

Tanner, GA, and M Steinhausen. 1976. 'Tubular obstruction in ischemia-induced acute renal failure in the rat', *Kidney international. Supplement*, 6: S65.

Tariq, Mohammad, Christudas Morais, Samia Sobki, Mohammed Al Sulaiman, and Khader Abdullah, A.L. (2000). 'Effect of lithium on cyclosporin induced nephrotoxicity in rats'. *Renal Failure*, 22: 545–60.

Tchounwou Paul, B., Yedjou Clement, G. Patlolla Anita, K. and Sutton Dwayne, J. (2012). 'Heavy metal toxicity and the environment.' *In*: *Molecular, Clinical and Environmental Toxicology* (Springer).

Testa Roberto, Anna Rita Bonfigli, Stefano Genovese, Valeria De Nigris and Antonio Ceriello (2016). 'The possible role of flavonoids in the prevention of diabetic complications'. *Nutrients*, 8: 310.

Tirkey Naveen, Sangeeta Pilkhwal, Anurag Kuhad and Kanwaljit Chopra (2005). 'Hesperidin, a citrus bioflavonoid, decreases the oxidative stress produced by carbon tetrachloride in rat liver and kidney'. *BMC Pharmacology*, 5: 2.

Tsai Pei-Yi, Shuk-Man Ka, Jia-Ming Chang, Hsiang-Cheng Chen, Hao-Ai Shui, Chen-Yun Li, Kuo-Feng Hua, Wen-Liang Chang, Jiann-Jyh Huang and Sung-Sen Yang (2011). 'Epigallocatechin-3-gallate prevents lupus nephritis development in mice *via* enhancing the Nrf2 antioxidant pathway and inhibiting NLRP3 inflammasome activation'. *Free Radical Biology and Medicine*, 51: 744–54.

Tune Bruce, M. (1997). 'Nephrotoxicity of beta-lactam antibiotics: Mechanisms and strategies for prevention'. *Pediatric Nephrology*, 11: 768–72.

Turgut Faruk, Omer Bayrak, Ferhat Catal, Reyhan Bayrak, Ali Fuat Atmaca, Akif Koc, Ali Akbas, Ali Akcay and Dogan Unal (2008). 'Antioxidant and protective effects of silymarin on ischemia and reperfusion injury in the kidney tissues of rats'. *International Urology and Nephrology*, 40: 453–60.

Vasavada Nina and Rajiv Agarwal (2005). 'Role of oxidative stress in diabetic nephropathy', *Advances in Chronic Kidney Disease*, 12: 146–54.

Venkatesan, R.S., Mohamed Sadiq, A., Suresh Kumar, J., Raja Lakshmi, G. and Vidhya, R. (2010). 'Effect of Morin on mercury chloride induced nephrotoxicity', *Ecoscan*, 4: 193–96.

Vessal Ghazal, Masoumeh Akmali, Parisa Najafi, Mahmood Reza Moein and Mohammad Mahdi Sagheb (2010). 'Silymarin and milk thistle extract may prevent the progression of diabetic nephropathy in streptozotocin-induced diabetic rats'. *Renal Failure*, 32: 733–39.

Vijayaprakash Shanmugam, Kulanthaivel Langeswaran, Subbaraj Gowtham Kumar, Rajendran Revathy and Maruthaiveeran Periyasamy Balasubramanian (2013). 'Nephro-protective significance of kaempferol on mercuric chloride induced toxicity in Wistar albino rats'. *Biomedicine & Aging Pathology*, 3: 119–24.

Vinayagam Ramachandran, and Baojun Xu (2015). 'Antidiabetic properties of dietary flavonoids: A cellular mechanism review'. *Nutrition & Metabolism*, 12: 60.

Vincenti Matthew, P. (2001). 'The matrix metalloproteinase (MMP) and tissue inhibitor of metalloproteinase (TIMP) genes: Transcriptional and posttranscriptional regulation, signal transduction and cell-type-specific expression'. *Matrix Metalloproteinase Protocols*, pp. 121–48.

Wang Guo Guang, Xiao Hua Lu, Wei Li, Xue Zhao and Cui Zhang (2011). 'Protective effects of luteolin on diabetic nephropathy in STZ-induced diabetic rats'. *Evidence-Based Complementary and Alternative Medicine*, 2011.

Waz Wayne, R., Van Liew Judith, B. and Feld, Leonard G. (1998). 'Nitric oxide metabolism following unilateral renal ischemia/reperfusion injury in rats'. *Pediatric Nephrology*, 12: 26–29.

Widemann Brigitte, C. and Adamson Peter, C. (2006). 'Understanding and managing methotrexate nephrotoxicity'. *The Oncologist*, 11: 694–703.

Widemann Brigitte, C., Stefan Schwartz, Nalini Jayaprakash, Robbin Christensen, Ching Hon Pui, Nikhil Chauhan, Claire Daugherty, King Thomas, R., Rush Janet, E. and Howard Scott, C. (2014). 'Efficacy of glucarpidase (carboxypeptidase g2) in patients with acute kidney injury after high dose methotrexate therapy'. *Pharmacotherapy: The Journal of Human Pharmacology and Drug Therapy*, 34: 427–39.

Yan Ning, Li Wen, Rui Peng, Hongmei Li, Handeng Liu, Huimin Peng, Yan Sun, Tianhui Wu, Lei Chen and Qingrui Duan (2016). 'Naringenin ameliorated kidney injury through Let-7a/TGFBR1 signaling in diabetic nephropathy'. *Journal of Diabetes Research*, 2016.

Yao Xin, Kessarin Panichpisal, Neil Kurtzman and Kenneth Nugent (2007). 'Cisplatin nephrotoxicity: A review'. *American Journal of the Medical Sciences*, 334: 115–24.

Yousef Mokhtar, I., Omar Sahar, A.M., El-Guendi Marwa, I. and Abdelmegid Laila, A. (2010). 'Potential protective effects of quercetin and curcumin on paracetamol-induced histological changes, oxidative stress, impaired liver and kidney functions and haematotoxicity in rat'. *Food and Chemical Toxicology*, 48: 3246–61.

Zou Peimei, Jian Song, Bei Jiang, Fei Pei, Binbin Chen, Xiangdong Yang, Guangyi Liu and Zhao Hu. (2014). 'Epigallocatechin-3-gallate protects against cisplatin nephrotoxicity by inhibiting the apoptosis in mouse'. *Int. J. Clin. Exp. Pathol.*, 7: 4607–16.

Zuscik Michael, J., Pateder Dhruv, B., Edward Puzas, J., Schwarz Edward, M. Rosier Randy, N. and O'Keefe Regis, J. (2002). 'Lead alters parathyroid hormone related peptide and transforming growth factor β 1 effects and AP 1 and NF κKB signaling in chondrocytes'. *Journal of Orthopaedic Research*, 20: 811–18.

11

Anti-allergic Mechanisms of Flavonoids

DHAMODHARAN BAKKIYARAJ[1*]

ABSTRACT

Allergy can be defined in simple terms as the excess action or reaction of our own immune system against certain substances referred as allergens. Allergic reactions induce chemical mediators like histamine, cytokines and various other pro-inflammatory molecules in turn triggering inflammation either at local or systemic level. Allergy related diseases include anaphylaxis, asthma, hay fever and atopic dermatitis, and shows symptoms like runny nose, red eyes and improper breath apart from the other symptoms associated with inflammation such as pain, fever, itching, reddening and swelling. Flavonoids being one of the widely consumed phytochemicals, have major impact on cellular functions. Besides their multifaceted role as antimicrobial, antioxidant, anti-cancer, anti-fungal agents etc., flavonoids also have the potential to inhibit allergic and inflammatory responses. The mechanisms by which flavonoids inhibit allergic responses are known to some extent and the most probable ones are by inhibiting the synthesis and release of histamine and other cytokines, inhibiting the production of pro-inflammatory mediators thus preventing allergic inflammation, preventing degranulation by stabilizing the mast cells and basophils, and by regulating the transcription factors and various enzymes involved in inflammation. This chapter summarizes various anti-allergic mechanisms adapted by different flavonoids in detail.

Key words: Flavonoids, Anti-allergic, Allergy, Anti-inflammatory, Anti-histamines, INOS, COX-2

[1]Centre for Food Technology, Anna University, Chennai – 600113, TN, India
**Corresponding author*: E-mail: bakkya@gmail.com

1. INTRODUCTION

Allergy is a complex biological process triggered by the host's immune machinery in response to foreign substances. The agents that cause or induce allergy are called allergens and the people with inherited ability to develop allergic response are called atopic. Approximately about 25% of the people in developed nations are prone to ailments associated with allergy like anaphylaxis, hay fever, eczema and asthma[1]. Changes in our diet has been called as one of the environmental factors responsible for increased incidence and severity of allergy and associated diseases. Allergy develops inflammatory symptoms like redness, edema, hives, etc. in addition to site specific symptoms like asthma (lung), allergic rhinitis (nasal cavity) and conjunctivitis (eyes). Substances that are known to cause allergy are dust mites, pets, pollen, insects, moulds, foods especially sea foods and few vegetables, and medicines. Allergic or atopic disorders in most instances are not fatal except in certain individuals who develop a potentially fatal systemic allergic reaction, called anaphylaxis, upon exposure to allergens very rapidly[1].

Commonly used anti-allergic drugs include administration of antihistamines, corticosteroids, adrenaline, non-steroidal anti-inflammatory drugs (NSAIDs), etc. with great success, yet they do have side effects while used for longer run. Hence, the focus has shifted to natural products especially from dietary sources with potential anti-allergic and anti-inflammatory potentials. The anti-inflammatory properties of flavonoids have gained special attention in recent times as they were highly significant while having no deleterious effects.

Flavonoids comprise a group of naturally occurring phenolic compounds and are abundantly found in varied plant sources like vegetables, fruits, flowers, as well as in cocoa, tea and wine[2]. Flavonoids are reported to display diverse bioactive potentials like antibacterial, antiviral, cytotoxic, anti-aging, hepato- and cardioprotective, anti-diabetic, anti-thrombogenic, anti-atherogenic activities, anti-cancer, antioxidant, anti-radical scavenging, anti-allergic and anti-inflammatory properties[3-5]. Flavonoids have been reported to interfere with the functions of mast cells and basophils in turn inhibiting the production of cytokines, expression of CD40 ligand and release of chemical mediators and pro-inflammatory substances like histamines[6,7].

2. ANTI-ALLERGIC DRUGS

Several synthetic and semi-synthetic anti-allergic drugs with different modes of actions are available to treat allergic reactions and associated inflammatory responses. Anti-allergic drugs available as of now for public use are given in Table 1.

Table 1: Anti-allergic drugs available in market

Sl. no.	*Mode of action*	*Drugs*
1.	Antihistamines	Cetirizine, Levocetirizine, Clemastine, Fexofenadine, Loratadine, Brompheniramine, Chlorpheriramine, Diphenhydramine, Hydroxyzine, Carbinoxamine, Naphazoline, Ketotifen fumarate, Pheniramine, Azelastine, Emedastine
2.	Mast cell stabilizers	Cromolyn, Lodoxamide, Nedocromil, Pemirolast
3.	Corticosteroids	Beclomethasone dipropionate, Budesonide, Ciclesonide, Flunisolide, Fluticasone furoate, Fluticasone propionate, Prednisone, Prednisolone, Cortisol, Methylprednisolone
4.	Leukotriene inhibitor	Montelukast, Zafirlukast, Zyflo
5.	Topical immunomodulators	Tacrolimus, Pimecrolimus

Besides the above said antiallergic drugs, NSAIDs (Aspirin, Diclofenac, Indomethacin, Celebrex, Ibuprofen, Naproxen, etc.) were also used for controlling the allergic inflammation. Though the above said drugs have the ability to display rapid relief, there are several side effects associated with most them ranging as simple as drowsiness, insomnia to weight gain, increased blood pressure, oto-, cardio- and hepato-toxicity in certain cases.

3. FLAVONOIDS WITH ANTI-ALLERGIC PROPERTIES

Several flavonoids from diverse sources have been reported with the potential to inhibit allergic responses both *in vitro* and *in vivo*. Flavonoids with anti-allergic and anti-inflammatory potentials along with their sources are listed in Table 2.

3.1. Anti-allergic Mechanisms of Flavonoids

The anti-allergic properties of flavonoids have been attributed to their ability to inhibit various cellular functions like production and release of cytokines by the mast cells and basophils, stabilizing the mast cells thus preventing degranulation – a process that releases the cytokines and pro-inflammatory mediators, inhibiting the CD40 ligand-receptor interactions, blocking histamine production and its interaction with receptors, inhibition of pro-inflammatory enzymes, inhibition of nitric oxide (NO) production, etc.[6,7].

3.1.1. *Inhibition of mast cell/basophil activation and cytokine release*

Mast cells and basophils of the immune machinery were shown responsible for producing high affinity IgE receptor (FcεRI) that plays crucial role in allergic inflammation by releasing histamine and cysteinyl leukotrienes, cytokines and chemokines[26]. Flavonoids were well known for their ability

Table 2: Flavonoids with anti-allergic and anti-inflammatory properties

Sl. no.	*Flavonoid*	*References*
1.	Apigenin	(6, 8)
2.	Methoxyflavone compounds	(9)
3.	Quercetin	(10-12)
4.	Kaempferol	(10)
5.	Luteolin	(13, 14)
6.	Hydroxyflavones	(6)
7.	Fustin, Scutellarein, Ombuin, Diosmetin, Ayanin, Galangin, Morin, Chrysin, Rhamnetin, Astragalin, Gossypin, Phloridzin, Phloretin	(6, 11, 15)
8.	Rhein	(16)
9.	Naringenin	(17, 18)
10.	Anthocyanin	(19)
11.	Fisetin, Rutin, Myricetin, Amentoflavone	(11, 15)
12.	Isoquercetin	(20)
13.	Gallocatechin gallate, Epigallocatechin gallate, Epigallocatechin, Epicatechin gallate, Catechin,	(21)
14.	Hesperidin, Diosmin	(22)
15.	Baicalein	(14)
16.	Daidzein, Genistein, Isorhamnetin	(23)
17.	Silybin	(24)
18.	Cirsiliol	(25)

to inhibit the activation of high-affinity IgE receptor (FcεRI) expressing mast cells and basophils thus inhibiting the synthesis of leukotriene or other chemical mediators besides blocking histamine release (Fig. 1)[27,28]. Allergic diseases are characterized by the over expression of IgE in response to allergens. Interactions of CD40 ligand with CD40 receptor and the action of Interleukin (IL)-4 or IL-13 on B cells are indispensable for the differentiation

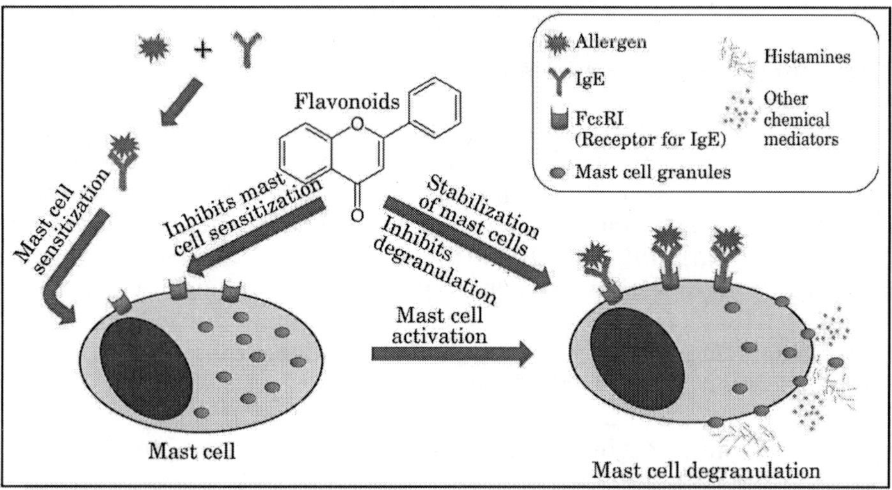

Fig. 1: Mechanism of action of flavonoids inhibiting the release of histamines and cytokines

of B cells into IgE producing cells. Th2 cells, basophils and mast cells are the cells responsible for producing the above said signals like CD40 ligand, IL-4 and IL-13, thus explaining their immaculate role in allergic reactions[29]. Luteolin, apigenin and fisetin strongly inhibited the IL-4 and IL-13 synthesis by basophils[13,30], IL-4 and TNF-α synthesis in rat mast cells[31] and CD40 ligand expression in basophils[13].

Naringenin, a flavanone type of flavonoid rich in grapes, inhibits the release of Th2 cytokines like IL-4, IL-5 and IL-13 by the CD4 T cells thus preventing allergic responses[17]. Total flavonoids with two anthocyanins (cyanidin-3-O-glucoside and cyanidin-3-O-rutinoside) as major components effectively inhibited the pro-inflammatory cytokines such as IL-1β, Tumor necrosis factor (TNF) -α and Interferon (IFN)-γ apart from inhibiting the production of nitric oxide (NO) in mice model[19].

Flavonoids like fisetin, quercetin and rutin were reported to down regulate the expression of genes and subsequent production of proinflammatory cytokines such as TNF-α, IL-1β, IL-6 and IL-8. Similarly, myricetin inhibited the cytokines TNF-α and IL-6 with no action on others. Inhibition of nuclear translocation of NF-κB, NF-κB/DNA binding and NF-κB dependent gene reporter assayprovide direct evidence that the activation of NF-κB has been stifled upon treatment with fisetin, myricetin and rutin[11,32]. Quercetin has also been shown to regulate the equilibrium between Th1 and Th2 cells through *in vivo* studies, thus inhibiting the allergic responses in murine model of asthma[33,34]. Luteolin, ayanin, apigenin and fisetin were found to be the potent inhibitors of IL-4 production. Luteolin effectively inhibited the production of IL-4, IL-13, CD40 ligand expression as well as phosphorylation of c-Jun and DNA binding activity of activator protein (AP)-1 in activated basophils[13,35].

3.1.2. *Inhibition of histamine release*

Histamine which is stored in the granules of basophils and mast cells, acts as a chemical mediator in allergic response, and its concentration directly correlates to the severity of the allergic reactions and the extent of inflammation. Histamine is produced by the decarboxylation of histidine by L -histidine decarboxylase (HDC), in the presence of pyridoxal-5'-phosphate as cofactor[36]. The activity of HDC is regulated by cytokines such as IL-1, IL-3, IL-12, IL-18, GM-CSF, macrophage-colony stimulating factor, TNF-α, and calcium ionophore[37,38]. Among the 4 Histamine receptors (H1-H4), H1 and H2 receptors play crucial roles in histamine mediated allergic responses in most cases especially in asthma, allergic rhinitis and urticaria[39]. Antigen-specific T_H1 and T_H2 cells were also regulated by the histamine[40].

Agents inhibiting histamines are called anti-histamines and were shown to have promising effect in controlling allergic inflammation. The mechanism of anti-histamines could be any of the following: competitive inhibition of the histamine receptors; direct inhibition of histamine production or its release; inhibition of degranulation or mast cell stabilization; inhibition or scavenging of cytokines required for the production of histamines. Several flavonoids like Quercetin, Luteolin, Amentoflavone, Flavone, Apigenin, Fisetin, Kaempferol, Myricetin, Rutin and Cromoglicate have been reported with anti-histamine properties[11,15]. The anti-histamine activity of the flavonoid fraction extracted from *Bryophyllum calycinum* (Crassulaceae) has also been reported, though there is no clue on the identity of the active flavonoid present in the fraction[41]. Epigallocatechin gallate, a flavonoid derivative found rich in green tea also has the potential to inhibit histamine release from basophils[42]. Study on cultured mammalian cell lines has showed that quercetin, luteolin and baicalein strongly inhibited the release of histamine, leukotrienes, prostaglandin D2 and granulocyte macrophage-colony stimulating factor (GM-CSF). Quercetin, Kaempferol and luteolin have the potential to inhibit the activation of mast cells by interfering with the activation of protein kinase C and Ca^{2+} uptake[14,27,43,44].

3.1.3. *Inhibition of inducible nitric oxide synthase (iNOS)*

Nitric oxide (NO) concentrations are found to be at higher levels during inflammation and has been shown to have both pro-inflammatory and regulatory effects. There are three nitric oxide synthase (NOS) enzymes namely endothelial NOS (eNOS), neuronal NOS (nNOS) and inducible NOS (iNOS), which catalyze the production of NO. The enzyme iNOS is of major importance as it is found responsible for the production of NO in large amounts and for extended period. In addition, iNOS is an inducible enzyme that could be induced by various cytokines and bacterial products resulting in inflammatory response during allergic conditions[45-47].

Although it has been known from late 1990s that flavonoids can inhibit the production of NO and NO mediated inflammation[48, 49], the precise mechanism behind such action has been delineated much later. A detailed study analyzing the effects of 36 different naturally occurring flavonoids has revealed that daidzein, genistein, isorhamnetin, flavone, kaempferol, quercetin, naringenin and the anthocyanin pelargonidin have the potential to inhibit the expression of iNOS and thus reducing the concentration of NO in a dose dependent manner. Analysis at transcript level provided insights that the active compounds inhibited the activation of nuclear factor (NF)-κB, a key transcription factor for the iNOS enzyme. In addition, few flavonoids like genistein, kaempferol, quercetin and daidzein also inhibited the activation of another transcription factor of iNOS, the signal transducer and activator of transcription 1 (STAT-1) (Fig. 2)[23,50].

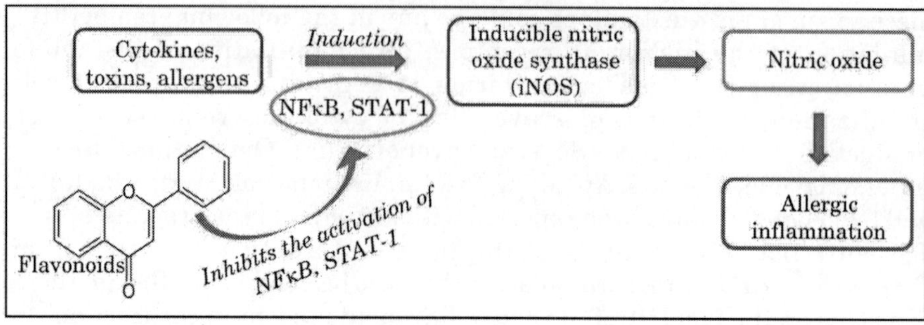

Fig. 2: Mechanism of action of flavonoids inhibiting inducible nitric oxide synthase

3.1.4. *Inhibition of pro-inflammatory enzymes*

Enzymes like cyclooxygenase-2 (COX-2) and 5-lipoxygenase (5LO) play important roles as pro-inflammatory enzymes causing allergic inflammation. COX-2 is imperative for the synthesis of prostaglandin and its up-regulation directly increased the release of prostaglandin during inflammation and allergy[51]. COX-2 is an inducible enzyme that gets induced by cytokines and various other pro-inflammatory molecules including mitogens in contrast to its isoform (COX-1) that is expressed constitutively in mammalian tissues and involved in homeostatic synthesis of prostanoid. COX-2 has been the target for anti-inflammatory drugs of the group NSAIDs. Off-target binding of NSAIDs has been observed resulting in immunomodulatory effects and side effects. Quercetin and Kaempferol were reported to inhibit the expression of COX-2 in macrophages[14]. Luteolin inhibited lipopolysaccharide induced COX-2 protein expression[52]. Myricetin effectively suppressed the lipoteichoic acid induced IL-1β and COX-2 expression in cultured human fibroblasts[53]. Apigenin, a flavone class of flavonoid, blocks the activation of the NF-κB signalling system by effectively inhibiting the function of LPS inducible kinases[54].

Quercetin, quercetagetin, kaempferol-3-Ogalactoside and scutellarein have the potential to suppress cysteinyl leukotriene synthesis by inhibiting the enzymes phospholipase (PL) A2 and 5LO[55,56]. A flavonoid, cirsiliol (3', 4', 5-trihydroxy-6,7-dimethoxy flavone) has been reported with 5LO inhibitory activity from rat basophils and the same has been shown to block the release of cysteinyl leukotrienes from guinea pig lung[25]. Flavonoids such as apigenin, luteolin, 3,6-dihydroxy flavones, fisetin, kaempferol, quercetin, and myricetin inhibit the release of hexosaminidase from mast cells[57].

3.1.5. *Other mechanisms*

Regulating the expression of genes involved in synthesis of pro-inflammatory mediators has been attributed as one of the anti-allergic mechanisms of flavonoids. Flavonoids target the NF-kB signalling pathway and regulate the expression of transcription factors like STAT-1 and IRF-1. Kaempferol reportedly inhibits the activation of STAT-1 by inhibiting the activation of Janus kinase 3 (JAK-3)[58].

Flavonoids were also shown to inhibit the functionalities of many kinases including those such as Lyn and Syk tyrosine kinases, Mitogen activated protein kinases (MAPK), Phosphatidylinositol 3 kinase (PI3), Protein kinase C (PKC), etc. (Fig. 3). Cross linking of IgE-allergen complex to the FcεRI triggers a series of phosphorylation reactions initiated by the tyrosine kinase Lyn that activates its counterpart Syk. Phosphorylation of Syk stimulates the other kinases PI3, MAPK and PLC. PI3 subsequently activates Rac/Rho GTPases and p38 MAPK, which involve in the production of cytokines like IL-4 and IL-13. Activated GTPases affects the cytoskeleton structures facilitating the process of degranulation. In addition, activated GTPases activate P44/42 MAPK that plays crucial role in the synthesis of cysteinyl leukotrienes. Different flavonoids have the potential to inhibit various steps in the above-mentioned pathways, where, Lyn and Syk, PI3 and p44/42 MAPK are the major targets. Protein kinase C (PKC) has also been reported to play a crucial role in diacyl glycerol mediated production of cytokines and degranulation of mast cells and basophils, and it has been shown to get inactivated by the flavonoids such as luteolin and quercetin.

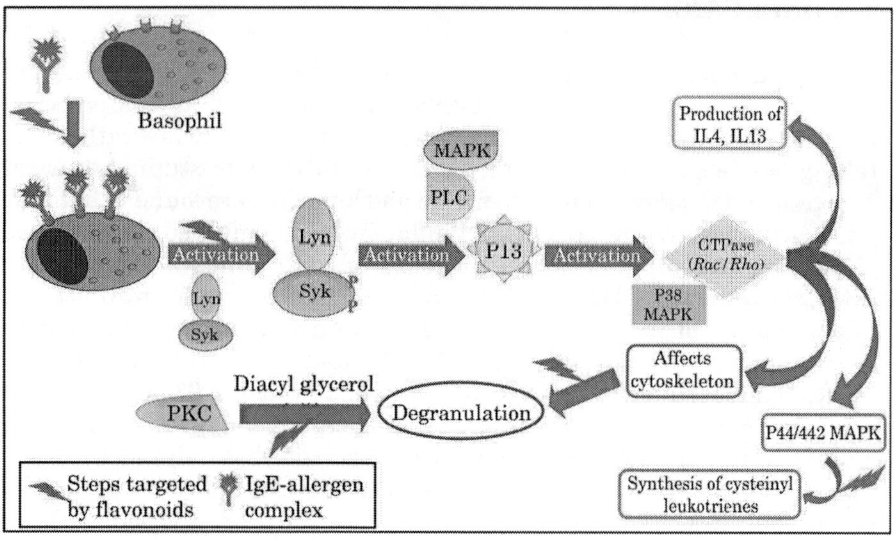

Fig. 3: Mechanism of action of flavonoids inhibiting various regulatory networks

Flavan-3-ol (procyanidins) present in the apple effectively repressed the expression of genes producing chemokines like IP-10, CXCL10 and other pro-inflammatory enzymes like COX-2 and CYP3A4[59]. Flavonoids such as luteolin, rutin and quercetin have been reported to inhibit the permeation of antigen in cultured monolayer of cells, thus providing clues that they could prevent the contact of antigens with receptors, in turn preventing sensitization of immune cells[60].

Naringenin chalcone, a flavonoid found rich in the peel of tomatoes, has been found to inhibit the production of IL-4 and IL-5 thus preventing the accumulation or recruitment of eosinophils[17]. Inhibition of intracellular proteases has been reported as one of the plausible mechanisms of actions exhibited by flavonoids. Epigallocatechin gallate and myricetin inhibited the proteases in turn resulting in reduced allergic responses[61,62].

Quercetin significantly inhibits the activity of membrane transport adenosine triphosphatases (ATPases) including the calcium-dependent ATPase, which is involved in calcium efflux from the cells. Though the flavonoids are not known for their direct inhibitory action against ATPases, the plausible mechanism of such action could be, facilitating the translocation of ions consequently reducing the uptake of ATP[63]. Several flavonoids like apigenin, luteolin, baicalein, quercetin, kaempferol and myricetin at their lower doses inhibit the activation of the aryl hydrocarbon receptor (Ahr) - a transcriptional factor that responds to planar aromatic hydrocarbons (*eg.* dioxins). In contrary, higher concentrations of daidzein, naringenin and baicalein induce Ahr activation[64].

4. CONCLUSIONS

Dietary flavonoids are part of almost every vegetable which we eat and they play vital roles in regulating various cellular processes. Anti-allergic properties of flavonoids are of high interest as it turns 'food to medicine' rather than taking 'medicines as food'. Among all the flavonoids studies thus far, quercetin, kaempferol, apigenin, fisetin and luteolin were found to be highly effective in controlling allergy and inflammation compared to the others. Hindering the production and release of histamines and cytokines, interference with CD40 ligand – receptor interactions, inhibition of degranulation of mast cells, blocking the functions of pro-inflammatory enzymes like iNOS, COX-2, 5LO and PLA2 are the molecular mechanisms involved in anti-allergic properties of various flavonoids. Though there are evidences providing information on the anti-allergic mechanisms of flavonoids, still there is room for unravelling further information by analyzing the effects of flavonoids at systemic level in contrast to studies monitoring a single or set of genes. Research on flavonoids with proven anti-allergic potentials has to be taken up to the next level by developing them as working drug formulations for further trials and subsequent applications.

ACKNOWLEDGEMENT

Financial assistance provided through UGC's Dr. DS. Kothari Postdoctoral Fellowship Scheme has been gratefully acknowledged. Infrastructure

Facilities and support provided by Prof. S. Meenakshisundaram at the Centre for Food Technology, Anna University has been thankfully acknowledged.

REFERENCES

[1] Galli, S.J., Tsai, M. and Piliponsky, A.M. (2008). The development of allergic inflammation. *Nature,* 454(7203): 445–54.

[2] Rathee, P., Chaudhary, H., Rathee, S., Rathee, D., Kumar, V. and Kohli, K. (2009). Mechanism of action of flavonoids as anti-inflammatory agents: A review. *Inflamm Allergy Drug Targets*, 8(3): 229–35.

[3] Havsteen, B.H. (2002). The biochemistry and medical significance of the flavonoids. *Pharmacol Ther.*, 96(2–3): 67–202.

[4] Robak, J. and Gryglewski, R.J. (1996). Bioactivity of flavonoids. *Pol. J. Pharmacol.*, 48(6): 555–64.

[5] Russo, A., Acquaviva, R., Campisi, A., Sorrenti, V., Di Giacomo, C., Virgata, G., Barcellona, M.L. and Vanella, A. (2000). Bioflavonoids as antiradicals, antioxidants and DNA cleavage protectors. *Cell Biol. Toxicol.*, 16(2): 91–8.

[6] Kawai, M., Hirano, T., Higa, S., Arimitsu, J., Maruta, M., Kuwahara, Y., Ohkawara, T., Hagihara, K., Yamadori, T., Shima, Y., Ogata, A., Kawase, I. and Tanaka, T. (2007). Flavonoids and related compounds as anti-allergic substances. *Allergol Int.*, 56(2): 113–23.

[7] Tanaka, T. (2014). Flavonoids for allergic diseases: Present evidence and future perspective. *Curr. Pharm. Des.*, 20(6): 879–85.

[8] Choi, J.-R., Lee, C.-M., Jung, I.D., Lee, J.S., Jeong, Y.-I., Chang, J.H., Park, H.-J., Choi, I.-W., Kim, J.-S., Shin, Y.K., Park, S.N. and Park, Y.-M. (2009). Apigenin protects ovalbumin-induced asthma through the regulation of GATA-3 gene. *Int. Immunopharmacol.*, 9(7-8): 918–24.

[9] Tewtrakul, S., Subhadhirasakul, S. and Kummee, S. (2008). Anti-allergic activity of compounds from *Kaempferia parviflora*. *J. Ethnopharmacol.*, 116(1): 191–3.

[10] Kim, M., Lim, S.J., Kang, S.W., Um, B.H., Nho, C.W. (2014). Aceriphyllum rossii extract and its active compounds, quercetin and kaempferol inhibit IgE-mediated mast cell activation and passive cutaneous anaphylaxis. *J. Agric. Food Chem.*, 62(17): 3750–8.

[11] Park, H.H., Lee, S., Son, H.Y., Park, S.B., Kim, M.S., Choi, E.J., Singh, T.S., Ha, J.H., Lee, M.G., Kim, J.E., Hyun, M.C., Kwon, T.K., Kim, Y.H. and Kim, S.H. (2008). Flavonoids inhibit histamine release and expression of proinflammatory cytokines in mast cells. *Arch. Pharm. Res.*, 31(10): 1303–11.

[12] Sato, A., Zhang, T., Yonekura, L. and Tamura, H. (2015). Antiallergic activities of eleven onions (*Allium cepa*) were attributed to quercetin 4-glucoside using QuEChERS method and Pearson's correlation coefficient. *J. Funct Foods.*, 14: 581–9.

[13] Hirano, T., Higa, S., Arimitsu, J., Naka, T., Ogata, A., Shima, Y., Fujimoto, M., Yamadori, T., Ohkawara, T., Kuwabara, Y., Kawai, M., Matsuda, H., Yoshikawa, M., Maezaki, N., Tanaka, T. and Kawase, I. (2006). Luteolin, a flavonoid, inhibits AP-1 activation by basophils. *Biochem. Biophys. Res. Commun.,* 340(1): 1–7.

[14] Kimata, M., Shichijo, M., Miura, T., Serizawa, I., Inagaki, N. and Nagai, H. (2000). Effects of luteolin, quercetin and baicalein on immunoglobulin E-mediated mediator release from human cultured mast cells. *Clin. Exp. Allergy*, 30(4): 501–8.

[15] Amellal, M., Bronner, C., Briancon, F., Haag, M., Anton, R., Landry, Y. (1985). Inhibition of mast cell histamine release by flavonoids and biflavonoids. *Planta Med.*, 51(1): 16–20.

[16] Singh, B., Nadkarni, J.R., Vishwakarma, R.A., Bharate, S.B., Nivsarkar, M. and Anandjiwala, S. (2012). The hydroalcoholic extract of *Cassia alata* (Linn.) leaves and

its major compound rhein exhibits antiallergic activity *via* mast cell stabilization and lipoxygenase inhibition. *J. Ethnopharmacol.*, 141(1): 469–73.
[17] Iwamura, C., Shinoda, K., Yoshimura, M., Watanabe, Y., Obata, A. and Nakayama, T. (2010). Naringenin chalcone suppresses allergic asthma by inhibiting the type-2 function of CD4 T Cells. *Allergol Int.*, 59(1): 67–73.
[18] Yamamoto, T., Yoshimura, M., Yamaguchi, F., Kouchi, T., Tsuji, R., Saito, M., Obata, A. and Kikuchi, M. (2004). Anti-allergic activity of naringenin chalcone from a tomato skin extract. *Biosci Biotechnol Biochem.*, 68(8): 1706–11.
[19] Chen, H., Pu, J., Liu, D., Yu, W., Shao, Y., Yang, G., Xiang, Z. and He, N. (2016). Anti-inflammatory and antinociceptive properties of flavonoids from the fruits of Black Mulberry (*Morus nigra* L.). *PLoS ONE*, 11(4): e0153080.
[20] Hirano, T., Kawai, M., Arimitsu, J., Ogawa, M., Kuwahara, Y., Hagihara, K., Shima, Y., Narazaki, M., Ogata, A., Koyanagi, M., Kai, T., Shimizu, R., Moriwaki, M., Suzuki, Y., Ogino, S., Kawase, I. and Tanaka, T. (2009). Preventative effect of a flavonoid, enzymatically modified isoquercitrin on ocular symptoms of Japanese cedar pollinosis. *Allergol Int.*, 58(3): 373–82.
[21] Ohmori, Y., Ito, M., Kishi, M., Mizutani, H., Katada, T. and Konishi, H. (1995). Antiallergic constituents from oolong tea stem. *Biol. Pharm. Bull.*, 18(5): 683–6.
[22] Damon, M., Flandre, O., Michel, F., Perdrix, L., Labrid, C. and Crastes de Paulet, A. (1987). Effect of chronic treatment with a purified flavonoid fraction on inflammatory granuloma in the rat. Study of prostaglandin E2 and F2 alpha and thromboxane B2 release and histological changes. *Arzneimittel forschung,* 37(10): 1149–53.
[23] Hamalainen, M., Nieminen, R., Vuorela, P., Heinonen, M. and Moilanen, E. (2007). Anti-inflammatory effects of flavonoids: Genistein, kaempferol, quercetin, and daidzein inhibit STAT-1 and NF-kappaB activations, whereas flavone, isorhamnetin, naringenin, and pelargonidin inhibit only NF-kappaB activation along with their inhibitory effect on iNOS expression and NO production in activated macrophages. *Mediators Inflamm.*, 2007: 45673.
[24] Cho, J.Y., Kim, P.S., Park, J., Yoo, E.S., Baik, K.U., Kim, Y.K. and Park, M.H. (2000). Inhibitor of tumor necrosis factor-alpha production in lipopolysaccharide-stimulated RAW264.7 cells from *Amorpha fruticosa*. *J. Ethnopharmacol.*, 70(2): 127–33.
[25] Yoshimoto, T., Furukawa, M., Yamamoto, S., Horie, T. and Watanabe-Kohno, S. (1983). Flavonoids: Potent inhibitors of arachidonate 5-lipoxygenase. *Biochem. Biophys. Res. Commun.*, 116(2): 612–8.
[26] Stone, K.D., Prussin, C. and Metcalfe, D.D. (2010). IgE, mast cells, basophils, and eosinophils. *J. Allergy Clin. Immunol.*, 125(2 Suppl 2): S73–80.
[27] Fewtrell, C.M. and Gomperts, B.D. (1977). Quercetin: A novel inhibitor of Ca^{2+} influx and exocytosis in rat peritoneal mast cells. *Biochim. Biophys. Acta*, 469(1): 52–60.
[28] Middleton, Jr. E., Kandaswami, C. and Theoharides, T.C. (2000). The effects of plant flavonoids on mammalian cells: Implications for inflammation, heart disease, and cancer. *Pharmacol Rev.*, 52(4): 673–751.
[29] Yanagihara, Y. (2003). Regulatory mechanisms of human ige synthesis. *Allergol Int.*, 52(1): 1–12.
[30] Hirano, T., Higa, S., Arimitsu, J., Naka, T., Shima, Y., Ohshima, S., Fujimoto, M., Yamadori, T., Kawase, I. and Tanaka, T. (2004). Flavonoids such as luteolin, fisetin and apigenin are inhibitors of interleukin-4 and interleukin-13 production by activated human basophils. *Int. Arch. Allergy. Immunol.*, 134(2): 135–40.
[31] Mastuda, H., Morikawa, T., Ueda, K., Managi, H. and Yoshikawa, M. (2002). Structural requirements of flavonoids for inhibition of antigen-Induced degranulation, TNF-alpha and IL-4 production from RBL-2H3 cells. *Bioorg Med. Chem.,* 10(10): 3123–8.
[32] Serafini, M., Peluso, I. and Raguzzini, A. (2010). Flavonoids as anti-inflammatory agents. *Proc. Nutr. Soc.*, 69(3): 273–8.

[33] Park, H.J., Lee, C.M., Jung, I.D., Lee, J.S., Jeong, Y.I., Chang, J.H., Chun, S.H., Kim, M.J., Choi, I.W., Ahn, S.C., Shin, Y.K., Yeom, S.R. and Park, Y.M. (2009). Quercetin regulates Th1/Th2 balance in a murine model of asthma. *Int. Immunopharmacol.*, 9(3): 261–7.

[34] Weng, Z., Zhang, B., Asadi, S., Sismanopoulos, N., Butcher, A., Fu, X., Katsarou-Katsari, A., Antoniou, C. and Theoharides, T.C. (2012). Quercetin is more effective than cromolyn in blocking human mast cell cytokine release and inhibits contact dermatitis and photosensitivity in humans. *PLoS ONE*, 7(3): e33805.

[35] Higa, S., Hirano, T., Kotani, M., Matsumoto, M., Fujita, A., Suemura, M., Kawase, I. and Tanaka, T. (2003). Fisetin, a flavonol, inhibits TH2-type cytokine production by activated human basophils. *J. Allergy Clin. Immunol.*, 111(6): 1299–306.

[36] Endo, Y. (1982). Simultaneous induction of histidine and ornithine decarboxylases and changes in their product amines following the injection of *Escherichia coli* lipopolysaccharide into mice. *Biochem Pharmacol.*, 31(8): 1643–7.

[37] Kubo, Y. and Nakano, K. (1999). Regulation of histamine synthesis in mouse CD4+ and CD8+ T lymphocytes. *Inflamm. Res.*, 48(3): 149–53.

[38] Szeberenyi, J.B., Pallinger, E., Zsinko, M., Pos, Z., Rothe, G., Orso, E., Szeberenyi, S., Schmitz, G., Falus, A. and Laszlo, V. (2001). Inhibition of effects of endogenously synthesized histamine disturbs *in vitro* human dendritic cell differentiation. *Immunol Lett.*, 76(3): 175–82.

[39] White, M.V. (1990). The role of histamine in allergic diseases. *J. Allergy. Clin. Immunol.*, 86(4 Pt 2): 599–605.

[40] Akdis, C.A. and Blaser, K. (2003). Histamine in the immune regulation of allergic inflammation. *J. Allergy Clin. Immunol.*, 112(1): 15–22.

[41] Nassis, C.Z., Haebisch, E.M. and Giesbrecht, A.M. (1992). Antihistamine activity of *Bryophyllum calycinum. Braz. J. Med. Biol. Res.*, 25(9): 929–36.

[42] Matsuo, N., Yamada, K., Shoji, K., Mori, M., Sugano, M. (1997). Effect of tea polyphenols on histamine release from rat basophilic leukemia (RBL-2H3) cells: The structure-inhibitory activity relationship. *Allergy,* 52(1): 58–64.

[43] Lee, E.J., Ji, G.E. and Sung, M.K. (2010). Quercetin and kaempferol suppress immunoglobulin E-mediated allergic inflammation in RBL-2H3 and Caco-2 cells. *Inflamm Res.*, 59(10): 847–54.

[44] Pearce, F.L., Befus, A.D. and Bienenstock, J. (1984). Mucosal mast cells. III. Effect of quercetin and other flavonoids on antigen-induced histamine secretion from rat intestinal mast cells. *J. Allergy Clin. Immunol.*, 73(6): 819–23.

[45] Alderton, W.K., Cooper, C.E. and Knowles, R.G. (2001). Nitric oxide synthases: Structure, function and inhibition. *Biochem. J.,* 357(Pt 3): 593–615.

[46] Bogdan, C. (2001). Nitric oxide and the immune response. *Nat. Immunol.*, 2(10): 907–16.

[47] Korhonen, R., Lahti, A., Kankaanranta, H. and Moilanen, E. (2005). Nitric oxide production and signaling in inflammation. *Curr Drug Targets Inflamm Allergy,* 4(4): 471–9.

[48] Kim, H., Kim, Y.S., Kim, S.Y. and Suk, K. (2001). The plant flavonoid wogonin suppresses death of activated C6 rat glial cells by inhibiting nitric oxide production. *Neurosci Lett.*, 309(1): 67–71.

[49] Liang, Y.C., Huang, Y.T., Tsai, S.H., Lin-Shiau, S.Y., Chen, C.F. and Lin, J.K. (1999). Suppression of inducible cyclooxygenase and inducible nitric oxide synthase by apigenin and related flavonoids in mouse macrophages. *Carcinogenesis,* 20(10): 1945–52.

[50] Kim, A.R., Cho, J.Y., Zou, Y., Choi, J.S. and Chung, H.Y. (2005). Flavonoids differentially modulate nitric oxide production pathways in lipopolysaccharide-activated RAW264.7 cells. *Arch. Pharm. Res.*, 28(3): 297–304.

[51] Chacon, P., Vega, A., Monteseirin, J., El Bekay, R., Alba, G., Perez-Formoso, J.L., Msartinez, A., Asturias, J.A., Perez-Cano, R., Sobrino, F. and Conde, J. (2005).

Induction of cyclooxygenase-2 expression by allergens in lymphocytes from allergic patients. *Eur. J. Immunol.*, 35(8): 2313–24.

[52] Harris, G.K., Qian, Y., Leonard, S.S., Sbarra, D.C. and Shi, X. (2006). Luteolin and chrysin differentially inhibit cyclooxygenase-2 expression and scavenge reactive oxygen species but similarly inhibit prostaglandin-E2 formation in RAW 264.7 cells. *J. Nutr.*, 136(6): 1517–21.

[53] Gutiérrez-Venegas, G., Luna, O.A., Ventura-Arroyo, J.A. and Hernández-Bermúdez, C. (2013). Myricetin suppresses lipoteichoic acid-induced interleukin-1β and cyclooxygenase-2 expression in human gingival fibroblasts. *Microbiol Immunol.*, 57(12): 849–56.

[54] Middleton, Jr. E. and Kandaswami, C. (1992). Effects of flavonoids on immune and inflammatory cell functions. *Biochem Pharmacol.*, 43(6): 1167–79.

[55] Gil, B., Sanz, M.J., Terencio, M.C., Ferrandiz, M.L., Bustos, G., Paya, M., Gunasegaran, R. and Alcaraz, M.J. (1994). Effects of flavonoids on *Naja naja* and human recombinant synovial phospholipases A2 and inflammatory responses in mice. *Life Sci.*, 54(20): PL333–8.

[56] Lee, T.P., Matteliano, M.L. and Middleton, Jr. E. (1982). Effect of quercetin on human polymorphonuclear leukocyte lysosomal enzyme release and phospholipid metabolism. *Life Sci.*, 31(24): 2765–74.

[57] Cheong, H., Ryu, S.Y., Oak, M.H., Cheon, S.H., Yoo, G.S. and Kim, K.M. (1998). Studies of structure activity relationship of flavonoids for the anti-allergic actions. *Arch. Pharm. Res.*, 21(4): 478–80.

[58] Tanaka, T. (2013). Flavonoids as complementary medicine for allergic diseases: Current evidence and future prospects. *OA Alternative Medicine,* 1(2): 11.

[59] Jung, M., Triebel, S., Anke, T., Richling, E. and Erkel, G. (2009). Influence of apple polyphenols on inflammatory gene expression. *Mol. Nutr. Food Res.*, 53(10): 1263–80.

[60] Kobayashi, S., Watanabe, J., Fukushi, E., Kawabata, J., Nakajima, M. and Watanabe, M. (2003). Polyphenols from some foodstuffs as inhibitors of ovalbumin permeation through caco-2 cell monolayers. *Biosci Biotechnol Biochem.*, 67(6): 1250–7.

[61] Nauta, A.J., Engels, F., Knippels, L.M., Garssen, J., Nijkamp, F.P., Redegeld, F.A. (2008). Mechanisms of allergy and asthma. *Eur. J. Pharmacol.*, 585(2–3): 354–60.

[62] Noguchi, Y., Fukuda, K., Matsushima, A., Haishi, D., Hiroto, M., Kodera, Y., Nishimura, H. and Inada, Y. (1999). Inhibition of Df-protease associated with allergic diseases by polyphenol. *J. Agric. Food Chem.*, 47(8): 2969–72.

[63] Fewtrell, C.M. and Gomperts, B.D. (1977). Effect of flavone inhibitors of transport ATPases on histamine secretion from rat mast cells. *Nature,* 265(5595): 635–6.

[64] Amakura, Y., Tsutsumi, T., Sasaki, K., Nakamura, M., Yoshida, T. and Maitani, T. (2008). Influence of food polyphenols on aryl hydrocarbon receptor-signaling pathway estimated by *in vitro* bioassay. *Phytochemistry,* 69(18): 3117–30.

12

Beneficial Effect of Flavonoids on Neurodegenerative Disorders – Old and New Challenges

NATARAJAN SUGANTHY[1]*

ABSTRACT

Increase in aging population is one of the major risk factor for the incidence of neurodegenerative disorders such as Alzheimer's disease, Parkinson's disease, multiple sclerosis, amyotrophic lateral sclerosis, and Huntington disease in 21st century. Several cellular and molecular events such as oxidative stress, mitochondrial dysfunction, deposition of aggregated proteins, neuro-inflammation and activation of apoptotic factors were considered as causative factors leading to neurodegeneration. Therefore, drugs with multipotent action against diverse targets are essential for the treatment of neurodegenerative disorder. Flavonoids are a group of ubiquitous, low-molecular-weight plant polyphenolic compounds, widely distributed in fruits, vegetables and beverages. In traditional and oriental medicine flavonoid rich nutraceuticals have been used for improving cognitive function and preventing neurodegenerative disorders in humans. Several preclinical and clinical studies have shown that flavonoids and their metabolites reduced cognitive decline and neuronal dysfunction via its antioxidant, anti-inflammatory, anti-stress, immunomodulatory and anti-aging effect. Elucidation of molecular mechanism illustrated that flavonoids exhibited neuroprotective effect by interacting with neurosignalling cascade such as phosphoinositide 3-kinase (PI 3-kinase), Akt / protein kinase B (Akt / PKB), tyrosine kinases, protein kinase C (PKC), and mitogen activated protein kinase (MAP kinase), which are involved in apoptosis, neuronal survival and differentiation. In addition, flavonoids have also been reported to induce angiogenesis, thereby promoting new nerve cell growth in the hippocampus.

[1] Department of Nanoscience and Technology, Science Campus, Alagappa University, Karaikudi, Tamil Nadu, India.

**Corresponding author*: E-mail: suganthy.n@gmail.com

Recent reports have shown that regular uptake of flavonoids rich food reduced the risk of age related neurodegenerative disorders, extending their life span. The present review focuses on summarizing the recent findings on the neuroprotective effect of flavonoids, its mechanism of action and its possible roles in the prevention of neurodegenerative disorders, which might provide new insight for the treatment of neurological disease.

***Key words*:** Neurodegenerative disorders, Flavonoids, Oxidative stress, Inflammation, Cognitive function, Neurogenesis.

ABBREVIATIONS

NDDS – Neurodegenerative disorders, AD – Alzheimer's disease, PD – Parkinson disease, HD – Huntington's disease, ALS – Amyotrophic lateral sclerosis disease, AChE – Acetylcholinesterase, BuChE – Butyrylcholinesterase, PSEN – Presenilin, TLR – Toll like receptor, iNOS – Nitric oxide synthase, APP – Amyloid precursor protein, Aβ – Beta amyloid peptide, GSK-3β – Glycogen synthase kinase 3β, CDK5 – Cyclin-dependant kinase, NFT – Neurofibrillary tangles (NFT), TNF-α – Tumor necrosis factor alpha, IL-1β – Interleukin 1 beta, IL-6 – Interleukin-6, IF-γ – Interferon gamma, CREB – cAMP response element-binding protein, BDNF – Brain-derived neurotrophic factor, NGF – Neuronal growth factor, α Syn – Alpha-synuclein, EGCG – Epigallocatechin gallate, PI3 kinase – phosphoinositide 3-kinase, Akt/PKB – Akt/protein kinase, PKC – protein kinase C, MAPK – mitogen activated protein kinase.

1. NEURODEGENERATIVE DISORDERS

Increase in life expectancy of populations in developed countries is considered as one of the leading cause for high incidence rate of age-related illnesses such as neurodegenerative diseases (NDDs). In developed countries NDDs is considered as fourth highest source of overall disease burden in terms of human suffering and economic cost. Neurodegenerative diseases are multifactorial debilitating disorders of nervous system affecting approximately 30 million people worldwide. Etymologically "neuro" refers to nerve cells (*i.e.,* neurons), and "degeneration," refers to the process of losing structure or function in tissues or organs. Neurodegenerative disorders are described as heterogeneous group of disorders characterized by progressive degeneration and/or death of neurons in the central and peripheral nervous system resulting in problems with movement (ataxias) or mental functioning (dementia) (Kovacs, 2016). Scientific evidences demonstrated that proteins with altered physicochemical properties, mostly misfolded protein play a central role in the pathogenesis of NDDS; hence NDDS are termed commonly as conformational disease. In addition impairment of protein elimination pathways such as Ubiquitin-proteasome and autophagy-lysosome pathways also have greater influence in the pathogenesis of NDDs (Ross and Poirier, 2004; Nijholt *et al.,* 2011). Neurodegenerative disorders includes Alzheimer's disease (AD), Parkinson's disease (PD) and PD-related disorders Prion disease, Motor neuron diseases

(MND), Huntington's disease (HD), amyotrophic lateral sclerosis disease (ALS), Spinocerebellar ataxia (SCA) (Armstrong, 2012). Among these long term progressive NDDS such as AD, PD, HD and ALS are the most prevalent and mainly focused disorders, which are caused as a result of misfolding and dysfunctional trafficking of proteins. In addition, several interrelated cellular and molecular events like impaired mitochondrial function, altered voltage-dependant anion channels and lipid rafts, oxidative stress, neuroinflammatory process, activation of apoptotic factors along with normal brain aging were considered as main causative factors leading to neuronal dysfunction and death in NDDs (Ramanan and Saykin, 2013). Despite of the fact that each disease has its own molecular mechanism and clinical manifestations, certain pathways, which occurs concurrently such as protein misfolding and aggregation, free radical formation and oxidative stress, metal dyshomeostasis, mitochondrial dysfunction and phosphorylation impairment (Fig. 1) are considered as general pathways for therapeutic interventions of these disorders (Kovacs, 2016; Ahmed *et al.,* 2016). Inspite of the progress in understanding the pathogenesis of neurodegenerative diseases, the treatment of these disorders still remain obscure. Neurodegenerative disorder commences very early in life, while the symptoms emerge in later stage, hence early diagnosis and appropriate therapeutic strategies are necessary to stop the progression of disease.

1.1. Focus on Pathogenesis of Neurodegenerative Disorders

1.1.1. *Alzheimer's disease*

Alzheimer disease (AD) is the most common cause of dementia and one of the leading sources of morbidity and mortality in the aging population, affecting more than 36 million people worldwide. Clinically AD is characterized by gradual memory loss, a decline in cognitive function and deterioration of physical activities affecting basic bodily functions (Alzheimer's Association, 2016). Genetic factors such as mutation of amyloid precursor protein gene (APP) and presenilin genes (PSEN1, 2) together with aging and environmental risk factors leads to the incidence of AD. Altered metabolism of APP by α and β secretase leads to formation of hydrophobic Aβ (1-42) peptide, which in the presence of transition metal ions such as Cu^{2+} and Fe^{2+} aggregates as β-amyloid (Aβ) plaques at the synaptic junction, disrupting functional receptors, causing synaptic dysfunction. Aggregation of Aβ peptide in the synaptic cleft induces secondary pathogenesis such as oxidative stress mediated damage, alters the function of transmembrane protein, thereby disturbing calcium homeostasis leading to mitochondrial dysfunction and neuronal death (Korolev, 2014). Enhanced intracellular calcium level activates glycogen synthase kinase 3β, cyclin-dependant kinase (*e. g.,* GSK-3β and CDK5) promoting hyperphosphorylation of tau protein leading to the formation of neurofibrillary tangles (NFT) impairing the axonal transport. β-amyloid plaques in the synapse and NFT

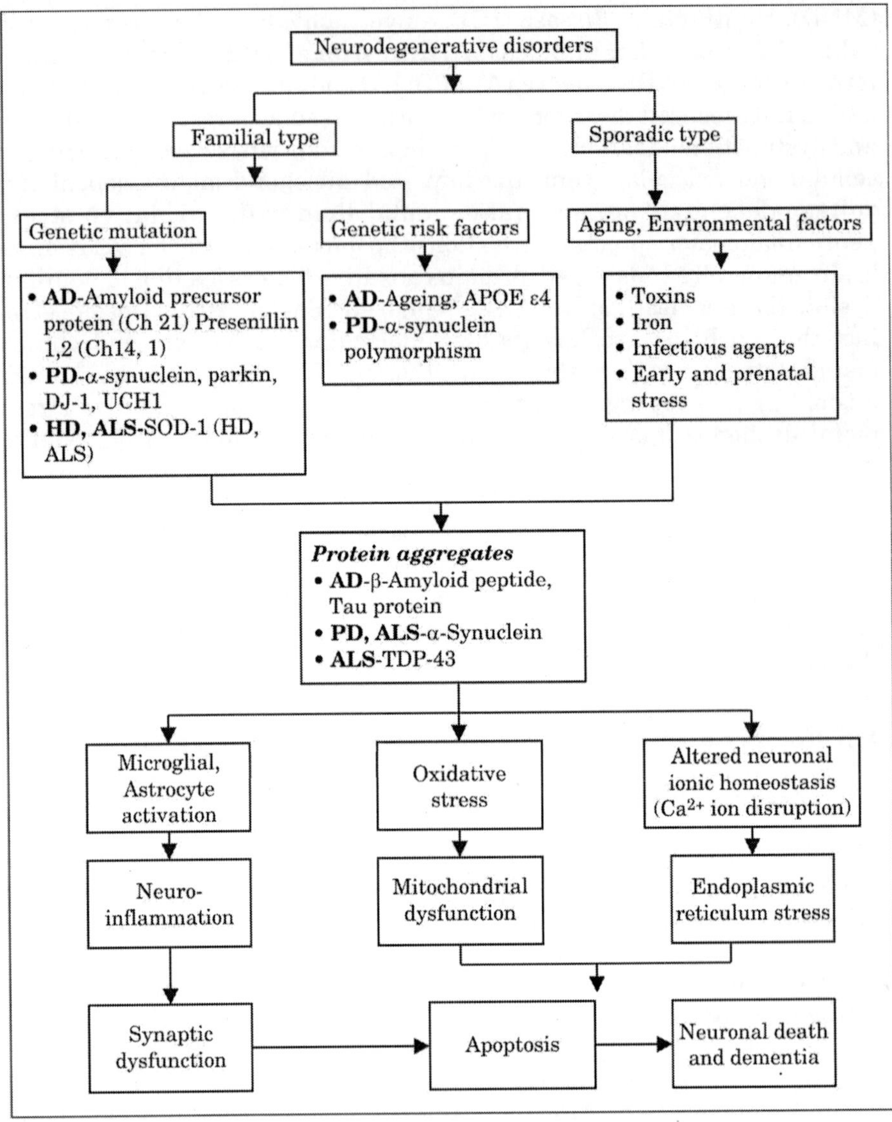

Fig. 1: Overview of Neurodegenerative disorders

in the axon activates microglial cells and astrocytes inducing neuroinflammation by activating pro-inflammatory cytokines through the upregulation of nuclear factor kappa B (NF-κB), mitogen activated protein kinase (MAPK) and C-Jun-N-terminal kinase (JNK) (Kumar *et al.*, 2015). Plaques and tangles are present mainly in brain regions involved in learning, memory and emotional behaviours such as the entorhinal cortex, hippocampus, basal forebrain and amygdale, hence activities of daily life are affected. Not only the Cholinergic and Glutamatergic neurons are affected, the serotonergic and Norepinephrine neurons are also damaged. Since several etiological factors and multiple pathways are involved in the pathogenesis of AD, multipotent drug can only acts as disease-modifying agent for the treatment of AD (Folch *et al.*, 2014).

1.1.2. *Parkinson's disease*

Parkinson's disease (PD) is chronic debilitating neurodegenerative movement disorder characterized by the selective degeneration of neurons such as dopaminergic neurons in the substantia nigra of the midbrain and other monoaminergic neurons in the brain stem. PD is characterized by the changes that occur in motor function like bradykinesia, rigidity, postural instability and rest tremor, although myriad non-motor manifestations are increasingly recognized. Familial autosomal dominant PD is caused due to point mutations or increased gene dosage of the α-synuclein gene *via* a gain-of-function mechanism, while mutation in gene encoding parkin, DJ-1 or PINK 132 causes recessive early-onset PD *via* loss-of-function mechanism. Sporadic PD is caused due to aging and environmental risk factors such as plant-derived toxins, bacterial and viral infection, exposure to organic solvents and toxic pollutants (Schapira *et al.*, 2009). Pathogenesis of PD is a multifactorial cascade of events involving both cell autonomous (inside the degenerating neurons) and non-cell autonomous mechanism (outside the degenerating neurons). In cell-autonomous mechanism, mutation in parkin, DJ-1 or PINK 132 gene and dysregulation of transcriptional coactivator PG1-a alters mitochondrial bioenergetic's which leads to enhanced calcium conductance into the cell driven by L-type calcium $Ca_V1.3$ channel. Increased intracellular calcium induces the production of ROS leading to oxidative stress mediated mitochondrial dysfunction. Mutation in either Parkin or PINK 1 gene hampers the clearance of damaged mitochondria leading to neuronal death. Non cell-autonomous mechanism involves prion like behavior of misfolded protein and neuroinflammation (Schapira and Jenner, 2011). The pathological hallmark represents the presence of Lewy bodies and Lewy neurit is composed of α-synuclein deposits in the substantia nigra pars compacta where melanized neurons degenerate. Transfer of α-synuclein from affected neuron to healthy neuron is called prion like process, which on accumulation in synaptic junction impairs the neuronal excitability, enhances neuroinflammation by inducing the expression of pro-inflammatory mediators like tumor necrosis factor alpha (TNF-α), interleukin 1 beta (IL-1β), interleukin-6 (IL-6) and interferon gamma (IFN-γ) ultimately leading to degeneration of dopminergic neurons of substantia nigra pars compacta (Xu and Pu, 2016). Neuronal loss in PD is not restricted to substantia nigra, other neurons like cholinergic neurons, serotonergic neurons and noradnergic neurons are also affected. Multifactorious cascade of pathogenic events in PD illustrated that single therapeutic intervention is ineffective for treatment of PD.

1.1.3. *Huntington disease (HD)*

Huntington disease is a progressive neurodegenerative disorder which onsets in the middle age (30-50) years and last for 17-20 years. HD is an autosomal dominant disorder caused by elongated Cysteine-adenosine-guanine (CAG) repeat in the short arm of chromosome 4p16.3 in the huntingtin gene encoding for polyglutamine tract in the N-terminus of protein called huntingtin, which is widely present in the cytoplasmic surface of synaptic vesicles, microtubule and mitochondria. The wild-type contain a CAG repeat encoding for polyglutamine stretch of 6-26 in the protein, while in HD the CAG repeat exceeds 40 leading to the formation for abnormal huntingtin protein, which accumulates to form neuronal intranuclear inclusions leading to neuronal death specifically in basal ganglia and cortex (Ross and Tabrizi, 2011). Several pathogenic mechanism including excitotoxicity, oxidative stress, impaired energy metabolism and apoptosis are involved in the neuronal dysfunction and subsequent loss of neurons. Nuclear symptoms of HD include disturbances in motor, cognitive and psychiatric functions followed by weight loss, circadian rhythm disturbances and autonomous nervous system dysfunction. Progression of disease depends on life style ultimately leading to pneumonia and death (Labbadia and Morimoto, 2013).

1.1.4. *Amyotrophic lateral sclerosis*

Most common degenerative disease preferentially causing progressive loss of motor neurons responsible for controlling voluntary muscle movement like chewing, walking, breathing and talking. ALS affects the upper motor neurons present in the brain causing spasticity and lower motor neurons in spinal cord and brain stem leading to muscle weakness, muscle *atrophy* (shrinkage of muscles) and twitching. ALS is incurable and the survival period is 3 years, which can be extended on treatment (Salameh *et al.*, 2015). Mutations in the copper/zinc superoxide dismutase 1 (*SOD1*) gene encoding antioxidant protein, leads to 20% of familial ALS. Prion like propagation of misfolded protein SOD1 and 43 KDa transactive responses DNA binding protein (TDP-43) causes degeneration of motor neurons. Pathogenic mechanism leading to death of motor neurons include glutamate excitotoxicity, oxidative stress owing to mutation in superoxide dismutase gene (SOD-1), mitochondrial damage, alteration in Ca^{2+} homeostasis (Kiernan *et al.*, 2011). As most of these neurodegenerative disorders share common pathways, drugs with multi-targeting ability, which intervene these pathways can prevent the progression and severity of these disorders.

1.1.5. *Multiple sclerosis*

Multiple sclerosis (MS) is a chronic autoimmune inflammatory neurological disorder of the CNS affecting 2.5 million people worldwide.

MS attacks the myelinated axons destroying the myelin and axons leading to deterioration of neurons in the white and gray matter. Etiological factors causing MS in not clear, but it appears to involve combination of genetic susceptibility and a non-genetic trigger, such as a virus, metabolism and environmental factors which acts together resulting in a self-sustaining autoimmune disorder that leads to recurrent immune attacks on the CNS. Clinical symptoms vary depending on the type of neurons affected and extend of damage. Neuropathological of MS includes neurologic dysfunction including optic neuritis and transverse myelitis (Torkildsen *et al.,* 2015).

1.1.6. *Human prion disease*

Human prion diseases are one of the deadliest neurodegenerative disorders including Kuru, Creutzfeldt-Jakob disease, Gerstmann-Sträussler-Scheinker syndrome and fatal familial insomnia. Prion diseases result from the conformational conversion of a normal cellular prion protein (PrPC) into an abnormal misfolded pathological form (PrPSc) which on accumulation in the CNS resulted in progressive neuronal degeneration and vacuolation (Head, 2013).

Neurodegenerative diseases are characterized by different structural and pathologic conditions, which require variety of targets and more efficient methods for their treatment. Till date, no effective treatment is available for NDDs and the currently available drugs are symptom oriented, with severe side effect and limited efficacy. Hence search for multipotent drug with novel preventive strategies from natural medicinal plants has gained attention as potential neuroprotective agents. The present review provides an overview on the scientific literature concerning with the neuroprotective effects of flavonoids for the prevention or treatment of NDDS.

2. FLAVONOIDS- SOURCE AND CLASSIFICATION

Flavonoids are hydrophilic polyphenols found ubiquitously in plants contributing to wide range of colors such as orange, blue and purple for fruits, flowers and leaves. Flavonoids are synthesized in plants *via* photosynthetic process as defensive mechanism against oxidative stress induced by reactive oxygen species (ROS). More than 8000 different flavonoids were identified, which are widely distributed in fruits, grains, nuts, black tea and vegetables. Flavonoids acts as major phytoconstituent of medicinal plants used for the treatment of various life threatening disorders like cancer and neurodegenerative disorders (Table 1).

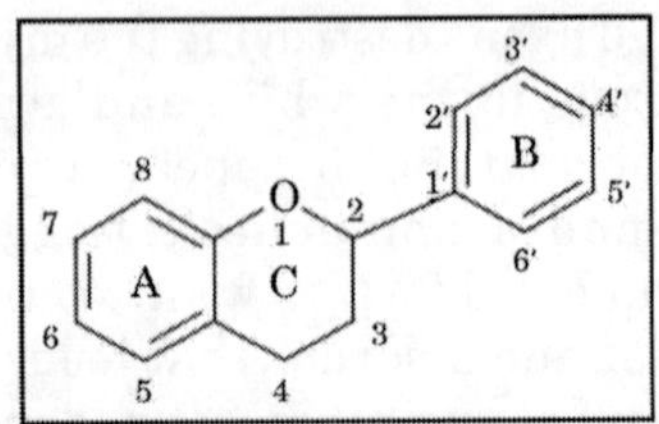

Fig. 2: Basic structure of Flavonoids

Table 1: Dietary Flavonoids Classification, Source and Cholinesterase inhibitory activity

Flavonoids	*Source*	*Substituent groups*			*AChE*	*BuChE*	*References*
		OH	OCH_3	*Other groups*			
Flavones							
Luteolin	Celery, broccoli, green pepper, parsley, spinach, basil	5,7, 3',4'			17.3 ± 2.0[a]	37.2[a]	Conforti *et al.*, 2010
Chrysin	*Passiflora incarnata*, honey	5,7			74.9 ± 1.1[a]	ND	Xie *et al.*, 2014
Baicalein	*Scutellaria baicalensis*	5,6,7			11 ± 1.4[a]	ND	Xie *et al.*, 2014
Baicalin	*Scutellaria baicalensis*	5,6		7-β-D-Glucuronide	204.1 ± 16.5[a]	ND	Xie *et al.*, 2014
Apigenin	Parsley celery other spices such as rosemary, oregano, thyme, basil and coriander, chamomile, cloves, Lemon balm, artichokes and spinach, peppermint Red wine & Licorice	5,7,4''			34.43 ± 2.41[a]	29.11 ± 1.49[a]	Choi *et al.*, 2014
7,8 dihyroflavone	*Godmania aesculifolia, Tridax procumbes, and primula* tree leaves	7,8			314.3 ± 10.2[a]	ND	Xie *et al.*, 2014
Flavanone							
Hesperidin	*Citrus* fruits like *Citrus sinensis*, lemon and tangelos	5,7,3'	4'		27.3 ± 1.2[b]	17.3 ± 4.2[b]	Senol *et al.*, 2016
Naringenin	Grapefruit, oranges, tomatoes (skin] and in water mint	5,7,4'			143.6 ± 16.2[a]	ND	Xie *et al.*, 2014
Leufolins A	*Leucas urticifolia*	5,7,4'	6-*O*-[(2*E*)-3-(4-hyd-		74.5 ± 0.2[a]	1.6 ± 0.98[a]	Atia-tun-Noor *et al.*, 2007

Table 1: (*Contd...*)

Table 1: (*Contd...*)

Flavonoids	*Source*	*Substituent groups*			*AChE*	*BuChE*	*References*
		OH	*OCH_3*	*Other groups*			
			roxyphenyl) prop-2-enoyl]-β-D-glucopyranosyl at 4'				
Leufolin B	*Leucas urticifolia*	6,8,4'	6-*O*-[(2*E*)-3-(4-hydroxyphenyl)prop-2-enoyl]-β-D-glucopyranosyl at 4'		72.3 ± 0.03[a]	3.6 ± 1.7[a]	Atia-tun-Noor *et al.*, 2007
Flavonols							
Kaempferol	Fruits, green vegetables, green tea and in medicinal plants like *Aloe vera, Hypericum perforatum, Moringa oleifera, Rosmarinus officinalis*	3,5,7, 4'			0.9 ± 0.2[c]	0.7 ± 0.1[c]	Szwajgier, 2015
Quercetin	Apples, *Citrus* fruits, onions, parsley, red wine and tea	3,5,7, 3',4'			0.9 ± 0.2[c]	1.9 ± 0.1[c]	Szwajgier, 2015
Quercitrin	*Citrus* fruits, apples, onions, parsley, sage, tea, and red wine, olive oil and berries	5,7,3, 4		3-O-Rhamnoside	94.5 ± 3.8[a]	ND	Xie *et al.*, 2014
Myricetin	Vegetables, fruits, nuts, berries, tea, red wine.	3,5,7, 3',4', 5'			1.4 ± 0.1[c]	0.4 ± 0.0[c]	Szwajgier, 2015
Myricitrin	*Myrica cerifera, Myrica esculenta, Nymphaea lotus, N. odorata*	5,7, 3',4', 5'		3-O-Rhamnoside	228.6 ± 12.3	ND	Xie *et al.*, 2014
Fisetin	Strawberries, Apples, Persimmons, onions,	3,7, 3',4'			336.4 ± 4.3[a]	90 ± 10[d]	Xie *et al.*, 2014; Katalinic *et al.*, 2014

Table 1: (*Contd...*)

Table 1: (*Contd...*)

Flavonoids	*Source*	*Substituent groups*			*AChE*	*BuChE*	*References*
		OH	*OCH_3*	*Other groups*			
	cucumbers						
Rutin	Mulberry, Cranberries, Buckwheat, Asparagus	3,7, 3′,4′		3-a-L-Rham-1, 6 D-Glc	186.6 ± 16.3[a]	ND	Xie *et al.*, 2014
Isoflavones							
Formononetin	Red clover, Leguminosae plants	7	4′		481.5 ± 19.9[a]	ND	Xie *et al.*, 2014
Daidzin	*Pueraria lobata*, Soyabean leaves	4′		7-Glucoside	8.8 ± 1.5[b]	ND	Xie *et al.*, 2014
Daidzein	Soyabeans and soya products	7, 4′			18.4 ± 2.9[b]	ND	Xie *et al.*, 2014
Genistein	Lupin, Fava beans, Soybeans, Kudzu, *Psoralea*, Coffee	5,7,4′			389 ± 9.4[a]	65.7 ± 1.24[b]	Xie *et al.*, 2014; Orhan *et al.*, 2007
Puerarin	*Radix pueraria*	7, 4′		8-C-glucoside	571.2 ± 34.9[a]	ND	Xie *et al.*, 2014
Flavanols							
(+)- Catechin	Tea, red grapes				36.13 ± 0.0[e]	20.02 ± 0.02[e]	Suganthy *et al.*, 2015
Epigallocatechin-3-gallate	Cocoa beverages and chocolate				0.0096[a]		Okello *et al.*, 2012
Flavanonols							
Taxifolin	Milk thistle, Red onion	3,5,7, 3′,4′			133.1[a]		Ding *et al.*, 2013
Silymarin	*Silybum marianum*				ND	51.4 ± 1.05[b]	Orhan *et al.*, 2007
Silibinin	*Silybum marianum*				245 ± 49[a]	530 ± 22[a]	Duan *et al.*, 2015
Anthocyanidins							
Cynadinin	Red and Blue Berries	3,5,7, 32,42			0.7 ± 0.0[c]	1.4 ± 0.2[c]	Szwajgier, 2015
Delphinidin	Cranberries, Concord grapes, Pomegranates, Bilberries	3,5,7, 32,42, 52			0.4 ± 0.0[c]	1.4 ± 0.1[c]	Szwajgier, 2015
Petunidin	Chokeberries Saskatoon berries, *Vitis vinifera*	3,5,7, 32,42, 52	2 ± 0.0[c]		1.8 ± 0.11[c]	–	Szwajgier, 2015

[a] IC_{50} in mM; [b] % of inhibition (concentration), [c] inhibition activity in terms of mM of serine; [d] Ki value mM

Flavonoids are fifteen carbon skeleton aglycone compounds consisting of two benzene rings (A and B) linked through heterocyclic pyrane ring (C) (Fig. 2). Flavonoids are widely classified into flavones (*e.g.*: apigenin, chrysin and luteolin), flavonones (hesperetin, and naringenin), flavanonols (Silibinin,

Silymarin, Taxifolin, Pinobanksin), isoflavones (Genistein, Daidzein, Glycetin, Formanantine), flavonols (Rutin, Quercetin, Kaempferol, Myricetin, isoquercitrin) and Flavan-3-ols (catechin and Epigallocatechin gallate) anthocyanidins (Kumar and Pandey, 2013). Naturally flavonoids exist as aglycones, glycosides and methylated derivatives. Flavonoids within class differ in the substitution of ring A and B, while different classes of flavonoids vary based on their substitution in ring C. Flavonoids are often hydroxylated in positions 3, 5, 7, 2, 3', 4', 5 and in glycosides the glycosidic linkage occurs normally at position 3 or 7 (Heim *et al.,* 2002). Pharmacological actions of flavonoids depend on the biological fate of flavonoids in gastrointestinal tract, liver and cells. Ingested flavonoids undergoes hydrolysis and oxidation in the small intestine (oxidative metabolism), then transported to liver *via*, hepatic portal vein, where it undergoes conjugation and detoxification to form glucuronides, sulfates and O-methylated derivatives. These metabolites are transported to targeted cells and tissues, excreted to bile and eliminated *via* urine and/or feces. The aglycones that reach the colon undergo microbial degradation and reabsorption. Blood brain permability of flavonoids depends upon the lipohilicity of the compound *i.e.,* less polar O-methylated derivaties show high BBB permeability when compared to more polar flavonoid glucuronides (Thilakarathna and Rupasinghe, 2013). Besides its potent antioxidant activity, flavonoids were reported for its broad pharmacological activities such as antiviral, antibacterial, antiatheroscleorotic, antiallergic, antiplatelet, antiinflammatory, antioxidant, antidiabetic, antiapoptotic, anticancer, anti-inflammatory, immune booster, antiaging and neuroprotective effects (Agarwal *et al.,* 2011; Sangeetha *et al.,* 2016). Traditionally, flavonoid rich nutraceuticals have been used as food supplements to enhance the cognitive function and prevent neurodegenerative disorders in human (Keservani *et al.,* 2016). Moreover scientific evidences illustrated the beneficial effect of flavonoids in overcoming oxidative stress related diseases such as cancer, atherosclerosis, and asthma, neurodegenerative disease like PD and AD in human (Sandhar *et al.,* 2011; Busch *et al.,* 2015). Multiple target action of flavonoids in brain has attracted the attention of researchers as potential therapeutic agents in the treatment of neurodegenerative disorder. Source of widely distributed dietary flavonoids are illustrated in Table 1. The present review emphasizes the protective and preventive functions of flavonoids in neurodegenerative diseases through its antioxidant, anticholinergic, antiinflammatory activitis and by modulating neurosignaling pathways.

3. MULTIPOTENT NEUROPROTECTIVE EFFECT OF FLAVONOIDS

3.1. Anticholinergic Effect of Flavonoids

Memory impairment in neurodegenerative disorders are caused due to deficiency in the level of acetylcholine (ACh) the cholinergic neurotransmitter affecting neurotransmission in brain cortical and hippocampal region, which are mainly involved in learning and memory (Jahn, 2013). According to cholinergic hypothesis inhibition of acetylcholinesterase (AChE) increases the level of acetylcholine improving the cholinergic function in dementia specifically AD patients. BuChE the predominant cholinesterase in the glial cells cleaves ACh similar to that of AChE and its level increases to 85% in later stage of AD (Mesulam *et al.,* 2002). Hence in order to restore the level of ACh in the synaptic junction, inhibition of both AChE and BuChE is essential. Current symptomatic treatment available for AD and other related dementia's include cholinesterase inhibitors *i.e.,* both AChE and BuChE inhibitors (Raina *et al.,* 2008). In addition scientific evidences illustrated that AChE plays a major role in the acceleration of amyloid plaque associated neurodegeneration, while BuChE promotes the maturation of benign plaques leading to neuronal degeneration. Inhibition of ChE not only restores the level of ACh in the brain, but also prevents the aggregation of β-amyloid peptide (Dinamarca *et al.,* 2010; Carvajal and Inestrosa, 2011). At present FDA approved cholinesterase inhibitors like donepezil, rivastigmine, galantamine and tacrine are widely used for the management of AD, which possessed severe side effects and least therapeutic efficacy (Yiannopoulou and Papageorgiou, 2013). Hence, extensive researches are underway in search for novel AChE inhibitors from natural sources. Plenty of phytochemicals belonging to class of alkaloids, curcumins, stilbenes and flavonoids from natural sources exhibited potent AChE inhibiton, among which flavonoid attracted much interest due to its low toxicity and high cholinesterase inhibitory activity (D'Onofrio *et al.,* 2016). The inhibitory activity of flavonoids against AChE and BuChE are listed in Table 1.

3.1.1. *Structure activity relationship*

AChE is a complex protein comprising of α/β hydrolase fold containing a deep groove called gorge and the active site is present below the gorge. In AChE the catalytic triad in the active site is Ser200-His440-Glu327, while Try 341, Tyr 72 and Tyr124 form the peripheral anionic site, which modulates the entry of small molecules like substrate or inhibitors into the active site (Dvir *et al.,* 2010). AChE inhibitory activity of flavonoids depends on the structure of flavonoids, generally flavones and flavonols showed strong inhibitory activity, when compared to isoflavones, which might be due to the fact that higher affinity of flavones and flavonols towards AChE increases the chance to entire the catalytic gorge. Hydroxylation of ring A and B and the position of –OH gp in the ring determine the inhibitory efficacy of flavonoids. Presence of –OH gp in 5th position of fisetin and 6th position of baicalein of ring A increases the inhibitory activities by 20.3 and 6.8 fold when compared to chrysin. However, presence of –OH gp in 42 and 52 position of ring B in chrysin and quercetin hardly influences the inhibitory activities illustrating the fact that –OH gp in ring A play a crucial role in AChE inhibition. Results were further substantiated by docking studies, which illustrated that -OH gp of flavonoids forms hydrogen bond with active site residues of AChE. Luteolin exhibited greater binding effect with higher inhibitory activity when compared to apigenin. Glycosylation and hydrogenation of C2-C3 double bond in conjugation with 4-oxo-group decreases the binding affinity and inhibitory activity of flavonoids against AChE. In addition the presence of 4'-OMe group and 7-O sugar moiety is necessary for AChE inhibition. In flavones and flavanones the presence of pyrrolidin-1-ylmethyl in C42 plays important role in AChE inhibitory activity. C6 and C7-OMe groups and presence of piperidin, pyrrolidin or ethylamino derivates at C32 or C42 position of isoflavone showed increased inhibitory activity (Xie *et al.*, 2014). Overall the substituent in flavones, isoflavone and chalcone derivatives acts as most promising drug candidates for AD. In the case of BuChE the catalytic traid is Ser 198, Glu 325, His 438. Substrate binds to the Asp 70 of the pheripheral anionic site and slides down the active site gorge (Trp82) and rotates horizontal for hydrolysis by Ser 198. Inhibitory activity of flavonoids depends on the number of –OH group and their position in phenyl ring. Docking studies illustrated that flavonoids bind to BuChE active site by multiple π–π interaction and hydrogen bonds (Katalinic *et al.*, 2014).

In addition to dietary flavonoids, many plant extracts rich in flavonoid content exhibited potent AChE and BuChE inhibitory activity. Geranylated flavonoids identified in the methanolic fruit extract of *Paulownia tomentosa* exhibited dual cholinesterase inhibitory activity (Hanáková *et al.*, 2015). The flavonols like sophoflavescenol, icaritin, demethylanhydroicaritin, 8-C-lavandury1 kaempferol and kaempferol present in *Sophora flavescens* exhibited potent AChE inhibitory activity with IC_{50} values of 8.37, 6.47, 6.67, 5.16 and 3.31 µM, respectively (Jung *et al.*, 2011). Nine flavonoids isolated from methanolic root extract of *Morus lhou* (Moraceae) exhibited both AChE and BuChE inhibition. Among the flavonoids, 5'-geranyl-4'-methoxy- 5,7,2'-trihydroxyflavone exhibited highest inhibition (IC_{50} = 10.95 µM), while 5'-geranyl-5,7,2',4'- tetrahydroxyflavone, kuwanon U, kuwanon E, morusin, cyclomorusin, neocyclomorusin and kuwanon C exhibited moderate inhibition with IC_{50} value ranging 16.21–36.4 µM (Kim *et al.*, 2011). Three Prenylated flavonols isolated from ethanolic root extract of *Broussonetia papyrifera* elicited cholinesterase inhibitory activity against human erythrocyte AChE with IC_{50} values of 0.82, 3.1 and 2.7 µM, respectively (Ryu *et al.*, 2012). Isoorientin and isovitexin isolated from flowers and rhizomes of *Iris pseudopumila* (Iridaceae) exhibited potent AChE activity with IC_{50} value of 26.8 and 36.4 µM respectively (Murray *et al.*, 2013). Dual cholinesterase activity of flavonoids plays a key role in attenuating the cholinergic deficit in AD and other related neurodegenerative disorders.

3.2. Role of Flavonoids in Combating Oxidative Stress

Brain the vital organ consumes 20% of the total oxygen intake and high glucose level for their normal functioning, which makes them highly susceptible for free radical formation. Presence of rich source of polyunsaturated fatty acid, transition metal ions Fe^{2+}, Cu^{2+}, Zn^{2+}, low antioxidant surveillance and regenerative capacity, makes the neural cells vulnerable to ROS mediated damage, with enhanced susceptibility in aged brain. Increased level of ROS and insufficient antioxidants provokes the pathogenesis of ND including ALS, AD, PD and HD (Kim *et al.,* 2015). ROS overload in neuronal cells causes oxidation of lipids, proteins and DNA generating byproducts highly toxic to blood lymphocytes and macrophages. Acrolein (oxidatively modified lipids) inhibits glutamate and glucose uptake, blocks neuronal ion transporters, activates c-Jun and MAPkinase pathway leading to cellular apoptosis. Protein oxidation dysregulates antioxidant enzymes involved in balancing oxidative status in cellular system. Enhanced ROS level provoked increased influx of intracellular calcium which in turn leads to activation of glutamate receptors causing glutamate excitotoxicity and apoptosis in HD, AD, PD and ALS. Moreover aging alters metal metabolism leading to accumulation of redox metals (Cu^{2+}, Fe^{2+} and Zn^{2+}), which makes the brain highly susceptible to oxidative stress mediated neurodegenerative disorders (Gandhi *et al.,* 2012). Scientific reports illustrated that antioxidants overcoming upstream oxidative stress (attenuates free radical generation, modualtes metal-neuronal protein interaction and promotes normal metal homoeostasis) and downstream oxidative stress (neuroinflammation) (Uttara *et al.,* 2009; Feng and Wang, 2012) have been proved as effective alternative tool to overcome ROS mediated neuronal damage. The potential beneficial health effect of flavoniods in overcoming neurodegenerative disease is mainly due to its rich antioxidant property. The antioxidant property of flavonoids depends upon the position of functional groups in their nuclear structure. Total number of hydroxyl groups and their position influences the mechanism of antioxidant activity such as radical scavenging and metal ion chelating ability (Prochαzková *et al.,* 2011). Flavonoids attenuates oxidative stress by one of the following mechanism such as:

- ***Direct free radical scavenger:*** Flavonoids effectively scavenges free radicals by donating hydrogen atom or electrons. Structure activity relationship illustrate that number and position of OH groups (Orthodihydroxy group in ring B and 2, 3-double bond in conjugation with a 4-oxo in ring C) determines the antioxidant activity of flavonoids. Polymerization of flavonoid monomer enhances the antioxidant capacity *e.g.*: proanthocyanidins, the catechin polymer exhibited potent antioxidant activity when compared to catechin alone due to increase in the number of –OH groups (Procházková *et al.,* 2011). However, glycosylation reduces their antioxidant activity, when compared to aglycones *e.g.,* Quercetin on glycosylation showed significant reduction in superoxide scavenging ability and reducing power (Rice-Evans *et al.,* 1996). Flavonols like quercetin and myricetin were found to be the most free radical scavengers among the flavonoids (Heim *et al.,* 2002).

- ***Activates antioxidant enzymes:*** Flavonoids activates electrophile responsive element (EpRE), a set of regulatory genes encoding phase II detoxifying enzymes, thereby enhancing the level of phase II detoxifying enzymes like NAD(P)H-quinone oxidoreductase, glutathione Stransferase, and UDP-glucuronosyl transferase the major defense antioxidant enzymes in combating oxidative stress (Lee-Hilz *et al.,* 2006). Flavones and flavanones methoxylated at the 5-position of the A-ring are reported as inducers of the cytoprotective NAD(P) H:quinone-oxidoreductase 1 (NQO1) (Tsuji *et al.,* 2013).
- ***Metal chelating activity:*** Flavonoids effectively chelates metal ions like iron and copper, thereby preventing the formation of free radicals. Catechol moiety in ring B, 3-hydroxyl and 4-oxo groups of ring C and the 4-oxo and 5-hydroxyl groups between the C and A rings of flavonoids were involved in metal chelation (Pietta, 2000). Quercetin acts as potent iron chelating and stabilizing agent, while morin effectively chelates Cd^{3+} exhibiting strong antioxidant activity under *in vitro* condition (Kopacz *et al.,* 2003). Myricetin and quercetin showed potent Cu^{2+} and Fe^{3+} chelating effect due to the presence of ortho-catechol group, the 5-hydroxyl and the 4-oxo groups the chelating site for Cu^{2+} and Fe^{3+} (Mira *et al.,* 2002).
- ***Reduction of α-tocopheryl radicals*:** α-tocopherol the cellular antioxidant acts as prooxidant effectively protecting the cell membrane against oxidative damage. Flavonoids stabilizes α-tocopheryl radical by donating hydrogen atom, which in turn prevents the oxidation of lowdensity lipoprotein in cell membrane (Hirano *et al.,* 2001).
- ***Inhibits xanthine oxidases:*** Flavonoids inhibit enzymes involved in the formation of superoxide ($O_2\bullet^-$) radical like xanthine oxidase and protein kinase C. Structure activity relationship studies revealed that planar flavones and flavonols with 7 hydroxyl group like chrysin, luteolin, kaempferol, quecetin, myricetin and isorhamnetin inhibition xanthine oxidase with IC_{50} value ranging rom 0.42 to 5.02 μM and the mode of inhibition is mixed type inhibition, when compared to nonplanar isoflavones and anthocyanidins (Lin *et al.,* 2015).
- ***Mitigates oxidative stress induced by nitric oxide*:** Flavonoids mitigates NO mediated oxidative stress either by directly scavenging NO radicals or by inhibiting the expression of iNOS the enzyme involved in NO production. Presence of 2, 3-double bond with 4-oxo group and 3, 5, 4′ - trihydroxyl group played crucial role in inhibiting NO production. Apigenin, diosmetin, and luteolin the naturally occurring flavones exhibited potent NO inhibitory activity. Quercetin reduced ischemia–reperfusion injury by inhibiting iNOS activity.

Flavonoids also effectively scavenged peroxynitrite directly and their activity is related to 32, 4′-catechol arrangement, followed by an unsubstituted 3-hydroxyl group (Heim *et al.,* 2002; Choi *et al.,* 2002).

- ***Enhances the antioxidant properties of low molecular antioxidants*:** Several studies illustrated that flavonoids like EGCG, genistein, Kaempferol, Apigenin and Anthocyanin exhibited neuroprotective effect against oxidative stress induced toxicity in AD model system (PC12, SH-SY5Y and Neuro 2a cells) by lowering ROS, inhibiting lipid peroxidation and GSSH formation through its antioxidant activity (Zeng *et al.,* 2004; Wang *et al.,* 2001; Liu *et al.,* 2010). Flavonoids in *Ginkgo biloba* extract attenuated oxidative stress mediated damage in hippocampal cells treated Aβ peptides and H_2O_2 (Bastianetto *et al.,* 2000). Apigenin ameliorates AD-associated learning and memory impairment *via* inhibiting oxidative stress, and improving the activity of antioxidative enzyme SOD and glutathione peroxidase (Zhao *et al.,* 2013).

3.3. Protective Effect of Flavonoids Against Neuroinflammation

The CNS is an immune privileged organ in which the immune responses is partially dependent on the blood–brain barrier (BBB), which limits the entry of circulating immune cells in the healthy brain. Inflammatory process a double edged sword in CNS is an innate or adaptive immune response against diverse insults, designed to remove noxious agents and to inhibit their detrimental effects. In neurodegenerative diseases, inflammation is considered as driving force triggered by the accumulation of proteins with abnormal conformations or by signals emanating from injured neurons leading to neuropathologies (Glass *et al.,* 2010). Microglial cells are resident brain cells existing in deactivated phenotype in healthy brain, which on sensing signals initiate inflammatory responses that are further amplified by astrocytes (Lull and Block, 2010). Inflammatory mediators such as abnormal protein deposits of Aβ (AD), α-synuclein (PD), mutant SOD1 (ALS), and myelin peptide (MS) on recognition by Toll like receptor (TLR4) activates microglial cells secrete inflammatory mediators such as TNF-α, IL-1β, which in turn induces secondary inflammatory response like activation of complement components, acute phase protein and iNOS expression. Uncontrolled activation of iNOS in glial cells constitutes a critical event in inflammatory-mediated neurodegeneration. Activation of MAPK signaling leads to the induction of pro-inflammatory transcription factors (STAT-1, NF-κB), mediating the production of amplifiers and effectors, such as cytokines and Interleukins (*e.g.,* TNF-α, IL-1β, IL-6, ROS and NO) leading to neuroinflammation (Spencer *et al.,* 2012). Crosstalk between microglia and astrocytes led to the amplification of inflammation and release of ATP by necrotic neurons, which in turn activates microglia independent of the original inducing molecules required to initiate inflammatory responses

(Chen *et al.,* 2016). Overall it is hypothesized that specific inducers associated with ND converge to activate cascade of events culminating in neuronal damage that underpins NDDs like AD, MS, PD and ALS (Spencer *et al.,* 2011). Antiinflammatory agents which inhibit microglial activation and associated cytokine release, iNOS expression, NO production and NADPH oxidase activity might attenuate inflammation induced neuronal death. Multiple evidences suggest that dietary flavonoids exert neuroprotective effect by inhibiting activation of microglia the key mediator of inflammatory processes in CNS. Possible mechanisms by which flavonoids attenuates neuroinflammation are (i) attenuating the release of cytokines such as IL-1β and TNF-α in activated microglia (ii) suppressing NF-κB and iNOS expression and subsequent NO production in activated glial cells (iii) inhibiting NADPH oxidase and subsequent ROS production in activated glial cells (iv) inhibiting the phosphorylation of p38-MAPK thereby down regulating of pro-inflammatory transcription factors such as NF-κB, AP-1 (Vauzour *et al.,* 2008). Flavonoid-rich blueberry extracts inhibited NO, IL-1β and TNF-α production in activated microglia cells (Lau *et al.,* 2007). Flavonol quercetin (Chen *et al.,* 2005), flavones such as wogonin (Chun *et al.,* 2005), baicalein (Hwang *et al.,* 2008) Apigenin, (Zhang *et al.,* 2014) Chrysin (Ha *et al.,* 2008), the flavanols catechin and epigallocatechin gallate (EGCG) (Li *et al.,* 2004a), and the isoflavone genistein (Wang *et al.,* 2005) attenuated microglial/ astrocyte mediated neuroinflammation by inhibiting expression of iNOS and cyclooxygenase (COX-2), NO production, cytokine release, and NADPH oxidase activation with subsequent reduction in the generation of ROS in astrocytes and microglia.. Icarrin attenuated inflammation by inhibiting TAK1/IKK/NF-κB, JNK and p38 pathway leading to reduction in level of NO, PGE-2, ROS, TNF-α, IL-6, IL-1β, iNOS and COX-2 (Xu *et al.,* 2010). Quercetin widely occurring flavonols inhibited inflammatory response in endotoxin stimulated BV-2 microglial cells by inhibiting ERK, JNK, p38, AKT, Src, Janus kinase-1, Tuk2IKK, NF-κB, AP-1 and STAT-1, iNOS expression reducing the level of NO, increasing Hemeoxygenase level and disruption of accumulated lipid rafts (Kao *et al.,* 2010). Fisetin activates ERK pathway leading to phophorlyation of CREB enhancing memory in rat hippocampus (Maher *et al.,* 2006). Fisetin inhibits inflammation in LPS-stimulated BV-2 microglial cells by blocking the phosphorylation of p38 MAPkinase (Zheng *et al.,* 2008), while the flavones luteolin inhibits microglial activation by inhibiting JNK signaling pathway inhibiting the production of cytokine IL-6. Flavanones, naringenin blocks the phosphorylation of p38 MAPK and STAT-1 inhibiting iNOS expression and NO production in neuronal glial cocultures and BV-2 microglial cells (Chao *et al.,* 2010).

3.4. Flavonoids Reduces Glutamate Mediated Excitotoxicty

L-Glutamate is the predominant excitatory neurotransmitter of mammalian central nervous system necessary for normal synaptic function. Glutamate released from the presynaptic terminals binds to the ionotropic/G-protein coupled receptor in the post synaptic terminal mediating excitatory transmission, which gets terminated by the uptake of glutamate by the excitatory aminoacid transporter in glial cells and astrocytes around the synapse. Excess level of L- glutamate causes over-activation of postsynaptic neurons leading to condition called neuronal excitotoxicity the major mechanism leading to progressive neurodegenerative disorders such as AD and PD. Glutamate excitotoxicity causes increased influx of ca^{2+}, alteration in MMP, increased production of ROS leading to death of neurons and glial cells (Matute *et al.,* 2002). Drugs with glutamate receptor antagonistic activity, antioxidant capacity and metal chelating activity can help in overcoming oxidative damage and ameliorate disease progression. Reports have shown that, flavonoids attenuate glutamate induced excitotoxicity *via* its antioxidant potential. Flavonoids such as patuletin, nepetin, and axillarin isolated from butanol extract of *Inula britannica* showed protective effect against oxidative stress induced by glutamate in primary cultures of rat cortical cells by restoring antioxidant status of the cells and Ca^{2+} homeostasis (Kim *et al.,* 2002). Kaempferol 3-O--D-(200-Oacetyl-600-(E)-p-coumaroyl)-glucopyranoside (2"-acetyltiliroside) was isolated from the methanolic stem extract of *Agrimonia eupatoria* showed a neuroprotective effect against glutamate-induced toxicity in HT22 cells (Lee *et al.,* 2010). Proanthocyanidin trimer isolated from water soluble cinnamon extract attenuates post ischemic excitotoxicity of glutamate in C6 glial cells (Panickar *et al.,* 2012). Nicotiflorin and rutin enhanced the survival rate of retinal ganglion cell (RGC) by inhibiting caspase-3 blocking the induction of calpain during oxidative stress (Nakayama *et al.,* 2011). Myricetin attenuated glutamate induced toxicity by modulating NMDAR phosphorylation leading to reduction in glutamate induced intracellular Ca^{2+} load, inhibits ROS level and activation of caspase-3 (Shimmyo *et al.,* 2008). Grape seed proanthocyanidin extract (GSPE) attenuated glutamate-induced excitotoxicity by reducing the calcium signals and NO in cultured rat hippocampal neurons (Ahn *et al.,* 2011). Luteolin protected rat brains from Kainic-induced excitotoxic damage by reducing glutamate levels, mitigating inflammation, and enhancing Akt activation in the hippocampus (Lin *et al.,* 2016). Hesperidin and Apigenin attenuated glutamate neurotoxicity induced by 4- aminopyridine in rat hippocampal nerve terminals and murine cerebellar and cortical cell cultures by inhibiting glutamate release and elevation of cytosolic free Ca^{2+} level (Chang *et al.,* 2015; Losi *et al.,* 2004). EGCG reduced glutamate induced calcium increase by inhibiting ionotropic Ca^{2+} influx, promoting viability of PC12 cells treated with glutamate (Lee *et al.,* 2004). Quercetin exhibited protective effect against glutamate induced toxicity in HT22 cells by dowregulating intracellular ROS level, glutamate mediated Ca^{2+} influx, apoptotic marker, suppressing the phosphorylation of MAPKinase thereby increasing the cell survival (Yang *et al.,* 2013).

3.5. Effect of Flavonoids in Learning, Memory and Cognitive Performance

Scientific reports illustrated that regular consumption of food rich in flavonoids improved cognitive ability. Ability to cross blood brain barrier and interact directly with brain innate architecture might be responsible for the memory enhancement capacity of flavonoids. Studies have shown that flavonoids helps to overcome memory deficits associated with normal aging and other neurodegenerative associated disorders like AD, PD and VD (Spencer *et al.,* 2009; Krishnaveni, 2012). MAPK and PI3 kinase pathways play crucial role in mechanism behind learning and memory storage in the hippocampus and cortex of the brain. Flavonoids have the potential to enhance memory and learning by activating MAPKinases such as ERK and PKB/Akt, increasing the expression of transcription factor cAMP response element-binding protein (CREB) leading to the production of neurotrophins BDNF required for neuronal survival, differentiation, and function enhancing short and long term memory (Schroeter *et al.,* 2002; Spencer *et al.,* 2003; Schroeter *et al.,* 2007). Studies suggest that flavonoids particularly isoflavones like genistein improves neurocognitive function in post menopausal women. In addition animal studies also showed positive effect in improving cognitive function with the intake of isoflavones, which might be due to its ability to mimic oestrogen activity in brain (Casini *et al.,* 2006). Studies have shown that isoflavones also modulates the synthesis of acetylcholine and neurotrophic factor like BDNF, NGF in hippocampus and frontal cortex (Lee *et al.,* 2004). Blue berries rich in anthocyanins effectively reversed aged related neuronal deficits in motor function and working memory, improved object recognition and short term memory, long term reference memory in aged rats (Goyarzu *et al.,* 2004; Williams *et al.,* 2008). Flavonoid rich extract of *Ginkgo biloba* induces positive effects on memory, learning and concentration with prominent effect on brain activity in animals such as senescent mice and humans suffering from cognitive impairment (Hoffman *et al.,* 2004; Shif *et al.,* 2006). *Ginkgo biloba* extract promotes cognitive effects *via* reducing the level of ROS, increasing cerebral blood flow, modulating brain fluidity and interacting with muscarinic cholinergic system, protecting striatal dopaminergic system (Cohen-Salmon *et al.,* 1997). Fruits rich in flavonols like quercetin and rutin and fisetin are beneficial in reversing the course of neuronal and behavioural changes on aging. Intake of Flavanol (-)-epicatechin in combination with exercise enhanced spatial memory in rats by enhancing angiogenesis and increasing neuronal spine density in the dentate gyrus of the hippocampus, upregulating genes associated with learning in the hippocampus (van Praag *et al.,* 2007). In addition, (-)- epicatechin induced ERK1/2 and CREB activation in cortical neurons with subsequent increase in CREB regulated proapoptotic gene expression enhancing the survival rate of cortical neurons (Schroeter *et al.,* 2007). Fisetin rich in strawberries improved long-term potentiating and object recognition in mice by activating ERK and CREB pathway promoting neurogenesis (Maher *et al.,* 2006). Hesperetin capable of activating ERK1/2 signaling in cortical neurons (Vauzour *et al.,* 2007) and flavanols such as EGCG restores both protein kinase C and ERK1/2 activities in 6-hydroxy dopamine toxicity and serum deprived neurons (Reznichenko *et al.,* 2005). Quercetin has been reported to attenuate behavioral and cognitive impairment in several neurodegenerative diseases including Parkinson's disease (Sriraksa *et al.,* 2012), Alzheimer's disease, and chronic cerebral ischemia models. Quercetin improved cognitive deficits by reducing Aβ plaques, amerliorating mitochondrial dysfunction, activates AMP protein kinase, enhances learning and memory in transgenic Alzheimer's disease animal models (APPswe/PS1dE9) (Wang *et al.,* 2014).

3.6. Flavonoids Modulates Sirtuins in Age Related Neurodegenerative Disorders

Mammalian sirtuin (SIRT) proteins belongs to class III histone deacetylases comprising of seven members (SIRT 1–7), which play important role in regulating metabolism, stress responses and longevity in both prokaryotes and Eukaryotes (Carafa *et al.,* 2016). SIRT1 is ubiquitously expressed in neurons of hippocampus and hypothalamus primarily localized in the nucleus (Zakhary *et al.,* 2010). SIRT1 mainly linked with neuronal survival, neuropathology and expression of BDNF exhibiting potent neuroprotective effect (Zakhary *et al.,* 2010). Several reports have shown that SIRT1 knockout results in exacerbation of the pathology, while its re-expression displays neuroprotective effects. SIRT1 expression blocked Aβ peptide formation in primary Tg2576 neuronal cultures (Qin *et al.,* 2006), and enhanced longevity in transgenic *Caenorhabditis elegans* – NL5901 (Nazir *et al.,* 2013). Activation of SIRT-1 cause inhibition of Aβ peptide, attenuation of apoptosis and repression of multiple pro-apoptotic transcription factors, hence compounds which activate SIRT1 can act as neuroprotective agent (Gräff *et al.,* 2013). Very few scientific evidences regarding the SIRT 1 modulatory effect of flavonoids are reported. Quercetin has been reported to activate SIRT-1 dependent pathway, blocking the release of inflammatory cytokines thereby preventing demylination of neurons in multiple sclerosis (Hendriks *et al.,* 2003). Quercetin also exhibits antiaging effect and neuroprotective effect by activating SIRT1 regulated stress regulators (de Boer *et al.,* 2006). Myricetin activated SIRT1 exhibiting potential in MS treatment (Hong *et al.,* 2012).

3.7. Flavonoids and Autophagy Related Proteins

Autophagy is a lysosomal degradative process used to recycle aged cellular constituents and eliminate damaged organelles and protein aggregates. The functional integrity of the CNS depends on the basal autophagy process a protective mechanism involving removal of accumulated damaged organelles and misfolded protein in the neurons (Nixon, 2013). Mutations in the gene regulating autophagic processes lead to neurodegeneration, hence agents stimulating autophagy acts as neuroprotective agent. Flavonoids like hesperetin and hesperidin regulated Aβ stimulated autophagy in insulin stimulated neuronal cells treated high glucose, improving cognitive function (Huang *et al.*, 2012). Kaempferol protected SH-SY5Y and primary neuronal cells from rotenone toxicity through the activation of autophagy (Park *et al.*, 2011). Quercetin exhibited neuroprotection by activating autophagy processes in schwann cells treated with high glucose (Qu *et al.*, 2014) and in *C. elegans* induced with Aβ (1–42) neurotoxicity (Regitz *et al.*, 2014).

3.8. Flavonoids Modulates Abnormal Protein Aggregation

Abnormal protein folding and self-assembly comprising of proteinaceous inclusion bodies in many brain regions are the major causatives of several neurodegenerative disorders like AD, PD, ALS and HD. Protein folding and aggregation depends on the posttranslational modifications (PTMs), such as phosphorylation, glycosylation and ubiquitination. In most of neurodegenerative disorders, phosphorylation of protein plays a key role in aggregation and toxicity (Salazar and Höfer, 2009).

3.8.1. *Blocking alpha-synuclein fibrillisation*

Alpha-synuclein (α-Syn) the synuclein protein is primarily found in neural tissue in the neocortex, hippocampus and cerebellum essential for the supply of synaptic vesicles in presynaptic terminals and regulate the release of dopamine controlling voluntary and involuntary movements (Oueslati, 2016). S129 the main component of α-Syn on phosphorylation by protein kinase such as G-protein coupled receptor kinases, casein kinases (CK) and the polo like kinases (PLKs) intiates aggregation of α-Syn causing defects in synaptic vesicle homeostasis and neurotransmission. α-Syn the principle component of Lewy bodies (LBs), are the major causatives to PD and other disorders collectively known as synucleinopathies. Aggregated forms of α-Syn forming inclusions are found in substantia nigra of PD patients and patients suffering from other synucleinopathies, such as dementia with LBs (DLB), multiple system atrophy, and Hallervorden-Spatz disease (Anderson *et al.*, 2006). Flavonoids have been reported for its ability to prevent aggregation of α-synuclein and disaggregate the preformed fibrils into monomers and nonpathogenic oligomers. The ability of flavonoids to inhibit α-synuclein fibrillation depends on the vicinal dihydroxyphenyl moiety and the number of hydroxyl groups (Meng *et al.*, 2010). The antioxidant activities of flavonoids were generally correlated with their *in vitro* inhibitory effects on α-Syn fibrillation (Meng *et al.*, 2009). Quercetin interacts with α-Syn covalently forming quercetin-α-syn adducts increasing hydrophilicity preventing fibrilliation. Quercetin also effectively disaggregates the preformed fibrils through the protein/quercetin interaction, detaching into stable oligomers (Zhu *et al.,* 2013). Flavonoids with low molecular weight having three vicinal hydroxyl groups like Baicalein, Myricetin, EGCG, Tricetin and luteolin effectively interferes with aggregation of α-synuclein to oligomers, as well as disaggregates preformed oligomer to monomers with IC_{50} value ranging around 1 mM (Meng *et al.,* 2010). Sructure–activity analysis of flavonoids illustrated that compounds with (i) aromatic recognition elements allow non-covalent binding to the amyloidogenic core of the αS monomer/oligomer preventing aggregation and (ii) hydroxyl groups (three > two > one –OH groups on the same ring structure) will be effective in hindering the progress of the self-assembly process of -α-synclein monomer and also destabilizes the preformed -α-synclein oligomers (Meng *et al.,* 2010; Caruana *et al.,* 2011). Baicalein undergoes auto-oxidation to form quinones, which in turn forms Schiff base with lysine side chain in α-synuclein inhibiting fibrillation process. With respect to disaggregation process baicalein intercalates into the α-sheet fibrils with its many hydrogen bond donor/ acceptors, causing both endo and exodisaggregation (Zhu *et al.,* 2004).

3.8.2. *Prevention of Tau pathology*

Tau proteins are microtubule associated proteins necessary for the stabilization of neuronal microtubules, providing the tracks for intracellular transport (Avila *et al.,* 2004). Tau protein on hyperphosphorylation detaches from microtubules, depolymerizes microtubules, self aggregates due to its hydrophobicity forming neurofibrillary tangles (NFT), activating inflammatory cascade, ultimately leading to neuronal death (Tai *et al.,* 2012). Glycogen synthase kinase 3β (GSK3β) and heat shock protein 70 (HSP 70) play a crucial role in the phosphorylation of tau protein (Gong and Iqbal, 2008). Formed NFT are widely distributed in hippocampal and frontal cortex region of brain leading to cognitive dysfunction and neurodegeneration in AD and other related tauopathies. Drugs which block aggregation of tau protein, modulate the activity of tau-effector proteins GSK3β, stabilize microtubules and inhibit HSP 70 were considered to be effective for the treatment of tauopathies (Karakaya *et al.,* 2012) Flavonoids prevent tau aggregation by blocking targets involved in tau phosphorylation. Quercetin attenuated tau hyperphosphorylation by effectively modulating PI3K/Akt/ GSK3β signaling pathway thereby inactivating GSK3β kinases with IC_{50} value of 2 mM and also through its anti HSP-70 activity (Johnson *et al.,* 2011). Myrecetin and epicatechin-5-gallate inhibited heparin induced tau formation (Taniguchi *et al.,* 2005). EGCG administration in Alzheimer transgenic mice modulates tau profiles, with suppression of sarkosyl-soluble phosphorylated Tau isoforms (Rezai-Zadeh *et al.,* 2008). Morin attenuated Aβ-induced Tau phosphorylation by inhibiting GSK-3β activity and protected human neuroblastoma cells against Aβ cytotoxicity. In addition, treatment of 3×Tg-AD mice with morin resulted in reductions in tau hyperphosphorylation and paired helical filament-like immunoreactivity in hippocampal neurons illustrating the fact that morin can act as potential therapeutic agent in tauopathies (Gong *et al.,* 2011). Tg2576 mouse model of AD fed with luteolin decreased soluble Aβ levels, reduced GSK-3β activity and disrupted PS1-APP association (Rezai-Zadeh *et al.,* 2011).

3.8.3. *Antiamyloidogenic effect of flavonoids*

Amyloid precursor proteins (APP) are transmembrane protein expressed in the central nervous system essential to maintain synaptic plasticity and neurons healthy. In healthy neurons APP is processed by α-secretase to form SAPPα through non-amyloidogenic pathway. Under diseased condition like AD, APP is cleaved by β and γ secretase resulting in the formation of Aβ (1-42) peptide, which tends to aggregates forming senile plaques and gets deposited in the synaptic junction disrupting neurotransmission (Serrano-Pozo *et al.,* 2011). Hence, development of drugs, which blocks amyloid production, inhibits Aβ aggregation and disaggregates the preformed fibrillary aggregates, can act as an effective therapeutic approach for AD treatment (Salloway *et al.,* 2008). Since β-secretase (BACE) and γ-secretase are the prime enzymes involved in the formation of Aβ peptide, compounds which inhibit both β-secretase and γ-secretase can act as effective antiamyloidogenic agent attenuating Aβ induced toxicity in AD. Anthocyanin-enriched bilberry and black currant extracts modulated APP processing and alleviated behavioral abnormalities in the APP/PS1 mouse model of AD (Vepsalainen *et al.,* 2013). Luteolin inhibits γ-secretase activity thereby reducing Aβ peptide generation in both human "Swedish" mutant APP transgene-bearing neuron-like cells and primary neurons (Shimmyo *et al.,* 2008). Green tea flavonoid EGCG reduced the level of Aβ in brain by activating ADAM10 (γ-secretase) promoting nonamyloidogenic pathway and inhibiting BACE1 blocking amyloidogenic process (Obregon *et al.,* 2006). EGCG similar to other flavonoids like myricetin, querctin inhibits the formation of Aβ fibrils and destabilizes the preformed mature fibrils by reinforcing the hydrophobic interaction between the aromatic rings with β-sheet structures of Aβ by hydrogen bonds. Dihydroxyl group of the B ring plays a key role in its anti-aggregation effect (Ehrnhoefer *et al.,* 2008; Jiménez-Aliaga *et al.,* 2011). SPR analysis and fluorescence spectroscopy studies showed that quercetin acts as class II inhibitors, which binds to the growing ends of Aβ inhibiting the binding of monomers blocking elongation (Hirohata *et al.,* 2007). Regitz *et al.* (2014) reported that quercetin inhibited the aggregation of Aβ (1–42) peptide and the associated paralysis in transgenic *C. elegans* (CL2006) by activating macroautophagy and proteasomal degradation pathways. Quercetin directly reduces the level of Aβ peptide by inhibiting BACE1 (Shimmyo *et al.,* 2008). *In silico* studies illustrated that flavonoids like kaempferol, quercetin, acacetin, apigenin and luteolin indirectly lowered the Aβ levels by inhibiting NF-κB activation, which in turn blocks the transcription of BACE1 enzyme (Paris *et al.,* 2011).

3.9. Flavonoids Modulating Neuronal Survival Signaling Pathways

Flavonoids exhibit neuroprotection against oxidative stress and neuronal injury by modulating cell survival signaling pathways such as protein kinase and lipid kinase, by altering the phosphorylation state of the target molecules and modulating the gene expression through activation of transcription factors (Mansuri *et al.,* 2014). Significant cell survival signaling pathways includes phosphatidylinositol-3 kinase/Akt (PI3K/Akt), mitogen-activated protein kinase (MAPK), tyrosine kinase, extracellular signal–regulated protein kinase (ERK), protein kinase C (PKC), while the cell death pathways include the p38 and c-Jun N-terminal kinase (JNK) (Mansuri *et al.,* 2014). Flavonoids such as EGCG (Na *et al.,* 2008) and hesperetin (Vauzour *et al.,* 2007), flavonoid-rich blueberry extract (William *et al.,* 2008), and the flavonoid baicalein (Zhang *et al.,* 2012) were reported to activate cell survival signaling pathways PI3K/Akt, ERK, and PKC in AD and PD model system attenuating the Aβ and 6OHDA toxicity under *in vitro* and *in vivo* conditions. Activation of pathways upregulates the antiapoptotic gene (Bcl2), inhibits proapoptotic genes (caspase 9 and caspase 3) and apoptosis signal-regulating kinase 1 (ASK1), and BclxL/Bcl2-associated death promoter (Bad) and BCL2-associated X protein (Bax) (Mansuri *et al.,* 2014). In addition flavonoids enhances the cell survival through the activation of CREB phosphorylation, increasing the amount of BDNF and NF-E2–related factor 2 (Nrf2)/heme oxygenase 1 (HO-1), enhancing the neuronal survival and antioxidant response element activity (Williams *et al.,* 2008). Flavonoids such as quercetin, EC, EGCG, Hesperetin, Luteolin, Myricetin, Genistein and Kaempferol inhibited p38 and JNK pathway in BV2 microglial cells and activated PKC, AKT/PKB, PI3K in neuronal cells, PC12 cells inhibiting neuroinflammation, improving cognitive function and attenuating oxidative stress mediated damage, improving mitochondrial function thereby exhibiting neuroprotective effect (Park *et al.*, 2011; Liu *et al.*, 2012). ECG and EGCG enhanced ERK1/2 activity in neuronal cells preventing oxidative stress mediated damage, apoptosis and improving brain function (Schroeter *et al.,* 2007; Levites *et al.,* 2002). Flavonol quercetin inhibits Akt/PKB signaling pathways inhibiting PI3-kinase activity (Spencer *et al.,* 2003). EGCG stimulates ERK and PI3K-dependent increase in CREB phosphorylation, upregulating GluR2 levels in cortical neurons and modulating neurotransmission, plasticity and synaptogenesis (Schroeter *et al.,* 2007). Feeding the blueberry diet for 12 weeks activates hippocampal PI3 kinase/Akt increasing the expression of proteins involved in maintaining neuronal morphology, including activity-regulated cytoskeletal-associated protein (Arc/Arg) (Williams *et al.,* 2008). Genistein protects the neurons from oxidative stress mediated cell death in Aβ treated neuronal cells by inhibiting the activation of p38, protecting neurons from cell death (Vallés *et al.,* 2008). Studies related to the neuroprotective effects of flavonoids against various *in vitro* and *in vivo* neurodegenerative model systems have been summarized in Table 2 and Fig. 3.

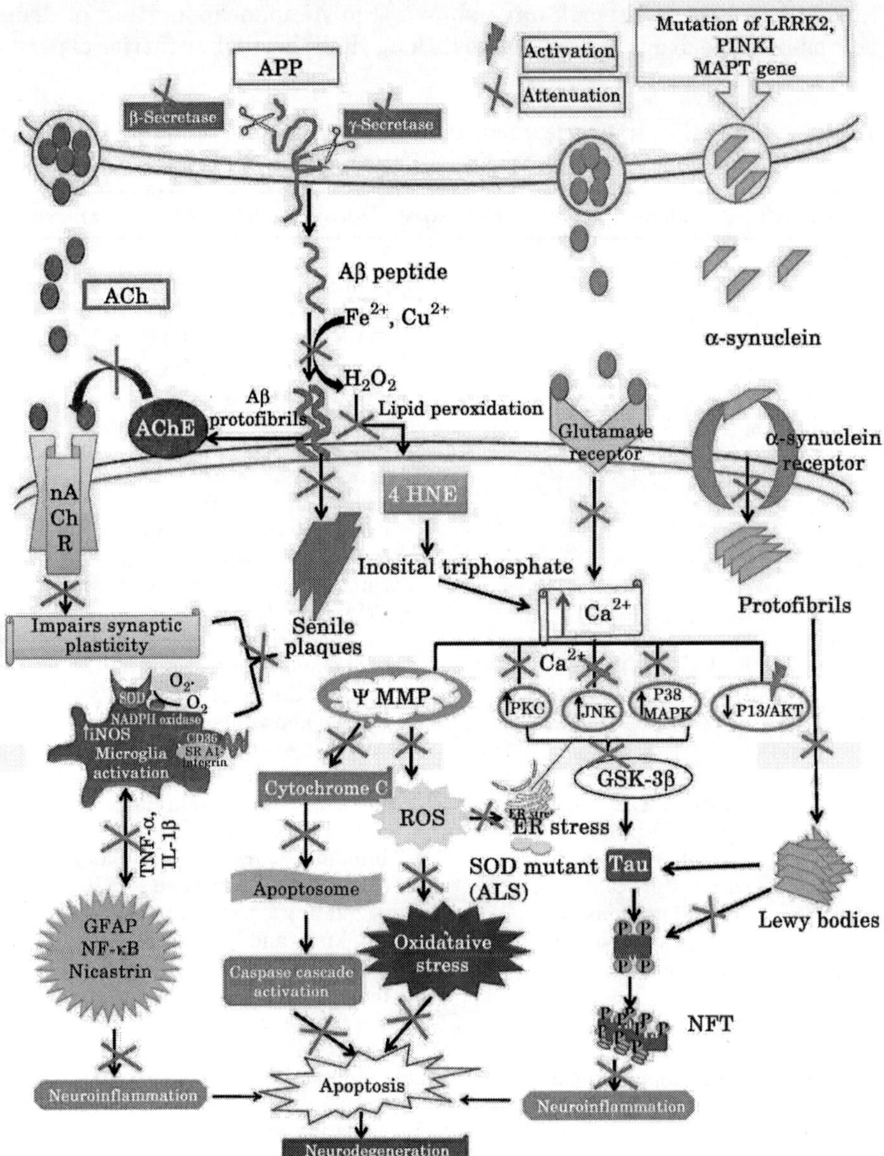

Fig. 3: Multitargeted neuroprotective action of flavonoids

3.10. Nanoencapsulated Flavonoids in the Treatment of Neurological Disorders

Drug accessibility to the central nervous system (CNS) is mainly limited by the blood–brain barrier (BBB), which restricts the selection of applicable compounds depending on their size and endothelial permeability (Chen and

Liu, 2012). Recent reports have shown that nanoencapsulation of drugs acts as effective drug carriers due to its long shelf life, higher carrier capacity,

Table 2: Studies illustrating neuroprotective effect of flavonoids in various *in vitro* and *in vivo* neurodegenerative model system

Flavonoids	*Model system*	*Exposure*	*Neuroprotective effects*	*References*
Alzheimer's disease				
Rutin	SH-SY5Y, BV-2 Microglial cells	Aβ (1-42)	Inhibits Aβ42 fibrillization and attenuate Aβ-induced cytotoxicity, inhibits the generation of ROS and RNS, reduces inducible iNOS activity, attenuates mitochondrial damage, enhances the level of antioxidant and modulates the production of proinflammatory cytokines by decreasing TNF-α and IL-1β	Wang *et al.*, 2012
Apigenin	Double transgenic mouse model (APP/PS1)		Ameliorated AD-associated memory impairment, reduced the Aβ plaque burden and inhibited oxidative stress mediated neuronal damage	Zhao *et al.*, 2013
	Murine HT2224 and human SH-SH5Y cell line		Reduced glutamate-induced Ca^{2+} signaling	
	Advent of induced pluripotent stem cell (iPSC) derived neurons from familial and sporadic AD patients		Inhibited neurite retraction and death by down regulating the release of cytokines and NO, attenuating Caspase3/7 mediated apoptosis, reducing the frequency of spontaneous Ca^{2+} signaling	Balez *et al.*, 2016
Quercetin	Mouse hippocampal cell line HT-22	Glutamate	Attenuates ROS production, prevents GSH oxidation andinhibits lipid peroxidation	Ishige *et al.*, 2016
	Human embryonic kidney (HEK) 293 cells	Aβ (1-42)	Inhibits fibrillation of Aβ peptide and destabilized the preformed mature fibrils.	Ono *et al.*, 2004
	HT22 murine neuroblastoma cells	Aβ (25-35)	Attenuates oxidative stress mediated cell damage	Kim *et al.*, 2005
	Triple-transgenic mouse model of AD (3×Tg-AD)		Reversed β-amyloidosis and tauopathy; reduced astrogliosis and microg-	Sabogal-Guáqueta

Table 2: (*Contd...*)

Table 2: (*Contd...*)

Flavonoids	*Model system*	*Exposure*	*Neuroprotective effects*	*References*
			liosis; enhanced memory and learning	*et al.*, 2015
	APP stable cell line (APP695-transfected SH-SY5Y)		Scavenges ROS radicals, inhibit BACE activity, Anti-aggregation and Dis aggregation ability of Aβ peptide; augments the intracellular GSH content and prevents lipid peroxidation	Jiménez-Aliaga *et al.*, 2011
Quercitrin	Hippocampal rat neurons	Aβ (25-35)	Enhanced cell viability; restored the antioxidant status of the cells treated with Aβ	Rattanajarasroj and Unchern, 2010
	In vitro cell free system		Antiradical scavenging activity with IC_{50} value of 3.0 ± 1.10 mM, inhibits lipid peroxidation with IC_{50} value of 7.33±1.16 m M	Li *et al.*, 2016
Luteolin,	Murine N_2a cells transfected with SweAPP and primary neuronal cells derived from Swe APP-overexpressing mice (Tg2576 model)		Reduced Aβ peptide level by attenuating g secretase APP processing, reduces GSK-3β activity preventing hyperphosphorylation of τ-protein, disrupts PS1-APP association	Rezai-Zadeh *et al.*, 2009
	SHSY5Y Cells	Zinc	Inhibits hyperphosphorylation of t protein	Zhou *et al.*, 2012
	Human brain microvascular endothelial cells (hBMECs) and human astrocytes (hAs)	Fibrillar Aβ (1-40)	Protects blood brain barrier preserving transendothelial electrical resistance, attenuated production of inflammatory mediators and cytokine like COX-2, TNF-α, IL-β, IL-6 and IL-8, inhibited P38 MAPKinase, downregulates phosphorylated inhibitory κB kinase (phosphor-IKK) levels, blocks nuclear factor κB (NF-κB) p65 nuclear translocation, and reduction of the release of inflammatory cytokines.	Zhang *et al.*, 2017
	Alzheimer's disease Rat model	Streptozotocin	Ameliorated the spatial learning and memory impairment	Wang *et al.*, 2016

Table 2: (*Contd...*)

Table 2: (*Contd...*)

Flavonoids	*Model system*	*Exposure*	*Neuroprotective effects*	*References*
Anthocyanins	APP/PS1 mouse model of ADRat fed with anthocyanins		Modulate APP processing and behavioral abnormalities	Vepsalainen *et al.*, 2013
			Activation of CREB with increase in the levels of BDNF in the hippocampus	Williams *et al.*, 2008
Nobiletin	Differentiated PC12 cells and cultured hippocampal neuronal cells		Activates ERK pathways, inhibits phosphodiesterase increases the level of CAMP leading to activation of protein kinase	Nagase *et a1.*, 2005
	APP-SL 7-5 transgenic (Tg) mice - APP695 harboring the double Swedish and London mutations		Attenuates Aβ induced memory impairment, Reduces Aβ plaques in hippocampus of transgenic mouse, Enhances cognitive memory by activation of ERK pathways	Onozuka *et al.*, 2008
EGCG	N_2a transfected with the human “Swedish” mutant APP; Primary neurons derived from Swedish mutant APP-overexpressing mice (Tg APPsw line 2576).		Promotes non-amyloidogenic activity by activating -secretase activity.	Rezai-Zadeh *et al.*, 2005
	In vitro cell free system	Aβ (1-42)	Inhibits fibrillogenesis by directly binding to nascent polypeptide, promotes degradation of Aβ aggregates to intermediate fibrils	Ehrnhoefer *et al.*, 2008
	Rat model	Colchicine	Inhibits AChE enhancing cognitive function, restores antioxidant status attenuating oxidative stress mediated damage	Bagchi, 2016
	AβPP/PS-1 (presenilin 1) double mutant transgenic mouse model		Restores the mitochondrial respiratory rates, MMP, ROS production, and ATP levels	Dragicevic *et al.*, 2011
	Senescence-accelerated mouse prone-8		Attenuated spatial learning and memory impairments, decreasing the level of Aβ (1–42) oligomers, enhancing the activity of PKA/CREB thereby up regulating synaptic plasticity	Li *et al.*, 2009
	Corticol neurons		Stimulates ERK and PI3 K-dependent enhancing	Schroeter *et al.*, 2007

Table 2: (*Contd...*)

Table 2: (*Contd...*)

Flavonoids	*Model system*	*Exposure*	*Neuroprotective effects*	*References*
			phosphorylation of CREB and upregulates GluR2 levels modulating neurotransmission, plasticity, and synaptogenesis.	
	Human astrocytoma, U373MG cells	Aβ (25-35)	Modulates MAPK signaling pathway	Singh *et al.*, 2017
	SH-SY5Y cells	Aβ (1-42)	Increases protein kinase activity and enhances the nonamyloidogenic pathway	Singh *et al.*, 2017
Hesperetin	Cortical neurons		Activates Akt/PKB signaling enhancing neuronal survival	Vauzour *et al.*, 2007
Morin	Human neuroblastoma cells		Attenuates Aβ induced hyperphosphorylation of tau protein preventing the formation of NFT and inflammation mediated neuronal death	Gong *et al.*, 2011
	3xTg-AD mice	Aβ	Decreased tau hyperphosphorylation in hippocampal neurons	
Naringenin	*In vitro* cell free system		Inhibits AChE inhibitory activity in concentration dependant manner	Heo *et al.*, 2004
	ICR mice	Scopolamine	Antiamnestic effect improving locomotor activity and spatial memory	
Kaempferol	Hippocampal neuronal cells (HT22)	Glutamate	Reduced the increased level of ROS preventing oxidative stress mediated neurotoxicity, Modulated the expression levels of apoptotic proteins, such as Bcl-2, Bid, apoptosis-inducing factor (AIF), and mitogen-activated protein kinase (MAPK).	Yang *et al.*, 2014
	PC12 cells and ICR mice	Aβ (1-42)	Inhibited ROS mediated lipid peroxidation *via* its antioxidant potential, attenuated impaired spatial working memory and enhanced learning and memory retention	Kim *et al.*, 2010
Myricetin	Rat primary cortical neurons	Aβ (1-42)	Inhibits aggregation of Aβ peptide from random coil to β-sheet structure, attenuates Caspase 3 and	Shimmyo *et al.*, 2008

Table 2: (*Contd...*)

Table 2: (*Contd...*)

Flavonoids	*Model system*	*Exposure*	*Neuroprotective effects*	*References*
			7 apoptotoic pathway, upregulates a-secretase and inhibits BACE1 activity thereby significantly reducing the level of Aβ 1-42 level	
	Rat	Streptozotocin	Increased the survival rate of hippocampal CA3 pyramidal neurons and improved learning and memory impairments	Ramezani *et al.*, 2016
Fisetin	Mice	Aβ (1-42)	Attenuates BACE1 activity, Aβ deposition and t hyperphosphorylation, reversed synaptic dysfunction, by increasing the level of presynaptic and postsynaptic protein, reversed Aβ induced memory dysfunction, Activated the expression of P13K/Akt/GSK3β signaling, attenuates inflammation, gliosis and neuronal apoptosis	Ahmad *et al.*, 2017
Parkinson's disease				
Rutin	PC12 neuronal cells	6-hydroxydopamine (6-OHDA)	Activates antioxidant enzymes (SOD, CAT, GPx, GSH and suppresses lipid peroxidation	Magalingam *et al.*, 2013
Apigenin	BV-2 murine microglia cell Line, cerebral artery-occlusion-induced focalischemia in mice	LPS, cerebral artery occlusion induced	Blocks the production of NO and PGE2; suppresses phosphorylation of p38 MAPKinase, c-JNK, Protecting neuronal cells from injury in middle cerebral artery occlusion	Ha *et al.*, 2008
Luteolin	Primary mesencephalic neuron-glial cells	LPS	Attenuates dopamine and tyrosine hydroxylase loss, inhibits activation of microglial cells and production of TNF-α, nitric oxide, and superoxide	Chen *et al.*, 2008
Kaempferol	SH-SY5Y cells and primary neurons	Rotenone	Stimulates mitochondrial turnover by autophagy	Filomeni *et al.*, 2012
Myricetin	Dopaminergic cell line MES23.5 cells	1-methyl-4-phenyl pyridinium (MPP)	Prevents cells loss and nuclear condensation, suppresses the production of ROS, restores	Zhang *et al.*, 2011

Table 2: (*Contd...*)

Table 2: (*Contd...*)

Flavonoids	*Model system*	*Exposure*	*Neuroprotective effects*	*References*
			mitochondrial membrane potential, increases the ratio of Bcl-1/Bax ratio, decrease caspase 3 activation, decreases MAP-Kinase and JNK phosphorylation	
Isoquercitrin	PC12 cells	6-OHDA	Stimulates antioxidant enzymes, attenuates lipid peroxidation	Magalingam *et al.,* 2014
Quercetin	Rat	Rotenone	Reduces cell loss in striatal dopamine, scavenges –OH radicals, upregulates mitochondrial complex-I enzymes	Karuppagounder *et al.,* 2013
Catechin	Rats	6-OHDA	Attenuates increase in rotational behavior; improves locomotor activity, restores GSH level, enhances dopamine and 3,4-dihydroxyphenylacetic acid	Teixeira *et al.,* 2013
(“)”Epigallocatechin 3-gallate	SH-SY5Y neuroblastoma cells	Serum deprived	Induces the beta tubulin IV and tropomysin 3 level, increases the levels of binding protein 14-3-3 gamma, inhibits the expression of prolyl-4-hydroxylase; immunoglobulin heavy chain binding protein and heat shock protein - 90β	Weinreb *et al.,* 2007
Hesperidin	Mice	6-OHDA	Prevents memory impairment, attenuates ROS level, restores enzymatic antioxidant level and dopamine level in striatum	Antunes *et al.,* 2014
Fisetin	BV-2 microglial cells	LPS	Attenuates the expression of gene encoding proinflammatory markers like TNF-α, iNOS, reducing the production of TNF-α, NO, PEG2. Suppresses IkB degradation, preventing translocation of NF-κB and phosphorylation of p38 MAPKs	Zheng *et al.,* 2008
Naringenin	SH-SY5YMice	6-OHDA	Enhances level of Nrf2 activating antioxidant response pathway. Atten-	Lou *et al.,* 2014

Table 2: (*Contd...*)

Table 2: (*Contd...*)

Flavonoids	*Model system*	*Exposure*	*Neuroprotective effects*	*References*
			uates oxidative mediated insult in dopaminergic neurons	
Proantho-cyanidin	Primary neuronal cells	Rotenonoe	Protects dopaminergic cell by rescuing mitocho-ndrial respiration	Strathearn *et al.*, 2014
Amyotrophic lateral sclerosis (ALS)				
Genistein	Heterozygous transgenic mice carrying the human SOD-1 (Familial ALS mice model)		Estrogen dependent ne-uroprotection, estrogen independent neuropro-tective effect *via* inhi-biting tyrosine kinase dependant signalling events interfering ROS mediated apoptotic events	Trieu and Uckun, 1999
EGCG	Transgenic ALS mice [B6SJLTg(SOD1-G93 A)] with mutated SOD gene		Delayed the symptom, onset and life span, pre-served more survival signals, and attenuated death signals.	Koh *et al.*, 2006
	SOD1-G93A transgenic mice		Increases the number of motor neurons, dimini-shes microglial activation by attenuating NF-kB, iNOS and caspase 3 expression	Xu *et al.*, 2006
	Spinal cord cultures from old Sprague Dawley rats	Threohyd-roxyaspa-rtate (THA)	Protects motor neurons and regulate glutamate levels	Yu *et al.*, 2010
Luteolin	PC12 cells	4-Hydrox-ynonenol	Exhibits cytoprotective effect by activating MAPK and Nrf2 signaling casc-ade, restored ER homeo-stasis, acts as potent ROS scavenger prev-enting oxidative stress	Wu *et al.*, 2015
Multiple Sclerosis				
Luteolin	PBMC, Mast cells, microglial cells and astrocytes Mast cells	Multiple sclerosis patients	Inhibits IL-1, TNF-α and metalloproteinase-9 (MMP-9) release from activated peripheral blood mononuclear cells (PBM Cs) from multiple sclerosis (MS) patient. Inhibits myelin phagocytosis by macrophages	Theoharides, 2009
EGCG	Hippocampal HT22 cell	Glutamate and tumor necrosis	Regeneration of hippoca-mpal axons and impro-ves neuronal survival,	Herges *et al.*, 2011

Table 2: (*Contd...*)

Table 2: (*Contd...*)

Flavonoids	*Model system*	*Exposure*	*Neuroprotective effects*	*References*
		factor related apoptosis inducing ligand (TRAIL) induced	attenuates production of ROS and NF-kB activation preventing inflammation mediated neuronal damage	
	Experimental autoimmune encephalomyelitis (EAE)		Blocks inflammation by inhibiting the release of TNF-α and prolifereation of T cells	Aktas *et al.*, 2009
	HepG2	Hypoxia	Activates silent mating type information regulation 2 homolog1 (SIRT1) suppressing neuroinflammation	Hong *et al.*, 2012
Quercetin	PBMC from multiple sclerosis patients		Controls immune response by modulating IL-1β and TNF-α	Sternberg *et al.*, 2008
Fisetin	Macrophages		Prevents phagocytosis of myelin sheath by macrophages by effectively scavenging the ROS required for phagocytosis	Hendricks *et al.*, 2003
Huntington disease				
EGCG	Htt exon 1 GFP fusion proteins GFP-HDQ25 and GFP-HDQ72	Rats	Inhibits huntingtin protein aggregation. Intake of EGCG (1,200 mg/day for 12 months) in HD patients enhanced cognitive memory	Ehrnhoefer *et al.*, 2006
	3-Nitropropionic acid		Attenuates memory impairment and enhanced the non-enzymatic level in neuronal cells	Kumar and Kumar, 2009
Fisetin	PC12 cells expressing mutant Httex1, Drosophila expressing mutant Httex1 and the R6/2 mouse model of HD		Enhances ERK activation and inhibits JNK signaling pathway inducing cell survival rate	Maher *et al.*, 2011
Quercetin	3-nitropropionic acid (3-NP)	HD rat model	Improved respiratory chain functions *via* the activation mitochondrial complex enzymes, attenuated lipid peroxidation *via* antioxidant status and improved neurobehavioral functions. Enhanced the expression of sirtuins (SIRT1) or peroxisome	Sandhir and Mehrotra, 2012

Table 2: (*Contd...*)

Table 2: *(Contd...)*

Flavonoids	*Model system*	*Exposure*	*Neuroprotective effects*	*References*
			proliferator-activated receptor gamma co-activator (PGC-1) increasing mitochondrial biogenesis	
Naringin	3-NP	HD rat model	Increased the expression of Nrf2 inducing the level of phase II antioxidant enzymes like NAD(P)H: quinone oxidoreductase-1, heme oxygenase-1, GST and gGCL. Attenuated the expression of pro-inflammatory mediators like TNF-α, COX-2 and iNOS synthase.	Gopinath and Sudhandiran, 2012
Hesperidin	3-NP	HD rat model	Inhibited changes in locomotor activity slightly increased cortical, striatal level, reduced MDA and catalase activity, decreased the number of iNOS positive cells preventing oxidative stress and inflmmation mediated neuronal death	Menze *et al.*, 2012

good safety profile, BBB permeability and sustained drug release. Although most of the flavonoids exhibit neuroprotective effect through its multitargeted action, its efficacy is restricted due to its poor water solubility, low oral bioavailability and poor BBB, hence current research are underway in encapsulating flavonoids. Several reports illustrated that nanoencapsulation of quercetin increased BBB permeability and its therapeutic efficacy. Nasal administration of liposome encapsulated quercetin in AD animal model attenuated the degeneration of neurons and cholinergic neurons in hippocampus, elevated the antioxidant activity, reduced the MDA level in hippocampal region (Phachonpai *et al.*, 2010). Another study illustrated that oral administration of nanoencapsulated quercetin in ischemia-reperfusion-induced young and aged Swiss Albino rats, downregulated iNOS and caspase-3 activities, improved neuronal count, enhanced the antioxidant status in different brain regions exhibited neuronal protection (Ghosh *et al.*, 2013). Nasal administration of microemulsion of morin (Cremophor EL, and PEG-400) in streptozotocin treated rats increased learning and memory, attenuated oxidative stress mediated neuronal damage (Sharma *et al.*, 2017).

4. CONCLUSIONS

Dietary flavonoids exhibits neuroprotective effect through its multipotent action within brain including ability to protect neurons against neurotoxin induced injury, ability to inhibit inflammation and potential to enhance cognitive function. Flavonoids mitigates oxidative stress mediated neuronal damage through its direct and indirect antioxidant ability coupled with metal chelating activity, which depends on the number of hydroxyl groups in the ring A and B of chemical structure backbone. Flavonoids attenuates inflammation mediated neuronal damage by down regulating the expression of proinflammatory cytokines and chemokines such as cyclooxygenase, TNF-α, IL-1β, IL-6, iNOS. Flavonoids stimulates neurogenesis by activating Sirutin (SIRT-1) and CREB pathway, thereby elevating the level of BDNF level essential for neurogenesis. Flavonoids not only effectively inhibit the aggregation of Aβ peptide and α-synuclein, but also disaggregates the preformed mature fibrils preventing the deposition of abnormal protein aggregates. Flavonoids effectively modulate the neuronal signalling cascades like PI3 K/Akt and MAP kinase pathways in the brain leading to an inhibition of apoptosis triggered by neurotoxic species and to a promotion of neuronal survival and differentiation. Overall the review illustrates the multiple faceted actions of flavonoids in neuroprotection. Several reports have shown that consumption of flavonoid-rich foods, such as berries and cocoa, limits neurodegeneration and prevents or reverses age-dependent deteriorations of cognitive function, however, the exact mechanism of action in unclear. As current research focuses on development of drugs capable of enhancing brain function, flavonoids may represent important precursor molecules in the quest to develop of a new generation of brain enhancing drugs. Flavonoids are ubiquitous secondary metabolites of plant matrices with multiple pharmacological activities and limited toxicity, which makes it considerable as potent nutraceutical agent. Despite of multipotent neuroprotective effect of flavonoids under *in vitro* and *in vivo* neurodegenerative model systems, its application in pharmaceutical field is limited due to its low water solubility, bioavailability, poor BBB permeability and instability. Future research needs to be focused on (1) improving drug delivery systems such as nanoencapasulation and microemulsion to enhance the bioavailability and blood brain permeability; (2) Clinical trials to ascertain the effective dose for the treatment of neurodegenerative disorders; (3) pharmacokinetic and dynamic study of flavonoids in the central nervous system using suitable model system (4) Up-to-date *in vivo* toxicity profiling to assess the neurotoxic effect.

REFERENCES

Agarwal, A.D. (2011). Pharmacological activities of flavonoids: A review. *IJPSN*, 4(2): 1394–1398.

Ahmad, A., Ali, T., Park, H.Y., Badshah, H., Rehman, S.U. and Kim, M.O. (2017). Neuroprotective effect of fisetin against amyloid-beta-induced cognitive/synaptic dysfunction, neuroinflammation, and neurodegeneration in adult mice. *Mol. Neurobiol.*, 54(3): 2269–2285. doi: 10.1007/s12035-016-9795-4.

Ahmed, R.M., Devenney, E.M., Irish, M., Ittner, A., Naismith, S., Ittner, L.M., Rohrer, J.D., Halliday, G.M., Eisen, A., Hodges, J.R. and Kiernan, M.C. (2016). Neuronal network disintegration: Common pathways linking neurodegenerative diseases. *J. Neurol. Neurosurg. Psychiatry.*, 0: 1–8. doi:10.1136/jnnp-2014-308350.

Ahn, S.-H., Jung Kim, H., Jeong, I., Hong, Y.J., Kim, M-J., Rhie, D-J., Jo, Y-H., Hahn, S.J. and Yoon, S.H. (2011). Grape seed proanthocyanidin extract inhibits glutamate-induced cell death through inhibition of calcium signals and nitric oxide formation in cultured rat hippocampal neurons. *BMC Neurosci*, 12: 78. doi: 10.1186/1471-2202-12-78.

Aktas, O., Prozorovski, T., Smorodchenko, A., Savaskan, N.E., Lauster, R., Kloetzel, P.M., Infante-Duarte, C., Brocke, S. and Zipp, F. (2004). Green tea epigallocatechin-3-gallate mediates T cellular NF-kappa B inhibition and exerts neuroprotection in autoimmune encephalomyelitis. *J. Immunol.*, 173: 5794–5800.

Alzheimer's Association (2016). Alzheimer's disease facts and figures. *Alzheimer's & Dementia*, 12(4).

Anderson, J.P., Walker, D.E., Goldstein, J.M., de Laat, R., Banducci, K., Caccavello, R.J., Barbour, R., Huang, J., Kling, K., Lee, M., Diep, L., Keim, P.S., Shen, X., Chataway, T., Schlossmacher, M.G., Seubert, P., Schenk, D., Sinha, S., Gai, W.P. and Chilcote, T.J. (2006). Phosphorylation of Ser-129 is the dominant pathological modification of alpha-synuclein in familial and sporadic Lewy body disease. *J. Biol. Chem.*, 281: 29739–29752.

Antunes, M.S., Goes, A.T.R., Boeira, S.P., Prigol, M. and Jesse, C.R. (2014). Protective effect of hesperidin in a model of Parkinson's disease induced by 6-hydroxydopamine in aged mice. *Nutrition*, 30(11–12): 1415–1422.

Armstrong, R.A. (2012). On the 'classification' of neurodegenerative disorders: Discrete entities, overlap or continuum? *Folia Neuropathol*, 50(3): 201–218.

Atia-tun-Noor Fatima, I., Ahmad, I., Malik, A., Afza, N., Iqbal, L., Latif, M., Khan, S.B. (2007). Leufolins A and B, potent butyrylcholinesterase-inhibiting flavonoid glucosides from *Leucas urticifolia*. *Molecules*, 12: 1447–1454.

Avila, J., Lucas, J.J., Perez, M. and Hernandez, F. (2004). Role of tau protein in both physiological and pathological conditions. *Physiol. Rev.*, 84: 361–384.

Bagchi, A. (2016). Protective effect of epigallocatechin-3-gallate (EGCG) the major tea polyphenolic, against intracerebroventricularly colchicine induced oxidative damage production in brain and cognitive dysfunction in mice. *J. Alzheimers. Dis. Parkinsonism*, 6: 4. doi 10.4172/2161-0460.1000250.

Balez, R., Steiner, N., Engel, M., Muñoz, S.S., Lum, J.S., Wu, Y., Wang, D., Vallotton, P., Sachdev, P., Connor, M., Sidhu, K., Münch, G. and Ooi, L. Neuroprotective effects of apigenin against inflammation, neuronal excitability and apoptosis in an induced pluripotent stem cell model of Alzheimer's disease. *Sci. Rep.*, 6: 31450. doi 10.1038/srep31450.

Bastianetto, S., Ramassamy, C., Doré, S., Christen, Y., Poirier, J. and Quirion, R. (2000). The *Ginkgo biloba* extract (EGb 761) protects hippocampal neurons against cell death induced by beta-amyloid. *Eur. J. Neurosci.*, 12: 1882–1890.

Busch, C., Burkard, M., Leischner, C., Lauer, U.M., Frank, J. and Venturelli, S. (2015). Epigenetic activities of flavonoids in the prevention and treatment of cancer. *Clin. Epigenetics.*, 10(7): 64. doi: 10.1186/s13148-015-0095-z.

Carafa, V., Rotili, D., Forgione, M., Cuomo, F., Serretiello, E., Hailu, G.S., Jarho, E., Lahtela-Kakkonen, M., Mai, A. and Altucci, L. (2016). Sirtuin functions and modulation: From chemistry to the clinic. *Clin. Epigenetics.*, 8: 61. doi: 10.1186/s13148-016-0224-3.

Caruana, M., Högen, T., Levin, J., Hillmer, A., Giese, A. and Vassallo, N. (2011). Inhibition and disaggregation of α-synuclein oligomers by natural polyphenolic compounds. *FEBS Letters*, 585: 1113–1120.

Carvajal, F.J. and Inestrosa, N.C. (2011). Interactions of AChE with Aβ aggregates in Alzheimer's brain: Therapeutic relevance of IDN 5706. *Front. Mol. Neurosci.*, 14(4): 19. doi: 10.3389/fnmol.2011.00019

Casini, M.L., Marelli, G., Papaleo, E., Ferrari, A., D'Ambrosio, F. and Unfer, V. (2006). Psychological assessment of the effects of treatment with phytoestrogens on postmenopausal women: A randomized, double-blind, crossover, placebo-controlled study. *Fertil Steril*, 85: 972–978.

Chang, C.Y., Lin, T.Y., Lu, C.W., Huang, S.K., Wang, Y.C., Chou, S.S.P. and Wang, S.J. (2015). Hesperidin inhibits glutamate release and exerts neuroprotection against excitotoxicity induced by kainic acid in the hippocampus of rats. *Neurotoxicology*, 50: 157–169.

Chen, H.Q., Jin, Z.Y., Wang, X.J., Xu, X.M., Deng, L. and Zhao, J-W. (2008). Luteolin protects dopaminergic neurons from inflammation-induced injury through inhibition of microglial activation. *Neurosci Letts.*, 448(2): 175–179.

Chen, S., Jiang, H., Wu, X. and Fang, J. (2016). Therapeutic effects of quercetin on inflammation, obesity, and type 2 diabetes. *Mediators Inflamm.*, 2016 (Article ID 9340637): 5. doi.org/10.1155/2016/9340637

Chen, Y. and Liu, L. (2012). Modern methods for delivery of drugs across the blood-brain barrier. *Adv. Drug Deliv. Rev.*, 64(7): 640–665.

Choi, J.S., Chung, H.Y., Kang, S.S., Jung, M.J., Kim, J.W., No, J.K. and Jung, H.A. (2002). The structure–activity relationship of flavonoids as scavengers of peroxynitrite. *Phytother. Res.*, 16: 232–235.

Choi, J.S., Islam, M.N., Ali, M.Y., Kim, E.J., Kim, Y.M. and Jung, H.A. (2014). Effects of C-glycosylation on anti-diabetic, anti-alzheimer's disease and anti-inflammatory potential of apigenin. *Food Chem. Toxicol.*, 64: 27–33.

Cohen-Salmon, C., Venault, P., Martin, B., Raffalli-Sébillea, M.-J., Barkatsa, M., Clostrec, F., Pardona, M-C., Christen, Y. and Chapouthie, G. (1997). Effects of *Ginkgo biloba* extract (EGb 761) on learning and possible actions on aging. *J. Physiol. Paris.*, 91: 291–300.

Conforti, F., Rigano, D., Formisano, C., Bruno, M., Loizzo, M.R., Menichini, F. and Senatore, F. (2010). Metabolite profile and *in vitro* activities of *Phagnalon saxatile* (L.) Cass. relevant to treatment of Alzheimer's disease. *J. Enzyme. Inhib. Med. Chem.*, 25(1): 97–104.

D'Onofrio, G., Sancarlo, D., Ruan, Q., Yu, Z., Panza, F., Daniele, A., Greco, A. and Seripa, D. (2016). Phytochemicals in the treatment of Alzheimer's disease: A systematic review. *Curr. Drug Targets*, 2016 [Epub ahead of print]

De Boer, V.C., de Goffau, M.C., Arts, I.C., Hollman, P.C. and Keijer, J. (2006). SIRT1 stimulation by polyphenols is affected by their stability and metabolism. *Mech. Ageing. Dev.*, 127: 618–627.

Dinamarca, M.C., Sagal, J.P., Quintanilla, R.A., Godoy, J.A., Arrazola, M.S. and Inestrosa, N.C. (2010). Amyloid-α-Acetylcholinesterase complexes potentiate neurodegenerative changes induced by the Aβ peptide. Implications for the pathogenesis of Alzheimer's disease. *Mol. Neurodegener*, 5: 4. doi: 10.1186/1750-1326-5-4.

Ding, X., Ouyang, M.A., Liu, X. and Wang, R.Z. (2013). Acetylcholinesterase inhibitory activities of flavonoids from the leaves of *Ginkgo biloba* against brown planthopper. *J. Chem.*, 2013 (Article ID 645086): p. 4. doi.org/10.1155/2013/645086.

Dragicevic, N., Smith, A., Lin, X., Yuan, F., Copes, N., Delic, V., Tan, J., Cao, C., Shytle, R.D. and Bradshaw, P.C. (2011). Green tea epigallocatechin-3-gallate (EGCG) and other flavonoids reduce Alzheimer's amyloid-induced mitochondrial dysfunction. *J. Alzheimers Dis.*, 26(3): 507–521.

Duan, S., Guan, X., Lin, R., Liu, X., Yan, Y., Lin, R., Zhang, T., Chen, X., Huang, J., Sun, X., Li, Q., Fang, S., Xu, J., Yao, Z. and Gu, H. (2015). Silibinin inhibits acetylcholinesterase activity and amyloid β peptide aggregation: A dual-target drug for the treatment of Alzheimer's disease. *Neurobiol Aging*, 36(5): 1792–1807.

Dvir, H., Silman, I., Harel, M., Rosenberry, T.L. and Sussman, J.L. (2010). Acetylcholinesterase: From 3D structure to function. *Chem. Biol. Interact*, 187(1–3): 10–22.

Ehrnhoefer, D.E., Bieschke, J., Boeddrich, A., Herbst, M., Masino, L., Lurz, R., Engemann, S., Pastore, A. and Wanker, E.E. (2008). EGCG redirects amyloidogenic polypeptides into unstructured, off-pathway oligomers. *Nat. Struct. Mol. Biol.*, 15: 558–566.

Feng, Y. and Wang, X. (2012). Antioxidant therapies for Alzheimer's disease. *Oxid. Med. Cell Longev*, 2012: 472932.

Filomeni, G., Graziani, I., De Zio, D., Dini, L., Centonze, D., Rotilio, G. and Ciriolo, M.R. (2012). Neuroprotection of kaempferol by autophagy in models of rotenone-mediated acute toxicity: Possible implications for Parkinson's disease. *Neurobiol Aging*, 33(4): 767–85.

Folch, J., Petrov, D., Ettcheto, M., Abad, S., Sánchez-López, E., Luisa García, M., Olloquequi, J., Beas-Zarate, C., Auladel, C. and Camins, A. (2016). Current research therapeutic strategies for alzheimer's disease treatment. *Neural Plasticity*, 2016 (8501693): 15. doi.org/10.1155/2016/8501693.

Gandhi, S. and Abramov, A.Y. (2012). Mechanism of oxidative stress in neurodegeneration. *Oxid. Med. Cell Longev.*, 2012 (Article ID 428010): 11. doi.org/10.1155/2012/428010.

Ghosh, A., Sarkar, S., Mandal, A.K. and Das, N. (2013). Neuroprotective role of nanoencapsulated quercetin in combating ischemia-reperfusion induced neuronal damage in young and aged rats. *PLoS ONE,* 8(4): e57735. doi.org/10.1371/journal.pone.0057735.

Glass, C.K., Saijo, K., Winner, B., Marchetto, M.C. and Gage, F.H. (2010). Mechanisms underlying inflammation in neurodegeneration. *Cell*, 140(6): 918–934.

Gong, C.X. and Iqbal, K. (2008). Hyperphosphorylation of microtubule-associated protein tau: A promising therapeutic target for Alzheimer disease. *Curr. Med. Chem.*, 15: 2321–2328.

Gong, E.J., Park, H.R., Kim, M.E., Piao, S., Lee, E., Jo, D-J., Chung, H.Y., Ha, N.C., Mattson, M.P. and Lee1, J. (2011). Morin attenuates tau hyperphosphorylation by inhibiting GSK3β. *Neurobiol Dis.*, 44(2): 223–230.

Gopinath, K. and Sudhandiran, G. (2012). Naringin modulates oxidative stress and inflammation in 3-nitropropionic acid-induced neurodegeneration through the activation of nuclear factor-erythroid 2-related factor-2 signalling pathway. *Neuroscience*, 27(227): 134–143.

Goyarzu, P., Malin, D.H., Lau, F.C., Taglialatela, G., Moon, W.D., Jennings, R., Moy, E., Moy, D., Lippold, S., Shukitt-Hale, B. and Joseph, J.A. (2004). Blueberry supplemented diet: Effects on object recognition memory and nuclear factor-kappa B levels in aged rats. *Nutr. Neurosci.*, 7: 75–83.

Gräff, J., Kahn, M., Samiei, A., Gao, J., Ota, K.T., Rei, D. and Tsai, L.H. (2013). A dietary regimen of caloric restriction or pharmacological activation of SIRT1 to delay the onset of neurodegeneration. *J. Neurosci.*, 33: 8951–8960.

Ha, S.K., Lee, P., Park, J.A., Oh, H.R., Lee, S.Y., Park, J.H., Lee, E.H., Ryu, J.H., Lee, K.R. and Kim, S.Y. (2008). Apigenin inhibits the production of NO and PGE2 in microglia and inhibits neuronal cell death in a middle cerebral artery occlusion-induced focal ischemia micemodel. *Neurochem Internat.,* 52(4–5): 878–886.

Hanáková, Z., Hošek, J., Babula, P., Dall'Acqua, S., Václavík, J. and Šmejkal, K.C. (2015). Geranylated flavanones from *Paulownia tomentosa* fruits as potential anti-inflammatory compounds acting *via* inhibition of TNF-α production. *J. Nat. Prod.*, 78(4): 850–863.

Head, M.W. (2013). Human prion diseases: Molecular, cellular and population biology. *Neuropathology*, 33(3): 221–236.

Heim, K.E., Tagliaferro, A.R. and Bobilya, D.J. (2002). Flavonoid antioxidants: Chemistry, metabolism and structure-activity relationships. *J. Nutri. Biochem.*, 13(10): 572–584.

Hendriks, J.J., de Vries, H.E., van der Pol, S.M., van den Berg, T.K., van Tol, E.A. and Dijkstra, C.D. (2003). Flavonoids inhibit myelin phagocytosis by macrophages; a structure activity relationship study. *Biochem. Pharmacol.*, 65: 877–885.

Heo, H.J., Kim, M.J., Lee, J.M., Choi, S.J., Cho, H.Y., Hong, B., Kim, H.K., Kim, E. and Shin, D.H. (2004). Naringenin from *Citrus junos* has an inhibitory effect on acetylcholinesterase and a mitigating effect on amnesia. *Dement Geriatr Cogn Diso*, 17: 151–157.

Herges, K., Millward, J.M., Hentschel, N., Infante-Duarte, C., Aktas, O. and Zipp, F. (2011). Neuroprotective effect of combination therapy of glatiramer acetate and epigallocatechin-3-gallate in neuroinflammation. *PLoS ONE*, 6(10): e25456. doi: 10.1371/journal.pone.0025456

Hirano, R., Sasamoto, W., Matsumoto, A., Itakura, H., Igarashi, O. and Kondo, K. (2001). Antioxidant ability of various flavonoids against DPPH radicals and LDL oxidation. *J. Nutr. Sci. Vitaminol.* (Tokyo), 47: 357–362.

Hirohata, M., Hasegawa, K., Tsutsumi-Yasuhara, S., Ohhashi, Y., Ookoshi, Y., Ono, Y., Yamada, M. and Naiki, H. (2007). The anti-amyloidogenic effect is exerted against Alzheimer's β-amyloid fibrils *in vitro* by preferential and reversible binding of flavonoids to the amyloid fibril structure. *Biochemistry*, 46: 1888–1899.

Hoffman, J.R., Donato, A. and Robbins, S.J. (2004). *Ginkgo biloba* promotes short-term retention of spatial memory in rats. *Pharmacol. Biochem. Behav.,* 77: 533–539.

Hong, K.S., Park, J.I., Kim, M.J., Kim, H.B., Lee, J.W., Dao, T.T., Oh, W.K., Kang, C.D. and Kim, S.H. (2012). Involvement of SIRT1 in hypoxic down-regulation of c-Myc and 5ØýÞ-catechin and hypoxic precondition effect of polyphenol. *Toxicol. Appl. Pharmacol.*, 259(2): 210–218.

Huang, S.M., Tsai, Y., Lin, J.A., Wu, C.H. and Yen, G.C. (2012). Cytoprotective effects of hesperetin and hesperidin against amyloid β-induced impairment of glucose transport through downregulation of neuronal autophagy. *Mol. Nutr. Food Res.*, 56(4): 601–609.

Hwang, P.A., Chien, S.Y., Chan, Y.L., Lu, M.K., Wu, C.H., Kong, Z.L. and Wu, C.J. (2011). Inhibition of lipopolysaccharide (LPS)-induced inflammatory responses by *Sargassum hemiphyllum* sulfated polysaccharide extract in RAW 264.7 macrophage cells. *J. Agri. Food Chem.*, 59: 2062–2068.

Ishige, K., Schubert, D. and Sagara, Y. (2001). Flavonoids protect neuronal cells from oxidative stress by three distinct mechanisms. *Free Radic. Biol. Med.*, 30: 433–446.

Jahn, H. (2013). A memory loss in Alzheimer's disease. *Dialogues Clin. Neurosci.*, 15(4): 4, 445–452.

Jiménez-Aliaga, K., Bermejo-Bescós, P., Benedí, J., Martín-Aragón, S. (2011). Quercetin and rutin exhibit antiamyloidogenic and fibril-disaggregating effects *in vitro* and potent antioxidant activity in APPswe cells. *Life Sci.*, 89: 939–945.

Johnson, J.L., Rupasinghe, S.G., Stefani, F., Schuler, M.A. and Gonzalez de Mejia, E. (2011). *Citrus* flavonoids luteolin, apigenin, and quercetin inhibit glycogen synthase kinase-3b enzymatic activity by lowering the interaction energy within the binding cavity. *J. Med. Food*, 14: 325–333.

Jung, H.A., Jin, S.E., Park, J.S. and Choi, J.S. (2011). Antidiabetic complications and anti-alzheimer activities of sophoflavescenol, a prenylated flavonol from *Sophora flavescens*, and its structure activity relationship. *Phytother. Res.*, 25: 709–715.

Kao, T-K., Ou, Y-C., Raung, S.-L., Lai, C-Y., Liao, S-L. and Chen, C-Y. (2010). Inhibition of nitric oxide production by quercetin in endotoxin/cytokine-stimulated microglia. *Life Sci.*, 86: 315–321.

Karakaya, T., Fußer, F., Prvulovic, D. and Hampel, H. (2012). Treatment options for tauopathies. *Curr. Treat Options Neurol.*, 14(2): 126–136.

Karuppagounder, S.S., Madathil, S.K., Pandey, M., Haobam, R., Rajamma, U. and Mohanakumar, K.P. (2013). Quercetin up-regulates mitochondrial complex-I activity to protect against programmed cell death in rotenone model of Parkinson's disease in rats. Neuroscience, 236: 136–148.

Kataliniæ, M., Rusak, G., Domaæinoviæ Baroviæ, J., Sinko, G., Jeliæ, D., Antoloviæ, R. and Kovarik, Z. (2014). Flavonoids as Inhibitors of Human BChE. *Food Technol. Biotechnol.*, 52 (1): 64–67.

Keservani, R.K., Sharma, A.K. and Kesharwani, R.K. (2016). Medicinal effect of nutraceutical fruits for the cognition and brain health. *Scientifica*, 2016 (Article ID 3109254): 10. doi.org/10.1155/2016/3109254.

Kiernan, M.C., Vucic, S., Cheah, B.C., Turner, M.R., Eisen, A., Hardiman, O., Burrell, J.R. and Zoing, M.C. (2011). Amyotrophic lateral sclerosis. *Lancet*, 377: 942–955.

Kim, G.H., Kim, J.E., Rhie, S.J. and Yoon, S. (2015). The role of oxidative stress in neurodegenerative diseases. *Exp. Neurobiol.*, 24(4): 325–340.

Kim, H., Park, B.S., Lee, K.G., Choi, C.Y., Jang, S.S., Kim, Y.H. and Lee, S.E. (2005). Effects of naturally occurring compounds on fibril formation and oxidative stress of b-amyloid. *J. Agric. Food. Chem.*, 53: 8537–8541.

Kim, J.K., Choi, S.J., Cho, H.Y., Hwang, H.J., Kim, Y.J., Lim, S.T., Kim, C.J., Kim, H.K., Peterson, S. and Shin, D.H. (2010). Protective effects of kaempferol (3,4',5,7-tetrahydroxyflavone) against amyloid beta peptide (Abeta)-induced neurotoxicity in ICR mice. *Biosci. Biotechnol. Biochem.*, 74(2): 397–401.

Kim, J.Y., Lee, W.S., Kim, Y.S., Curtis-Long, M.J., Lee, B.W., Ryu, Y.B., Park, K.H. (2011). Isolation of cholinesterase-inhibiting flavonoids from Morus lhou. *J. Agric. Food Chem.*, 59: 4589–4596.

Kim, S.R., Park, M.J., Lee, M.K., Sung, S.H., Park, E.J., Kim, J., Kim, S.Y., Oh, T.H., Markelonis, G.J. and Kim, Y.C. (2002). Flavonoids of *Inula britannica* protect cultured cortical cells from necrotic cell death induced by glutamate. *Free Radic Biol. Med.*, 32(7): 596–604.

Koh, S-H., Lee, S-M., Kim, H.Y., Lee, K.-Y., Lee, Y.J., Kim, H-T., Kim, J., Kim, M-H., Hwang, M.S., Song, C., Yang, K.-W., Lee, K.W., Kim, S.H. and Kim, O-H. (2006). The effect of epigallocatechin gallate on suppressing disease progression of ALS model mice. *Neurosci Letts*, 395: 103–107.

Kopacz, M. and KuŸniar, A. (2003). Complexes of cadmium (II), mercury (II) and lead (II) with quercetin-52 -sulfonic acid (QSA). *Pol. J. Chem.*, 77: 1777–1786.

Korolev, I.O. (2014). Alzheimer's disease: A clinical and basic science review. *M.S.R.J.*, 4: 24–33.

Kovas, G. (2016). Molecular pathological classification of neurodegenerative diseases: Turning towards precision medicine. *Int. J. Mol. Sci.*, 17: 189. doi: 10.3390/ijms1702018

Krishnaveni, M. (2012). Flavonoid in enhancing memory function. *J. Pharm. Res.*, 5(7): 3870–3874.

Kumar, A., Singh, A. and Ekavali (2015). A review on Alzheimer's disease pathophysiology and its management: An update. *Pharmacol Rep.*, 67(2): 195–203.

Kumar, P. and Kumar, A. (2009). Protective effects of epigallocatechin gallate following 3-nitropropionic acid-induced brain damage: Possible nitric oxide mechanisms. *Psychopharmacology,* 207(2): 257–270.

Kumar, S. and Pandey, A.K. (2013). Chemistry and biological activities of flavonoids: An overview. *Sci. World. J.*, 2013 (Article ID 162750): 16. doi.org/10.1155/2013/162750.

Labbadia, J. and Morimoto, R.I. (2013). Huntington's disease: Underlying molecular mechanisms and emerging concepts. *Trends Biomed Sci.*, 38(8): 378–385.

Lau, F.C., Bielinski, D.F. and Joseph, J.A. (2007). Inhibitory effects of blueberry extract on the production of inflammatory mediators in lipopolysaccharide-activated BV2 microglia. *J. Neurosci. Res.*, 85(5): 1010–1017.

Lee, J.H., Song, D.K., Jung, C.H., Shin, D.H., Park, J., Kwon, T.K., Jang, B.C., Mun, K.C., Kim, S.P., Suh, S.I. and Bae, J.H. (2004). (-)-Epigallocatechin gallate attenuates glutamate-induced cytotoxicity *via* intracellular Ca modulation in PC12 cells. *Clin. Exp. Pharmacol. Physiol.*, 31(8): 530–536.

Lee, K.Y., Hwang, L., Jeong, E.J., Kim, S.H., Kim, Y.C. and Sung, S.H. (2010). Effect of neuroprotective flavonoids of *Agrimonia eupatoria* on glutamate-induced oxidative injury to HT22 hippocampal cells. *Biosci Biotechnol Biochem.*, 74(8): 1704–1706.

Lee, Y.B., Lee, H.J., Won, M.H. *et al.* (2004). Soy isoflavones improve spatial delayed matching-to-place performance and reduce cholinergic neuron loss in elderly male rats. *J. Nutr.*, 134: 1827–1831.

Lee-Hilz, Y.Y., Boerboom, A.M.J.F., Westphal, A.H., van Berkel, W.J.H., Aarts, J.M.M.J.G. and Rietjens, I.M.C.M. (2006). Pro-oxidant activity of flavonoids induces EpREmediated gene expression. *Chem. Res. Toxicol.*, 19: 1499–1505.

Levites, Y., Amit, T., Youdim, M.B. and Mandel, S. (2002). Involvement of protein kinase C activation and cell survival/cell cycle genes in green tea polyphenol (-)-epigallocatechin 3-gallate neuroprotective action. *J. Biol. Chem.*, 277: 30574–3080.

Li, H., Wei, Y., Wang, Z. and Wang, Q. (2015). Application of APP/PS1 transgenic mouse model for Alzheimer's disease. *J. Alzheimers Dis. Parkinsonism*, 5: 3. doi:10.4172/2161-0460.1000201

Li, R., Huang, Y.-G., Fang, D. and Le, W.-D. (2004). Epigallocatechin gallate inhibits lipopolysaccharide-induced microglial activation and protects against inflammation-mediated dopaminergic neuronal injury. *J. Neurosci. Res.*, 78(5): 723–731.

Li, X., Jiang, Q, Wang, T., Liu, J. and Chen, D. (2016). Comparison of the antioxidant effects of quercitrin and isoquercitrin: Understanding the role of the 6''-OH Group. *Molecules*, 21: 1246. doi:10.3390/molecules21091246

Lin, S., Zhang, G., Liao, Y., Pan, J. and Gong, D. (2015). Dietary flavonoids as xanthine oxidase inhibitors: Structure-affinity and structure-activity relationships. *J. Agric. Food Chem.*, 9: 63(35), 7784-94.

Lin, T.Y., Lu, C.W. and Wang, S.J. (2016). Luteolin protects the hippocampus against neuron impairments induced by kainic acid in rats. *Neurotoxicology*, 55: 48–57. doi: 10.1016/j.neuro.2016.05.008.

Liu, L.L., Sheng, B.Y., Yan, Y.F., Gong, K., Ma, T., Zhao, N.M., Zhang, X.F. and Gong, Y.D. (2010). Protective effect of anthocyanin against the oxidative stress in neuroblastoma N2a cells. *Prog. Biochem. Biophys.*, 37: 779–785.

Losi, G., Puia, G., Garzon, G., de Vuono, M.C. and Baraldi, M. (2004). Apigenin modulates gabaergic and glutamatergic transmission in cultured cortical neurons. *Eur. J. Pharmacol.*, 502: 41–46.

Lou, H., Jing, X., Wei, X., Shi, H., Ren, D. and Zhang, X. (2014). Naringenin protects against 6-OHDA-induced neurotoxicity *via* activation of the Nrf2/ARE signaling pathway. *Neuropharmacology*, 79: 380–388.

Lull, M.E. and Block, M.L. (2010). Microglial activation and chronic neurodegeneration. *Neurotherapeutics*, 7(4): 354–365.

Magalingam, K.B., Radhakrishnan, A. and Haleagrahara, N. (2013). Rutin, a bioflavonoid antioxidant protects rat pheochromocytoma (PC-12) cells against 6-hydroxydopamine (6-OHDA)- induced neurotoxicity. *Inter. J. Mol. Med.*, 32(1): 235–240.

Magalingam, K.B., Radhakrishnan, A., Ramdas, P. and Haleagrahara, N. (2015). Quercetin glycosides induced neuroprotection by changes in the gene expression in a cellular model of Parkinson's disease. *J. Mol. Neurosci.*, 55(3): 609–617.

Maher, P., Akaishi, T. and Abe, K. (2006). Flavonoid fisetin promotes ERK-dependent long-term potentiation and enhances memory. *Proc. Natl. Acad. Sci. USA*, 103: 16568–16573.

Mansuri, M.L., Parihar, P., Solanki, I. and Parihar, M.S. (2014). Flavonoids in modulation of cell survival signalling pathways. *Genes Nutr.*, 9: 400.

Matute, C., Alberdi, E., Ibarretxe, G. and Sa´nchez-Go´mez, M.V. (2002). Excitotoxicity in glial cells. *Eur. J. Pharmacol.*, 447: 239–246.

Meng, X., Munishkina, L.A., Fink, A.L. and Uversky, V.N. (2009). Molecular mechanisms underlying the flavonoid-induced inhibition of alpha-synuclein fibrillation. *Biochemistry*, 48(34): 8206–8224.

Meng, X., Munishkina, L.A., Fink, A.L. and Uversky, V.N. (2010). Effects of various flavonoids on the α-synuclein fibrillation process. *Res. Parkinson's Dis.*, 2010 (Article ID 650794): 16. doi:10.4061/2010/650794.

Menze, E.T., Tadros, M.G., Abdel-Tawab, A.M. and Khalifa, A.E. (2012). Potential neuroprotective effects of hesperidin on 3-nitropropionic acid-induced neurotoxicity in rats. *Neurotoxicology*, 33(5): 1265–1275.

Mesulam, M., Guillozet, A., Shaw, P. and Quinn, B. (2002). Widely spread butyrylcholinesterase can hydrolyze acetylcholine in the normal and Alzheimer brain. *Neurobiol Dis.*, 9: 88–93.

Mira, L., Fernandez, M.T., Santos, M., Rocha, R., Florêncio, M.H. and Jennings, K.R. (2002). Interactions of flavonoids with iron and copper ions: A mechanism for their antioxidant activity. *Free Radic. Res.*, 36(11): 1199–208.

Murray, A.P., Faraoni, M.B., Castro, M.J., Alza, N.P. and Cavallaroa, V. (2013). Natural AChE Inhibitors from plants and their contribution to Alzheimer's disease therapy. *Curr. Neuropharmacol.*, 11: 388–413.

Na, H.K., Kim, E.H., Jung, J.H., Lee, H.H., Hyun, J.W. and Surh, Y.J. (2008) (")-Epigallocatechin gallate induces Nrf2-mediated antioxidant enzyme expression *via* activation of PI3K and ERK in human mammary epithelial cells. *Arch. Biochem. Biophys.*, 476: 171–177. doi: 10.1016/j.abb.2008.04.003.

Nagase, H., Yamakuni, T., Matsuzaki, K., Maruyama, Y., Kasahara, J., Hinohara, Y., Kondo, S., Mimaki, Y., Sashida, Y., Tank, A.W., Fukunaga, K. and Ohizumi, Y. (2005b). Mechanism of neurotrophic action of nobiletin in PC12D cells. *Biochemistry* 44: 13683–13691.

Nakayama, M., Aihara, M., Chen, Y.-N., Araie, M., Tomita-Yokotani, K. and Iwashina, T. (2011). Neuroprotective effects of flavonoids on hypoxia-, glutamate-, and oxidative stress–induced retinal ganglion cell death. *Mol. Vis.*, 17: 1784–1793.

Nazir, A. and Jadiya, P. (2013). Sirtuin mediated neuroprotection and its association with autophagy and apoptosis: Studies employing transgenic *C. elegans* model. *Mol. Neurodegenerat*, 8: 65. doi: 0.1186/1750-1326-8-S1-P65

Nijholt, D.A., De Kimpe, L., Elfrink, H.L., Hoozemans, J.J. and Scheper, W. (2011). Removing protein aggregates: The role of proteolysis in neurodegeneration. *Curr. Med. Chem.*, 18: 2459–76.

Nixon, R.A. (2012). The role of autophagy in neurodegenerative disease. *Nat. Med.*, 19: 983–997.

Obregon, D.F., Rezai-Zadeh, K., Bai, Y., Sun, N., Hou, H., Ehrhart, J., Zeng, J., Mori, T., Arendash, G.W., Shytle, D., Town, T. and Tan, J. (2006). ADAM10 activation is required for green tea (-)-epigallocatechin-3-gallate-induced alpha-secretase cleavage of amyloid precursor protein. *J. Biol. Chem.*, 281: 16419–16427.

Okello, E.J., Leylabi, R. and McDougall, J. (2012). Inhibition of acetylcholinesterase by green and white tea and their stimulated intestinal metabolites. *Food Funct.*, 3(6): 651–661.

Ono, K., Yoshiike, Y., Takashima, A., Hasegawa, K., Naiki, H. and Yamada, M. (2003). Potent anti-amyloidogenic and fibril-destabilizing effects of polyphenols *in vitro*: implications for the prevention and therapeutics of Alzheimer's disease. *J. Neurochem.*, 87: 172–181.

Onozuka, H., Nakajima, A., Matsuzaki, K., Shin, R.W., Ogino, K., Saigusa, D., Tetsu, N., Yokosuka, A., Sashida, Y., Mimaki, Y., Yamakuni, T. and Ohizumi, Y. (2008). Nobiletin, a citrus flavonoid, improves memory impairment and Abeta pathology in a transgenic mouse model of Alzheimer's disease. *J. Pharmacol. Exp. Ther.*, 326(3): 739–744.

Orhan, I., Senol, F.S., Kartal, M., Dvorska, M., Zemlicka, M., Smejkal, K., Mokry, P. (2009). Cholinesterase inhibitory effects of the extracts and compounds of *Maclura pomifera* (Rafin.) Schneider. *Food Chem. Toxicol.*, 47(8): 1747–1751.

Oueslati, A. (2016). Implication of alpha-synuclein phosphorylation at S129 in synucleinopathies: What have we learned in the last decade? *J. Parkinsons. Dis.*, 6(1): 39–51.

Panickar, K.S., Polansky, M.M., Graves, D.J., Urban, J.F. and Anderson, R.A. (2012). A procyanidin type a trimer from cinnamon extract attenuates glial cell swelling and the reduction in glutamate uptake following ischemia-like injury *in vitro*. *Neuroscience*, 202: 87–98.

Paris, D., Mathura, V., Ait-Ghezala, G., Beaulieu-Abdelahad, D., Patel, N., Bachmeier, C. and Mullan, M. (2011). Flavonoids lower Alzheimer's Aβ production *via* an NFêB dependent mechanism. *Bioinformation*, 6(6): 229–236.

Park, S.E., Sapkota, K., Kim, S., Kim, H. and Kim, S.J. (2011). Kaempferol acts through mitogen-activated protein kinases and protein kinase B/AKT to elicit protection in a model of neuroinflammation in BV2 microglial cells. *Br. J. Pharmacol.*, 164(3): 1008–1025.

Phachonpai, W., Wattanathorn, J., Muchimapura, S., Tong-Un, T. and Preechagoon, D. (2011). Neuroprotective effect of quercetin encapsulated liposomes: A novel therapeutic strategy against Alzheimer's disease. *Cold Spring Harb Perspect. Med.*, 1: a006189. doi: 10.1101/cshperspect.a006189

Pietta, P-G. (2000). Flavonoids as antioxidants. *J. Nat. Prod.*, 63(7): 1035–1042

Procházková, D., Boušová, I. and Wilhelmová, N. (2011). Antioxidant and prooxidant properties of flavonoids. *Fitoterapia,* 82(4): 513–523.

Qin, W., Yang, T., Ho, L., Zhao, Z., Wang, J., Chen, L., Zhao, W., Thiyagarajan, M., MacGrogan, D., Rodgers, J.T., Puigserver, P., Sadoshima, J., Deng, H., Pedrini, S., Gandy, S., Sauve, A.A. and Pasinetti, G.M. (2006). Neuronal SIRT1 activation as a novel mechanism underlying the prevention of Alzheimer disease amyloid neuropathology by calorie restriction. *J. Biol. Chem.*, 281: 21745–21754.

Qu, L., Liang, X.C., Gu, B. and Liu, W. (2014). Quercetin alleviates high glucose-induced Schwann cell damage by autophagy. *Neural Regen. Res.*, 9(12): 1195–1203.

Raina, P., Santaguida, P., Ismaila, A., Patterson, C., Cowan, D., Levine, M., Booker, L. and Oremus, M. (2008). Effectiveness of cholinesterase inhibitors and memantine for treating dementia: Evidence review for a clinical practice guideline. *Ann. Intern. Med.*, 148: 379.

Ramanan, V.K. and Saykin, A.J. (2013). Pathways to neurodegeneration: Mechanistic insights from GWAS in Alzheimer's disease, Parkinson's disease, and related disorders. *Am. J. Neurodegener. Dis.*, 2(3): 145–175.

Ramezani, M., Darbandi, N., Khodagholi, F. and Hashemi, A. (2016) Myricetin protects hippocampal CA3 pyramidal neurons and improves learning and memory impairments in rats with Alzheimer's disease. *Neural Regen Res.*, 11(12): 1976–1980.

Rattanajarasroj, S. and Unchern, S. (2010). Comparable attenuation of Aβ (25-35)-induced neurotoxicity by quercitrin and 17 beta-estradiol in cultured rat hippocampal neurons. *Neurochem Res.*, 35(8): 1196–1205.

Regitz, C., Dußling, L.M. and Wenzel, U. (2014). Amyloid-beta (Aβ 1–42)-induced paralysis in *Caenorhabditis elegans* is inhibited by the polyphenol quercetin through activation of protein degradation pathways. *Mol. Nutr. Food Res.*, 58(10): 1931–1940.

Rezai-Zadeh, K., Arendash, G.W., Hou, H., Fernandez F, Jensen M, Runfeldt, M., Shytle, R.D. and Tan, J. (2008). Green tea epigallocatechin-3-gallate (EGCG) reduces beta-amyloid mediated cognitive impairment and modulates tau pathology in Alzheimer transgenic mice. *Brain Res.*, 1214: 177–187.

Rezai-Zadeh, K., Douglas Shytle, R., Bai, Y., Tian, J., Hou, H., Mori, T., Zeng, J., Obregon, D., Town, T. and Tan, J. (2009). Flavonoid-mediated presenilin-1 phosphorylation reduces Alzheimer's disease beta-amyloid production. *J. Cell. Mol. Med.*, 13: 574–588.

Rezai-Zadeh, K., Gate, D., Gowing, G. and Town, T. (2011). How to get from here to there: Macrophage recruitment in Alzheimer's disease. *Curr. Alzheimer Res.*, 8(2): 156–163.

Reznichenko, L., Amit, T., Youdim, M.B. and Mandel, S. (2005). Green tea polyphenol (-)-epigallocatechin-3-gallate induces neurorescue of long-term serum-deprived PC12 cells and promotes neurite outgrowth. *J. Neurochem.*, 93: 1157–1167.

Rice-Evans, C.A., Miller, N.J. and Paganga, G. (1996). Structure–antioxidant activity relationships of flavonoids and phenolic acids. *Free Radic. Biol. Med.*, 20: 933–956.

Ross, C.A. and Poirier, M.A. (2004). Protein aggregation and neurodegenerative disease. *Nat. Med.*, 10: S10–S17.

Ross, C.A. and Tabrizi, S.J. (2011). Huntington's disease: From molecular pathogenesis to clinical treatment. *Lancet Neurol*, 10(1): 83–98.

Ryu, H.W., Curtis-Long, M.J., Jung, S., Jeong, I.Y., Kim, D.S., Kang, K.Y. and Park, K.H. (2012). Anticholinesterase potential of flavonols from paper mulberry (*Broussonetia papyrifera*) and their kinetic studies. *Food Chem.*, 132: 1244–1250.

Sabogal-Guáqueta, A.M., Muñoz-Manco, J.I., Ramírez-Pineda, J.R., Lamprea-Rodriguez, M., Osorio, E. and Cardona-Gómez, G.P. (2015). The flavonoid quercetin ameliorates Alzheimer's disease pathology and protects cognitive and emotional function in aged triple transgenic Alzheimer's disease model mice. *Neuropharmacology*, 93: 134–145.

Salameh, J.S., Brown, Jr. R.H. and Berry, J.D. (2015). Amyotrophic lateral sclerosis: Review. *Semin Neurol*, 35(4): 469–476.

Salazar, C. and Höfer, T. (2009). Multisite protein phosphorylation from molecular mechanisms to kinetic models. *FEBS J.*, 276: 3177–3198.

Salloway, S., Mintzer, J., Weiner, M.J. and Cummings, J.L. (2008). Disease-modifying therapies in Alzheimer's disease. *Alzheimer's Dement*, 4: 65–79.

Sandhar, H.K., Kumar, B., Prasher, S., Tiwari, P., Salhan, M. and Sharma, P. (2011). A review of phytochemistry and pharmacology of flavonoids. *IPS*, 1(1): 25–41.

Sandhir, R. and Mehrotra, A. (2013). Quercetin supplementation is effective in improving mitochondrial dysfunctions induced by 3-nitropropionic acid: Implications in Huntington's disease. *BBA-Mol. Basis Dis.,* 18323(3): 421–430.

Sangeetha, K.S.S., Umamaheswari, S., Reddy, C.U.M. and Kalkura, S.N. (2016). Flavonoids: Therapeutic potential of natural pharmacological agents. *Int. J. Pharm. Sci. Res.*, 7(10): 3924–3930.

Schapira, A.H. and Jenner, P. (2011). Etiology and Pathogenesis of Parkinson's Disease. *Movement Disorders*, 26(6): 1049–1055.

Schapira, A.H., Agid, Y., Barone, P., Jenner, P., Lemke, M.R., Poewe, W., Rascol, O., Reichmann, H. and Tolosa, E. (2009). Perspectives on recent advances in the understanding and treatment of Parkinson's disease. *Eur. J. Neurol.*, 16: 1090–1099.

Schroeter, H., Bahia, P., Spencer, J.P., Sheppard, O., Rattray, M., Cadenas, E., Rice-Evans, C. and Williams, R.J. (2007). (-)Epicatechin stimulates ERK-dependent cyclic AMP response element activity and up-regulates GluR2 in cortical neurons. *J. Neurochem.*, 101: 1596–1606.

Schroetera, H., Boyd, C., Spencer, J.P.E., Willaims, R.J., Cadenas, E. and Rice-Evans, C. (2002). MAPK signaling in neurodegeneration: Influences of flavonoids and of nitric oxide. *Neurobiol Aging,* 23(5): 861–880.

Senol, F.M., Ankli, A., Reich, E. and Orhan, I.E. (2016). HPTLC Finger-printing and cholinesterase inhibitory and metal-chelating capacity of various citrus cultivars and *Olea europaea. Food Technol Biotechnol*, 54(3): 275–281.

Serrano-Pozo, A., Frosch, M.P., Masliah, E. and Hyman, B.T. (2011). Neuropathological alterations in Alzheimer Disease. *Cold Spring Harb Perspect Med.*, 1: a006189. doi: 10.1101/cshperspect.a006189

Shif, O., Gillette, K., Damkaoutis, C.M., Carranoa, C., Robbins, S.J. and Hoffman, J.R. (2006). Effects of *Ginkgo biloba* administered after spatial learning on water maze and radial arm maze performance in young adult rats. *Pharmacol Biochem Behav*, 84: 17–25.

Shimmyo, Y., Kihara, T., Akaike, A., Niidome, T. and Sugimoto, H. (2008). Flavonols and flavones as BACE-1 inhibitors: Structure activity relationship in cell-free, cell-based and *in silico* studies reveal novel pharmacophore features. *Biochim Biophys Acta*, 1780: 819–825.

Singh, N.A., Mandal, A.K.A. and Khan, Z.A. (2016). Potential neuroprotective properties of epigallocatechin-3-gallate (EGCG). *Nutr. J.*, 15: 60. doi 10.1186/s12937-016-0179-4.

Spencer, J.P., Vafeiadou, K., Williams, R.J. and Vauzour, D. (2011). Neuroinflammation: Modulation by flavonoids and mechanisms of action. *Mol. Aspects. Med.*, 33(1): 83–97.

Spencer, J.P., Vauzour, D. and Rendeiro, C. (2009). Flavonoids and cognition: The molecular mechanisms underlying their behavioural effects. *Arch Biochem. Biophys.*, 492(1–2): 1–9.

Spencer, J.P.E. (2007). The interactions of flavonoids within neuronal signalling pathways. *Genes. Nutr.*, 2: 257–273.

Spencer, J.P.E., Rice-Evans, C. and Williams, R.J. (2003). Modulation of prosurvival Akt/PKB and ERK1/2 signalling cascades by quercetin and its *in vivo* metabolites underlie their action on neuronal viability. *J. Biol. Chem.*, 278: 34783–34793.

Sriraksa, N., Wattanathorn, J., Muchimapura, S., Tiamkao, S., Brown, K. and Chaisiwamongkol, K. (2012). Cognitive-enhancing effect of quercetin in a rat model of Parkinson's disease induced by 6-hydroxydopamine. *Evid. Based Complement Altern. Med.*, 2012 (823206): 9.

Sternberg, Z., Chadha, K., Lieberman, A., Hojnacki, D., Drake, A., Zamboni, P., Rocco, P., Grazioli, E., Weinstock-Guttman, B. and Munschauer, F. (2008). Quercetin and interferon-beta modulate immune Response(s) in peripheral blood mononuclear cells isolated from multiple sclerosis patients. *J. Neuroimmunol.*, 205(1–2): 142–147.

Sternberg, Z., Chadha, K., Lieberman, A., Hojnacki, D., Drake, A., Zamboni, P., Rocco, P., Grazioli, E., Weinstock-Guttman, B. and Munschauer, F. (2008). Quercetin and interferon-β modulate immune response(s) in peripheral blood mononuclear cells isolated from multiple sclerosis patients. *J. Neuroimmunol.*, 205(1–2): 142–147.

Strathearn, K.E., Yousef, G.G., Grace, M.H., Roy, S.L., Tambe, M.A., Ferruzzi, M.G., Wu, Q.L., Simon, J.E., Lila, M.2 and Rochet, J.C. Neuroprotective effects of anthocyanin- and proanthocyanidin-rich extracts in cellular models of Parkinson×s disease. *Brain. Res.*, 25(1555): 60–77.

Suganthy, N. and Devi, K.P. (2015). *In vitro* antioxidant and anti-cholinesterase activities of *Rhizophora mcronata*. *Pharm. Biol.*, 54(1): 118–129.

Szwajgier, D. (2015). Anticholinesterase activity of selected phenolic acids and flavonoids – interaction testing in model solutions. *Ann. Agri. Environ. Med.*, 22(4): 690–694.

Tai, H.C., Serrano-Pozo, A., Hashimoto, T., Frosch, M.P., Spires-Jones, T.L. and Hyman, B.L. (2012). The synaptic accumulation of hyperphosphorylated tau oligomers in Alzheimer disease is associated with dysfunction of the ubiquitin- proteasome system. *Am. J. Pathol.*, 181: 1426–1435.

Taniguchi, S., Suzuki, N., Masuda, M., Hisanaga, S., Iwatsubo, T., Goedert, M. and Hasegawa, M. (2005). Inhibition of heparin induced tau filament formation by phenothiazines, polyphenols, and porphyrins. *J. Biol. Chem.*, 280: 7614–7623.

Teixeira, M.D., Souza, C.M., Menezes, A.P., Carmo, M.R., Fonteles, A.A., Gurgel, J.P., Lima, F.A., Viana, G.S. and Andrade, G.M. (2013). Catechin attenuates behavioral neurotoxicity induced by 6-OHDA in rats. *Pharmacol Biochem Behav.*, 110: 1–7.

Theoharides, T.C. (2009). Luteolin as a therapeutic option for multiple sclerosis. *J. Neuroinflammation*, 6: 29. doi: 10.1186/1742-2094-6-29.

Thilakarathna, S.H. and Vasantha Rupasinghe, H.P. (2013). Flavonoid bioavailability and attempts for bioavailability enhancement. *Nutrients*, 5(9): 3367–3387.

Torkildsen, O., Myhra, K.M. and Bøa, L. (2015). Disease-modifying treatments for multiple sclerosis – A review of approved medications. *Eur. J. Neurol.*, 23(Suppl. 1): 18–27.

Trieu, V.N. and Uckun, F.M. (1999). Genistein is neuroprotective in murine models of familial amyotrophic lateral sclerosis and stroke. *Biochem. Biophys. Res. Commun*, 258: 685–688.

Tsuji, P.A., Stepheson, K.K., Wade, K.L., Liu, H. and Fahey, J.W. (2013). Structure-activity analysis of flavonoids: Direct and indirect antioxidant, and antiinflammatory potencies and toxicities. *Nutr. Cancer*, 65(7): 1014–1025.

Uttara, B., Singh, A.V. and Mahajan, Z.R. (2009). Oxidative stress and neurodegenerative diseases: A review of upstream and downstream antioxidant therapeutic options. *Curr. Neuropharmacol.*, 7: 65–74.

Vallés, S.L., Borrás, C., Gambini, J., Furriol, J., Ortega, A., Sastre, J., Pallardó, F.V. and Viña, J. (2008). Oestradiol or genistein rescues neurons from amyloid beta-induced cell death by inhibiting activation of p38. *Aging Cell*, 7: 112–118.

Van Praag, H., Lucero, M.J., Yeo, G.W., Stecker, K., Heivand, N., Zhao, C., Yip, E., Afanador, M., Schroeter, H., Hammerstone, J. and Gage, F.H. (2007). Plant-derived flavanol (-)epicatechin enhances angiogenesis and retention of spatial memory in mice. *J. Neurosci*, 27: 5869–5878.

Vauzour, D., Vafeiadou, K., Rice-Evans, C., Williams, R.J. and Spencer, J.P. (2007). Activation of pro-survival Akt and ERK1/2 signalling pathways underlie the anti-apoptotic effects of flavanones in cortical neurons. *J. Neurochem.*, 103: 1355–1367.

Vepsalainen, S., Koivisto, H., Pekkarinen, E., Makinen, P., Dobson, G., McDougall, G.J., Stewart, D., Haapasalo, A., Karjalainen, R.O., Tanila, H. and Hiltunen, M. (2013). Anthocyanin-enriched bilberry and blackcurrant extracts modulate amyloid precursor protein processing and alleviate behavioral abnormalities in the APP/PS1 mouse model of Alzheimer's disease. *J. Nutr. Biochem.*, 24: 360–370.

Wang, C.N., Chi, C.W., Lin, Y.L., Chen, C.F. and Shiao, Y.J. (2001). The neuroprotective effects of phytoestrogens on amyloid beta protein-induced toxicity are mediated by abrogating the activation of caspase cascade in rat cortical neurons. *J. Biol. Chem.*, 276: 5287–5295.

Wang, H., Wang, H., Cheng, H. and Che, Z. (2016). Ameliorating effect of luteolin on memory impairment in an Alzheimer's disease model. *Mol. Med. Rep.*, 13(5): 4215–4220.

Wang, S., Su, R., Nie, S., Sun, M., Zhang, J., Wu, D. and Moustaid-Moussa, N. (2014). Application of nanotechnology in improving bioavailability and bioactivity of diet-derived phytochemicals. *J. Nutr. Biochem.*, 25: 363–376.

Wang, S.W., Wang, Y.J., Su, Y.J., Zhou, W.W., Yang, S.G., Zhang, R., Zhao, M., Li, Y.N., Zhang, Z.P., Zhan, D.W. and Liu, R.T. (2012). Rutin inhibits β-amyloid aggregation and cytotoxicity, attenuates oxidative stress, and decreases the production of nitric oxide and proinflammatory cytokines. *NeuroToxicology*, 33: 482–490.

Wang, X., Chen, S., Ma, G., Ye, M. and Lu, G. (2005). Genistein protects dopaminergic neurons by inhibiting microglial activation. *Neuroreport*, 16(3): 267–270

Weinreb, O., Amit, T. and Youdim, M.B.H. (2007). A novel approach of proteomics and transcriptomics to study the mechanism of action of the antioxidant–iron chelator green tea polyphenol (-)-epigallocatechin-3-gallate. *Free Radic. Biol.*, 43(4): 546–556.

Williams, C.M., El Mohsen, M.A., Vauzour, D., Vauzour, D., Rendeiro, C., Butler, L.T., Ellis, J.A., Whiteman, M. and Spencer, J.P. (2008). Blueberry-induced changes in spatial working memory correlate with changes in hippocampal CREB phosphorylation and brainderived neurotrophic factor (BDNF) levels. *Free Radic Biol. Med.,* 45: 295–305.

Wu, P-S., Yen, J-H., Kou, M-C. and Wu, M-J. (2015). Luteolin and apigenin attenuate 4-hydroxy-2-nonenal-mediated cell death through modulation of UPR, Nrf2-ARE and MAPK pathways in PC12 cells. *PLoS ONE*, 10(6): e0130599. doi.org/10.1371/journal.pone.0130599.

Xie, Y., Yang, W., Chen, X. and Xiao, J. (2014). Inhibition of flavonoids on acetylcholine esterase: Binding and structure-activity relationship. *Food Funct*, (10): 2582–2589.

Xu, C-Q., Liu, B-J., Wu, J-F., Xu, Y-C., Duan, X-H., Cao, Y-X. and Dong, J-C. (2010). Icariin attenuates LPS-induced acute inflammatory responses: Involvement of PI3K/Akt and NF-êB signaling pathway. *Eur. J. Pharmacol.*, 642: 146–153.

Xu, L. and Pu, J. (2016). Alpha-synuclein in Parkinson's disease: From pathogenetic dysfunction to potential clinical application. *Parkinson's Disease*, 2016 (Article ID 1720621): 10. doi.org/10.1155/2016/1720621.

Xu, Z., Chen, S., Li, X., Luo, G., Li, L. and Le, W. (2006). Neuroprotective effects of (-)-epigallocatechin-3-gallate in a transgenic mouse model of amyotrophic lateral sclerosis. *Neurochem. Res.*, 31(10): 1263–1269.

Yang, E-J., Kim, G-S., Jun, M. and Song, K-S. (2010). Kaempferol attenuates the glutamate-induced oxidative stress in mouse-derived hippocampal neuronal HT22 cells. *Food Funct.*, 5(7): 1395–402. doi: 10.1039/c4fo00068d.

Yang, E-Y., Kim, G-S., Kim, J.A. and Song, K-S. (2013). Protective effects of onion-derived quercetin on glutamate-mediated hippocampal neuronal cell death. *Pharmacogn Mag.*, 9(36): 302–328.

Yiannopoulou, K.G. and Papageorgiou, S.G. (2013). Current and future treatments for Alzheimer's disease. *Ther. Adv. Neurol. Disord.*, 6(1): 19–33.

Yu, J., Jia, Y., Guo, Y., Chang, G., Duan, W., Sun, M., Li, B. and Li, C. (2010). Epigallocatechin-3-gallate protects motor neurons and regulates glutamate level. *FEBS Lett.*, 584: 2921–2925.

Zakhary, S.M., Ayubcha, D., Dileo, J.N., Jose, R., Leheste, J.R., Horowitz, J.M. and Torres, G. (2010). Distribution analysis of deacetylase SIRT1 in rodent and human nervous systems. *Anat. Rec.* (Hoboken), 293: 1024–1032.

Zeng, H., Chen, Q. and Zhao, B. (2004). Genistein ameliorates beta-amyloid peptide (25–35)-induced hippocampal neuronal apoptosis. *Free Radic. Biol. Med.*, 36: 180–188.

Zhang, J.-X., Xing, J-G., Wang, L-L., Jiang, H-L., Guo, S-L. and Liu, R. (2017). Luteolin inhibits fibrillary β-Amyloid1–40-Induced inflammation in a human blood-brain barrier model by suppressing the p38 MAPK-Mediated NF-κB signaling pathways. *Molecules*, 22: 334. doi:10.3390/molecules22030334.

Zhang, K., Ma, Z., Wang, J., Xie, A. and Xie, J. (2011). Myricetin attenuated MPP+-induced cytotoxicity by anti-oxidation and inhibition of MKK4 and JNK activation in MES23.5 cells. *Neuropharmacology,* 61(1–2): 329–335.

Zhang, X., Wang, G., Gurley, E.C. and Zhou, H. (2014). Flavonoid apigenin inhibits lipopolysaccharide-induced inflammatory response through multiple mechanisms in macrophages. *PLoS ONE*, 9(9): e107072. doi:10.1371/journal.pone.0107072

Zhang, Z., Cui, W., Li, G., Yuan, S., Xu, D., Hoi, M.P., Lin, Z., Dou, J., Han, Y. and Lee, S.M. (2012). Baicalein protects against 6-OHDA-induced neurotoxicity through activation of Keap1/Nrf2/HO-1 and involving PKCa and PI3K/AKT signalling pathways. *J. Agric. Food. Chem.*, 60: 8171–8182.

Zhao, L., Wang, J.L., Liu, R., Li, X.X., Li, J.F. and Zhang, L. (2013). Neuroprotective, anti-amyloidogenic and neurotrophic effects of apigenin in an Alzheimer's disease mouse model. *Molecules*, 18: 9949–9965.

Zheng, L.T., Ock, J., Kwon, B.-M. and Suk, K. (2008). Suppressive effects of flavonoid fisetin on lipopolysaccharide-induced microglial activation and neurotoxicity. *Inter. Immunopharmacol.*, 8(3): 484–494.

Zhou, F., Chen, S., Xiong, J., Li, Y. and Qu, L. (2012). Luteolin reduces zinc-induced tau phosphorylation at Ser262/356 in an ROS-dependent manner in SH-SY5Y cells. *Biol. Trace Elem. Res.,* 149: 273–279.

Zhu, M., Han, S. and Fink, A.L. (2013). Oxidized quercetin inhibits a-synuclein fibrillization. *Biochim. Biophysic. Acta.*, 1830: 2872–2881.

Zhu, M., Rajamani, S., Kaylor, J., Han, S., Zhou, F. and Fink, A.L. (2004). The Flavonoid baicalein inhibits fibrillation of α-synuclein and disaggregates existing fibrils. *J. Biol. Chem.*, 279(26): 26846–26857.

13

Flavonoids Are Multitargeted Hepatoprotective Agents: Insight into the Mechanisms of Action in Hepato-cellular Carcinoma

SARASWATHY S.D.[1*]

ABSTRACT

A large pool of dietary polyphenols more specifically flavonoids are the small molecules that has been studied widely for the treatment and prevention of human diseases including cancer. Most of the flavonoids commonly found in various vegetables, fruits and herbs are well known for their beneficial effects, long before their biochemical characterization. Moreover, flavonoids are multitargeted hepatoprotective agent since they possess antioxidant, anti-inflammatory and antiproliferative effects in a wide variety of cancer cells including liver. Many research groups have focused on their protective effects on hepatocellular carcinoma (HCC) both in vitro and in vivo studies. Flavonoids have been reported to prevent development of cancer by targeting multiple steps in the pathway of malignancy. Several lines of evidence suggest that flavonoids interfere with key proteins involved in various cell signaling pathways at multiple levels including cell cycle arrest, induction of apoptosis, proliferation and survival pathways. Flavonoids exert different biological effects against hepatocarcinogenesis; however the mechanism of action is yet to be disclosed. Collectively, multiple mechanisms are proposed to be involved in the pathogenesis HCC and in this chapter the literature available on the beneficial effects of several common flavonoids in the context of HCC and its molecular targets will be thoroughly discussed.

Key words: Hepatocellular carcinoma, Signaling, Apoptosis, Cell cycle, Flavonoids

[1] Department of Bio-Medical Science, Toxicology and Molecular Pathology Lab, Bharathidasan University, Tiruchirappalli - 620 024, Tamil Nadu, India.

**Corresponding author*: E-mail: sdswathi@yahoo.com

1. INTRODUCTION

Hepatocellular Carcinoma (HCC) normally develops as consequence of chronic liver disease of any etiology, and is considered as the fifth most common cancer in terms of global incidence (Parkin *et al.,* 2005). Its rate of occurrence has been steadily increasing in developing countries, with nearly 600,000 deaths each year globally (Parkin *et al.,* 2005). The most common risk factors for HCC development are chronic infection by virus, bacteria or chemical. Although, several etiological factors have been associated with HCC [*e.g.* hepatitis B virus (HBV) or hepatitis C virus (HCV) infection, aflatoxin B1exposure, tobacco, alcohol intake, non-alcoholic steatohepatitis etc.], cirrhosis is the predisposing condition for development of HCC (Anzola, 2004; Llovet *et al.,* 2003; El Serag and Rudolph, 2007; Soini *et al.,* 1996; Hashimoto *et al.,* 2004). Current standard practices for treatment of HCC include conventional chemotherapy, curative resection and liver transplantation.

Despite concerted efforts to improve the existing therapies, due to the asymptomatic nature of early HCC, the prognosis of cancer remains dismal (Blum, 2005). Several major cellular signaling pathways have been implicated in HCC, that are often accompanied by increased expression of several transcriptional factors that influence proliferation of cancerous cells by regulating cell cycle, suppressing apoptosis and inactivating tumor suppressor gene (Schirmacher *et al.,* 1992; Hickman *et al.,* 2002). Currently cytotoxic agents have limited therapeutic success in cancer; because they are highly expensive, toxic and are not very effective in changing the progress of the tumor growth. Many bioactive compounds have been identified from natural origin and one of the most interesting small molecules is flavonoids which are well known for several biological activities including antitumor activity. Unlike synthetic drugs, the selected natural products exhibit anticancer effect through induction of apoptosis by binding with death receptors and targeting multiple cellular signaling pathways including transcription factors, growth factors, protein kinases, tumor cell survival factors, inflammatory cytokines and angiogenesis that are often deregulated in cancers (Millimouno *et al.,* 2014). During the past decades, the anticancer activity of flavonoids from natural sources has been extensively investigated; still the underlying mechanisms remain unclear. Among them epigallocatechin-3-gallate, quercetin, genistsin, baicalein and silymarin can be highlighted. This review aims to summarize the anti-hepatic cancer effects of these flavonoids, unravel the underlying mechanisms of action with specific emphasis on major cellular signaling pathways with the hope of developing new treatment strategies.

2. FLAVONOIDS AS POTENTIAL ANTI-HEPATOCELLULAR CARCINOMA AGENTS

Although, many agents targeting signaling pathways are implicated in the pathogenesis of HCC and other cancers, dietary polyphenols have become not only important potential chemopreventive, but also therapeutic, natural agents. Prevention of cancer through dietary intervention recently has received an increasing interest, and polyphenols have been reported to interfere at the initiation, promotion and progression of cancer (Watson *et al.,* 2000; Garcia-Alonso *et al.,* 2006). Flavonoids represent a large class of at least 8000 phenolic compounds found in fruits, vegetables, roots, stems, flowers, red wine, herbs, tea, grain seeds etc (Bravo, 1998; Manach *et al.,* 2005). Flavonoids are a group of plant secondary metabolites with variable phenolic structures, reported to possess many pharmacological properties including cancer-preventive and anticancer effects (Rice-Evans *et al.,* 1996; Surh, 2003). There are seven subclasses of flavonoids including flavones, flavanols, flavanones, flavonols, isoflavones, flavonolignans and anthocyanidins (Ramos, 2007). The chemical activity of flavonoids is contributed due to the presence of phenolic hydroxyl group. In several studies, the chemopreventive effects of flavonoids like epigallocatechin-3-gallate (ECGC), quercetin, genistein and luteolin were analysed by *in vivo* and *in vitro* methods (Ramos *et al.,* 2005; Xia *et al.,* 2013). Furthermore, the anti-cancer effect of flavonoids have been found to be dose dependent and differs with cell type; studies on various cancer models have demonstrated that theses flavonoids interrupt the tumorigenesis process by acting on various intracellular signaling network molecules involved in the development of cancer which includes initiation, promotion and progression (Kim *et al.,* 2011). At the molecular level the pleiotropic actions of these flavonoids includes the modulation of main proteins involved in diverse cell signaling pathways linked to cell cycle arrest (cyclin D1 and cyclin-dependent kinases), apoptosis (caspases and Bcl-2 proteins), those regulated by transcription factors (NF-kB and AP-1), cell proliferation (EGF, ERK and MEK), survival pathways (PI3K and Akt) and inflammation (COX-2) and integration of different signals for the final chemopreventive or therapeutic effect (Yang *et al.,* 2001; Manson, 2003). However, the molecular mechanisms of action are not completely characterized and many features remains to be elucidated.

2.1 Role of Flavonoids in Cell Cycle Arrest

DNA damage in hepatic cancer typically leads to deregulated cell cycle, and uncontrolled cell proliferation. In cancer, the balance between cell growth and apoptosis is lost and alterations in the regulation of cell cycle have been described (Ahmad *et al.,* 2000; Chen *et al.,* 2004). Numerous studies have clearly demonstrated the role of intracellular signaling network molecules in the development of hepatocellular carcinoma (HCC) and chemopreventive effect of flavonoids play a key role in hindering and/or reversing the tumorigenesis (Fresco *et al.,* 2006). Dietary polyphenols can potentially affect and/or inhibit growth of tumour cells by perturbing the cell cycle specific proteins and thus are found to be anticarcinogens. Cyclins are well-studied cell cycle regulators and increase in cyclin D1 expression has been reported in a number of primary human tumors and cell lines (Favot *et al.,* 2003; Agarwal, 2000). Increased cyclin D1 expression has been shown in a number of primary human tumors and cell lines (Jung *et al.,* 2001). Besides, various oncogenes are associated with deregulation in cell proliferation, apoptosis, and cell survival, which ultimately cause cancerous growth. The 80 % dietary flavone inhibit HCC cell proliferation both *in vivo* and *in vitro via* arresting the cell cycle at G1 phase, increasing the expression of tumorsuppressor gene-coding proteins p53 and p21 and decreasing cyclin E and cyclins-dependent kinase (Cdk) 2 expression (Table 1).

Table 1: Effect of flavonoids on cell proliferation by cell cycle analysis.

Flavonoid	***Source/ Distribution***	***Model***	***Carcinogen/ Cell line***	***Molecular targets***
Epigallo-catechin 3-gallate	Green tea, red grapes and red wines	*In vitro*	HepG2; SMMC7721; Sk-Hep1 cells; Bel-7402	↓ cyclin D1, cyclin G1; ↓ S phase arrest
Genistein	Soybean and legumes	*In vitro*	HepG2; Sk-hep1 cells; HCC Bel 7402; Hep 3B/ nud mice; MHCC 97-H cells;	↓ cyclin D1, cyclin E; ↑ G0/G1 arrest; ↑ G2/M arrest; ↑ p53, p21, p27/ Cdk4; ↑ G0/G1 arrest, ↓ S phase arrest
Quercetin	Apple, tea, and wine	*In vitro*	HepG2;	↓ cyclin D1, cyclin E; ↑ p53, p21; ↓ Cdk2, Cdk 7; ↑ p16 mediated cell cycle arrest. ↑ G2/M phase arrest
Baicalein		*In vitro*	Bel-7404; HepJ5 cells; HepG2;	↑ G0/G1 arrest; ↑ G2/M arrest; ↓ cell proliferation
Silibinin	Milk thistle seed and plant	*In vitro*	HepG2; HepG2/Hep3B cell; HuH7	↓ cyclin D1↑ p21/Cdk4, ↑ p27/Cdk4 ↓ G1-S transition of the cell cycle, ↑G1 arrest in HepG2; ↑ G1 and G2M arrests in Hep3B cells; ↓ cyclin D1, D3 and E; ↓ Cdk2 , Cdk4
Oroxylin A	Roots of *Scutellaria baicalensis* Georgi or *S. radix*	*In vitro*	HepG2;	↑ G2/M phase arrest;

Several studies have shown that epigallocatechin-3-gallate (EGCG) present in green tea, red grapes has the ability to agitate cell cycle specific proteins and can effectively inhibit the cell proliferation in various *in vitro* tumor models (Nihal *et al.,* 2005). EGCG induced cell cycle arrest through cyclin D1 and cyclin G1 in HepG2 cells and human hepatocarcinoma cell lines (Bel7404/ADM; Bel7402/5-FU) respectively and S phase cell cycle arrest in SMMC7721 tumor cells (Lu *et al.,* 2007; Shen *et al.,* 2014; Tang *et al.,*

2008). Isoflavone genistein derived from soybean also affect HCC cell proliferation and invasion as a result of its effects on cell cycle progression. Down regulation of cyclin D1, cyclin E and Cdk 4 by genistein increased the percentage of cells in G0/G1phase and decreased those in S phase in sk-hep1 HCC cells, whereas in human hepatoma Bel 7402 cells cell cycle arrest was noted at both G0/G1 and G2/M phases (Gu *et al.,* 2005). Increased expressions of p53 and Cdk inhibitors p21 and p27 have also been observed by genistein treatment in HepG2 cells (Gu *et al.,* 2009). Moreover recent studies on the anti-carcinogenic properties of quercetin in *in vitro* and *in vivo* models have shown that quercetin block tumour growth and suppress the proliferation of hepatoma cells (Sudan and Rupasinghe, 2014; Dai *et al.,* 2016). Interestingly, quercetin disrupted the cell cycle arrest by increasing the expressions of p16 as well as p53 and p21 similar to genistein and prevents cell proliferation by arresting the cell cycle at G2/M phase followed by decrease in expressions of cyclin D1, Cdk2 and Cdk7. In combination with cisplatin, quercetin exhibit synergistic inhibitory effects on the growth of the HepG2 cells (Li *et al.,* 2014; Zhao *et al.,* 2014).

Additionally, baicalein, a key flavonoid isolated from roots of Chinese medicinal herb has been shown to demonstrate antiproliferative effects in several cancer cell lines. In this regard, treatment of Bel7404 with baicalein has led to G0/G1 phase arrest in a dose dependent manner, provoke G2/M cell cycle arrest in HepJ5 cells. Besides baicalein inhibit cell adhesion, invasion, migration and proliferation in human hepatoma cells (Zheng *et al.,* 2014; Chang *et al.,* 2002). Baicalein and silymarin suppressed HepG2 cell proliferation by increasing the ratio of cells in the G2M phase and decreasing those in S-phase, which were associated with up-regulation of tumor suppressors such as p53, p21, and p27 and downregulation of cyclin D1, cyclin E and Cdk4 (Chen *et al.,* 2009). Silibinin, extracted from the seeds and plant of milk thistle attenuated progression from G1 to the S transition phase cell cycle in HepG2 cells. Also, silibinin inhibited cell proliferation by perturbing expression of cell cycle proteins in two different HCC cell lines (Lah *et al.,* 2007; Varghese *et al.,* 2005). Furthermore, silibinin contributed to the growth inhibitory effect by arresting the cell cycle at G1 and G2/M phase through down regulation of cyclins D1, D3, E, Cdk2 and Cdk4 in HuH7, HepG2 and Hep3B human hepatoma cells. Induction of cyclin-dependent kinase inhibitor (CDIs; p21 and p27) has also been reported (Zhang *et al.,* 2013). Additionally, oroxylin A, a major bioactive flavone extracted from the roots of *S.baicalensis* Georgi or *S.radix* has been shown to exert chemopreventive activity in HCC and attenuated G2/M phase arrest of cell cycle (Hu *et al.,* 2006).

2.2 Role of Flavonoids on Cell Death or Apoptosis

Apoptosis is a process of programmed cell death accompanied by a complex cellular mechanism which has a crucial role in maintaining a healthy balance between cell survival and cell death, a relevant target in cancer-preventive approach. Apoptosis is a type of physiological self-destruction cascade which involves the active participation of tumor cells with certain distinct morphological changes. In addition, induction of apoptosis will stimulate endonuclease that involves double-strand DNA breaking and is one of the hallmarks of apoptotic cell death (Elmore, 2007). During the past decades, apoptosis induction has been recognized as a novel strategy for the identification of antitumor and chemopreventive agents (Philchenkov, 2004). *In vitro* studies have demonstrated that many dietary chemopreventive flavonoids including, epigallocatechin 3-gallate, genistein, quercetin, baicalein and silibinin effectively induce apoptosis and evoke their inhibitory effect on HCC (Jing *et al.,* 2011, Zhang *et al.,* 2015; Kuo *et al.,* 2009; Xu *et al.,* 2012b).

The apoptosis pathway can be subclassified as the mitochondria-mediated intrinsic pathway (activation of caspase-3 and caspase-9), the death receptor-induced extrinsic pathway, and apoptotic signaling evoked by endoplasmic reticulum (ER) stress. The intrinsic apoptotic pathway is a mitochondria-involved signaling cascade in which the cytochrome *c* released from the mitochondria to the cytosol binds to Apaf-1, resulting in proteolytic processing and activation of caspase-9. Activation of caspase-9 in turn activates caspase-3, thus initiating a cascade of additional caspase activations that culminates in apoptosis. In contrast to the intrinsic pathway caspase-8 is a major initiator caspase in the extrinsic apoptotic pathway (Duprez, 2009; Wu *et al.,* 2014).

In most of the apoptotic processes, caspase-3 an intracellular cysteine protease has been shown to play a pivotal role in the terminal, execution phase of apoptosis (Zhang *et al.,* 2010). Caspase activation is regulated by various cellular proteins, including inhibitor-of-apoptosis and Bcl-2 family proteins. The Bcl-2 family of proteins can be divided into two groups: anti-apoptotic proteins which include Bcl-2, Bcl-x_L, and Mcl-1 and pro-apoptotic proteins such as Bax, Bok and Bad that are critical regulators of the apoptotic pathways (Roth and Reed, 2002). Indeed, treatment with flavonoids activate the pre-existing apoptosis machinery and induce apoptosis *via* intrinsic pathway through Bcl-x_L down-regulation and release of cytochrome c to the cytosol and degradation of poly ADP-ribose polymerase (PARP), which precedes the onset of apoptosis (Scorrano and Korsmeyer, 2003).

For instance, EGCG significantly attenuated the proliferation and invasion of several hepatoma cells (HepG2, Sk-Hep, BEL-7402) and induced apoptosis partly through the mitochondrial pathway, which was consistent with a caspases-3, caspase-8 and caspase-9 activation, followed by increase in Bax/ Bcl-2 ratio (Table 2). Furthermore, EGCG was shown to delay growth of HepG2 cells through the inhibition of PI3K/Akt activity, as well as other Bcl-2 family members (Chen *et al.,* 2008; Shimizu *et al.,* 2008; Tsang and Kwok, 2010; Nishikawa *et al.,* 2006). Similarly, genistein a isoflavon present in *genista tinctoria* has also been shown to excite apoptosis both *in vitro* (human HCC cell lines) and *in vivo* (nude mice) *via*, activating protein related to programmed-cell death pathways such as caspases-3, caspases-9 and caspases-12, (Yeh *et al.*, 2007; Jiang *et al.*, 2010; Jin *et al.*, 2009) and shifting Bax/Bcl-2 ratio (Ma *et al.*, 2011). Moreover, activation of caspase-3 leads to the cleavage a number of proteins, such as procapases-8 as well as PARP. Although PARP is not essential for cell death, the cleavage of PARP is

Table 2: Effect of flavonoids on apoptosis pathway:

Flavonoid	*Model*	*Carcinogen/Cell line*	*Molecular targets*
Epigallo-catechin 3-gallate	*In vitro*	HepG2; SK-Hep1; SMCC-7721; BEL7402; HCCLM6	↑ apoptosis by↓ PI3K/AKT activity; ↑ caspase-3, caspase-8 and caspase-9 activity;
	In vivo	HLE cells/ BALB/nude mice	↓ Bcl-2 expression; ↓ Bcl-x_L ↓ c-myc
Genistein	*In vitro*	HepG2; Huh-7; SK-Hep1 cells; Hep 3B cells; MHCC 97-H cells;	↑ apoptosis *via* ↑ caspase-3, caspase-8, caspase-9 and caspase-12; ↑ Bax; ↓ Bcl-x_L ↓ Bcl-2, ↓ c-myc↑ cytochrome *c*; ↑ ROS;
	In vivo	Hep 3B/nude mice; HepG2 xenografts in BALB/c nude mice	↑ ER stress and↑ mitochondrial insult; ↑ ROS
Quercetin	*In vitro*	HepG2; Hepatoma SMCC-7721 cells; HA22T; HuH7; Hep3B2.1-7	↑ apoptotic cell death *via* ↓ anti-apoptotic proteins; Apoptosis independent of p53; ↑ apoptosis *via* ↑ caspase-3 and caspase-9; ↑ PARP (intrinsic mitochondrial pathway); ↑ ROS; ↑ oxidative stress; unbalance of Bcl-2 pro-apoptotic and antiapoptotic proteins; ↓ Bcl-x_L/Bcl-xS; ↑ Bax/Bcl-2
	In vivo	DEN-induced liver cancer in rat	
Baicalein	*In vitro*	HepG2; SMCC-7721; Bel-7402; HepJ5 cells;	↑ apoptosis (ER dependent)↑ apoptosis *via* ↑ caspase-3 and caspase-9 activity; ↑ cytochrome *c* release↓ Bcl-2 family expression; ↑ Bax/Bcl-2; ↑ Bax; ↑ caspase-3
	In vivo	HCC xenografts in mice; DEN-induced liver cancer in rat	
Silibinin	*In vitro*	HepG2; HuH7 cells;	↑ apoptotic index; ↓ survivin; ↑ caspase-3 and caspase-9; ↑ Bax; ↓ Bcl-2; ↑ ROS;
Oroxylin A	*In vitro*	HepG2 cells;	↑ apoptosis by MAC related ↑ PARP; ↓ PI3K/AKT signaling pathway; ↑ apoptosis *via* ↓ Bcl-2 ↓ procaspase-3, ↑ Bax protein
	In vivo	Transplanted H22 mice	
Luteolin	*In vitro*	HepG2 cells;	↑ cytochrome *c* release; ↑ apoptosis by Bax and Bak translocation to mitochondria; ↑ JNK; ↓ survivin, ↓ Bcl-x_L

another hallmark of apoptosis. One of the most abundant natural flavonoids, quercetin has been intensely studied to understand its chemopreventive effect. Treatment with quercetin caused DNA damage in HepG2 cell line and SMCC-7721 cells which appears to be primarily *via* a p53-dependent pathway whereas the DNA damaging effect of quercetin in HA22T; HuH7; Hep3B2.1-7 and TFK-1 cell lines (a human CC cell line) appears to be independent of p53 (Li *et al.,* 2014; Brito *et al.,* 2016). Quercetin stimulate apoptotic effects in all these hepatoma cells by activation of the caspase-dependent pathway, upregulating the expression of proapoptotic proteins such as Bax, down-regulating the expression of antiapoptotic Bcl-2 proteins, Bcl-x_L and increasing proteolytic fragmentation of PARP and intrinsic mitochondrial pathway indicating quercetin is a potential treatment option for liver cancer (Granado-Serrano *et al.,* 2006; Dai *et al.,* 2016; Lee *et al.,* 2015). In addition, the chemopreventive effect of quercetin has been demonstrated in DEN-induced hepatocarcinogesis in which it increased expression of cleaved caspase 3 and 9 inducing apoptosis whereas there is no alteration in cleaved caspase 8 (Vásquez-Garzón *et al.,* 2013). Moreover, quercetin induced apoptosis in HepG2 cells and liver cancer xenografts mouse model, in which the flavonoid increased the antitumor effects of doxorubicin (Chang *et al.,* 2009; Wang *et al.,* 2012).

In addition, apoptosis may also be induced by oxidative stress commonly associated with a previous increase of intracellular reactive oxygen species (ROS), which can act as signaling molecules to trigger the mitochondrial/ caspase apoptotic pathway, cytochrome c release, and caspase cascade (Li *et al.,* 2010). It has been now widely accepted that intracellular ROS play a vital role in cancer cell apoptosis. Flavonoids have been shown to induce ROS mediated apoptosis thus provoking DNA fragmentation and release of apoptogenic cytochrome *c* in cancerous hepatocytes (Seydi *et al.,* 2016). Silbinin derived from the milk thistle plant has been reported to exert hepatoprotective and antitumorigenic effects against various types of cancer, including HCC as evidenced not only by inhibition of cell viability, reductions in tumor cell adhesion and migration but also by stimulation of apoptotic index, caspase3 activity and ROS (Zhang *et al.,* 2013). In addition, baicalein exerted an antiproliferative effect on different hepatoma cells (SMCC-772; Bel-7402; HepJ5 cells), which was associated to apoptosis induction by activating caspase-3 and caspase-9 (Kuo *et al.,* 2009; Wang *et al.,* 2014b). It was previously shown that Baicalein inhibited cell proliferation and induced apoptosis in rat HCC and diverse cell lines (SMMC 7721; HepG2; L-02) in a dose- and time-dependent manner (Xu *et al.,* 2012b). Up-regulation of Bax/ Bcl-2 ratio has also been reported in HCC xenografts in mice together with increased levels of caspases-3 and caspase-9 (Liang *et al.,* 2012). Baicalein and silibinin have shown to increase the apoptotic index *via* cleavage of caspase-3 and -9, by downregulating the expression of Bcl-2 family of proteins, decreasing survivin and Bcl-x_L expression levels, increasing release of cytochrome *c* and cause cell death in HepG2 cells (Zhang *et al.,* 2013).

Additionally, treatment of HepG2 cells with oroxylin A, a natural mono-flavonoid extracted from Scutellariae radix led to apoptosis, enhanced expression of Bax and decreased expression of Bcl-2 (Hu *et al.,* 2006; Zhao *et al.,* 2010). Furthermore this flavonoid triggered the mitochondrial pathway of apoptosis in transplanted H22 mice by activating caspases-3 and -9, stimulating release of cytochrome c and increasing translocation of Bax/Bak to the mitochondria (Liu *et al.,* 2009; Zou *et al.,* 2012). In addition, investigation regarding the anticancer potential of luteolin, a natural flavonoid, suggested that luteolin induced apoptosis *via* the cytosolic release of cytochrome c and mechanisms involving mitochondrial translocation of Bax/Bak and activation of c-Jun N-terminal Kinase (JNK) in human hepatoma HepG2 cells (Lee *et al.,* 2005). Moreover, it has been reported that luteolin extracted from capsicum pepper induced apoptotic cell death, primarily *via* caspase-8 activation and decreased expressions of Bcl-x_L (Selvendiran *et al.,* 2006).

2.3 Role of Flavonoids on Tumorigenic Signaling in Hepatocarcinoma (Cell Survival or Cell Proliferation):

Flavonoids have been found to be powerful modulator of variety cellular signaling process likewise in a broad selection of human cancer. Recently much interest has been focused on the chemopreventive effects of flavonoids such as genistein, quercetin, epigallocatechin 3-gallate and curcumin since they interact with several signaling pathways and regulate cell survival or cell proliferation (Table 3). Alterations in numerous signaling pathways occur in cancer, and several specific pathways have been observed to be dysregulated in HCC. During different stages of cancer development the major signaling mediators downstream of the receptor tyrosine kinase phosphatidylinositol-3-kinase (PI3K), AKT/protein kinase B (PKB), members of the mitogen activated protein kinase (MAPK) family related to cellular proliferation and survival transduction pathways are activated (Villanueva *et al.,* 2007). PI3K is a family of ubiquitous signaling molecules plays a major role in malignant transformation. Protein kinase C (PKC) is a key regulator of cell growth and differentiation in mammalian cells and increased activity of PKC is believed to play an important role in tumor progression. Other predominant pathways involved in HCC pathogenesis include pathways regulating growth factor signaling such as the insulin-like growth factor (IGF), epidermal growth factor (EGF), platelet derived growth factor (PDGF), fibroblast growth factor (FGF) etc., (Whittaker *et al.,* 2010).

Numerous studies have shown the association between inflammation and cancer. Cyclooxygenase (COX)-2, NF-κB and tumor necrosis factor (TNF)-α are the key molecules involved in cancer inflammation since they influence angiogenesis and tumor microinvasion. Activation of NF- κB regulated gene products, promotes cellular proliferation, angiogenesis and invasion and subsequently inhibits apoptosis (Shishodia *et al.,* 2005). Moreover,

Table 3: Effect of flavonoids on cell survival or cell proliferation

Flavonoid	*Animal*	*Carcinogen/Cell line*	*Molecular targets*
Epigallo-catechin 3-gallate	*In vitro*	HepG2; SMMC7721; Sk-Hep1 cells; Bel-7402 & QGY-7703; Hep 3B; HuH7; cells; HLE cells	↓ NF-κB; ↓ EGFR; ↓ PI3K/Akt↓ CYP2E1; ↓ STAT-3 signaling; ↓ VEGF; ↓ ER(1)R; ↓ PGE(2); ↓ COX-2; ↓ IGF/IGF-1; p42/p44-MAPKinase; ↓ VEGF2; ↓ pVEGFR2 ↓ pERK; ↑ IGFBP-3; ↓ PI3/Akt/m TOR pathway and ↓ ERK1/2 signaling pathways
	In vivo	SD rats by thioacetamide; nude mouse xenograft model; BALB/c nude mice	↓ NF-κB; ↓ FGF2; ↓ VEGF2; ↓ p-VEGFR2; ↓ ERK/Akt
Genistein	*In vitro*	HepG2; Huh-7 and HA22T3	↓ NF-κB; ↓ MAPK, ↓ IκB ↓ PI3K/Akt, ↓ EGFR; ↓ COX-2, ↓ VEGF, ↓ p38MAPK and ↓ ERK
	In vivo	Hep 3B/nude mice;	
Quercetin	*In vitro*	HepG2;	↓ in major survival signals, ↓ Akt, ↓ERK; ↓ NF-κB; ↓ p38 MAPK; ↑ JNK, ↑ AP-1 regulation of survival/proliferation (AKT, ERK); ↓ PI3/Akt; ↓ PKCα and ↑ PKCδ
	In vivo	DEN-induced liver cancer in rats	↓ NF-κB;
Baicalein	*In vitro*	HepG2; H22, Bel-7404; MHCC97 H cells;	↓ AKT/mTOR pathway; ↓ p-AKT ↓ ERK pathway ↓ MEK1, ↓ ERK1/2; ↓ pIκB; ↓ pPKCα and p38 MAPK
	In vivo	DEN-induced liver cancer in rats; HCC xenografts in mice; BALB/c nude mice.	
Silibinin	*In vitro*	SNU761 cell line, Huh-BAT cell line; HepG2; Hep3B cell; HuH7 cells	↓ EGFR-dependent AKT signa ling; ↓ ERK1/2; ↓ mTOR/p70S6K/4E-BP1 signaling pathway; ↓ p-Akt production
	In vivo	HuH7 xeno grafts	↓ NF-κB content; ↓ p-ERK↑ PI3K-PTEN-Akt-mTOR and ↑ ERK pathways.
Oroxylin A	*In vitro*	HepG2; BALB/c nude mice	↓ AKT signaling; ↓ PI3K-PTEN-Akt-mTOR signaling pathway

accumulation of intracellular ROS triggers oxidative stress in the tumor microenvironment, leading to the increased activation of various oxidative stress-stimulated signaling molecules. It has been reported that ROS are the critical signal messengers for migration through MAPK pathway and adhesion (Chuang *et al.,* 2000).

Flavonoids are considered to be potential compounds for selectively blocking multiple signal transduction pathways. Several lines of evidence suggest that, depending on their structure, flavonoids may act as a potent inhibitors of several kinases involved in signal transduction pathway including protein kinase C (Gamet-Payrastre *et al.*, 1999; Hemström *et al.*, 2006) and tyrosine kinases (Agullo *et al.*, 1997). EGCG treatment resulted in suppression of NF-κB and phosphorylation of AKT in animal studies and various hepatoma cell lines. EGCG was demonstrated to exert its antiangiogenesis property through inhibition of growth factors receptors [epidermal growth factor receptor (EGFR), vascular endothelial growth factor receptor (VEGFR)-2] and related downstream signaling molecules including extracellular regulated kinase (ERK) and AKT (Shen *et al.*, 2014; Shimizu *et al.*, 2008).

The anticancer activity of genistein in several cancer cell types (HepG2; Huh-7; SK-Hep1cells; Hep 3B cells), has been attributed to the inhibition of ERK1/2, EGFR and VGEF. Moreover, it was found to inhibit the PI3K/AKT signaling pathway by down regulating signalling proteins including Akt, ERK, NF-κB and IκB. In this regard genestin suppressed cell invasion and inhibited cytosolic MMP-9 production in human hepatoma cells (HepG2, Huh-7, and HA22T) and murine embryonic liver cells (BNL CL2) by inhibiting activator protein (AP)-1 and NF-κB activity (Wang *et al.*, 2014a). Likewise, Quercetin prevented the progress of carcinogenesis through multifactorial pathway. Accordingly several studies have been conducted to investigate its chemopreventive ability in HCC using various *in vitro* and *in vivo* studies. In this regard, in human hepatoma HepG2 cells this bioactive flavonoid, inhibited NF-κB and led to the suppression of PI-3-Kinase/Akt and ERK cell proliferation pathways and induction of apoptosis (Granado-Serrano *et al.*, 2010). Interestingly the flavonol persuade apoptosis by the down regulation of p38, and MAPK kinase expressions whereas activated JNK in HepG2 cells. Quercetin also induced transactivation of AP-1 and PKCδ activity in transformed cells (Maurya and Vinayak, 2015). Similarly baicalein inhibited AKT/mTOR pathway as well as IGF 1-induced motility in hepatoma cells and *in vivo* HCC models which resulted in apoptosis and cell death. Furthermore, baicalein treatment dramatically decreased the levels of phosphorylation of MEK1 and ERK1/2 *in vitro* and *in vivo* (Chiu *et al.*, 2011) . Additionally it inhibited the expression of PKCα and decreased MAPK levels in hepatoma cell lines (Liang *et al.*, 2012).

In another study, silibinin was found to inhibit hypoxia-inducible factor 1 (HIF-1) transcriptional activity and reduce hypoxia-induced vascular endothelial growth factor (VEGF) in hepatoma (Hep3B) cells and this effect was potentiated in the presence of PI3K/Akt inhibitor (Garcia-Maceira and Mateo, 2009). Silibinin, also induced beneficial changes in various human hepatoma cells by inhibiting cell growth and proliferation, inducing cell cycle arrest and apoptosis. In the previously studies silibinin was correlated with decreased p-Akt production, indicating involvement of PTEN/PI(3)K/Akt and ERK pathways in its *in vivo* anti-HCC effects and was found to be a potent inhibitor of cell proliferation (Momeny, 2008; Lah *et al.*, 2007; Cui, 2009). Another natural flavonoid oroxylin A showed cytotoxicity in malignant HepG2 cells and causes inactivation of AKT signaling (Xu *et al.*, 2012a).

Also, investigation on oroxylin A induced Beclin 1-mediated autophagy in human hepatocellular carcinoma HepG2 cells and demonstrated that the induction was coupled with the suppressing of PI3K-PTEN-Akt-mTOR signaling pathway (Zou *et al.,* 2012).-This was the first report of oroxylin A in support of autophagy in promoting death of hepatocellular carcinoma cells.

3. CONCLUSIONS

Usage of targeted agents to inhibit multiple signaling pathways has emerged as a new paradigm for anticancer treatment. Flavonoids, isolated from natural sources have shown interesting anticancer activity against HCC both *in vivo* and *in vitro* models. The mechanisms by which flavonoids exhibit these beneficial properties appear to involve their interaction with diverse cellular signaling pathways and related machinery make it possible to act as an effective chemopreventive agent in hepatocarcinogenesis. Flavonoids can interfere at initiation, development and progression of HCC *via* modulation of different cellular signaling process *i.e.* block cell proliferation, promote cell cycle arrest, induce cell apoptosis and inhibit tumorigenic signaling. To conclude flavonoids play a major role in translational medicine and at present clinical translation is a major task for medical researchers. In addition, more extensive, optimized clinical trials are needed to fully evaluate the anticancer potential of flavonoids in terms of pharmokinetics and pharmodyanamic properties and interaction with other drugs.

REFERENCES

Agarwal, R. (2000). Cell signaling and regulators of cell cycle as molecular targets for prostate cancer prevention by dietary agents. *Biochem. Pharmacol.*, 60: 1051–9.

Agullo, G., Gamet-Payrastre, L., Manenti, S., Viala, C., Rémésy, C., Chap, H. and Payrastre, B. (1997). Relationship between flavonoid structure and inhibition of phosphatidylinositol 3-kinase: A comparison with tyrosine kinase and protein kinase C inhibition. *Biochem. Pharmacol.*, 53: 1649–57.

Ahmad, N., Cheng, P., Mukhtar, H. (2000). Cell cycle dysregulation by green tea polyphenol epigallocatechin-3-gallate. *Biochem. Biophys. Res. Commun.,* 275: 328–34.

Anzola, M. (2004). Hepatocellular carcinoma: Role of hepatitis B and hepatitis C viruses proteins in hepatocarcinogenesis. *J. Viral. Hepat.*, 11: 383–93.

Blum, H. (2005). Hepatocellular carcinoma: Therapy and prevention. *World J. Gastroenterol.*, 11: 7391–400.

Bravo, L. (1998). Polyphenols: Chemistry, dietary sources, metabolism, and nutritional significance. *Nutr. Rev.*, 56: 317–33.

Brito, A.F., Ribeiro, M., Abrantes, A.M., Mamede, A.C., Laranjo, M., Casalta-Lopes, J.E., Gonçalves, A.C., Sarmento-Ribeiro, A.B., Tralhão, J.G. and Botelho, M.F. (2016). New approach for treatment of primary liver tumors: The role of quercetin. *Nutr. Cancer.*, 68: 250–66.

Chang, W.H., Chen, C.H. and Lu, F.J. (2002). Different effects of baicalein, baicalin and wogonin on mitochondrial function, glutathione content and cell cycle progression in human hepatoma cell lines. *Planta Medica*, 68: 128–132.

Chang, Y.F., Hsu, Y.C., Hung, H.F., Lee, H.J., Lui, W.Y., Chi, C.W. and Wang, J.J. (2009). Quercetin induces oxidative stress and potentiates the apoptotic action of 2-methoxyestradiol in human hepatoma cells. *Nutr. Cancer*, 61: 735–45.

Chen, C.H., Huang, T.S., Wong, C.H., Hong, C.L., Tsai, Y.H., Liang, C.C., Lu, F.J. and Chang, W.H. (2009). Synergistic anti-cancer effect of baicalein and silymarin on human hepatoma HepG2 Cells. *Food Chem. Toxicol.*, 47: 638–644.

Chen, J.J., Ye, Z.Q. and Koo, M.W. (2004). Growth inhibition and cell cycle arrest effects of epigallocatechin gallate in the NBT-II bladder tumour cell line. *B.J.U. Int.*, 93: 1082–6.

Chen, X.L., Wang, Q., Cao, L.Q. *et al.* (2008). Epigallocatechin-3-gallate induces apoptosis in human hepatocellular carcinoma cells. *Zhonghua Yi Xue Za Zhi,* 88: 2524–8.

Chiu, Y.W., Lin, T.H., Huang, W.S. *et al.* (2011). Baicalein inhibits the migration and invasive properties of human hepatoma cells. *Toxicol. Appl. Pharmacol.*, 255: 316–26.

Chuang, S.M., Liou, G.Y. and Yang, J.L. (2000). Roles of JNK, p38 and ERK mitogen-activated protein kinases in the growth inhibition and apoptosis induced by cadmium. *Carcinogenesis*, 21:1491-500.

Cui, W., Gu, F. and Hu, K.Q. (2009). Effects and mechanisms of silibinin human hepatocellular carcinoma xenografts in nude mice. *World J. Gastroenterol.*, 15: 1943–1950.

Dai, W., Gao, Q., Qiu, J., Yuan, J., Wu, G. and Shen, G. (2016). Quercetin induces apoptosis and enhances 5-FU therapeutic efficacy in hepatocellular carcinoma. *Tumour. Biol.*, 37: 6307–13.

Duprez, L., Wirawan, E., Vanden Berghe, T. and Vandenabeele, P. (2009). Major cell death pathways at a glance. *Microbes Infect.*, 11: 1050–62.

Elmore, S. (2007). Apoptosis: A review of programmed cell death. *Toxicol. Pathol.*, 35: 495–516.

El-Serag, H.B. and Rudolph, K.L. (2007). Hepatocellular carcinoma: Epidemiology and molecular carcinogenesis. *Gastroenterology*, 132: 2557–76.

Favot, L., Martin, S., Keravis, T., Andriantsitohaina, R. and Lugnier, C. (2003). Involvement of cyclin-dependent pathway in the inhibitory effect of delphinidin on angiogenesis. *Cardiovasc Res.*, 59: 479–487.

Fresco, P., Borges, F., Diniz, C. and Marques, M.P. (2006). New insights on the anticancer properties of dietary polyphenols. *Med. Res. Rev.*, 26: 747–66.

Gamet-Payrastre, L., Manenti, S., Gratacap, M.P., Tulliez, J., Chap, H. and Payrastre, B. (1999). Flavonoids and the inhibition of PKC and PI 3-kinase. *Gen. Pharmacol.*, 32: 279–86.

Garcia-Alonso, J., Ros, G. and Periago, M.J. (2006). Antiproliferative and cytoprotective activities of a phenolic-rich juice in HepG2 cells. *Food Res. Int.*, 39: 982–91.

Garcia-Maceira, P. and Mateo, J. (2009). Silibinin inhibits hypoxia-inducible factor-1α and mTOR/p70S6K/4E-BP1 signaling pathway in human cervical and hepatoma cancer cells: Implications for anticancer theraphy. *Oncogene,* 28: 313–24.

Granado-Serrano, A.B., Martín, M.A., Bravo, l., Goya, L. and Ramos, S. (2006). Quercetin induces apoptosis *via* caspase activation, regulation of Bcl-2, and inhibition of PI-3-kinase/Akt and ERK pathways in a human hepatoma cell line (HepG2). *J. Nutr.*, 136: 2715–21.

Granado-Serrano, A.B., Martín, M.A., Bravo, l., Goya, L. and Ramos, S. (2010). Quercetin modulates NF-kappa B and AP-1/JNK pathways to induce cell death in human hepatoma cells. *Nutr. Cancer*, 62: 390–401.

Gu, Y., Zhu, C.F., Dai, Y.L., Zhong, Q. and Sun, B. (2009). Inhibitory effects of genistein on metastasis of human hepatocellular carcinoma. *World J. Gastroenterol.*, 15: 4952–4957.

Gu, Y., Zhu, C.F., Iwamoto, H. and Chen, J.S. (2005). Genistein inhibits invasive potential of human hepatocellular carcinoma by altering cell cycle, apoptosis, and angiogenesis. *World J. Gastroenterol.*, 11: 6512–7.

Hashimoto, E., Taniai, M., Kaneda, H., Tokushige, K., Hasegawa, K., Okuda, H. *et al.* (2004). Comparison of hepatocellular carcinoma patients alcoholic liver disease and nonalcoholic steatohepatitis. *Alcohol. Clin. Exp. Res.*, 28: 164S–68S.

Hemström, T.H., Sandström, M., Zhivotovsky, B. (2006). Inhibitors of the PI3-kinase/Akt pathway induce mitotic catastrophe in non-small cell lung cancer cells. *Int. J. Cancer.*, 1: 1028–38.

Hickman, E.S., Moroni, M.C and Helin, K. (2002). The role of p53 and pRB in apoptosis and cancer. *Curr. Opin. Genet. Dev.*, 12: 60–66.

Hu, Y., Yang, Y., You, Q.D. *et al.* (2006). Oroxylin A induced apoptosis of human hepatocellular carcinoma cell line HepG2 was involved in its antitumor activity. *Biochem Biophys Res. Commun.*, 351: 521–7.

Jiang, H., Ma,Y., Chen, X., Pan, S., Sun, B., Krissansen, G.W. and Sun, X. (2010). Genistein synergizes with arsenic trioxide to suppress human hepatocellular carcinoma. *Cancer Sci.*, 101: 975–83.

Jin, C.Y., Park, C., Kim, G.Y., Lee, S.J., Kim, W.J. and Choi, Y.H. (2009). Genistein enhances TRAIL-induced apoptosis through inhibition of p38 MAPK signaling in human hepatocellular carcinoma Hep3B cells. *Chem. Biol. Interact.*, 180: 143–50.

Jing, Yu., Yumin, Xu., Khaoustov, V. and Yoffe, B. (2011). Identification of components of grape powder with anti-apoptotic effects. *Toxicol. Ind. Health.*, 27: 19–28.

Jung, Y.J., Lee, K.H., Choi, D.W., Han, C.J., Jeong, S.H., Kim, K.C., Oh, J.W., Park, T.K. and Kim, C.M. (2001). Reciprocal expressions of cyclin E and cyclin D1 in hepatocellular carcinoma. *Cancer Lett.*, 168: 57–63.

Kim, B.R., Jeon, Y.K. and Nam, M.J. (2011). A mechanism of apigenin-induced apoptosis is potentially related to anti-angiogenesis and anti-migration in human hepatocellular carcinoma cells. *Food Chem. Toxicol.*, 49: 1626–32.

Kuo, H.M., Tsai, H.C., Lin, Y.L. Yang, J.S., Huang, A.C., Yang, M.D., Hsu, S.C., Chung, M.C., Gibson Wood, W. and Chung, J.G. (2009). Mitochondrial-dependent caspase activation pathway is involved in baicalein-induced apoptosis in human hepatoma J5 cells. *Int. J. Oncol.*, 35: 717–724.

Lah, J.J., Cui, W. and Hu, K.Q. (2007). Effects and mechanisms of silibinin human hepatoma cell lines. *World J. Gastroenterol.*, 13: 5299–305.

Lee, H.J., Wang, C.J., Kuo, H.C., Chou, F.P., Jean, L.F. and Tseng, T.H. (2005). Induction apoptosis of luteolin in human hepatoma HepG2 cells involving mitochondria translocation of Bax/Bak and activation of JNK. *Toxicol. Appl. Pharmacol.*, 203: 124–31.

Lee, RH., Cho, J.H., Jeon, Y.J., Bang, W., Cho, J.J., Choi, N.J., Seo, K.S., Shim, J.H. and Chae, J.I. (2015). Quercetin induces antiproliferative activity against human hepatocellular carcinoma (HepG2) cells by suppressing specificity protein 1 (Sp1). *Drug Dev. Res.*, 76: 9–16.

Li, S., Dong, P., Wang, J., Zhang, J., Gu, J., Wu, X., Wu, W., Fei, X., Zhang, Z., Wang, Y., Quan, Z. and Liu, Y. (2010). Icariin, a natural flavonol glycoside, induces apoptosis in human hepatoma SMMC-7721 cells *via* a ROS/JNK-dependent mitochondrial pathway. *Cancer Lett.*, 298: 222–30.

Li, Y., Duan, S., Jia, H., Bai, C., Zang, L. and Wang, Z. (2014). Flavonoids from tartary buckwheat induce G2/M cell cycle arrest and apoptosis in human hepatoma HepG2 cells. *Acta Biochimica et Biophysica Sinica*, 46: 460–70.

Liang, R.R., Zhang, S., Qi, J.A., Wang, Z.D., Li, J., Liu, P.J., Huang, C., Le, X.F., Yang, J. and Li, Z.F. (2012). Preferential inhibition of hepatocellular carcinoma by the flavonoid Baicalein through blocking MEK-ERK signaling. *Int. J. Oncol.*, 41: 969–78.

Liu, W., Mu, R., Nie, F.F., Yang, Y., Wang, J., Dai, Q.S., Lu, N., Qi, Q., Rong, J.J., Hu, R., Wang, X.T., You, Q.D. andGuo, Q.L. (2009). MAC-related mitochondrial pathway in oroxylin-A-induced apoptosis in human hepatocellular carcinoma HepG2 cells.*Cancer Lett.*,284: 198-207.

Llovet, J.M., Burroughs, A. and Bruix, J. (2003). Hepatocellular carcinoma. *Lancet*, 362: 1907–17.

Lu, L., Liu, H.M. and Tang, W.X. (2007). Effect of epigallocatechin 3-gallate on the invasiveness of hepatocarcinoma cells *in vitro*. *Zhonghya Gan Zang Bing Za Zhi*, 15: 825–827.

Ma, Y., Wang, J., Liu, L., Zhu, H., Chen, X., Pan, S., Sun, X. and Jiang, H. (2011). Genistein potentiates the effect of arsenic trioxide against human hepatocellular carcinoma: Role of Akt and nuclear factor-κB. *Cancer Lett.*, 301: 75–84.

Manach, C., Williamson, G., Morand, C., Scalbert, A. and Rémésy, C. (2005). Bioavailability and bioefficacy of polyphenols in humans. I. Review of 97 bioavailability studies. *Am. J. Clin. Nutr.*, 81(1 Suppl): 230S–242S.

Manson, M.M. (2003). Cancer prevention – the potential for diet to modulate molecular signaling. *Trends Mol. Med.*, 9: 11–8.

Maurya, A.K. and Vinayak, M. (2015). Anticarcinogenic action of quercetin by downregulation of phosphatidylinositol 3-kinase (PI3K) and protein kinase C (PKC) *via* induction of p53 in hepatocellular carcinoma (HepG2) cell line. *Mol. Biol. Rep.*, 42: 1419-29.

Millimouno, F.M., Dong, J., Yang, L., Li, J. and Li, X. (2014). Targeting apoptosis pathways in cancer and perspectives with natural compounds from mother nature. *Cancer Prev. Res.* (Phila)., 7: 1081–107.

Momeny, M., Khorramizadeh, M.R., Ghaffari, S.H. *et al.* (2008). Effects of silibinin on cell growth and invasive properties of a human hepatocellular carcinoma cell line, HepG-2, through inhibition of extracellular signal regulated kinase1/2 phosphorylation. *European Journal of Pharmacology,* 591: 13–20.

Nihal, M., Ahmad, N., Mukhtar, H. and Wood, G.S. (2005). Anti-proliferative and proapoptotic effects of (-)-epigallocatechin-3-gallate on human melanoma: Possible implications for the chemoprevention of melanoma. *Int. J. Cancer*, 114: 513–21.

Nishikawa, T., Nakajima, T., Moriguchi, M., Jo, M., Sekoguchi, S., Ishii, M., Takashima, H., Katagishi,T., Kimura, H., Minami, M., Itoh, Y., Kagawa, K. and Okanoue, T. (2006). A green tea polyphenol, epigalocatechin-3-gallate, induces apoptosis of human hepatocellular carcinoma, possibly through inhibition of Bcl-2 family proteins. *J. Hepatol.*, 44: 1074–82.

Parkin, D.M., Bray, F., Ferlay, J. and Pisani, P. (2005). Global Cancer Statistics, 2002. *CA Cancer J. Clin.*, 55: 74–108.

Philchenkov, A. (2004). Caspases: Potential targets for regulating cell death. *J. Cell. Mol. Med.*, 8: 432–44.

Ramos, S. (2007). Effects of dietary flavonoids on apoptotic pathways related to cancer chemoprevention. *J. Nutr. Biochem.*, 18: 427–42.

Ramos, S., Alía, M., Bravo, L. and Goya, L. (2005). Comparative effects of food-derived polyphenols on the viability and apoptosis of a human hepatoma cell line (HepG2). *J. Agric. Food Chem.*, 53: 1271–80.

Rice-Evans, C.A., Miller, N.J. and Paganga, G. (1996). Structure-antioxidant activity relationships of flavonoids and phenolic acids. *Free Radic Biol. Med.*, 20: 933–56. Erratum In: *Free Radic Biol. Med.*, 21: 417.

Roth, W. and Reed, J.C. (2002). Apoptosis and cancer: When BAX is TRAILing away. *Nat. Med.*, 8: 216–8.

Schirmacher, P., Held, W.A., Yang, D., Chisari, F.V., Rustum, Y. and Rogler, C.E. (1992). Reactivation of insulin-like growth factor II during hepatocarcinogenesis in transgenic mice suggests a role in malignant growth. *Cancer Res.*, 52: 2549–2556.

Scorrano, L. and Korsmeyer, S.J. (2003). Mechanisms of cytochrome c release by proapoptotic BCL-2 family members. *Biochem. Biophys Res. Commun.*, 304: 437–44.

Selvendiran, K., Koga, H., Ueno, T., Yoshida, T., Maeyama, M., Torimura, T., Yano, H., Kojiro, M. and Sata, M. (2006). Luteolin promotes degradation in signal transducer and activator of transcription 3 in human hepatoma cells: An implication for the antitumor potential of flavonoids. *Cancer Res.*, 66: 4826–34.

Seydi, E., Rasekh, H.R., Salimi, A., Mohsenifar, Z. and Pourahmad, J. (2016). Myricetin selectively induces apoptosis on cancerous hepatocytes by directly targeting their Mitochondria. *Basic Clin. Pharmacol. Toxicol.*, 119: 249–58.

Shen, X., Zhang, Y., Feng, Y., Zhang, L., Li, J., Xie, Y.A. and Luo, X. (2014). Epigallocatechin-3- gallate inhibits cell growth, induces apoptosis and causes S phase arrest in hepatocellular carcinoma by suppressing the AKT pathway. *Int. J. Oncol.*, 44: 791–796.

Shimizu, M., Shirakami, Y., Sakai, H., Tatebe, H., Nakagawa, T., Hara, Y., Weinstein, I.B. and Moriwaki, H. (2008). EGCG inhibits activation of the insulin-like growth factor (IGF)/IGF-1 receptor axis in human hepatocellular carcinoma cells. *Cance Lett.*, 262: 10–8.

Shishodia, S., Amin, H.M., Lai, R. and Aggarwal, B.B. (2005). Curcumin (diferuloylmethane) inhibits constitutive NF-kappaB activation, induces G1/S arrest, suppresses proliferation, and induces apoptosis in mantle cell lymphoma. *Biochem Pharmacol.*, 70: 700–713.

Soini, Y., Chia, S.C., Bennett, W.P., Groopman, J.D., Wang, J.S., De Benedetti, V.M. *et al.* (1996). An aflatoxin-associated mutational hotspot at codon 249 in the p53 tumor suppressor gene occurs in hepatocellular carcinoma from Mexico. *Carcinogenesis*, 17: 1007–1012.

Sudan, S. and Rupasinghe, H.P. (2014). Quercetin-3-O-glucoside induces human DNA topoisomerase II inhibition, cell cycle arrest and apoptosis in hepatocellular carcinoma cells. *Anticancer Res.*, 34: 1691–9.

Surh, Y.J. (2003). Cancer chemoprevention with dietary phytochemicals. *Nat. Rev. Cancer*, 3: 768–80.

Tang, H.H., Zhou, M. and Liang, G. (2008). Effect of epigallocatechin gallate on gene expression profiles of human hepatocellular carcinoma cell lines BEL7404/ADM and BEL7402/5-FU. *Ai Zheng*, 27: 1056–1064.

Tsang, W.P. and Kwok, T.T. (2010). Epigallocatechin gallate up-regulation of miR-16 and induction of apoptosis in human cancer cells. *J. Nutr. Biochem.*, 21: 140–146.

Varghese, L., Agarwal, C., Tyagi, A., Singh, R.P. and Agarwal, R. (2005). Silibinin efficacy against human hepatocellular carcinoma. *Clin. Cancer Res.*, 11: 8441–8.

Vásquez-Garzón, V.R., Macias-Péroz, J.R., Jiménez-García, M.N., Villegas, V., Fattel-Fazenta, S. and Villa-Treviño, S. (2013). The chemopreventive capacity of quercetin to induce programmed cell death in hepatocarcinogenesis. *Toxicol pathol.*, 41: 857–65.

Villanueva, A., Newell, P., Chiang, D.Y. *et al.* (2007). Genomics and signaling pathways in hepatocellular carcinoma. *Semin Liver Dis.*, 27: 55–76.

Wang, G., Zhang, J., Liu, L., Sharma, S. and Dong, Q. (2012). Quercetin potentiates doxorubicin mediated antitumor effects against liver cancer through p53/Bcl-xl. *PLoS ONE*, 7(12): Article ID e51764.

Wang, S.D., Chen, B.C., Kao, S.T., Liu, C.J. and Yeh, C.C. (2014a). Genistein inhibits tumor invasion by suppressing multiple signal transduction pathways in human hepatocellular carcinoma cells. *BMC Complementary Altern. Med.,* 14: 26.

Wang, Z., Jiang, C., Chen, W., Zhang, G., Luo, D., Cao, Y., Wu, J., Ding, Y. and Liu, B. (2014, 2014b). Baicalein induces apoptosis and autophagy *via* endoplasmic reticulum stress in hepatocellular carcinoma cells. *Biomed. Res. Int.*, Article ID. 732516. p. 13.

Watson, W.H., Cai, J. and Jones, D.P. (2000). Diet and apoptosis. *Annu. Rev. Nutr.*, 20: 484–505.

Whittaker, S., Marais, R. and Zhu, A.X. (2010). The role of signaling pathways in the development and treatment of hepatocellular carcinoma. *Oncogene,* 29: 4989–5005.

Wu, H., Che, X., Zheng, Q., Wu, A., Pan, K., Shao, A., Wu, Q., Zhang, J. and Hong, Y. (2014). Caspases: A molecular switch node in the crosstalk between autophagy and apoptosis. *Int. J. Biol. Sci.*, 10: 1072–83.

Xia, J.F., Gao, J.J., Inagaki, Y., Kokudo, N., Nakata, M. and Tang, W. (2013). Flavonoids as potential anti-hepatocellular carcinoma agents: Recent approaches using HepG2 cell line. *Drug Discov Ther.*, 7: 1–8.

Xu, M., Lu, N., Sun, Z., Zhang, H., Dai, Q., Wei, L., Li, Z., You, Q. and Guo, Q. (2012a). Activation of the unfolded protein response contributed to the selective cytotoxicity of oroxylin A in human hepatocellular carcinoma HepG2 cells. *Toxicol lett.*, 212: 113–25.

Xu, X.M., Yuan, G.J., Deng, J.J., Guo, H.T., Xiang, M., Yang, F., Ge, W. and Chen, S.Y. (2012b). Inhibition of 12-lipoxygenase reduces proliferation and induces apoptosis of hepatocellular carcinoma cells *in vitro* and *in vivo*. *Hepatobiliary Pancreat Dis. Int.*, 11: 193–202.

Yang, C.S., Landau, J.M., Huang, M.T. and Newmark, H.L. (2001). Inhibition of carcinogenesis by dietary polyphenolic compounds. *Annu Rev. Nutr.*, 21: 381–406.

Yeh, T.C., Chiang, P.C., Li, T.K., Hsu, J.L., Lin, C.J., Wang, S.W., Peng, C.Y. and Gu, J.H. (2007). Genistein induces apoptosis in human hepatocellular carcinomas *via* interaction of endoplasmic reticulum stress and mitochondrial insult. *Biochem Pharmacol.*, 73: 782–92.

Zhang, H.T., Luo, H., Wu, J., Lan, L.B., Fan, D.H., Zhu, K.D., Chen, X.Y., Wen, M. and Liu, H.M. (2010). Galangin induces apoptosis of hepatocellular carcinoma cells *via* the mitochondrial pathway. *World J. Gastroenterol.*, 16: 3377–84.

Zhang, S., Yang, Y., Liang, Z. *et al.* (2013). Silybin-mediated inhibition of notch signaling exerts antitumor activity in human hepatocellular carcinoma cells. *PLoS ONE*, 8: Article ID e83699.

Zhang, Y., Duan, W., Owusu, L., Wu, D. and Xin, Y. (2015). Epigallocatechin-3-gallate induces the apoptosis of hepatocellular carcinoma LM6 cells but not non-cancerous liver cells. *Int. J. Mol. Med.*, 35: 117–24.

Zhao, J.L., Zhao, J. and Jiao, H.J. (2014). Synergistic growth suppressive effects of quercetin and cisplatin on HepG2 human hepatocellular carcinoma cells. *Applied Biochemistry and Biotechnology*, 172: 784–791.

Zhao, L., Chen, Z., Wang, J., Yang, L., Zhao, Q., Wang, J., Qi, Q., Mu, R., You, Q.D. and Guo, Q.L. (2010).Synergistic effect of 5-fluorouracil and the flavanoidoroxylinA on HepG2 human hepatocellular carcinoma and on H22 transplanted mice. *Cancer Chemother.Pharmacol.*,65: 481-9.

Zheng, Y.H., Yin, L.H., Grahn, T.H.M., Ye, A.F., Zhao, Y.R. and Zhang, Q.Y. (2014). Anticancer effects of baicalein on hepatocellular carcinoma cells. *Phytotherapy Research,* 28: 1342–1348.

Zou, M., Lu, N., Hu, C., Liu, W., Sun, Y., Wang, X., You, Q., Gu, C., Xi, T. and Guo, Q. (2012). Beclin 1-mediated autophagy in hepatocellular carcinoma cells: Implication in anticancer efficiency of oroxylin A *via* inhibition of mTOR signaling. *Cell Signal.,* 24: 1722–32.

14

Isoflavonoids as Dietary Phytoestrogens in the Management of Postmenopausal Osteoporosis (PMO)

SOWMYA KUMAR[1] AND SREEPRIYA M.[1*]

ABSTRACT

Osteoporosis is a silently progressing and debilitating skeletal disease that affects mainly the women population in the postmenopausal age. Estrogen deficiency is the major risk factor in postmenopausal osteoporosis (PMO) and hence estrogen replacement therapy (ERT) is the gold standard for the treatment of the affected population. The major setback with ERT is that it is reported to increase the incidence of breast, uterine and endometrial cancers. Other anti-osteoporotic drug currently available in the market causes an array of painful side effects that limit the usage in the elderly population. Continued efforts to provide women with therapeutic options for the prevention and management of PMO with improved safety and tolerability has stimulated interest in the clinical development of Selective Estrogen Receptor Modulators (SERMs) which are a class of compounds that can have estrogen receptor agonistic or antagonistic activity depending on the target tissue. An ideal SERM with potential use against osteoporosis should have beneficial effects on the bone without stimulating the breast or endometrium. Phytoestrogens are plant-derived compounds with estrogen-like activity. It has been reported that phytoestrogens can act as selective estrogen receptor modulators and can be beneficial in the treatment of osteoporosis and phytoestrogen rich diets may help to prevent bone loss in ovariectomized animals. Isoflavonoids are a class of phytoestrogens that occur in different plants, especially legumes. Soy isoflavones and isoflavones from red clover are the major dietary sources of phytoestrogens that exert their effect through receptor dimerization and promote action depending on

[1] Department of Microbiology and Biotechnology, Bangalore University, Jnana Bharathi Campus, Bangalore – 560 056, Karnataka, India.

**Corresponding author*: E-mail: mpriya7@yahoo.com

the tissue and levels of endogenous estrogen. These are the best known source of dietary estrogens to prevent post menopausal osteoporosis by stimulating osteoblastic activity and inhibiting osteoclast formation. Hence phytoestrogen supplementation in the diet could be a safe alternative approach for the conventional estrogen replacement therapy in the management of PMO.

Key words: Phytoestrogens, Isoflavones, SERM, PMO, Osteoblast, Osteoclast

---

1. INTRODUCTION

Bone is a highly specialised tissue, made up of cells, vessels, and crystals of calcium compounds (hydroxyapatite) which provides a rigid framework for the body, protecting vital organs, acting as a site for attachment of muscles and housing the bone marrow (Florencio-Silva *et al.,* 2015). The structural components of the bone consist of extracellular matrix (largely mineralized), collagen, and cells. Bone matrix mainly consists of type I collagen fibers and noncollagenous proteins, which represent approximately 90% of the organic composition of the whole bone tissue (Boskey, 2013).

1.1. Bone Remodeling -The Continuous Process in Life

Bone undergoes constant remodeling through the action of bone forming osteoblasts and resorbing osteoclasts, which enable the faults such as microfractures to be repaired by their coordinated actions (Feng and McDonald, 2011). In a homeostatic equilibrium, resorption and formation are well balanced, that old bone is continuously replaced by new tissue and it adapts to mechanical load and strain (Fig. 1). The remodelling cycle consists of three consecutive phases: resorption, reversal, and formation. Resorption begins with the migration of partially differentiated mononuclear preosteoclasts to the bone surface where they form multinucleated osteoclasts (Qin, 2013). After the completion of osteoclastic resorption, there is a reversal phase when mononuclear cells appear on the bone surface. These cells prepare the surface for new osteoblasts to begin bone formation and provide signals for osteoblast differentiation and migration (Martin and Sims, 2014). The formation phase follows with osteoblasts placing down bone until the resorbed bone is completely replaced by new bone (Kini and Nandeesh, 2012). When this phase is complete, the surface is covered with flattened lining cells and a prolonged resting period begins until a new remodeling cycle is initiated (Delaisse, 2016).

1.2. Osteoblasts- The Bone Builders

Osteoblasts originate from multipotent mesenchymal stem cells (MSCs), which have the capacity to differentiate into osteoblasts, adipocytes,

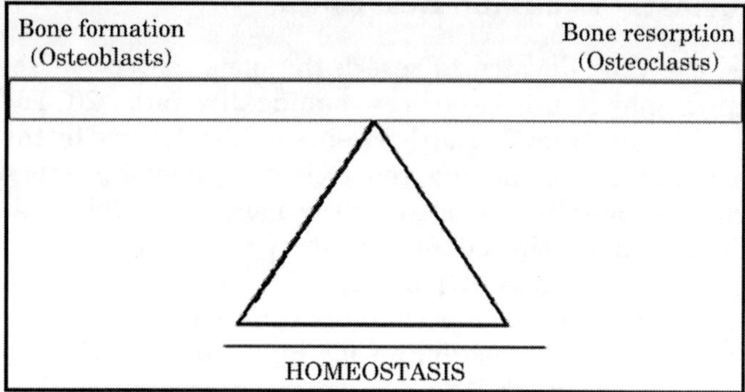

Fig. 1: Bone remodeling equilibrium managed by osteoblastic and osteoclastic actions

chondrocytes, myoblasts, or fibroblasts (Via, Frizziero and Oliva, 2012). The initial step of osteoblastogenesis is the commitment of MSCs towards an osteo/chondro-progenitor (Heino and Hentunen, 2008). Recent studies showed that Wnt10b (Wingless-int) not only shifts the commitment towards an osteo/chondro progenitor, but also inhibits preadipocyte commitment (Chen *et al.,* 2016). This is due to the suppression of the adipogenic transcription factors CCAAT enhancer binding protein γ (C/EBPα) and peroxisome proliferator- activated receptor gamma (PPARγ) along with an induction of transcription factors Runt-related transcription factor 2 (Runx2), distal-less homeobox 5 (Dlx5), and Osterix (Osx), the latter downstream of Runx2 (Baekand Baek, 2013). On the contrary, high levels of Wnt signalling in the presence of Runx2 promote osteoblastogenesis at the cost of chondrocyte differentiation. Committed pre-osteoblasts are identifiable as they express Alkaline Phosphatase (ALP), one of the earliest markers of osteoblast phenotype (Bilousova *et al.,* 2012). As the pre-osteoblasts terminate to proliferate, a key signaling event occurs for development of the large cuboidal differentiated osteoblasts (Rutkovskiy, Stenslokken, and Vaage, 2016). The active osteoblast is highly enriched in ALP and secretes bone matrix proteins such as collagen I and several non-collagenous proteins including osteocalcin, osteopontin, osteonectin and bone sialoprotein II (BSPII) (Clarke, 2008). Usually, ALP and the type 1 parathyroid receptor (PTH1R) are early markers of osteoblast progenitors that increase as osteoblasts mature and deposit matrix, but decline again as osteoblasts become osteocytes (Ono *et al.,* 2012), whereas osteocalcin is a late marker that is up-regulated only in post-proliferative mature osteoblasts associated with mineralized osteoid. The principal function of the osteoblasts is to synthesize the proteins of the bone matrix and to bring about the process of calcification. Indeed, several evidences report a crucial role of osteoblasts in osteoclast biology by expressing and/or secreting key molecules that in turn regulate osteoclastogenesis and bone resorption (Glorieux and Moffatt, 2012).

1.3. Osteoclasts- The Bone Resorbers

Osteoclasts, the cells devoted to resorb the bone matrix, arise from the monocyte/macrophage lineage (Charles and Aliprantis, 2014). They are multinucleated cells (from four up to twenty nuclei) formed by the fusion of mononuclear precursors. Starting from totipotent hematopoietic stem cells, the transcription factor PU.1, along with the macrophage colony stimulating factor (M-CSF) drive the commitment of a common progenitor for macrophages and osteoclasts. In particular, M-CSF stimulates proliferation of osteoclast precursors and upregulates RANK expression, while PU.1 positively regulates the transcription of c-Fms, the M-CSF receptor. With the appearance of c-Fms and RANK receptors, the precursors become fully committed to an osteoclast lineage (Takahashi, Udagawa and Suda, 2014). RANKL pathway is mandatory for osteoclast differentiation and function, although it is not the only player for osteoclastogenesis (Lee *et al.,* 2016).

Differentiated, multinucleated osteoclasts need to adhere to the bone matrix and diverge in order to resorb bone (Hassanpour *et al.,* 2014). Indeed, two principal domains can be identified on the osteoclast plasma membrane: the basolateral and the apical domains, which also differ in their function (Breton and Brown, 2013). In the apical domain, it is possible to identify a specialized membrane that is the ruffled border, characterized by several folding and representing the resorbing organ. One of the earliest events of osteoclast activity is to degrade the inorganic component of the bone matrix that is the alkaline salts of bone mineral hydroxyapatite (Barrere, van Blitterswijk and De Groot, 2006). This can be obtained by the release of protons into the area to be resorbed, called resorption lacuna. This function also requires sealing the underlined bone matrix, which is obtained through a cytoskeletal rearrangement and the subsequent formation of the actin ring (Georgess *et al.,* 2014). This is a circumferential structure that surrounds the ruffled membrane and isolates the acidified resorptive microenvironment from the extracellular space. It is formed by several dynamic and dot-like structures called podosomes, each of them consisting of an actin core surrounded by the avb3 integrin and associated cytoskeletal proteins such as vinculin, α-actinin and talin (Winograd-Katz *et al.,* 2014). As previously reported, the initial step of bone resorption is the release of protons in the compartment between the osteoclast and the bone surface through an electrogenic proton pomp called vacuolar type ATPase, which is present both in intracellular vesicles as well as in the ruffled border. The production of protons is ensured by the activity of the carbonic anhydrase II (CA II), which catalyses hydration of CO_2 thus forming carbonic acid (H_2CO_3). H_2CO_3 in turn dissociates to protons (H^+) and bicarbonate ions (HCO_3^-). H^+ are then secreted into the resorption lacuna, while HCO_3^- are extruded *via* an electro neutral chloride/bicarbonate exchanger in the basolateral membrane. Moreover, the chloride ion (Cl^-) that enters the cell in exchange of HCO_3^- are transported into the resorptive microenvironment through a chloride channel, thus generating HCl. Dissolution of mineral crystals allows the digestion of the bone matrix organic component that is performed by matrix metalloproteinases (MMPs) and lysosomal cathepsins (Marcoline *et al.,* 2016).

1.4. Osteoporosis - The Brittle Bone Disease

Osteoporosis is a progressive, debilitating metabolic bone disease characterized by low bone mass and weakening of bone structure that causes bone fragility (Fig. 2) and increases the risk of fractures. Individuals with osteoporosis are at high risk of suffering fractures that can often be physically debilitating and potentially lead to a downward spiral in physical and mental health thereby significantly affecting the life expectancy and quality of life in the elderly population (Leali *et al.,* 2011). Generalized osteoporosis is the most common form of the disease, affecting and damaging most of the skeleton. Osteoporosis can also occur in localized parts of the skeleton because of predisposing medical conditions that reduce muscle forces on the bone, such as limb paralysis.

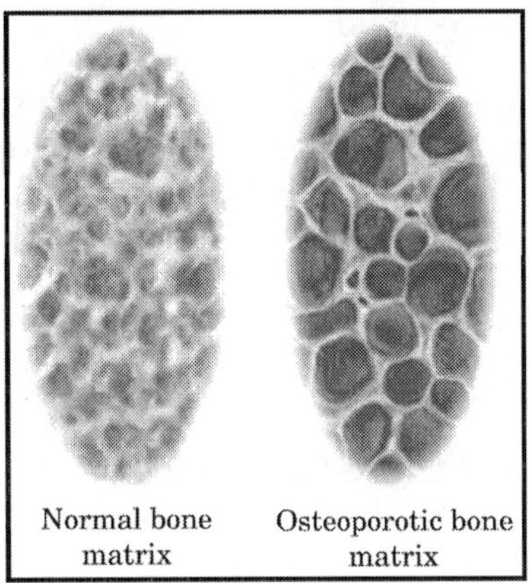

Fig. 2: Illustrates normal bone matrix and osteoporotic bone matrix

2. TYPES OF OSTEOPOROSIS

2.1. Primary Osteoporosis:

Primary osteoporosis is mainly a disease of the aged population, the result from the collective impact of bone loss and deterioration of bone structure that occurs naturally as people age (Hendrickx, Boudin and Hul, 2015). This form of osteoporosis is sometimes referred to as age-related osteoporosis. Since postmenopausal women are at greater risk, the term "*postmenopausal osteoporosis*" is frequently used to refer to this condition.

Younger individuals (including children and young adults) seldom get primary osteoporosis, although it can occur on rare occasions. This infrequent form of the disease is sometimes referred to as "*idiopathic osteoporosis*", since in many cases the exact cause of the disease is not known, or "*idiopathic*" (Peris *et al.,* 2008)

2.2. Idiopathic Juvenile Osteoporosis:

There are several types of idiopathic osteoporosis that can affect both children and adolescents, although the occurrence is quite rare (Khalid and Khoshhal, 2011). Juvenile osteoporosis affects children between the ages of 8 and 14 due to which over a period of several years, bone growth is impaired. The condition may be relatively mild, or severe depending on the underlying cause of the problem. The disease almost always goes into remission at the time of puberty with a resumption of normal bone growth. Patients with slight or modest forms of the disease may be left with a curvature of the spine (kyphosis) and short stature, but those with a more severe form of the disease may be debilitated for life (Bacchetta *et al*, 2013).

2.3. Secondary Osteoporosis

Secondary osteoporosis can occur at any age and the symptoms and extent of damage are similar to that of primary osteoporosis. It occurs due to prevailing medical conditions like hyperparathyroidism, hyperthyroidism, or leukemia. Secondary osteoporosis can also be drug-induced, the best example being chronic administration of high dose of corticosteroids, thyroid replacement therapy or usage of aromatase inhibitors (used in the treatment of breast cancer).

3. POSTMENOPAUSAL OSTEOPOROSIS - NATIONAL AND GLOBAL INCIDENCE

Postmenopausal osteoporosis is the most prevalent form of osteoporosis that is considered as a global health concern next to cardiovascular disease and cancer. It imposes enormous social and economic burdens on the governments worldwide by incapacitating and debilitating the affected individuals for the rest of their life. Currently, it is estimated that over 200 million people suffer from this disease worldwide (Vijayakumar and Busselberg, 2016). The numbers are increasing in leaps and bounds and as per the estimate made by the expert groups of Asian audits 2009, the estimated number of osteoporosis patients in India was approximately 26 million in 2003. As per the survey conducted in 2013, sources estimate that 50 million people in India are either osteoporotic or have low bone mass which puts them at a considerable risk for developing osteoporosis in future. By 2020, India is expected to be the osteoporotic capital of the world with maximum number of individuals affected with osteoporosis.

3.1. Pathogenesis of Postmenopausal Osteoporosis

3.1.1. *Role of estrogen on bone*

Estrogen deficiency is the most critical factor in the pathogenesis of osteoporosis in women. Postmenopausal women, whose estrogen levels naturally decline, are at the highest risk for developing the disease. Estrogen regulates bone turnover in both sexes, and is also critical for epiphyseal closure in puberty in men as well as women (Khosla, Melton, Riggs, 2011). In fact, estrogen has a greater effect than androgen in inhibiting bone resorption in men, although androgen may still play a role (Manolagas, O'Brien and Almeida, 2013). Estrogen may also be important in the acquisition of peak bone mass in men. Moreover, osteoporosis in older men is more closely associated with low estrogen than with low androgen levels (Sutton, Dian, Guy, 2011). Estrogen (E) deficiency is associated with large increases in bone resorption caused by increased osteoclast (OC) numbers (due to enhanced OC formation and reduced OC apoptosis) and by increased OC activity (Okman-Kilic., 2015). Since the demonstration in 1988 that bone cells contain functional estrogen receptors, progress on elucidating the molecular basis of estrogen action has been rapid, albeit controversial and incomplete. Early studies on estrogen's role in bone metabolism focused on the role of the proinflammatory cytokines - IL-1, IL-6, TNF-α, growth factors like granulocyte macrophage colony-stimulating factor, macrophage colony-stimulating factor (M-CSF), and prostaglandin-E2 (PGE2) (Singh *et al.*, 2012). These factors increase bone resorption, mainly by increasing the pool size of pre-OCs in bone marrow, and are downregulated by estrogen. Ovariectomy induced increases in the number of OCs are attenuated or prevented by measures that impair the synthesis of or response to IL-1, IL-6, TNF-α, or PGE2 (Eghbali-Fatourechi *et al.*, 2003).

3.1.2. *Role of Calcium and Vitamin D*

Under normal physiological conditions, calcium balance in the body is maintained predominantly by two factors: parathyroid hormone (PTH) and calcitriol (1, 25-dihydroxyvitamin D). PTH regulates short-term plasma calcium concentrations by dipping into bone reserves. Vitamin D strategically maintains the total calcium pool of the body (Milivojac *et al.*, 2015). The active hormonal form, 1, 25 dihydroxy vitamin D (calcitriol), is not only necessary for optimal intestinal absorption of calcium and phosphorus, but also exerts a tonic inhibitory effect on parathyroid hormone (PTH) synthesis, so that there are dual pathways that can lead to secondary hyperparathyroidism (Fleet and Schoch, 2010). Vitamin D deficiency and secondary hyperparathyroidism can contribute not only to accelerated bone loss and increasing fragility (Sindhu *et al.,* 2016), but also to neuromuscular impairment that can increase the risk of falls (Thacher and Clarke, 2011). Increased PTH levels are associated with increased mortality in the frail elderly, independent of bone mass and vitamin D status. The precise mechanisms underlying this relationship have not yet been determined.

3.1.3. *The Role of RANKL and other cytokines*

The long-sought osteoblast-derived paracrine effector of osteoclast (OC) differentiation has been identified as the receptor activator of NF-kB ligand (RANKL, also called OC differentiating factor), which is expressed by stromal-osteoblast lineage cells (Grimaud *et al.*, 2003). Contact between these cells and cells of the OC lineage allows RANKL to bind its physiologic receptor, RANK, potently stimulating all aspects of OC function (Novack, 2011). In response to RANKL signalling, OC differentiation and activity increases, and OC apoptosis decreases. Indeed, RANKL is both necessary and sufficient for OC formation, provided that permissive concentrations of M-CSF are present (Mori *et al.,* 2013). The stromal osteoblast lineage cells also secrete osteoprotegerin (OPG), a soluble decoy receptor that neutralizes RANKL. Estrogen increases OPG and decreases M-CSF and RANK. Part of the effect on this signalling system may be indirect, acting through estrogen responsive intermediaries. Thus, IL-1 and TNF-α increase RANKL, OPG and M-CSF, whereas PGE2 increases RANKL and decreases OPG (Kim *et al.,* 2009). Estrogen has not yet been shown to regulate RANKL directly. It has been reported that increased production of TNF-α by T cells in bone marrow mediates the increased bone resorption and bone loss in ovariectomized (OVX) mice. These authors show that ovariectomy induced bone loss can be prevented by administering either estrogen, TNF-α binding protein, or an inactivating antibody specific for TNF-α, and that bone loss does not occur in OVX, T cell- deficient animals. Both RANKL and TNF-α independently activate the NF-κB and Janus Kinase (JNK) intracellular signalling pathways in OC lineage cells, and this convergence explains the additive effects of the two cytokines (Pacifici, 2010). While MCSF and RANKL are essential for physiologic OC renewal, TNF-α plays a key causal role in the bone loss associated with estrogen deficiency.

3.2. Diagnosis

Low bone mass has been shown to be the biggest risk factor for fragility fractures; thus, the World Health Organization (WHO) has defined osteoporosis by Bone Mineral Density (BMD) measurement, based on values derived from Dual-energy X-ray Absorptiometry [DEXA] (Blake and Fogelman, 2007). Besides BMD, that only partly explains bone quality, other abnormalities occur in the skeleton that contributes to fragility that may be better estimated by a quantitative assessment of macrostructural and microstructural characteristics. The imaging techniques play a central role in the evaluation of bone status by a) fracture diagnosis and characterization and b) bone quality assessment. The commonly used imaging modalities to assess bone mass and macrostructure are X-ray, DEXA and quantitative computed tomography; an indirect evaluation of the bone mass and microstructure uses ultrasonography (D'Elia *et al.*, 2009).

4. THERAPY OF OSTEOPOROSIS

4.1. Dietary and Exercise Therapy:

Osteoporosis is a preventable and treatable condition. Main aim of the therapy is to increase peak bone mass by diet and exercise which is a primary prevention strategy. Secondary prevention strategy is to prevent bone loss by the use of drugs. Supplementation with calcium and vitamin D through diet and physical activity/therapy are considered as non drug therapies (Bhutani and Gupta, 2013). Adequate calcium intake is an important prerequisite to attain normal bone growth but will not prevent accelerated bone loss after menopause. Major active metabolite of vitamin D, 1, 25-dihydroxycholecalciferol is derived 80% from the conversion of 7-dehydrocholesterol by UV light and 20% from the diet, in particular blue fish and dairy products. The vitamin D precursor is liposoluble and settles mostly in the adipose tissue. The free quota is converted in the liver into 25- hydroxycholecalciferol [25 (OH) D], the major circulating vitamin D metabolite, whose levels are the most reliable index of vitamin D status. 25 (OH) D is converted into the active metabolite in the kidney, through a complex homeostatic mechanism involving parathyroid hormone (PTH), serum calcium and phosphorus levels. Vitamin D receptors are ubiquitous and are especially abundant in osteoblasts, chondrocytes, hepatocytes, parathyroid cells, and muscle cells (Bernabei *et al.*, 2014). The major actions of vitamin D in the context of bone homeostasis include the regulation of calcium metabolism by increasing intestinal absorption and renal reabsorption, and the stimulation of the synthesis of bone proteins such as osteocalcin by osteoblasts (Eisman and Bouillon, 2014). The daily vitamin D allowance ranges from 1, 500 IU (healthy adults) to 2, 300 IU (elderly with low calcium intake). Physical activity is highly effective in attenuating the age-related bone mass loss (Marques, Mota and Carvalho, 2012). Weight bearing exercise like walking (rather than swimming) contributes to the development and maintenance of bone mass. Exercise in the elderly is beneficial in increasing blood supply to muscle, bone and neural tissue (Marenzana and Arnett, 2013).

4.2. Pharmacological Therapies

There are two types of medications prescribed for osteoporosis. The therapy is aimed at reducing bone loss to produce secondary gains in mass or directly stimulating increase in bone mass (Varenna *et al.*, 2013). Some commonly used medications for osteoporosis are

4.2.1. *Fluoride*

Fluoride is used to treat established osteoporosis. It stimulates the osteoblasts and causes an increase in cancellous bone mass. However at high doses, it leads to a disease called Fluorosis resulting in fragile bones. Recent studies have shown that it actually increases the rate of non-vertebral fractures (Kleerekoper and Mendlovic, 1993) Gastrointestinal side effects and arthralgias are the main adverse effects associated with fluoride.

4.2.2. *Anabolic steroids*

Anabolic steroids are used to treat early menopause associated osteoporosis in the elderly by obtaining appositive calcium balance (Ferrucci *et al.*, 2014). Anabolic steroids can increase bone mass but long term usage is limited by side effects such as virilisation, as well as adverse effects on lipid and carbohydrate metabolism and liver function

4.2.3. *Parathyroid hormone*

Recombinant PTH (teriparatide) is a potential therapeutic stimulator of bone formation. It has been shown to increase bone mass when given in low doses (Kwon and Kim, 2016). But long term use (more than one year) is not advised and usage is contraindicated in patients with osteosarcoma.

4.2.4. *Calcitonin*

Calcitonin is a long chain polypeptide hormone used principally in established osteoporosis because it decreases bone loss by inhibiting bone resorption by a direct inhibitory action on the activity of osteoclasts (Keller *et al.*, 2014). Also, it prevents trabecular bone loss during the first few years after the menopause, but, is rarely used prophylactically because it has to be given parenterally. Nasal sprays are also available.

4.2.5. *Bisphosphonates*

Bisphosphonates are a class of drugs which reduce bone loss and vertebral fracture rate during the early years of administration in established postmenopausal osteoporosis (Sim and Ebeling, 2013). But usage is associated with several side effects including gastrointestinal problems and thromboembolic events.

4.2.6. *Estrogen replacement therapy (ERT)*

Hormone replacement therapy with estrogen decreases the occurrence of all osteoporosis-related fractures, including vertebral and hip fractures, even in women not at a high risk of fracture. Based on evidence of effectiveness, cost and safety, standard ERT should be considered one of the first-line therapies for the prevention and treatment of fractures in postmenopausal women (Gambacciani and Levancini, 2014). Estrogen replacement therapy (ERT) is effective in the prevention of bone loss in early menopause, but it also is accompanied by several adverse effects including uterine bleeding and hyperplasia. Indeed, estrogens are combined with low-dose progestins to prevent estrogen-induced endometrial cancer. However, there is evidence that the use of estrogen, with or without progestin, increases the risk of breast cancer. This potential drawback, in combination with the low compliance to HRT, has stimulated interest in the research on alternatives to the classical HRT with estrogen.

5. SELECTIVE ESTROGEN RECEPTOR MODULATORS (SERMS)-POTENTIAL ALTERNATIVES TO ERT

SERMs are a class of compounds that interact with intracellular ERs in target organs as estrogen receptor agonists and antagonists. They include chemically diverse molecules that lack the steroidal structure of estrogens, but possess a tertiary structure that allows them to bind to ER. For many years these compounds were classified simply as estrogen agonists or antagonists, but several experimental and clinical observations have led to rethink this classification with the development of the concept of "selective estrogen receptor modulation" (Maximov, Lee and Jordan *et al.,* 2013). The mechanism of action of SERM class of compounds relies on their tissue-selective estrogen receptor agonist or antagonist activity during their interaction with the estrogen receptor. These properties encompass a certain level of molecular and functional complexity. The estrogen receptor has two subunits (α and β chains), and SERMs interact with either of these subunits, and from this interaction, there is a certain level of target-site specificity and tissue specificity. This differential behaviour of SERMs depends on elicitation of varying signaling properties from the estrogen receptor that is tissue specific, and such effects have profound physiological effects which are not dictated at the DNA level. Regarding bone loss and osteoporosis, the action of SERMs on the estrogen receptor affects bone homeostasis by down modulating the activity of osteoclasts in a transforming growth factor-β3-dependent manner and thereby reducing bone resorption. This in turn helps in the prevention and management of osteoporosis (Nelson, Wardell, McDonnell, 2013).

Tamoxifen-like triphenylethylene derivatives are the recently identified class of SERMs found to possess pro/anti estrogenic effects. Clinical data from phase II/III clinical trials in women with advanced breast cancer have been published with four triphenylethylene tamoxifen-like compounds (toremifene, droloxifene, idoxifene and TAT-59). Pre-clinical data had suggested a better modulation of the estrogen receptors by these compounds compared with the antiestrogen tamoxifen thereby implicating that these compounds may prove safer or form a class of more effective anti-estrogens for the treatment of breast cancer (Martinkovich *et al.,* 2014).

5.1. Mycoestrogens

Mycoestrogens are estrogens produced as secondary metabolites of fungi. The well known class of mycoestrogens are zearalenone (ZEN) and its metabolites primarily produced by the mould *Fusarium* growing on a variety of crops. These are resorcyclic acid lactones (Bucheli *et al.*, 2008; Bakos *et al.*, 2013) and belong to a structurally diverse class of mycotoxins. After digestion by animals, ZEN is known to be rapidly metabolized into different metabolites mainly to α-zearalenol (α-ZEL) or β-zearalenol (β-ZEL) and concentration ratios of different metabolites vary among species (Molina-Molina *et al.*, 2014).

The toxin produces agonistic as well as antagonistic effect on the estrogen receptor (17β-estradiol) and thus exhibits distinct estrogenic properties with varying effect on reproductive system in several species of animals. Ingestion of ZEN and its other derivatives by humans might contribute to decreased resistance to infectious agents and neoplasm, and these compounds may function as unrecognized etiological factor of immune dysfunction diseases (Zain, 2011). The mycotoxin causes hepatocellular adenomas in female mice and pituitary adenomas in both male and female mice. Moreover, ZEN drastically reduced the number and motility of live spermatozoa in adult male albino mice and also affects the reproduction of animals at the level of changes in the function of the reproductive organs, even at the level of gametes-oocytes and spermatozoa (Sambuu *et al.*, 2011). In addition to this in females, ZEN caused an increased size of the uterus and mammary glands, swelling of the vulva and hatching the birth canal in rats, mice and guinea pigs. Reduction in fertility, damage to the reproductive tract, vaginal prolapse, increased embryonic re-absorption, changes in weight of adrenal, thyroid, pituitary glands, changes in serum levels of progesterone and 17β-estradiol were also reported by various workers (Husain *et al.*, 2014).

5.2. Phytoestrogens

Phytoestrogens are a group of natural compounds that exert estrogenic activity and are used for the treatment of menopausal disorders. Phytoestrogenic compounds occur in many different plants, mainly in legumes. Soy is the major dietary source of phytoestrogens but it contains a smaller number of estrogenically active substances compared to red clover.

Phytoestrogens are broadly classified into Isoflavones, lignans and coumestans. They are contained in high concentrations in red clover and in soybean and can be absorbed from nutrients in the gut. Red clover contains the isoflavones genistein, daidzein, biochanin A and formononetin (Fig. 3), whereas soy only contains two of these compounds (genistein and daidzein) and additionally glycitein (Patisaul and Jefferson, 2010).

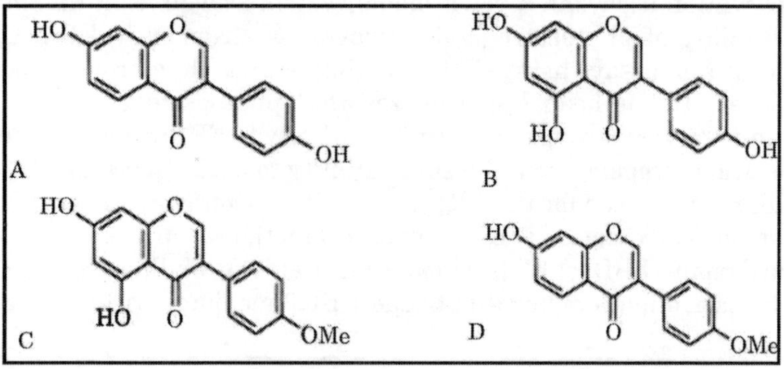

Fig. 3: Chemical structure of isoflavones (A) Formononetin (B) Biochanin A (C) Daidzein (D) Genistein

6. MECHANISM OF ACTION OF ISOFLAVONES ON BONE METABOLISM

Isoflavones are subclass of flavonoids found mainly in leguminous plants. The chemical structures of some isoflavones are similar to 17 β estradiol, hence such compounds can bind to estrogen receptors (ER) and modulate downstream estrogenic effects. Estrogen receptors α and β are nuclear receptors that can act as transcription factors for the expression of estrogen regulated genes. Binding of isoflavones to estrogen receptors may either result in partial activation of the receptor (agonistic effect) or the displacement of an estrogen molecule, thus reducing receptor activation [antagonisitic effect] (Bucar, 2013).

The distribution of estrogen receptors ER α and ER β are different in various tissues. ER α is abundantly seen in the reproductive tissues like uterus; breast whereas bone has a greater amount of ER β (Paterni *et al.*, 2014). Phytoestrogens including isoflavones derived from redclover show their beneficial effects on humans' in many different ways and exert their molecular action on a variety of tissues and cell types. The classical genomic effects of phytoestrogens expressing estrogenic or anti-estrogenic effects on ER α or ER β as well as on the other nuclear receptors are most obvious, but nongenomic effects of phytoestrogens may also be very important. They comprise effects such as the regulation of protein activity, cell cycle regulation and antioxidant activity. Nongenomic effects lead to an altered activity of certain proteins, whereas genomic effects lead to a change in the quantity of proteins whose expression is under the control of the estrogen receptors.

Isoflavones are weak ER α agonists and potent ER β agonists, because they mediate transcriptional activation or repression selectively with ER β. They have been shown to bind to both estrogen receptors in competition binding assays and reported to induce transactivation of reporter genes in transactivation assays in a yeast model system as well as in mammalian cells. Binding of phytoestrogens, however, is stronger to ER β and in transactivation assays using ER β, a higher equivalent estrogenic activity is achieved. It has been hypothesized that phytoestrogens exert their estrogenic activity through their higher affinity to ER β whereas synthetic and natural estrogens have the same affinity to both ER α and ER β. The molecular mechanism for the ER β-selectivity of isoflavones is not yet fully understood. The creation of an activation function-2 surface in the ligand binding domain (LBD) of ER β seems to facilitate the binding of coregulators to the transcription complex that triggers ER β mediated pathways (Fig. 4).

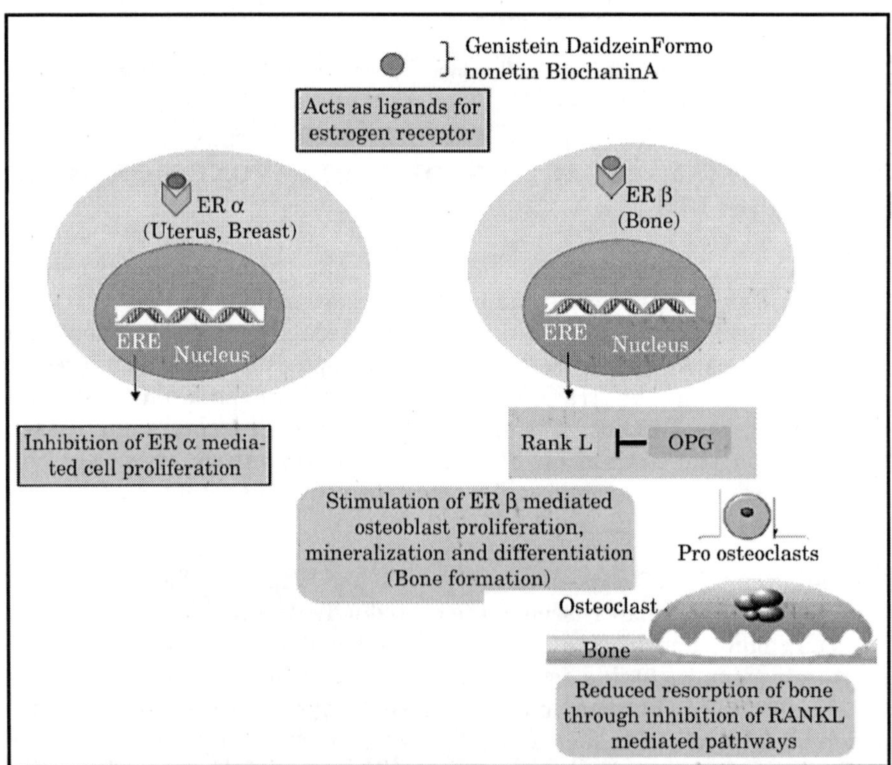

Fig. 4: Molecular mechanisms for the SERM like actions of isoflavones

Further, isoflavones are more potent at triggering transcriptional repression compared with activation. Stimulation of ER β-mediated genes and the potent repression of ER α-mediated genes could be the reason for the low incidence of menopausal symptoms, breast and endometrial cancer, osteoporosis and cardiovascular disease in countries with a isoflavone-rich diet. This selective recruitment of coregulators by both estrogen receptors has also been investigated by Warnmark *et al.* (2001). They reported that the mammalian mediator subunit TRAP220 is differentially bound by ER β, which is due to the ER binding motif of TRAP220.Also these workers, confirmed that an activation function-2 surface mediates selective binding of phytoestrogens to the estrogen receptor.

Not only the incidence of breast and endometrial cancer is lower in countries with a diet rich in isoflavones, but also the prostate cancer rate is lower than in Western countries. This suggests that isoflavones besides their estrogenicity also has beneficial effects on androgen receptor related diseases and in managing symptoms of andropause (male equivalent of menopause wherein reduction in testosterone levels are noted). A study from our laboratory implicated the beneficial effects of supplementation with phytoestrogens formononetin and biochanin A to prevent drug-induced bone loss in male rats. Chronic exposure of the rats to glucocorticoids resulted in thinning of the femur bone as evidenced by reduced radio opacity during X-ray imaging analysis. Co-treatment with formononetin and biochanin-A during glucocorticoid administration was able to prevent this thinning of the femur which was substantiated by increased radio opacity during X-ray imaging (Fig. 5). The results could be of significance as it implicated that irrespective of the sexes, phytoestrogens could exhibit their osteoprotective effects. In competitive radio ligand binding assays phytoestrogens showed binding to Androgen Receptor (AR). Affinities of red clover isoflavone extracts for AR were higher than those of soy isoflavone preparations. The molecular mechanism of the anti-androgenic effect of isoflavones on androgen mediated gene expression is not yet clear. It might occur either through inhibition of AR or androgen-controlled genes, through blocking of the receptor or through a combination of these events. In animal models it was shown that doses of dietary genistein comparable to the serum levels of humans consuming an isoflavone-rich diet down-regulate the expression of androgen and both estrogen receptors in the rat prostate (Boam., 2015). This could lead to a reduced sensitivity towards circulating androgens and thereby prevent an enlargement of the prostate. Another report showed that inhibition of Prostate specific antigen (PSA) production in the human prostate cancer cell line LNCap by genistein occurs via a transcriptional mechanism. A decrease of AR protein and AR–mRNA levels as well as a decrease in binding to the ARE in the PSA promoter could be observed. However, the molecular mechanism of action is not yet fully understood (Mohmoud *et al.,* 2013). Another study performed in Long–Evans rats fed with a diet containing a high level of soy phytoestrogens showed a down-regulation of AR in the prostate (Lonergan and Tindall, 2011) In this study, an altered prostate growth through binding of phytoestrogens to ER

RANK/OPGNF-κB pathway of osteoclastogenesis. Karieb and Fox (2014) reported that genistein, daidzein, and coumestrol significantly reduce the RANKL/OPG mRNA expression ratio in human osteoblasts, and zinc sulphate augmented the reducing effect. Low-dose genistein treatment (at 107 or 104 mol/L) for 48 h significantly increased the expression of osteogenic markers alkaline phosphatase (ALP) and OCN as well as OPG, but decreased the expression of RANKL and the RANKL/OPG ratio in cultured osteoblasts isolated from rat mandibular condyle. Genistein directly inhibits TNFα-induced osteoclastogenesis and bone resorption by suppressing the expression of c-Fos and NFATc1, two main transcription factors upregulated by NF-kB (Karieb and Fox, 2011). Furthermore, as a tyrosine kinase inhibitor and thus blocking the tyrosine kinase-NF-kB pathway for osteoclast activation, genistein inhibits the actions of IL-1 in the activation of osteoclasts and expression of cathepsin K protein, a key protease secreted by osteoclasts for bone resorption. Apart from the aforementioned ER pathway for its osteogenic effect and RANKL/ RANK/OPG NF-kB pathway for its anti-osteoclastogenic effect, how genistein exerts its osteogenic effects remain largely unknown. It is clearly understood that the transcriptional pathways induced by isoflavones genistein, daidzein, formononetin and biochanin A are distinct from those triggered by estrogens. Irrespective of their different mechanisms of action, their selectivity towards estrogen receptor beta in comparison with estrogen receptor alpha could be the prime factor contributing for their selective estrogen receptor modulation property. This SERM like property of these phytoestrogenic isoflavones could be the crucial determinant for their bone selective agonistic actions (due to increased affinity to ERβ) and their breast/uterine antagonistic actions (due to decreased affinity to ERα) unlike estrogens. Synthetic estrogens could be beneficial in managing postmenopausal symptoms and bone loss but increases the incidence of breast/uterine cancers due to their binding affinities to estrogen receptor α. Thus dietary isoflavones like genistein, daidzein, formononetin and biochanin A could form important class of selective estrogen receptor modulators that can have immense applications in the management of postmenopausal symptoms and bone loss and can serve as potent alternatives to conventional estrogen replacement therapy.

7. CONCLUSIONS

Selective estrogen receptor modulation by isoflavones of dietary origin is an important therapeutic strategy that could have potential applications in the future in the management of progressive diseases like osteoporosis, breast and uterine cancer. As they are of dietary origin, they form an important class of compounds called "Diet based disease modifying agents" that could have better tolerability and safety in women as against the current therapeutic options available for the treatment of these diseases. Such diet based modulators finds applications not only in the therapy of the disease but also as prophylactic agents in the prevention of diseases owing to their tissue selective agonistic/antagonistic properties. Regular substitution of diets rich in phytoestrogenic isoflavones could help in preventing osteoporosis in a risk prone population (women in perimenopause, women with early menopause owing to ovariectomy, patients on long term therapy with glucocorticoids and women with a family history of breast and uterine cancer). Avenues are wide open for these compounds to be explored as effective antiosteoporotic/anticancer agents. With the current scenario existing in the Indian population (increased prevalence of osteoporosis in both sexes and early onset of the disease) and India predicted to be the osteoporotic capital of the world by 2020, such nutrition based disease prevention strategies gain considerable attention in drug discovery and development programmes.

REFERENCES

An, K.C. (2016). Selective estrogen receptor modulators. *Asian Spine Journal,* 10(4): 787–791.

Bacchetta, J., Wesseling-Perry, K., Gilsanz, V., Gales, B., Pereira, R.C. and Salusky, I.B. (2013). Idiopathic juvenile osteoporosis: A cross-sectional single-centre experience with bone histomorphometry and quantitative computed tomography. *Pediatric Rheumatology,* 11: 6.

Baek, K. and Baek, J.H. (2013). The transcription factors myeloid Elf-1-like gactor (MEF) and distal-less homeobox 5 (Dlx5) inversely regulate the differentiation of osteoblasts and adipocytes in bone marrow. *Adipocyte,* 2(1): 50–54.

Bakos, K., Kovacs, R., Staszny, A., Sipos, D.K., Urbanyi, B., Muller, F. *et al.* (2013). Developmental toxicity and estrogenic potency of zearalenone in zebrafish (*Danio rerio*). *Aquat. Toxicol.,* 15: 136–137.

Barrere, F., van Blitterswijk, C.A. and de Groot, K. (2006). Bone regeneration: Molecular and cellular interactions with calcium phosphate ceramics. *International Journal of Nanomedicine,* 1(3): 317–332.

Bernabei, R., Martone, A.M., Ortolani, E., Landi, F. and Marzetti, E. (2014). Screening, diagnosis and treatment of osteoporosis: A brief review. *Clinical Cases in Mineral and Bone Metabolism,* 11(3): 201–207.

Bhutani, G. and Gupta, M.C. (2013). Emerging therapies for the treatment of osteoporosis. *Journal of Mid-Life Health,* 4(3): 147–152.

Bilousova, G. and Roop, D.R. (2014). Induced pluripotent stem cells in dermatology: Potentials, advances, and limitations. *Cold Spring Harbor Perspectives in Medicine,* 4(11): a015164.

Blake, G.M. and Fogelman, I. (2007). The role of DXA bone density scans in the diagnosis and treatment of osteoporosis. *Postgraduate Medical Journal,* 83(982): 509–517.

Boam, T. (2015). Anti-androgenic effects of flavonols in prostate cancer. *Cancer Medical Science,* 9: 585.

Boskey, A.L. (2013). Bone composition: Relationship to bone fragility and antiosteoporotic drug effects. *Bonekey Reports,* 2: 447.

Breton, S. and Brown, D. (2013). Regulation of luminal acidification by the V-ATPase. *Physiology* (Bethesda), 28(5): 318–329.

Bucar, F. (2013). Chap 2 phytoestrogens in plants: With special reference to isoflavones, isoflavones: Chemistry, analysis, function and effects. The Royal Society of Chemistry Publising, pp. 14–27.

Bucheli, T.D., Wettstein, F.E., Hartmann, N., Erbs, M., Vogelgsang, S., Forrer, H.R. *et al.* (2008). Fusarium Mycotoxins: Overlooked aquatic micropollutants? *J. Agric. Food Chem.*, 56(3): 1029–1034.

Charles, J.F. and Aliprantis, A.O. (2014). Osteoclasts: More than 'bone eaters'. *Trends in Molecular Medicine,* 20(8): 449–459.

Chen, Q., Shou, P., Zheng, C., Jiang, M., Cao, G., Yang, Q. *et al.* (2016). Fate decision of mesenchymal stem cells: Adipocytes or osteoblasts? *Cell Death and Differentiation,* 23(7): 1128–1139.

Clarke, B. (2008). Normal bone anatomy and physiology. *Clinical Journal of the American Society of Nephrology,* 3: S131–139.

D'Elia, G., Caracchini, G., Cavalli, L. and Innocenti, P. (2009). Bone fragility and imaging techniques. *Clinical Cases in Mineral and Bone Metabolism,* 6(3): 234–246.

Delaisse, J.M. (2016). The reversal phase of the bone-remodeling cycle: Cellular prerequisites for coupling resorption and formation. *Bonkey Reports,* 5: 856.

Eghbali-Fatourechi, G., Khosla, S., Sanyal, A., Boyle, W.J., Lacey, D.L. and Riggs, B.L. (2003). Role of RANK ligand in mediating increased bone resorption in early postmenopausal women. *J. Clin. Invest.*, 111: 1221–1230.

Eisman, J.A. and Bouillon, R. (2014). Vitamin D: Direct effects of vitamin D metabolites on bone: Lessons from genetically modified mice. *Bonekey Reports,* 3: 499.

Feng, X. and McDonald, J.M. (2011). Disorders of bone remodeling. *Annual Review of Pathology*, 6: 121–145.

Ferrucci, L., Baroni, M., Ranchelli, A. *et al.* (2014). Interaction between bone and muscle in older persons with mobility limitations. *Current Pharmaceutical Design*, 20(19): 3178–3197.

Fleet, J.C. and Schoch, R.D. (2010). Molecular mechanisms for regulation of intestinal calcium absorption by vitamin D and other factors. *Critical Reviews in Clinical Laboratory Sciences*, 47(4): 181–195.

Florencio-Silva, R., Sasso, G.R., Sasso-Cerri, E., Simoes, M.J. and Cerri, P.S. (2015). Biology of bone tissue: Structure, function, and factors that influence bone cells. *BioMed Research International,* 2015: 421746.

Gambacciani, M. and Levancini, M. (2014). Hormone replacement therapy and the prevention of postmenopausal osteoporosis. *Przegla"d Menopauzalny = Menopause Review,* 13(4): 213–220.

Georgess, D., Machuca-Gayet, I., Blangy, A. and Jurdic, P. (2014). Podosome organization drives osteoclast-mediated bone resorption. *Cell Adhesion & Migration,* 8(3): 192–204.

Glorieux, F.H. and Moffatt, P. (2013). Osteogenesis imperfecta, an ever–expanding conundrum. *Journal of Bone and Mineral Research,* 28(7): 1519–1522.

Grimaud, E., Soubigou, L., Couillaud, S., Coipeau, P., Moreau, A., Passuti, N. *et al.* (2003). Receptor activator of nuclear factor êB Ligand (RANKL)/Osteoprotegerin (OPG) ratio is increased in severe osteolysis. *The American Journal of Pathology,* 163(5): 2021–2031.

Hassanpour, S., Jiang, H., Wang, Y., Kuiper, J.W.P. and Glogauer, M. (2014). The Actin binding protein adseverin regulates osteoclastogenesis. *PLoS ONE,* 9(10): e109078.

Heino, T.J. and Hentunen, T.A. (2008). Differentiation of osteoblasts and osteocytes from Mesenchymal stem cells. *Current Stem Cell Research & Therapy,* 3(2): 131–145.

Hendrickx, G., Boudin, E. and Van Hul, W. (2015). A look behind the scenes: The risk and pathogenesis of primary osteoporosis. *Nature Reviews Rheumatology,* 11(8): 462–474.

Husain, A.S., Thalij, K.M. and Dheeb, B.I. (2014). Effects of interaction between aflatoxins (AFs) and functional materials FM in the hematological, biochemical parameters and enzyme activity in rats. *Egypt. Acad. J. Biolog. Sci.*, 6(2): 17–22.

Jiang, Y., Gong, P., Madak-Erdogan, Z. *et al.* (2013). Mechanisms enforcing the estrogen receptor β-selectivity of botanical estrogens. *The FASEB Journal,* 27(11): 4406–4418.

Karieb, S. and Fox, S. (2011). Phytoestrogens directly inhibit TNF-α-induced bone resorption in RAW264.7 cells by suppressing c-fos-induced NFATc1 expression. *J. Cell Biochem.*, 112(2): 476–87.

Karieb, S. and Fox, S. (2014). Zinc modifies the effect of phyto-oestrogens on osteoblast and osteoclast differentiation *in vitro*. *British Journal of Nutrition,* 108(10): 1736–1745.

Keller, J., Catala-Lehnen, P., Huebner, A.K., Jeschke, A., Heckt, T., Lueth, A. *et al.* (2014). Calcitonin controls bone formation by inhibiting the release of sphingosine 1-phosphate from osteoclasts. *Nature Communications*, 5: 5215.

Khalid, I. (2011). Khoshhal, childhood osteoporosis. *Journal of Taibah University Medical Sciences,* 6(2): 61–67.

Khosla, S., Melton, L.J. and Riggs, B.L. (2011). The unitary model for estrogen deficiency and the pathogenesis of osteoporosis: Is a revision needed? *Journal of Bone and Mineral Research,* 26(3): 441–451.

Kim, H., Choi, H.K., Shin, J.H. *et al*. (2009). Selective inhibition of RANK blocks osteoclast maturation and function and prevents bone loss in mice. *The Journal of Clinical Investigation,* 119(4): 813–825.

Kini, U. and Nandeesh, B.N. (2012). Physiology of Bone Formation, Remodeling, and Metabolism. *In*: Fogelman *et al*. (*eds*.), Radionuclide and Hybrid Bone Imaging, Springer-Verlag Berlin Heidelberg. pp. 29–57.

Kleerekoper, M. and Mendlovic, D.B. (1993). Sodium fluoride therapy of postmenopausal osteoporosis. *Endocr. Rev.,* 14(3): 312–323.

Kwon, Y.D. and Kim, D.Y. (2016). Role of teriparatide in medication-related osteonecrosis of the jaws (MRONJ). *Dent. J.*, 4: 41.

Leali, P.T., Muresu, F., Melis, A., Ruggiu, A., Zachos, A. and Doria, C. (2011). Skeletal fragility definition. *Clinical Cases in Mineral and Bone Metabolism,* 8(2): 11–13.

Lee, K., Chung, Y.H., Ahn, H., Kim, H., Rho, J. and Jeong, D. (2016). Selective regulation of MAPK signaling mediates RANKL-dependent osteoclast differentiation. *International Journal of Biological Sciences,* 12(2): 235–245.

Lonergan, P.E. and Tindall, D.J. (2011). Androgen receptor signaling in prostate cancer development and progression. *Journal of Carcinogenesis*, 10: 20.

Manolagas, S.C., O'Brien, C.A. and Almeida, M. (2013). The role of estrogen and androgen receptors in bone health and disease. *Nature Reviews Endocrinology,* 9(12): 699–712.

Marcoline, F.V., Ishida, Y., Mindell, J.A., Nayak, S. and Grab, M. (2016). A mathematical model of osteoclast acidification during bone resorption. *Bone.*, 93: 167–180.

Marenzana, M. and Arnett, T.R. (2013). The key role of the blood supply to bone. *Bone Research,* 1(3): 203–215.

Marques, E.A., Mota, J. and Carvalho, J. (2012). Exercise effects on bone mineral density in older adults: A meta-analysis of randomized controlled trials. *Age,* 34(6): 1493–1515.

Martin, T.J. and Sims, N.A. (2014). Coupling the activities of bone formation and resorption: A multitude of signals within the basic multicellular unit. *Bonekey Reports*, 3: 481.

Martinkovich, S., Shah, D., Planey, S.L. and Arnott, J.A. (2014). Selective estrogen receptor modulators: Tissue specificity and clinical utility. *Clinical Interventions in Aging,* 9: 1437–1452.

Maximov, P.Y., Lee, T.M. and Jordan, V.C. (2013). The discovery and development of selective estrogen receptor modulators (SERMs) for clinical practice. *Current Clinical Pharmacology,* 8(2): 135–155.

Milivojac, T., Raseta, N., Aksentic, V. and Grabez, M. (2015). Impact of vitamin D deficiency on fluctuation of calcium and parathyroid hormone levels in post menopausal osteoporosis. *SportLogia,* 11(1): 18–33.

Mohmoud, A.M., Zhu, T., Parray, A., Siddiqui, H.R., Saleem, M. *et al*. (2013). Differential effects of genistein on prostrate cancer cells depend on mutation status of androgen receptor. Ed. *Plos ONE*, 8(10): e78479.

Molina-Molina, J.M., Real, M., Jimenez-Diaz, I., Belhassen, H., Hedhili, A., Torne, P. *et al.* (2014). Assessment of estrogenic and anti-androgenic activities of the mycotoxin zearalenone and its metabolites using *in vitro* receptor-specific bioassays. *Food Chem. Toxicol.*, 74: 233–239.

Mori, G., D'Amelio, P., Faccio, R. and Brunetti, P. (2013). The interplay between the bone and the immune system. *Clinical and Developmental Immunology*, 720504: 16.

Nelson, E.R., Wardell, S.E. and McDonnell, D.P. (2013). The molecular mechanisms underlying the pharmacological actions of estrogens, SERMs and oxysterols: Implications for the treatment and prevention of osteoporosis. *Bone.*, 53(1): 42–50.

Novack, D.V. (2011). Role of NF-κB in the skeleton. *Cell Research,* 21: 169–182.

Ono, N., Nakashima, K., Schipani, E., Hayata, T., Ezura, Y., Soma, K. *et al.* (2012). Constitutively active PTH/PTHrP receptor specifically expressed in osteoblasts enhances bone formation induced by bone marrow ablation. *Journal of Cellular Physiology,* 227(2): 408–415.

Pacifici, R. (2010). The immune system and bone. *Archives of Biochemistry and Biophysics*, 503(1): 41–53.

Paterni, I., Granchi, C., Katzenellenbogen, J.A. and Minutolo, F. (2014). Estrogen Receptors Alpha (ERα) and Beta (ERβ): Subtype-selective ligands and clinical potential. *Steroids,* 10: 13–29.

Patisaul, H.B. and Jefferson, W. (2010). The pros and cons of phytoestrogens. *Frontiers in Neuroendocrinology,* 31(4): 400–419.

Peris, P., Ruiz-Esquide, V., Monegal, A., Alvarez, L., Martínez de Osaba, M.J., Martínez-Ferrer, A. *et al.* (2008). Idiopathic osteoporosis in premenopausal women. Clinical characteristics and bone remodelling abnormalities. *Clin. Exp. Rheumatol.*, 26(6): 986–91.

Pisani, P., Renna, M.D., Conversano, F. *et al.* (2016). Major osteoporotic fragility fractures: Risk factor updates and societal impact. *World Journal of Orthopedics*. 7(3): 171–181.

Qin, Q.H. (2013). Mechanics of Cellular Bone Remodeling: Coupled Thermal, Electrical, and Mechanical Field Effects. CRC Press.

Radominska-Pandya, A., Bratton, S.M., Redinbo, M.R. and Miley, M.J. (2010). The crystal structure of human UDP-glucuronosyltransferase 2B7 C-terminal end is the first mammalian UGT target to be revealed: The significance for human UGTs from both the 1A and 2B families. *Drug Metabolism Reviews,* 42(1): 133–144.

Rutkovskiy, A., Stenslokken, K.O. and Vaage, I.J. (2016). Osteoblast Differentiation at a Glance. *Medical Science Monitor Basic Research,* 22: 95–106.

Sambuu, R., Takagi, M., Namula, Z., Otoi, T., Shiga, S., Rodrigues dos Santos, R. *et al.* (2011). Effects of exposure to zearalenone on porcine oocytes and sperm during maturation and fertilization *in vitro*. *Journal of Reproduction and Development,* 57(4): 547–550.

Shanle, E.K. and Xu, W. (2011). Endocrine disrupting chemicals targeting estrogen receptor signaling: Identification and mechanisms of action. *Chemical Research in Toxicology*, 24(1): 6–19.

Sim, IeW. and Ebeling, P.R. (2013). Treatment of osteoporosis in men with bisphosphonates: Rationale and latest evidence. *Therapeutic Advances in Musculoskeletal Disease,* 5(5): 259–267.

Sindhu, Y.U., Navyar, A.S., Siddhartha, K., Kartheeki, B. and Bhargavi, D. (2016). Osteoporosis: Current state and need for screening with the help of oral health physicians. *Indian J. Health Sci. Biomed. Res.*, 9: 251–7.

Singh, A., Mehdi, A.A., Srivastava, R.N. and Verma, N.S. (2012). Immunoregulation of bone remodelling. *International Journal of Critical Illness and Injury Science,* 2(2): 75–81.

Somjen, D., Katzburg, S., Sharon, O., Grafi-Cohen, M., Knoll, E., Stern, N. *et al.* (2011). *Journal of Cellular Biochemistry,* 112: 625–632.

Sutton, R.A.L., Dian, L. and Guy, P. (2011). Osteoporosis in men: An under recognized and undertreated problem. *BCMJ,* 53(10): 535–540.

Takahashi, N., Udagawa, N. and Suda, T. (2014). Vitamin D endocrine system and osteoclasts. *Bonekey Rep.*, 3: 495.

Thacher, T.D. and Clarke, B.L. (2011). Vitamin D Insufficiency. *Mayo Clinic Proceedings,* 86(1): 50–60.

Tulay Okman-Kilic. (2015). Estrogen Deficiency and Osteoporosis, Advances in Osteoporosis, PhD. Yannis Dionyssiotis (*ed.*), In Tech. 10: 5772/59407.

Varenna, M., Bertoldo, F., Di Monaco, M., Giusti, A., Martini, G. and Rossini, M. (2013). Safety profile of drugs used in the treatment of osteoporosis: A systematical review of the literature. *Reumatismo*, 65(4): 143–166.

Via, A.G., Frizziero, A. and Oliva, F. (2012). Biological properties of mesenchymal Stem Cells from different sources. *Muscles, Ligaments and Tendons Journal,* 2(3): 154–162.

Vijayakumar, R. and Busselberg, D. (2016). Osteoporosis: An under-recognized public health problem. *Journal of Local and Global Health Science*, 2.

Warnmark, A. *et al.* (2001). Differential recruitment of the mammalian mediator subunit TRAP220 by estrogen receptors ERalpha and ERbeta. *J. Biol. Chem.*, 276: 23397–23404.

Winograd-Katz, S.E., Fassler, R., Geiger, B. and Legate, K.R. (2014). The integrin adhesome: From genes and proteins to human disease. *Nat. Rev. Mol. Cell Biol.*, 15(4): 273–288.

Wuttke-Seidlova, D., Becker, T., Cristoffel, V., Jarry, H. and Wuttke, W. (2003). Silymarin is a selective estrogen receptor beta (ER beta) agonist and has estrogenic effects in the metaphysis of the femur but no antiestrogenic effects in the uterus of ovariectomized rats. *J. Steroid Biochem. Mol. Biol.*, 86(1): 179–188.

Zain, M.E. (2011). Impact of mycotoxins on humans and animals. *Journal of Saudi Chemical Society*, 2011; 15(2):129-144.

Subject Index

Rs7 2,495